THE SELF AND ITS BRAIN

Titles by Karl Popper
available from Routledge

THE OPEN SOCIETY AND ITS ENEMIES VOLUME I

THE OPEN SOCIETY AND ITS ENEMIES VOLUME II

THE POVERTY OF HISTORICISM

THE LOGIC OF SCIENTIFIC DISCOVERY

CONJECTURES AND REFUTATIONS

UNENDED QUEST

THE OPEN UNIVERSE

QUANTUM THEORY AND THE SCHISM IN PHYSICS

REALISM AND THE AIM OF SCIENCE

IN SEARCH OF A BETTER WORLD

KNOWLEDGE AND THE BODY-MIND PROBLEM

THE MYTH OF THE FRAMEWORK

THE LESSON OF THIS CENTURY

THE WORLD OF PARMENIDES

ALL LIFE IS PROBLEM SOLVING

THE SELF AND ITS BRAIN

An Argument for Interactionism

KARL POPPER AND JOHN C. ECCLES

Routledge
Taylor & Francis Group
LONDON AND NEW YORK

First published in 1977 by
Springer-Verlag, Berlin, Heidelberg, London, New York.
This edition first published in 1983 by
Routledge

2 Park Square, Milton Park, Abingdon, Oxfordshire, OX14 4RN

Simultaneously published in the USA and Canada
by Routledge

711 Third Avenue, New York, NY 10017

Routledge is an imprint of the Taylor and Francis Group, an informa business

First issued in hardback 2015

British Library Cataloguing in Publication Data
A catalogue record for this book is available from the British Library

Library of Congress Cataloging in Publication Data
A catalogue record for this book is available from the Library of Congress

ISBN 978-0-415-05898-8 (pbk)
ISBN 978-1-138-13149-1 (hbk)

To our wives

Each waking day is a stage dominated for good or ill, in comedy, farce or tragedy by a *dramatis persona,* the 'self', and so it will be until the curtain drops.

C. S. Sherrington, 1947.

Only human beings guide their behaviour by a knowledge of what happened before they were born and a preconception of what may happen after they are dead: thus only human beings find their way by a light that illumines more than the patch of ground they stand on.

Peter B. Medawar and Jean S. Medawar, 1977.

Preface

The problem of the relation between our bodies and our minds, and especially of the link between brain structures and processes on the one hand and mental dispositions and events on the other is an exceedingly difficult one. Without pretending to be able to foresee future developments, both authors of this book think it improbable that the problem will ever be solved, in the sense that we shall really understand this relation. We think that no more can be expected than to make a little progress here or there. We have written this book in the hope that we have been able to do so.

We are conscious of the fact that what we have done is very conjectural and very modest. We are aware of our fallibility; yet we believe in the intrinsic value of every human effort to deepen our understanding of ourselves and of the world we live in. We believe in humanism: in human rationality, in human science, and in other human achievements, however fallible they are. We are unimpressed by the recurrent intellectual fashions that belittle science and the other great human achievements.

An additional motive for writing this book is that we both feel that the debunking of man has gone far enough – even too far. It is said that we had to learn from Copernicus and Darwin that man's place in the universe is not so exalted or so exclusive as man once thought. That may well be. But since Copernicus we have learned to appreciate how wonderful and rare, perhaps even unique, our little Earth is in this big universe; and since Darwin we have learned more about the incredible organization of all living things on Earth, and also about the unique position of man among his fellow creatures.

These are some of the points on which the two authors of the book agree. But we also disagree on a number of important points. We hope that these points will become clear in our recorded dialogue which forms Part III of the book.

However, it may be well to mention at once one important difference between the authors: a difference in religious belief. One of us (Eccles) is a believer in God and the supernatural, while the other (Popper) may be described as an agnostic. Each of us not only deeply respects the position of the other, but sympathizes with it.

This difference of opinion should be quite immaterial in our discussion of some of the problems, especially of the purely scientific ones, but it obtrudes in our discussion of problems of a more philosophical nature. Thus one of us is inclined to defend the idea of the survival of the human soul as does Socrates in Plato's *Phaedo,* while the other inclines towards an agnostic position more like that of Socrates in Plato's *Apology*. And, although we are both evolutionists, Eccles believes that the gulf between animal consciousness and human self-consciousness is wider than Popper thinks it to be. However, we do agree on many important points, such as a distrust of solutions which are very simple. We suspect that there are deep riddles to be solved. Our main thesis – psychophysical interactionism – will be discussed at length in the book. Here we wish to mention just one or two points of method.

Among these, we agree on the importance of a presentation that strives for clarity and simplicity. Words should be used well and carefully (we have certainly not everywhere succeeded in this); but their meaning should never, we think, become a topic of discussion or be permitted to dominate the discussion, as happens so often in contemporary philosophical writing. And although it is sometimes useful to indicate in which of its various senses we use a word, it is not possible to do so by defining it, since every definition must make essential use of undefined terms. Where practicable, we have used non-technical terms in preference to technical ones.

However, to put it in a nutshell, what we are interested in is not the meaning of terms but the truth of theories; and this truth is largely independent of the terminology used.

Something may be said in this connection about our use of the terms "soul", "mind", "self", "consciousness of self", and so on. We have in the main avoided the word "soul" because in the English language it has strong religious connotations. It is not quite the same with the words *"Seele"*, *"anima"*, *"psyche"*. The word "mind" is used as in ordinary language (for example "I made up my mind"). We have tried to avoid its philosophical connotations: what is important is not to prejudge the issue by the terminology used.

It may be mentioned that we have decided not to refer to parapsychology, of which neither of us has had any direct experience.

This book may be described as an attempt in interdisciplinary co-operation. One of us (Eccles) is a brain scientist who was led into this field of research by his life-long interest in the brain-mind problem. The other (Popper) is a philosopher who throughout his life has been dissatisfied with the prevailing schools of philosophy and deeply interested in science. Both are dualists or even pluralists, and interactionists. Their co-operation was inspired by the hope of learning from each other.

The P (Popper) and E (Eccles) chapters form Parts I and II of the book. They were written independently, partly in the Villa Serbelloni, and partly later, during the two years that have elapsed since. Part III is based on the taped recording of a dialogue that was carried on from day to day as indicated by the dates and times. It spontaneously flowed from the many discussions that we had while walking in the lovely grounds of the Villa Serbelloni; especially from discussions of problems on which we disagreed. We have decided to present it more or less in its original form. (However, we cut out in the end some of the topics from our dialogue because they were afterwards treated at length in our respective chapters; though this may in some cases have been at the cost of continuity.) The dialogue shows that some of our views changed in the light of criticisms that arose in different guises from day to day.

KARL R. POPPER
JOHN C. ECCLES

Acknowledgements

We wish to express our thanks firstly to Doctor Ralph Richardson and Doctor Jane Allen of the Rockefeller Foundation (Bellagio Study and Conference Center) for arranging the invitation to the Center. Doctor William Olson, the Director of the Center and Mrs Olson provided wonderful hospitality in the most attractive of Academic havens, the Villa Serbelloni on Lago di Como. For the month of September 1974 we were guests there with our wives. The venue was ideal for wandering and talking between the discipline of writing our respective chapters, and eventually the developing peripatetic dialogue was recorded in daily taped sessions to form Part III of this book.

J. C. E.
K. R. P.

The influence on my sections of discussions with Sir John Eccles – especially of the long discussion of 1974 which was recorded and is now reproduced in this book – will be apparent. He has, in addition, made critical comments on my sections, and suggested several important improvements. So have Sir Ernst Gombrich, and also my wife, who typed and criticized in detail several versions of the manuscript.

Jeremy Shearmur who, thanks to the generosity of the Nuffield Foundation, is my Research Assistant, was immensely helpful. He carefully scrutinized an earlier version. He criticized the presentation of my arguments, and made many suggestions for remedies. He also made important positive contributions, which I have acknowledged at the relevant places. I would also like to thank Mrs. P. Watts for her work on typing the final manuscript, and David Miller for his help with the proofs.

K. R. P.

Without the example, encouragement and criticism of Sir Karl Popper I would not have dared to express my ideas on the brain-mind problem in the manner evident in the philosophical sections of my chapters. I wish to express my thanks to my wife, Helena, for her valuable comments on the manuscript and for composing many of the illustrations as well as for much of the typing. Most of this manuscript was completed during my Buffalo period. My assistant, Miss Virginia Muniak, made a specially notable contribution by her typing from the 12 hour taped recording of our dialogues (Part III). Miss Tecla Rantucci gave most valuable assistance in the construction of some of the figures and with her expert photography.

I wish to express my grateful thanks to the many neuroscientists named below for so kindly allowing the reproduction of figures from their publications and in some cases for providing me with figures for reproduction: Drs G. Allen, T. Bliss, A. Brodal, A. Gardner

Medwin, N. Geschwind, G. Gray, A. Hein, R. Held, D. Hubel, E. Jones, H. Kornhuber, B. Libet, B. Milner, T. Powell, R. Sperry, J. Szentágothai, C. Trevarthen, N. Tsukahara, and T. Wiesel.

J.C.E.

Our association with the publishers has not been in the characteristic mode of a purely business relationship. Dr. Heinz Götze, President of Springer-Verlag, has taken a deep personal interest through the long incubation period of over two years and has been wonderfully helpful to both of us. Once the manuscript was finally submitted at the end of March, 1977, the efficiency of his staff, notably Miss Monika Brendel and Mr. Kurt Teichmann, has resulted in a publication in just six months, which is remarkable for a book of this size and complexity.

K.R.P.
J.C.E.

Contents

PART I by Karl R. Popper

Part I

Chapter P1 Materialism Transcends Itself

1. Kant's Argument

Two things, says Kant near the end of his *Critique of Practical Reason,*[1] fill his mind with always new and increasing admiration and respect: the starry heavens above him, and the moral law within him. The first of these two things symbolizes for him the problem of our knowledge about the physical universe,[2] and the problem of our place in this universe. The second pertains to the invisible self, to the human personality (and to human freedom, as he explains). The first annihilates the importance of a man, considered as a part of the physical universe. The second raises immeasurably his value as an intelligent and responsible being.

I think that Kant is essentially right. As Josef Popper-Lynkeus once put it, every time a man dies, a whole universe is destroyed. (One realizes this when one identifies oneself with that man.) Human beings are irreplaceable; and in being irreplaceable they are clearly very different from machines. They are capable of enjoying life, and they are capable of suffering, and of facing death consciously. They are selves; they are ends in themselves, as Kant said.

This view seems to me incompatible with the materialist doctrine that men are machines.

In the present introductory chapter, my aim is to open up a number of problems, and to emphasize the importance of some things which should, perhaps, give the materialist or the physicalist pause. At the same time, I wish to do justice to the great historical achievements of materialism. But I wish to make clear, at once, that it is not my intention to raise any "what is" questions, such as "What is mind?" or "What is matter?". (In fact, the need to avoid "what is" questions will turn out to be one of my major points.) It is

---

1 Immanuel Kant [1788], *Beschluß* (pp. 281 – 285).

2 For Kant, this knowledge was summed up by astronomical theory by Newtonian mechanics, including the theory of gravitation.

still less my intention to *answer* such questions. (That is, I am not offering what is sometimes called an "ontology".)

2. Men and Machines

The doctrine that men are machines, or robots, is a fairly old one. Its first clear and forceful formulation is due, it seems, to the title of a famous book by La Mettrie, *Man a Machine* [1747]; though the first writer to play with the idea of robots was Homer.[1]

Yet machines are clearly not ends in themselves, however complicated they may be. They may be valuable because of their usefulness, or because of their rarity; and a certain specimen may be valuable because of its historical uniqueness. But machines become valueless if they do not have a rarity value: if there are too many of a kind we are prepared to pay to have them removed. On the other hand, we value human lives in spite of the problem of over-population, the gravest of all social problems of our time. We respect even the life of a murderer.

It must admitted that, after two world wars, and under the threat of the new means for mass destruction, there has been a frightening deterioration of respect for human life in some strata of our society. This makes it particularly urgent to reaffirm in what follows a view from which we have, I think, no reason to deviate: the view that men are ends in themselves and not "just" machines.

We can divide those who uphold the doctrine that men are machines, or a

---

[1] La Mettrie did not deny the existence of conscious experience. He also reacted strongly to Descartes's doctrine that animals (though not men) are mere automata. (See section 56, below.)

There are two passages in Book 18 of the *Iliad* in which "Hephaestus, the famous craftsman" is described as a creator of robot-like machines. (The term "robot" was introduced by Karel Čapek.) In the first of these passages Hephaestus is at work constructing something like automatic waiters (or tea waggons). In the second passage he is assisted in his work by clever girls whom he has forged of gold, a metal possessed of peculiar powers. The first passage (373 – 377) may be translated:

> Three-legged tables he was constructing, twenty in all, to
> Stand round the wall of his well-built hall. To these he had fitted
> Wheels wrought of gold, so that they could run by themselves to the banquet
> Of the gods, at his wish, and back home, leaving everyone staggered.

Here is the second passage (417 – 420):

> Handmaidens, fashioned of gold, gave ready support to their master.
> Looking like genuine girls they proved their keen understanding
> By their intelligent speech, their proficient and skilful performance.

(In the last two lines one might perhaps find traces of Homer's reading of Gilbert Ryle.)

similar doctrine, into two categories: those who deny the existence of mental events, of personal experiences, or of consciousness; or who say perhaps that the question whether such experiences exist is of minor importance and may be safely left open; and those who admit the existence of mental events, but assert that they are "epiphenomena" – that everything can be explained without them, since the material world is causally closed. But whether they belong to the one category or the other, both must neglect, it seems to me, the reality of human suffering, and the significance of the fight against unnecessary suffering.

Thus I regard the doctrine that men are machines not only as mistaken, but as prone to undermine a humanist ethics. However, this very reason makes it all the more necessary to stress that the great defenders of that doctrine – the great materialist philosophers – were, nevertheless, almost all upholders of humanist ethics. From Democritus and Lucretius to Herbert Feigl and Anthony Quinton, materialist philosophers have usually been humanists and fighters for freedom and enlightenment; and, sad to say, their opponents have sometimes been the opposite. Thus just because I regard materialism as mistaken – just because I do not believe that men are machines or automata – I wish to stress the great and indeed vital role which the materialist philosophy has played in the evolution of human thought, and of humanist ethics.

3. Materialism Transcends Itself

Materialism as a philosophic movement has been an inspiration to science. It has created two of the oldest and still most important of scientific research programmes, two opposed traditions, which merged only very recently. The one is the Parmenidean theory of the *plenum,* which developed into the continuity theory of matter and which has led with Faraday and Maxwell, Riemann, Clifford, and, in our own time, with Einstein, Schrödinger and Wheeler, to the field theory of matter, and to quantum geometrodynamics. The other is the atomism of Leucippus, Democritus, Epicurus and Lucretius, which has ultimately led to modern atomic theory, and to quantum mechanics.

Yet both these research programmes have to some extent transcended themselves. Both research programmes started from the theory that matter, in the sense of something extended in space, or occupying space (or parts of space), was ultimate; essential; substantial: an essence or substance neither capable of further explanation nor in need of it, and thus a principle in terms of which everything else had to be, and could be, explained. This view of matter was first superseded by Leibniz and Boscovich (see section 51 below). Modern physics contains *explanatory theories* of matter, and of the properties of matter, such as the property of occupying space (once called the property of "impenetrability"), or the properties of elasticity, of cohesion, and of the "states" of matter (or the "states of aggregation": solid, liquid, or gaseous). In thus *explaining matter* and its properties modern physics transcended the original programme of materialism. In fact it was physics itself which produced by far the most important arguments against classical materialism.

I will briefly summarize the most important of these arguments. (See also sections 47–51, below.) The classical materialism of Leucippus or Democritus, like the later theories of Descartes or of Hobbes, assumes that matter or body or "extended substance" fills parts of space or perhaps the whole of space, and that a body can *push* another body. Push, or impact, becomes the explanation of causal interaction ("action by contact"). The world is a clockwork mechanism of bodies which push each other like cogwheels.

This theory was first transcended by Newtonian gravitation, which was (1) pull, not push and (2) action at a distance rather than action by contact. Newton himself found this absurd;[1] but he and his successors (especially Lesage[2]) were unsuccessful in their attempts to explain gravitational pull as due to push. However, this first breach in the armour of classical materialism was repaired by an extension of the idea of materialism: gravitational pull was accepted by later Newtonians as an "essential" property of matter, neither capable nor in need of further explanation.[3]

One of the most important events in the history of the self-transcendence of materialism was J. J. Thomson's discovery of the electron which he (and H. A. Lorentz) diagnosed as a tiny splinter of the atom. Thus the atom – by definition the indivisible – could be divided. This was bad; but one could adjust oneself to it by regarding the atoms as systems of smaller charged material particles, electrons and protons, which could be regarded as very small charged bits of matter.

The new theory could *explain* the push between pieces of matter (the "impenetrability of matter") by the electrical repulsion of equally charged particles (the electron shells of the atoms). This was convincing, but it

---

[1] See my [1963(a)] p. 106 (text to note 20 to chapter 3), and section 48, below.

[2] See my [1963(a)] p. 107 (note 21 to chapter 3).

[3] More about the role of Newton's theory in the decline of essentialism may be found in section 51, below.

destroyed the idea that push was "essential", depending on the essential space-filling property of matter, and that push was the model of all physical causal action. Other elementary particles are now known which cannot be interpreted as charged (or uncharged) bits of matter – matter in the sense of materialism – for they are *unstable:* they disintegrate. Moreover, even stable particles like electrons can be pairwise annihilated, with the production of photons (light quanta); and they can be created, out of a photon (a gamma ray). But light is not matter, though we may say that light and matter are forms of energy.

Thus the law of conservation of matter (and of mass) had to be given up. Matter is not "substance", since it is not conserved: it can be destroyed, and it can be created. Even the most stable particles, the nucleons, can be destroyed by collision with their anti-particles, when their energy is transformed into light. Matter turns out to be highly packed energy, transformable into other forms of energy; and therefore something of the nature of a *process*, since it can be converted into other processes such as light and, of course, motion and heat.

Thus one may say that the results of modern physics suggest that we should give up *the idea of a substance or essence.*[4] They suggest that there is no self-identical entity persisting during all changes in time (even though bits of matter do so under "ordinary" circumstances); that there is no essence which is the persisting carrier or possessor of the properties or qualities of a thing. The universe now appears to be not a collection of things, but an interacting set of events or processes (as stressed especially by A. N. Whitehead).

A modern physicist thus might well say that physical things – bodies, matter – have an atomic structure. But atoms have a structure in their turn, a structure that can hardly be described as "material", and certainly not as "substantial": with the programme of explaining the structure of matter, physics had to transcend materialism.

This whole development beyond materialism was a result of research into the structure of matter, into atoms, and thus a result of the materialist research programme itself. (This is why I am speaking of the self-transcendence of materialism.) It has left the importance and the reality of matter and of material things – atoms, molecules, and structures of molecules – un-

[4] There is, of course, the fact that contemporary physics operates with the conjecture that the amount of energy in a closed system is conserved. But this does not mean that we need, in physics, something like a substance: the theory of Bohr, Kramers and Slater [1924] assumed that only in the statistical average was energy conserved. Bohr made a similar suggestion years later, before Pauli's conjecture of the existence of the neutrino; and Schrödinger [1952] also suggested a similar theory. This shows that physicists were quite ready to discard the one and only property of energy in which it resembles a substance, and that there is no *a priori* necessity behind this idea.

scathed. One might even say that it has led to a gain in reality. For as the history of materialism and especially of atomism shows, the reality of matter was regarded as dubious not only by idealist philosophers such as Berkeley and Hume but even by physicists such as Mach, at the very time of the rise of quantum theory. But since 1905 (Einstein's paper on the molecular theory of Brownian motion), things began to look different; and even Mach changed his mind at least temporarily,[5] not long before his death, when he was shown on a scintillation screen the flashes due to alpha particles, the fragments of disintegrating radium atoms. Atoms were accepted as really "real", one might say, when they ceased to be "atomic": when they ceased to be indivisible bits of matter; when they acquired a structure.

Thus the physical theory of matter may be said to be no longer materialist, even though it has retained much of its original character. It still operates with particles (although these are no longer confined to "bits of matter"), but it has added fields of forces, and various forms of radiating energy. But it is now becoming a *theory* of matter, a theory that explains matter by assumptions about non-material (although certainly not mental) entities. As J.A. Wheeler [1973] puts it: "Particle physics is not the right starting point for particle physics. Vacuum physics is."[6]

Materialism has thus transcended itself. The view that animals and men are machines in a mechanical sense, a view that was originally inspired by the title of La Mettrie's book *Man a Machine* (see section 56, below), has been replaced by the view that animals and men are electrochemical machines.

The change is important. Yet for reasons stated at the beginning of the chapter, this modern version of the theory that men are machines appears to me (though perhaps one step nearer to the truth) no more acceptable than the old mechanistic version of materialism.

Many modern philosophers who hold this view (especially U. T. Place, J. J. C. Smart and D. M. Armstrong) call themselves "materialists", thereby giving the term "materialism" a meaning which somewhat differs from its earlier meaning. Others who hold very similar views, and especially the view that men are machines, call themselves "physicalists", a term due, so far as I know, to Otto Neurath. (So does Herbert Feigl, who regards the existence of human consciousness as one of the most important problems of philosophy.)

Terminology is of course quite irrelevant. But we must not overlook one thing: criticism of the old materialism, even if conclusive, is not necessarily applicable to the prevailing physicalistic version of materialism.

---

[5] See Blackmore [1972], pp. 319–24.

[6] John Archibald Wheeler [1973], p. 235. As Wheeler points out (p. 229), this important idea can be traced back to William Kingdon Clifford [1873], [1879], [1882].

4. Remarks on the term "Real"

In general I try to avoid "what is" questions, and even more "what do you mean by" questions, because they seem to me prone to produce the danger of substituting verbal problems (or problems about meaning) for real ones. Yet in this section I will deviate from this principle[1] and discuss briefly the use or meaning of a term – the term "real", which has been used in the previous section (where I said that atoms were accepted as "real" when they ceased to be "atomic").

I suppose that the most central usage of the term "real" is its use to characterize material things of ordinary size – things which a baby can handle and (preferably) put into his mouth. From this, the usage of the term "real" is extended, first, to bigger things – things which are too big for us to handle, like railway trains, houses, mountains, the earth and the stars; and also to smaller things – things like dust particles or mites. It is further extended, of course, to liquids and then also to air, to gases and to molecules and atoms.

What is the principle behind the extension? It is, I suggest, that the entities which we conjecture to be real should be able to exert a causal effect upon the *prima facie* real things; that is, upon material things of an ordinary size: that we can explain changes in the ordinary material world of things by the causal effects of entities conjectured to be real.

However, there is then the further question of whether or not these entities, conjectured to be real, actually exist.

Many people were reluctant to accept that atoms existed, but atoms were widely admitted to exist after Einstein's theory of Brownian motion. Einstein proposed the well-testable theory that small particles suspended in a liquid (whose movements are visible through a microscope, and therefore "real") moved as a result of the random impacts of the moving molecules of the liquid. He conjectured that the then still invisibly small molecules exerted *causal effects* upon those very small yet "ordinary" real things. This provided good reasons for the reality of molecules, and then further of atoms.

Mach, who did not like to work with conjectures, became (for a time at least) convinced of the existence of atoms by the observable evidence of the physical effects of their disintegration. And the existence of atoms became common knowledge when the artificial disintegration of atoms caused the destruction of two populated cities.

---

[1] Even though I am doing here something like raising a "what is" question, I am not doing "meaning analysis". Behind my discussion of the word "real" there is a *theory:* the theory that matter exists, and that this fact is *crucially* important, but that some other things which interact with matter, such as minds, exist also; see below. (See also Plato, *Sophist,* 247d–e, 248c.)

However, the question of accepting such evidence is not quite straightforward. While no evidence can be conclusive, we seem to be inclined to accept something (whose existence has been conjectured) as actually existing if its existence is corroborated; for example, by the discovery of effects that we would expect to find if it did exist. However, we may say that this corroboration indicates, first, that *something* is there; at least the fact of this corroboration will have to be explained by any future theory. Secondly, the corroboration indicates that the theory that involves the conjectured real entities may be true, or that it may be near to the truth (that it has a good degree of verisimilitude). (It is perhaps better to talk of the truth or verisimilitude of theories than of the existence of entities, because the existence of the entities is part of a theory or conjecture.)

If we keep these reservations in mind, there is no reason why we should not say, for example, that atoms and also electrons and other elementary particles are now accepted as really existing; say, because of their causal effects on photographic emulsions. We accept things as "real" if they can causally act upon, or interact with, ordinary real material things.

It has to be admitted, though, that real entities can be concrete or abstract in various degrees. In physics we accept forces and fields of forces as real, because they act upon material things. But these entities are more abstract, and perhaps also more conjectural or hypothetical, than are the ordinary material things.

Forces and fields of forces are attached to material things, to atoms, and to particles. They are of a dispositional character: they are dispositions to interact. Thus they may be described as highly abstract theoretical entities; yet as they interact in a direct or indirect way with ordinary material things, we accept them as real.

To sum up, I share with old-fashioned materialists the view that material things are real, and even the view that, for us, solid material bodies are the paradigms of reality. And I also share with the modern materialists or physicalists the view that forces and fields of forces, charges, and so on – that is, theoretical physical entities other than matter – are also real.

Moreover, though I conjecture that we take, in early childhood, our idea of reality from material things, I do not suggest that material things are in any sense "ultimate". On the contrary, having learned about physical forces, events, and processes, we may discover that material things, especially solids, are to be interpreted as very special physical processes, in which molecular forces play a dominant role.

5. Materialism, Biology, and Mind

Materialism is a great movement and a great tradition not only in physics, but also in biology. We do not know much about the origin of life on earth, but it looks very much as if life originated with the chemical synthesis of giant self-reproducing molecules, and that it evolved through natural selection, as materialists would assert, following Darwin.

Thus it seems that in a material universe something new can emerge. Dead matter seems to have more potentialities than merely to produce dead matter. In particular, it has produced minds – no doubt in slow stages – and in the end the human brain and the human mind, the human consciousness of self, and the human awareness of the universe.

Thus I share with the materialists or physicalists not only the emphasis on material objects as the paradigms of reality, but also the evolutionary hypothesis. But our ways seem to part when evolution produces minds, and human language. And they part even more widely when human minds produce stories, explanatory myths, tools and works of art and of science.

All this, so it seems, has evolved without any violation of the laws of physics. But with life, even with low forms of life, problem-solving enters the universe; and with the higher forms, purposes and aims, consciously pursued.

We can only wonder that matter can thus transcend itself, by producing mind, purpose, and a world of the products of the human mind.

One of the first products of the human mind is human language. In fact, I conjecture that it was the very first of these products, and that the human brain and the human mind evolved in interaction with language.

6. Organic Evolution

In order to understand this interaction better, we should look at an aspect of the theory of natural selection which is sometimes neglected.

Natural selection is often seen as the result of an interaction between blind chance working from within the organism (mutation) and external forces upon which the organism has no influence. The aims and the preferences of the organism do not seem to come in at all, except as products of natural selection. The theories of Lamarck or Butler or Bergson, according to which an animal's preferences or aims can influence its evolution, seem to clash with Darwinism, by bringing in the inheritance of acquired characteristics.

This view is mistaken, as a number of people seem to have found independently, especially the two Darwinians, J. M.Baldwin and C. Lloyd Morgan, who called their theory "organic evolution".[1]

The theory of organic evolution starts from the fact that all organisms, but especially the higher organisms, have a more or less varied repertoire of behaviour at their disposal. By adopting a new form of behaviour the individual organism may change its environment. Even a tree may push a root into a fissure between two rocks, force the rocks apart, and thus get access to soil of a chemical composition differing from that of its immediate surroundings. More significantly, an animal may adopt a preference for a new kind of food consciously, as the result of trial and error. This means changing its environment to the extent that new aspects of the environment take on a new biological (ecological) significance. In this way, individual preferences and skills may lead to the selection, and perhaps even to the construction, of a new ecological niche by the organism. By this individual action, the organism may "choose", as it were, its environment;[2] and it may thereby expose itself and its descendants to a new set of selection pressures, characteristic of the new environment. Thus the activity, the preferences, the skill, and the idiosyncrasies of the individual animal may indirectly influence the selection pressures to which it is exposed, and with it, the outcome of natural selection.

To take a well-known example. According to Lamarck it was the preference for browsing among the higher branches of trees which led the ancestors of the giraffe to stretch their necks, and which led, through the inheritance of acquired characteristics, to our giraffe. According to modern Darwinism (the "synthetic theory") this explanation is indeed unacceptable, because acquired characteristics are not inherited. Yet this does not mean that the actions, preferences and choices of the giraffe's ancestors did not play a decisive (though indirect) role in its evolution. On the contrary, they created a new environment for its descendants, with new selection pressures; and these led to the selection of long necks.

Up to a point, one can even say that preferences are often decisive. It is much more likely that a new feeding habit leads, by natural selection (and by way of accidental mutations), to new anatomical adaptations, than that accidental anatomical changes enforce new feeding habits. For changes

---

[1] An important contribution to the history of the idea of organic evolution may be found in Sir Alister Hardy's great book, *The Living Stream* [1965].

[2] While I personally believe that animals and men make genuine choices, a materialist might, of course, choose to interpret such choices and preferences as being ultimately no more than the outcome of randomness and of selective filters. It is, however, not my concern here to argue this issue.

which are not adapted to the habits of the organism would hardly be of positive value in its struggle for life.

Darwin himself wrote: "... it would be easy for natural selection to adapt the structure of the animal to its changed habits ...". However, he continued: "It is ... difficult to decide, and immaterial for us, whether habits generally change first, and structures afterwards; or whether slight modifications of structure lead to changed habits; both probably often occurring almost simultaneously."[3] I agree that both cases occur, and that in both it is natural selection which works on the genetic structure. Still, I think that in many cases, and in some of the most interesting cases, habits change first. These are the cases called "organic evolution".

I disagree with Darwin, however, when he says that the question is "immaterial for us". I think it matters a lot. Evolutionary changes that start with new behaviour patterns – with new preferences, new purposes of the animal – not only make many adaptations better understandable, but they re-invest the animal's subjective aims and purposes with an evolutionary significance. Moreover, the theory of organic evolution makes it understandable that the mechanism of natural selection becomes more efficient when there is a greater behavioural repertoire available. Thus it shows the selective value of a certain innate behavioural freedom – as opposed to behavioural rigidity which must make it more difficult for natural selection to produce new adaptations. And it may become more understandable how the human mind emerged. As Sir Alister Hardy hints (in the subtitle of his book *The Living Stream*), this "restatement" of the Darwinian theory can elucidate "its relation to the spirit of man". We could say that in choosing to speak, and to take interest in speech, man has chosen to evolve his brain and his mind; that language, once created, exerted the selection pressure under which emerged the human brain and the consciousness of self.

These points are, I think, of some significance for the mind-body problem. For, as suggested in section 4 above, not only do we conjecture something to be real if it is capable of affecting physical objects, but we are inclined to accept that it exists if these effects are corroborated. The points discussed in this section – the way in which our choices, our thoughts, our plans and our actions lead to a situation which in its turn has its repercussions upon us, including the evolution of the human brain – suggest that, in the evolution

[3] Charles Darwin [1859], chapter VI, "On the Origin and Transitions of Organic Beings with Peculiar Habits and Structure". The passage quoted in the text is the version to be found in the fifth and subsequent editions. See Morse Peckham (ed.) [1959], chapter VI, sentences 92 and 93 (p. 332 of this variorum edition).

and in the behaviour of the higher animals, especially of man, there is some evidence for the existence of conscious experience. These points constitute a problem for those who deny that consciousness exists, and even for those who admit that consciousness exists but claim that the physical world is causally self-contained (see chapter P3).

7. Nothing New Under the Sun. Reductionism and "Downward Causation"

One of the oldest of philosophical dogmas is summed up by the saying (of Ecclesiastes) "There is no new thing under the sun". In a way, this is also implied by materialism, especially by the older forms of atomism and even of physicalism. Materialists hold – or held – that matter is eternal and that all change consists in the motion of bits of matter, and in the consequent changes of their arrangements. Physicists as a rule hold that the physical laws are eternal. (There are exceptions, such as the physicists Paul Dirac and John Archibald Wheeler; see Wheeler's [1973].) It is indeed difficult to think otherwise, since what we call the laws of physics are the results of our search for invariants. Thus even if a supposed law of physics should turn out to be variable, so that (say) one of the apparently fundamental physical constants should turn out to change in time, we should try to replace it by a new invariant law that specifies the rate of change.

The view that there is no new thing under the sun is, in a way, involved in the original meaning of the word "evolution": to evolve means to unroll; and evolution meant originally the unrolling of what is there already: what is there, *preformed,* is to be made manifest. (To develop, similarly, means to unfold what is there.) This original meaning may be said to be now superseded, at least since Darwin, though it still seems to play its role in the world-view of some materialists or physicalists.

Today some of us have learnt to use the term "evolution" differently. For we think that evolution – the evolution of the universe, and especially the evolution of life on earth – has produced new things: *real novelty.* My thesis in this section is that we should be more clearly aware of this real novelty.

According to present physical theory, it seems that the expanding universe created itself many billion years ago with a big bang. The story of evolution suggests that the universe has never ceased to be creative, or "inventive", as Kenneth G. Denbigh suggests.[1]

---

[1] See Kenneth G. Denbigh [1975]. G. H. Lewes' [1874–79] term is "emerging".

The usual materialist and physicalist view is that all the possibilities which have realized themselves in the course of time and of evolution must have been, potentially, preformed, or pre-established, from the beginning. This is either a triviality, expressed in a dangerously misleading way, or a mistake. It is trivial that nothing can happen unless permitted by the laws of nature and by the preceding state; though it would be misleading to suggest that we can always know what is excluded in this way. But if it is suggested that the future is and always was foreseeable, at least in principle, then this is a mistake, for all we know, and for all that we can learn from evolution. Evolution has produced much that was not foreseeable, at least not for human knowledge.

Some people think that there was, from the beginning, something like mind, something psychical, inherent in matter; though this became sentience and consciousness only very much later, in the evolution of the higher animals. This is the theory of "panpsychism": everything (every material thing) has a soul, or something like a forerunner or a rudiment of a soul (see also section 19 below).

The motivation of these views, whether materialist or panpsychist, is, I think, "There is no new thing under the sun" or "Out of nothing, nothing can emerge". The great philosopher Parmenides taught this, 2,500 years ago, and he deduced from it that change is impossible, so that change must be an illusion. The founders of atomic theory, Leucippus and Democritus, followed him in so far as they taught that what exists are only unchanging atoms, and that they move in the void, in empty space. The only possible changes are thus the movements, collisions, and recombinations of atoms, including the very fine atoms which constitute our souls. And some of the most important of living philosophers (such as Quine) teach that there can be only physical entities, and that there are no mental events or mental experiences. (Some others compromise and admit that there are mental experiences, but say that these are, in some sense, physical events, or that they are "identical" with physical events.)

As against all these views I suggest that the universe, or its evolution, is creative, and that the evolution of sentient animals with conscious experiences has brought about something new. These experiences were first of a more rudimentary and later of a higher kind; and in the end that kind of consciousness of self and that kind of creativity emerged which, I suggest, we find in man.

With the emergence of man, the creativity of the universe has, I think, become obvious. For man has created a new objective world, the world of the products of the human mind; a world of myths, of fairy tales and scientific theories, of poetry and art and music. (I shall call this "World 3", in contradistinction to the physical World 1 and the subjective or psychological World 2; see section 10 below.) The existence of the great and unquestionably creative works of art and of science shows the creativity of man, and with it of the universe that has created man.

What I here describe by the word "creative" is described by Jacques Monod [1970], [1975] when he speaks of the unpredictability of the emergence of life on earth, of the unpredictability of the various species, and especially of our own human species: ". . . we were unpredictable before we appeared", he says. ([1975], p. 23.)

In using the admittedly vague idea of creative evolution or emergent evolution I have at least two different kinds of fact in mind. First there is the fact that in a universe in which there once existed (according to our present theories) no elements other than, say, hydrogen and helium, no theorist who knew the physical laws then operative and exemplified in this universe could have predicted all the properties of the heavier elements not yet emerged, or that they would emerge; or all the properties of even the simplest compound molecules, such as water. Secondly, there appear to be at the very least the following stages in the evolution of the universe, some of which produce things with properties that are altogether unpredictable or emergent: (1) The production of the heavier elements (including isotopes), and the emergence of liquids and of crystals. (2) The emergence of life. (3) The emergence of sentience. (4) The emergence (together with human language) of the consciousness of self and of death (or even of the human cerebral cortex). (5) The emergence of the human language, and of theories of the self and of death. (6) The emergence of such products of the human mind as explanatory myths, or scientific theories, or works of art.

It may be useful, for various reasons (especially for comparison with Table 2: see below) to arrange some of these cosmic evolutionary stages in the following Table 1.

World 3 (the products of the human mind)	(6) Works of Art and of Science (including Technology) (5) Human Language. Theories of Self and of Death
World 2 (the world of subjective experiences)	(4) Consciousness of Self and of Death (3) Sentience (Animal Consciousness)
World 1 (the world of physical objects)	(2) Living Organisms (1) The Heavier Elements; Liquids and Crystals (0) Hydrogen and Helium

Table 1: Some Cosmic Evolutionary Stages

It is obvious that much has been omitted from this table, and that it is greatly oversimplified. However, it has the advantage of summing up very briefly what seem to be some of the greatest events of creative evolution or of emergent evolution.

Against the acceptance of the view of emergent evolution there is a strong intuitive prejudice. It is the intuition that, if the universe consists of atoms or elementary particles, so that all things are structures of such particles, then every event in the universe ought to be explicable, and in principle predictable, in terms of *particle structure* and of *particle interaction.*

Thus we are led to what has been called *the programme of reductionism.* In order to discuss it, I shall make use of the following Table 2.

(12)	Level of ecosystems
(11)	Level of populations of metazoa and plants
(10)	Level of metazoa and multicellular plants
(9)	Level of tissues and organs (and of sponges?)
(8)	Level of populations of unicellular organisms
(7)	Level of cells and of unicellular organisms
(6)	Level of organelles (and perhaps of viruses)
(5)	Liquids and solids (crystals)
(4)	Molecules
(3)	Atoms
(2)	Elementary particles
(1)	Sub-elementary particles
(0)	Unknown: sub-sub-elementary particles?

Table 2: Biological Systems and their Parts

The reductionist idea behind this table is that the events or things on each level should be explained in terms of the lower levels.

Let me first point out in criticism of this Table 2 that it ought to be far more complex: it should show, at least, some branches like a tree. Thus it is clear that (6) and (7) are far from homogeneous. Moreover, the entities in level (8) are in no sense parts of the entities in level (9).

Yet what happens in (9) – say, to the lungs of an animal or man suffering from tuberculosis – may indeed be partly explained in terms of (8). Moreover, (10) may be an ecosystem (environment) of (8), or part of an ecosystem of (8). All this shows a certain disorder in our table. (It would be easy to construct a table in which these difficulties are not as obvious as in Table 2; but they would be there all the same: the biosystem is not intrinsically organized in a neat stepwise hierarchy.)

However, let us forget about these difficulties and turn to a consideration of the intuitive idea that the events and things on one of the higher levels can be explained in terms of what happens on the lower levels; more especially, that what happens to a whole can be explained by way of explaining the structure (the arrangement) and the interaction of its parts.

This reductionist idea is interesting and important; and whenever we can explain entities and events on a higher level by those of a lower level, we can speak of a great scientific success, and can say that we have added much to our understanding of the higher level. As a *research programme,* reductionism is not only important, but it is part of the programme of science whose aim is to explain and to understand.

However, do we really have good reasons to hope that a reduction to the lowest levels will be achieved? Paul Oppenheim and Hilary Putnam who have given ([1958], p. 9) a table somewhat similar to Table 2, have claimed that we have good reasons not only for accepting a reductionist *research programme* and for expecting *further successes* along this path (with this I fully agree), but also for expecting or believing that *the programme will finally succeed.* On this latter point I disagree: I do not think that there are any examples of a successful and complete reduction (perhaps with the exception of the reduction of Young and Fresnel's optics to Maxwell's electromagnetic field theory – see note 2 below – a reduction which does not exactly fit Table 2). Moreover, I do not think that Oppenheim and Putnam ever discuss the difficulties, inherent for example in the upper region of our Table 1, such as the difficulty of reducing to psychology, and then to biology, the ups and downs of the British Trade Deficit and its relations to the British Net National Income. (I owe this example to Sir Peter Medawar who in his [1974], p. 62, speaks of the reducibility of the "foreign exchange deficit".) Oppenheim and Putnam (*op. cit.,* p. 11) refer to a famous passage, also quoted by Medawar ([1969], p. 16; [1974], p. 62), in which J. S. Mill claims the reducibility of sociology to human psychology. But they do not discuss the weaknesses of this argument of Mill's (which I pointed out in my [1945(c)], chapter 14; [1958(i)], chapter 4).

In fact, even the often referred to reduction of chemistry to physics, important as it is, is far from complete, and very possibly incompletable. Some properties of molecules (mainly of simple two-atom molecules) such as some molecular spectra, or the crystal system of diamond and graphite, have been explained in terms of atomic theory; but we are far removed indeed from being able to claim that all, or most, properties of chemical compounds can be reduced to atomic theory, even though what might be called the "*reduction in principle*" of chemistry to physics is highly suggestive.[2] In fact, the five lower levels of Table 2 (which more or less agree with those of the Table of Oppenheim and Putnam) can be used to show that we have reason to regard this kind of intuitive reduction programme as clashing with some results of modern physics.

For what this Table 2 suggests may be characterized as the principle of "upward causation". This is the principle that causation can be traced in our Table 2 from a lower level to a higher level, but never *vice versa*: that what happens on a higher level can be explained in terms of the next lower level, and ultimately in terms of elementary particles and the relevant physical laws. It appears at first that the higher levels cannot act on the lower ones.

But the idea of particle-to-particle or atom-to-atom interaction has been superseded by physics itself. A diffraction grating or a crystal (belonging to level (5) of our Table 2) is a spatially very extended complex (and periodic) structure of billions of molecules; but it interacts as a whole extended periodic structure with the photons or the particles of a beam of photons or of particles. Thus we have here an important example of *"downward causation"*, to use an expression of D. T. Campbell's [1974]. That is to say, the whole, the macro structure, may, *qua* whole, act upon a photon or an elementary particle or an atom. (The particle beam in question may have as low an intensity as we choose.)

Other physical examples of downward causation — of macroscopic structures on level (5) acting upon elementary particles or photons on level (1) — are lasers, masers, and holograms. And there are also many other macro structures which are examples of downward causation: every simple arrangement of negative feedback, such as a steam engine governor, is a macroscopic structure that regulates lower level events, such as the flow of the molecules that constitute the steam.

Downward causation is of course important in all tools and machines which are designed for some purpose. When we use a wedge, for example, we do not arrange for the action of its elementary particles, but we use a structure, relying on it to guide the actions of its constituent elementary particles to act, in concert, so as to achieve the desired result.

---

[2] "Explanation in principle" is critically discussed by F. A. von Hayek [1955]; see his [1967], pp. 11 ff. "Reduction in principle" is a special case of it.

The comparatively most successful reduction of which I know is that of the Young-Fresnel optics to Maxwellian theory. Yet (1) this theory was developed later than the Young-Fresnel theory of optics, and (2) neither the "reduced" theory nor the reducing theory were complete: the theories of emission and absorption — quantum mechanics and quantum-electrodynamics — were (and partly are) still missing. Another important example of an incomplete reduction is statistical mechanics. For a fuller discussion of reduction, see my paper [1974(z_2)].

Stars are undesigned, but one may look at them as undesigned "machines" for putting the atoms and elementary particles in their central region under terrific gravitational pressure, with the (undesigned) result that some atomic nuclei fuse and form the nuclei of heavier elements; an excellent example of downward causation, of the action of the whole structure upon its constituent particles.

(Stars, incidentally, are good examples of the general rule that things are processes. Also, they illustrate the mistake of distinguishing between "wholes" – which are "more than the sum of their parts" – and "mere heaps": a star is, in a sense, a "mere" accumulation, a "mere heap" of its constituent atoms.[3] Yet it is a process – a dynamic structure. Its stability depends upon the dynamic equilibrium between its gravitational pressure, due to its sheer bulk, and the repulsive forces between its closely packed elementary particles. If the latter are excessive, the star explodes. If they are smaller than the gravitational pressure, it collapses into a "black hole".)

The most interesting examples of downward causation are to be found in organisms and in their ecological systems, and in societies of organisms. A society may continue to function even though many of its members die; but a strike in an essential industry, such as the supply of electricity, may cause great suffering to many individual people. An animal may survive the death of many of its cells, and the removal of an organ, such as a leg (with the consequent death of the cells constituting the organ); but the death of the animal leads, in time, to the death of its constituent parts, cells included.

I believe that these examples make the existence of downward causation obvious; and they make the complete success of any reductionist programme at least problematic.

Peter Medawar (in his [1974]; compare also his [1969], pp. 15–19) critically discusses reduction, using the following Table 3.

(4) Ecology/Sociology
(3) Biology
(2) Chemistry
(1) Physics

Table 3: Customary Table of Reduction

[3] It is a "heap" like a "heap of sand" or a "heap of stones"; see note 2 to section 8.

Medawar suggests that the true relation of the higher to the lower of these subjects is not simply one of logical reducibility, but rather comparable to the relation between the subjects mentioned in Table 4.

(4) Metrical (Euclidean) Geometry
(3) Affine Geometry
(2) Projective Geometry
(1) Topology

Table 4: Various Geometries

The fundamental relation between the higher geometrical disciplines listed in Table 4 and the lower ones is not quite easy to describe, but it is certainly not one of reducibility. For example, metrical geometry, especially in the form of Euclidean geometry, is only very partially reducible to projective geometry, even though the results of projective geometry are all valid in a metrical geometry embedded in a language rich enough to employ the concepts of projective geometry. Thus we may regard metrical geometry as an *enrichment* of projective geometry. Similar relations hold between the other levels of Table 4. The enrichment is partly one of concepts, but mainly one of theorems.

Medawar suggests that the relations between consecutive levels of Table 3 may be analogous to those of Table 4. Thus chemistry may be regarded as an enrichment of physics; which explains why it is partly though not wholly reducible to physics; and similarly the higher levels of Table 3.

Thus the subjects in Table 4 are clearly *not reducible* to the ones on lower levels, even though the lower levels remain, in a very clear sense, valid within the higher levels, and even though they are somehow contained in the higher levels. Moreover, *some* of the propositions on the higher levels are reducible to the lower levels.

I find Medawar's remarks highly suggestive. They are, of course, only acceptable if we give up the idea that our physical universe is deterministic – that physical theory, together with the initial conditions prevalent at some given moment, *completely* determine the state of the physical universe at any other moment. (See the discussion of Laplace in the next section.) If we accept this physicalist determinism, then Table 4 cannot be regarded as analogous to Table 3. If we reject it, Table 4 can serve as a key to Table 3, and also to Table 1.

8. Emergence and its Critics

The idea of "creative" or "emergent" evolution (to which I have alluded in section 7) is very simple, if somewhat vague. It refers to the fact that in the course of evolution new things and events occur, with unexpected and indeed unpredictable properties; things and events that are new, more or less in the sense in which a great work of art may be described as new.

This unpredictability has been questioned, however, by the critics of emergence. The challenge has come in the main from three sides: from the determinists; from the classical atomists; and from the upholders of a theory of capacities or potentialities.

(1) The most famous formulation of the determinist's point of view is due to Laplace ([1819]; [1951], pp. 4–5): "We ought . . . to regard the present state of the universe as the effect of its anterior state and as the cause of the one which is to follow. Assume . . . an intelligence which could know all the forces by which nature is animated, and the states at an instant of all the objects that compose it; . . . for [this intelligence], nothing would be uncertain; and the future, as the past, would be present to its eyes." If this Laplacean determinism is accepted, nothing whatever can be unpredictable in principle. So evolution cannot be emergent.

The passage quoted from Laplace is from the Introduction to his *Philosophical Essays on Probability*. Its function there is to make quite clear that the theory of probability – as seen by Laplace – is concerned with events of which we have *subjectively* insufficient knowledge, and not with *objectively* indeterminate or chancelike events: *these do not exist.* (Note that Laplacean determinism does not allow *any* exceptions: the assertion that there are any objectively chancelike events at all is tantamount to indeterminism, even if these chancelike events should be rare exceptions.)

The deterministic thesis is intuitively fairly convincing – if we neglect our own voluntary movements – as long as atoms are regarded as indivisible rigid bodies (even though Epicurus introduced an indeterministic atomism). But the introduction of composite atoms, and subatomic particles such as the electrons, suggested another possibility: the idea that atomic and molecular collisions may not be of a deterministic character. This seems to have been first broached in our time by Charles Sanders Peirce, who stressed that we have to assume objective chance in order to understand the diversity of the universe, and by Franz Exner.[1] The reply to Laplace is, in brief, that modern

[1] See Erwin Schrödinger ([1957], chapter VI, p. 133). These remarks of Schrödinger's come from a lecture delivered in 1922. Schrödinger says there (pp. 142f.) that Exner discussed these ideas – perhaps in a lecture? – in 1919. In chapter III of the same book (p. 71), Schrödinger

physics assumes that there are objectively chancelike events, and objective probabilities or propensities.

(2) From the atomist's point of view, all physical bodies and all organisms are nothing but structures of atoms. (See Table 2 in the preceding section 7.) Thus there can be no novelty except a *novelty of arrangement.* Given the precise arrangement of the atoms it should in principle be possible, the argument goes, to derive, or to predict, all the properties of every new arrangement from a knowledge of the "intrinsic" properties of the atoms. Of course, our human knowledge of the properties of the atoms as well as of their precise arrangement will in general be insufficient for this kind of prediction. But in principle, this knowledge can be improved; and so, the argument goes, we must agree that the novel arrangement and its results are predictable in principle.

A partial reply to the atomist was given in the preceding section 7. The main point of the reply is that new atomic arrangements may lead to physical and chemical properties which are not derivable from a statement describing the arrangement of the atoms, combined with a statement of atomic theory. Admittedly, some such properties have been successfully derived from physical theory, and these derivations are highly impressive; yet it seems that the number and complexity of both the different molecules and their properties are unlimited and that they may far transcend the possibilities of deductive explanation. Some important properties, foremost among them some of the properties of DNA, are well understood on the basis of the atomic structure; yet although the progress made is most impressive, we are very far – some would say infinitely far – from deriving or predicting even the majority of the properties of the infinitely varied macro-molecules from first principles.

(3) A third argument (which may be described as a weak form of "preformationism") is perhaps less clear but nevertheless intuitively appealing. It is closely related to the two preceding arguments; and it may be expounded as follows. If something new seems to emerge in the course of the evolution of the universe – a new chemical element (that is, a new structure of atomic nuclei), or a new compound molecule, or a living organism, or human speech, or conscious experience – then the physical particles or structures involved must have possessed beforehand what we may call the "disposition" or "possibility" or "potentiality" or "capacity" for producing the new properties, under appropriate conditions. In other words, the possibility or potentiality of entering into the new combination or structure, and the possibility

gives 1918 as the date of Exner's lecture, and in Schrödinger's address [1929] he says that Exner discussed the matter in his lectures *published* in 1919. (On Peirce, see my [1972(a)], chapter 6, pp. 212–13.)

or potentiality of producing thereby the apparently unpredictable or emergent new property, must have been there before the event; and sufficient knowledge of this inherent or hidden possibility or potentiality should have allowed us in principle to predict the new evolutionary step, and the new property. Thus evolution cannot be creative or emergent.

If this third argument is applied, more especially, to the problem of the (apparently emergent) evolution of mind or of conscious experience, then it leads to the doctrine of panpsychism (which will be more fully discussed in section 19).

It seems to me interesting that the arguments (1) to (3) here outlined have been marshalled quite recently against the idea of emergent evolution by the great *Gestalt* psychologist and philosopher, Wolfgang Köhler ([1960]; [1961], pp. 15–32).

At the time when he wrote this paper Köhler had been concerned with the problem of emergence and with the mind-body problem for more than forty years: forty years earlier he had published a very original book on *The Physical Gestalten at Rest and in the Stationary State* ([1920]; not, to my knowledge, translated into English). In this book he attempted to counter the arguments of his former teacher, the psychologist Carl Stumpf, who was an opponent of materialism and of psycho-physical parallelism, and a supporter of interaction and of emergent evolution. Köhler had also been a student of Max Planck, the great physicist and determinist; and Köhler's book of 1920 showed considerable insight into physics. I read it as a student, shortly after its publication, and it made a great impression on me. Its implicit central thesis may be stated as follows: materialism and an epiphenomenalist parallelism are not refuted by the existence of mental "wholes" or of *"Gestalten"*; for *Gestalten* can occur, and can often be fully explained, within physics. (A simple example is a soap bubble.[2]) No doubt this line of thought led Köhler to demand, forty years later, that *all* wholes (living organisms, *Gestalt* experiences) should be physically explained.[3]

However, the arguments (1) to (3) are based on classical physics and its apparently deterministic character. There is no allusion in Köhler's [1960] to the fact that the new atomic theory – quantum mechanics – has jettisoned

---

[2] Even a heap of stones has a *Gestalt* in Köhler's sense (although I do not think that Köhler was aware of this fact); see my [1944(b)], p. 129, [1957(g)], p. 83. I there distinguished a whole in the sense of a *Gestalt* from a whole in the sense of a totality, and I denied that we can know any object in the sense of knowing the totality of its properties. See also dialogue X.

[3] It is interesting that Köhler ([1961], p. 32) is led close to panpsychism; but he rightly comes to the conclusion that panpsychism is not fully compatible with his materialist position: ". . . if [panpsychism] were true it would . . . show that the [physical] scientists have not given us an adequate description of nature" (that is, of the nature of atoms).

strict determinism. It has enriched physics by introducing *objective probability statements* into the theory of elementary particles and atoms. As a consequence of this, we ought to abandon Laplacean determinism. Indeed, many of the former strictly causal statements of classical physics about macroscopic objects have been re-interpreted as probability statements that assert probabilities close to 1. Causal explanation has been at least partly replaced by probabilistic explanation.

Now if we take into account the change from classical (Newtonian) physics to modern atomic physics, with its objective probabilities or propensities, then we find that a full defence of the idea of emergent evolution against criticisms like those of Köhler's (1) to (3) is at our disposal. We can admit that the world does not change in so far as certain universal laws remain invariant. But there are other important and interesting lawlike aspects – especially probabilistic propensities – that do change, depending upon the changing situation. Thus my answer to Köhler is simple. There can be invariant laws *and* emergence; for the system of invariant laws is not sufficiently complete and restrictive to prevent the emergence of new lawlike properties.

Probability became important in physical theory mainly with the molecular theory of heat and of gases and, in the twentieth century, with atomic theory.

At first, the role played by probability in physics was interpreted subjectively, according to the interpretation of Laplace. Physical events were assumed to be objectively fully determined. It was only due to our subjective lack of knowledge concerning the precise positions and velocities of molecules or atoms or elementary particles that we had to use probabilistic rather than strict deterministic methods. This subjectivist interpretation of probability was adhered to by physicists for a long time. Einstein adhered to it (see his letter to me printed at the end of my [1959(a)], and my comments there on p. 457, third paragraph); Heisenberg inclined towards it; and even Max Born, the founder of the statistical interpretation of wave mechanics, seemed sometimes to adopt it. However, with the announcement by Rutherford and Soddy [1902] of their famous law of radioactive decay, an alternative interpretation presented itself: that radioactive atomic nuclei were breaking up *"spontaneously"*: that each atomic nucleus had a *tendency or propensity* to disintegrate, dependent upon its structure. This tendency or propensity can be measured by the *"half-life"*, a constant characteristic of the structure of the radioactive nucleus. It is the length of time needed for one half of any given number of nuclei (of a given structure) to decay. The objective constancy of the half-life, and its dependence upon the nuclear structure, show that there is an objective and constant measurable tendency or propensity of the nucleus, dependent upon its structure, to break up within any chosen unit of time.[4]

In this way, the situation in physics leads to the assumption of *objective probabilities* or probabilistic *propensities* in physics. This is an idea without which, I suggest, modern atomic physics (quantum mechanics) is hardly understandable. But it is far from univerally accepted among physicists: the older, subjective theory of Laplace, from which the propensity interpretation should be sharply distinguished, still lingers on. (I have long upheld the thesis that the strange role played by "the observer" in some interpretations of quantum mechanics can be explained as a residue of the subjectivist interpretation of probability theory, and that all this can and should be given up.[5])

There are several reasons indicating that objective probabilistic propensities may be regarded as generalizations of causal situations, and causal situations as special cases of propensities. (See my [1974(c)], section 37.) It is however important to realize that statements asserting probabilities or propensities other than 0 or 1 cannot be derived from causal laws of a deterministic type (together with initial conditions) or from laws asserting that a certain type of event always happens in a certain situation. A probabilistic conclusion can be derived only from probabilistic premises; for example, premises about equal propensities. But it is possible, on the other hand, to derive statements asserting propensities equal to, or approaching, 0 or to 1 – and therefore of causal character – from typically probabilistic premises.

As a consequence, we can say that a typical propensity statement, such as a statement of the propensity of a certain unstable nucleus to disintegrate, cannot be derived from a universal law (of the causal type) plus initial conditions. On the other hand, the *situation* in which an event takes place may greatly influence a propensity; for example, the arrival of a slow neutron in the immediate neighbourhood of a nucleus may influence the propensity of the nucleus to capture the neutron and subsequently to disintegrate.

---

[4] This is perhaps the strongest argument in favour of what I have called *"the propensity interpretation of probability in physics"*. See my [1957(e)], [1959(a)], and [1967(k)]; also my reply to Suppes in [1974(c)]. The propensity is the *weighted disposition (Verwirklichungstendenz)* of a thing *in a certain situation* to assume a certain property or state.

As the example of radioactive nuclei shows, propensities may be irreversible: they may determine a direction of time (the "arrow of time"). Some propensities, however, may also be reversible: the Schrödinger equation (and thus quantum mechanics) is reversible with respect to time, and the propensity of an atom in a certain state s_1 to make a transition to state s_2 by absorbing a photon will in general be equal to the propensity to make the reverse transition by emitting a photon.

[5] See for example my [1967(k)]; see also note 1 above and text.

In order to illustrate the significance of the situation for the probability or propensity of an event to take place, let us consider the tossing of a penny. We may say that if the penny is not biased, its probability of falling "heads up" will be equal to $^1/_2$. But assume that we toss the penny over a table with cracks or slots in it which are pointing in different directions, designed to catch a penny upright. Then its propensity to fall "heads up" may be considerably less than $^1/_2$, although it will still be equal to its propensity to fall "tails up",[6] for the propensity of the penny to stay upright will have changed from zero to some positive value (say, to three per cent).

The situation is very similar if we consider the propensity of a hydrogen atom, taken at random, to become part of a certain macro-molecule (say, of a nucleic acid): the presence or the absence of a catalyst (an enzyme) may make a great difference – like the presence or the absence of slots in the table used in tossing the penny. The probability or propensity will be zero for a hydrogen atom, taken at random anywhere in the universe. The probability or propensity may be quite considerable for a hydrogen atom within an organism and in the immediate neighbourhood of an appropriate enzyme.

I suggest that this idea of the situational dependence of the probability or propensity of some interesting event can throw some light on the problems of evolution and emergence.

Among the most important emergent events according to present day cosmological views are perhaps the following. (They correspond to points (1) to (5) of Table 1, p. 16 above.)

(a) The "cooking" of the heavier elements (other than hydrogen and helium which are assumed to have existed from the first big bang).

(b) The beginning of life on earth (and perhaps elsewhere).

(c) The emergence of consciousness.

(d) The emergence of the human language, and of the human brain.

Of these events (a), the emergence of the elements, looks predictable rather than emergent. It looks as if we could in principle explain the cooking of the elements by the tremendous pressures in the centre of a huge star. At first glance, the properties of the new elements may also look predictable rather than emergent, if we remember the regularities of the periodic table of the elements, regularities which have been largely explained, with the help of Pauli's exclusion principle and of other principles of quantum theory. However, what would have to be explained is not only the table of the elements, but the sequence of the atomic nuclei – the isotopes – with their characteristic properties. To these properties belong, especially, the degree of

[6] See my [1957(e)] where this example is briefly mentioned on p. 89.

stability or instability of the atomic nucleus; and this means, for unstable nuclei, the probability or propensity of their radioactive disintegration. The propensity of a nucleus to disintegrate (measured by its half-life) is among the most characteristic properties of a radioactive isotope. It changes from isotope to isotope, varying from less than a millionth of a second to more than a million years, though it is constant for all nuclei of the same structure. Although a great amount is known about nuclear structure – we know that the stability of the nucleus depends strongly on its symmetry properties – it very much looks as if the *precise* value of the half-life of a nucleus would have to remain for ever an emergent property, a property unpredictable from the properties of its constituents.[7]

As to (b), the origin of life, I have already said that the probability or propensity of any atom, taken at random in the universe, to become (within a chosen unit of time) part of a living organism, has always been and still is indistinguishable from zero. It certainly was zero before the emergence of life; and even on the assumption that there are many planets in the universe capable of sustaining life, the probability in question must still be immeasurably small.

Jacques Monod [1970] writes: "Life appeared on earth: what, *before the event,* were the chances that this would occur?" And he gives good reasons for replying that the probability was "virtually zero".[8] The reasons are that, even if a naked gene, synthesised by chance, were to find itself in a soup of enzymes, the probability would be zero that the enzymes – highly complex and highly specialized molecules – would just fit the gene so as to help it in its two main functions: the production of new enzymes, *and* in its own replication; functions for which precisely fitting enzymes are required. (Monod estimates that about 50 different enzymes are needed for the purpose; by the principle "one gene, one enzyme", this would raise the number of genes needed also to about 50. But the original system is likely to have been far more primitive.)

Even if in the case of the origin of the elements we can give some explanation of how it may have happened, it seems that we cannot give an explanation for the origin of life; for a probabilistic explanation must work

[7] Another emergent property seems to be the propensity of certain molecules to form crystals capable of reflecting light of a certain wavelength: the emergence of coloured surfaces. The optical properties of a complex crystal – of a spatially extended complex periodic or aperiodic arrangement of molecules – and thus the properties of spectral analysers, may also be not fully predictable from the properties of single atoms and photons, although those of simple and highly symmetrical arrangements are predictable, and although much about the structure of highly complex molecules can be deduced from their X-ray spectrograms.

[8] See Jacques Monod, [1970], p. 160; [1971], p. 144; [1972], p. 136.

with probabilities near to 1, and cannot work with probabilities near to zero – to say nothing of probabilities virtually equal to zero. (See my [1959 (a)], sections 67–8.)

The amount of knowledge recently acquired about genes and enzymes, and what appear to be minimum conditions of life, is staggering. Nevertheless, it is just this detailed knowledge which suggests that the difficulties in the way of an *explanation* of the origin of life may be insuperable – even though we have some idea of the conditions necessary for this event to happen. Much speaks in favour of the view that the event was unique.

Under the circumstances, many of the properties of living organisms may be unpredictable – emergent. (Among them are properties of their development.) So are the properties of new species which arise in the course of evolution.

As to (c), it is difficult to say anything about the emergence of consciousness. We have here theories which are radically opposed to each other. Two of them are: panpsychism, which says that even atoms have an inner life (of a very primitive kind); and that form of behaviourism which denies conscious experiences even to man. Both views avoid the problem of the emergence of consciousness.[9] Then there is the Cartesian view that consciousness arises only with man, and that animals are inanimate automata; a view which is clearly pre-evolutionary. I suggest that we have reason to accept the view that there are lower and higher stages of consciousness. (Think of dreams.) If the fact that animals cannot speak is a sufficient reason to deny consciousness to them, it would also be a sufficient reason to deny it to babies at an age before they learn to speak. Moreover, there is good evidence in favour of the theory that higher animals dream (*pace* Malcolm and Wittgenstein).

The most reasonable view seems to be that consciousness is an emergent property of animals arising under the pressure of natural selection (and therefore only after the evolution of a mechanism of reproduction). How early its antecedents arise, and whether there are somewhat similar states in plants, seem to me questions which, while interesting, are perhaps for ever unanswerable. It seems worth mentioning, however, that the great biologist H. S. Jennings [1906] reported that the observation of the behaviour of the amoeba created in him the strong impression that it was conscious. He saw symptoms of activity and of initiative in its behaviour. Indeed, if a free-moving animal is to use this freedom, it has to be an active explorer of its

[9] There is also a queer egocentric version of behaviourism which allows consiousness only to the ego: only to oneself, but not to anybody else: a psychistic form of solipsism. See chapter 9 of Sidney Hook [1960], [1961].

environment. Its senses are not merely passive receptors of information, but it uses them actively as "perceptual systems", "to pick up information", as J. J. Gibson [1966] emphasizes. But the perceptual systems are not enough: there is a centre of activity, of curiosity, of exploration, of planning; there is an explorer, the animal's mind.

Thus we can speculate on the conditions of the emergence of consciousness. But it is clearly something new, and unpredictable: it emerges.

As to (d), the human brain is estimated to contain ten thousand million neurons, interconnected by means of perhaps a thousand times this number of synapses; and this incredibly complex system is in almost constant agitation. It has been suggested by F. A. von Hayek ([1952], p. 185) that it must be impossible for us ever to explain the functioning of the human brain in any detail since "any apparatus . . . must possess a structure of a higher degree of complexity than is possessed by the objects" which it is trying to explain. Monod, referring to this kind of argument, points out that we are still "far . . . from that ultimate border of knowledge".[10] How did the brain emerge? We can only guess. My guess is – see section 5 above – that it was the emerging human language which created the selection pressure under which the cerebral cortex emerged, and with it, the human consciousness of self.

Of the three arguments against emergence stated at the beginning of this section, I have more or less answered, I think, the arguments from determinism and from atomism. But the third argument is still to be answered – the argument that the physical parts constituting a new structure (like an organism) must possess beforehand the possibility or potentiality or capacity for producing the new structure in question. Thus a full knowledge of the pre-existing possibilities or potentialities would have enabled us to predict the properties of the new structure which therefore must, in principle, be predictable rather than emergent.

The answer to this can be found, I think, if we replace the classical ideas of possibility or potentiality or capacity or force by their new version – by probability or propensity. As we have seen, the first emergence of a novelty such as life may change the possibilities or propensities in the universe. We might say that the newly emergent entities, both micro and macro, change the propensities, micro and macro, in their neighbourhood. They introduce new possibilities or probabilities or propensities into their neighbourhood:[11] they create *new fields of propensities,* as a new star creates a new field of gravitation. The assimilation of inanimate matter by an organism has zero possibility

---

[10] Monod [1970], p. 162; [1971], p. 146; [1972], p. 137.

[11] A suggestion similar to this may be found in R. A. Fisher [1954], pp. 91–2.

or probability if it is outside the field of the organism. Within such a field it may become highly probable. (As I have tried to show in [1974 (c)], section 37, a formal analysis in terms of propensities can be given of causal *and* probabilistic explanations of events, analogous to the way in which we use forces – gravitational, or electromagnetic – in classical physics.)

There is a striking illustration of the radical manner in which the early evolution of life on earth may have changed the conditions and the probabilities or propensities of the occurrence of events that constitute the later evolution. I am alluding to the theory of A. I. Oparin and J. B. S. Haldane according to which oxygen was absent in the early atmosphere of the earth and that it appeared later, as a result of the activity of photosynthetic molecules like chlorophyll. Evolutionary events, impossible and unforseeable before, may then happen as a matter of course.

This is my reply to Köhler's claim [1960] that the very idea of evolution necessarily implies a "postulate of invariance" which he formulates as follows: "While evolution took place, the basic forces, the elementary processes, and the general principles of action remain the same as they had always been, and still are, in inanimate nature. As soon as . . . any new elementary process or any new principle of action were discovered in some organism, the concept of evolution in its strict sense would become inapplicable."[12] That may be so. But while the invariances may continue to hold for elementary physical entities (atoms, inanimate structures) sufficiently distant from the newly emerged structures, new types of events may become the rule within the fields of the newly emerged structures; for with these emerge new propensities, and new probabilistic explanations.[13]

---

[12] Wolfgang Köhler [1960]; see [1961], pp. 23f. It is interesting that the whole discussion seems to go back to the early ninteenth century discussion of catastrophism in geology which, no doubt, Thomas Huxley had in mind when he said things very similar to these remarks of Köhler's. See his [1893], p. 103, where he writes: "The doctrine of evolution . . . postulates the fixity of the rules of operation of the causes of motion in the material universe . . . the orderly evolution of physical nature out of one substratum and one energy implies that the rules of action of that energy should be fixed and definite." More recently the constancy of natural laws has been challenged by some dialectical materialists such as David Bohm [1957].

[13] An interesting objection to this argument has been raised by Jeremy Shearmur: even if we admit propensities, we do not escape the idea of preformation — we just have several preformationist possibilities instead of one. My reply is that we may have an *infinity* of open possibilities, and this means giving up preformationism; and this infinity of possible propensities may still rule out infinitely many logical possibilities. Propensities may rule out possibilities: in this consists their lawlike character.

I suggested something like this many years ago, in an attempt to explain the world view of the propensity interpretation of probability in my still unpublished *Postscript*. The *infinity* of the inherent possibilities or propensities is important, since a probabilistic doctrine of preformation does not otherwise differ sufficiently from a deterministic doctrine of preformation.

9. Indeterminism; the Interaction of Levels of Emergence

The "natural" view of the universe seems to be indeterministic: the world is the intentional product, the work of the gods, or of God; in Homer, of very arbitrary gods. The Platonic demiurge is a craftsman;[1] and this may still carry over to Aristotle's unmoved mover. Aristotle's view is still indeterministic in this sense; this is particularly important since he had an elaborate theory of *causes*. But the most important of his causes was the *final cause*. It was *purpose* that moved the world; that made it move nearer to its aim, its end, its "perfection"; that made it better. This shows that the Aristotelian idea of a final cause cannot be described as a (determining) cause in our sense. It is "soul", either animal soul or human or divine reason, which is the principle of movement. Only the movement of the heavens is completely lawful and rational. The events of the sub-lunary world are influenced but not fully determined by the lawful changes of the season, but they are also subject to other final causes; and there is no suggestion that these can be completely summed up by invariant laws, least of all by mechanical laws. For Aristotle, cause is not mechanical, and the future is not fully determined by laws.

The founders of determinism, Leucippus and Democritus, were also founders of atomism and of mechanical materialism. Leucippus said (DK B2)[2]: "Nothing occurs at random or without cause; but everything occurs according to reason, and by necessity." For Democritus, time is not cyclical but infinite, and worlds come for ever into being and pass away: "The causes of things . . . have no beginning, but from infinite time back, and foreordained by necessity, are all things that have existed, that are now, and that are still to come." (DK A39.) And Diogenes Laertius reports about the teaching of Democritus (IX, 45): "All things happen according to necessity; for the whirl is the cause of the genesis of all things, and this he calls necessity." Aristotle (*De generatione animalium,* 789b2) complains that Democritus did not know a final cause: "Democritus omitted the final cause and so he refers all the operations of nature to necessity." Aristotle (*Physics* 196a24) further complains that according to Democritus (for he seems to be meant) our heavens and all the worlds are ruled by chance (and not only by necessity); but "chance" does not seem to mean here randomness, but the absence of a purpose, of a final cause.[3]

---

[1] For Plato's indeterminism see the passage from the *Phaedo,* quoted below in section 46.

[2] DK = Diels & Kranz [1951–2].

[3] Compare Cyril Bailey [1928], pp. 140f. Also DK, A69. Bailey (pp. 142f.) argues, perhaps correctly, that "chance" meant for Democritus those objective mechanical causes which, subjectively, are "unaccessible to man". (Objective randomness was introduced into atomism much later, by Epicurus's theory of "swerve".)

Democritus viewed all things as generated by a whirl of atoms: the atoms impinged on each other; they pushed each other along; and they also pulled each other, since some of them had hooks through which they could get entangled and form filaments. (Cp. DK A66; and Aëtius I 26,2.[4]) The atomist view of the world was utterly mechanical. But this did not prevent Democritus from being a great humanist (see sections 44 and 46, below).

Determinism of a more or less mechanistic character remained the dominant view of science down to my own day. The great names in modern times are Hobbes, Priestley, Laplace, and even Einstein. (Newton was an exception.) Only with quantum mechanics, with Einstein's probabilistic interpretation of the amplitude of light waves, with Heisenberg's interpretation of his indeterminacy formulae, and especially with Max Born's probabilistic interpretation of Schrödinger's wave amplitudes, did physics become indeterministic.

In order to discuss the ideas of indeterminism and determinism, I introduced in 1965 (see my [1972(a)], chapter 6) the metaphor of *clouds* and *clocks*. For the ordinary man, a cloud is highly unpredictable and, indeed, indeterminate: the vagaries of the weather are proverbial. By contrast, a clock is highly predictable and, indeed, a perfect clock is a paradigm of a mechanical and determinist material system.

Taking clouds and clocks to start with as paradigms of indeterminist and determinist systems we can formulate the view of a determinist, such as a Democritean atomist, as follows:

All physical systems are, in reality, clocks.

Thus the whole world is a clockwork of atoms pushing each other along like the cogs of a cogwheel. Even the clouds are parts of the cosmic clockwork; though owing to the complexity and practical unpredictability of the molecular movements in them, they may create in us the illusion that they are not clocks, but undetermined clouds.

Quantum mechanics, especially in Schrödinger's form, has had important things to say about this matter. It says, indeed, that the electrons form a *cloud* round the atomic nucleus, and that the positions and velocities of the various electrons within this cloud are indeterminate and therefore indeterminable. More recently, the subatomic particles have in their turn been diagnosed as complex structures; and David Bohm [1957] has discussed the possibility that there may be an infinity of such hierarchic layers. (The level 0 in Table 2 in section 7 would be supported by negative levels.) This, if true, would make

[4] See H. Diels (ed.) *Doxographi Graeci* [1929].

the idea of a thoroughly deterministic cosmos based upon atomic clocks impossible.

However this may be, the interpretation of the atomic nucleus as a system of particles in rapid motion and of the surrounding electrons as an electron cloud is sufficient to destroy the old atomistic intuition of a mechanical determinism. The interaction between atoms or between molecules has a *random* aspect, a *chance* aspect; "chance" not only in the Aristotelian sense in which it is opposed to "purpose", but chance in the sense in which it is subject to the objective probabilistic theory of random events, rather than to anything like exact mechanical laws.

Thus the thesis that all physical systems including clouds, are, in reality, clocks, has turned out to be mistaken. According to quantum mechanics we have to replace it by the opposite thesis, as follows:

All physical systems, including clocks, are, in reality, clouds.

The old mechanism turns out to be an illusion, created by the fact that sufficiently heavy systems (systems consisting of a few thousands of atoms, such as the big organic macromolecules, and heavier systems) interact *approximately* according to the clockwork laws of classical mechanics, provided they do not react with each other chemically. Systems of crystals – the solid physical bodies which we handle in ordinary tools like our watches and clocks, and which constitute the main furniture of our environment – do behave approximately (but only approximately) like mechanical deterministic systems. This fact is, indeed, the source of our mechanistic and deterministic illusions.

Each cogwheel of our watches is a structure of crystals, a lattice of molecules held together, like the atoms in the molecules, by electrical forces. It is strange, but it is a fact, that it is electricity which underlies the laws of mechanics. Moreover, each atom and each molecule vibrates, with amplitudes depending on the temperature (or *vice versa*); and if the cogwheel gets hot, the clockwork will stop because the cogs expand. (If it gets hotter still it will melt.)

The interaction between heat and the watch is very interesting. On the one hand, we can regard the temperature of the watch as defined by the average velocity of its vibrating atoms and molecules. On the other hand, we can heat or cool the watch by putting it in contact with hot or cold surroundings. According to present theory temperature is due to the movement of the individual atoms; at the same time it is something on a level different from that of individual atoms in motion – a holistic or emergent level – since it is defined by the *average* velocity of *all* the atoms.

Heat behaves very much like a fluid ("caloric"), and we can *explain* the laws of this behaviour by an appeal to the way in which an increase or decrease in the velocity of an atom – or a group of atoms – spreads to neighbouring atoms. This explanation can be described as a "reduction": it reduces the holistic properties of heat to the properties of motion of the atoms or molecules. Yet the reduction is not complete; for new ideas have to be used – the ideas of *molecular disorder* and of *averaging*; and these are, indeed, ideas on a new holistic level.[5]

The levels can *interact* with each other. (This is an important idea for mind-brain interactionism.) For example, not only does the movement of each single atom influence the movements of the neighbouring atoms; but also the *average* velocity of a *group* of atoms influences the *average* velocity of the neighbouring *groups* of atoms. It thereby influences (and herein lies the interaction of the levels, including "downward causation") the velocities of many individual atoms in the group. Which individual atoms we cannot say without investigating the details of the lower level.

Any change in the higher level (temperature) will thus influence the lower level (the movement of individual atoms). The opposite also holds. Yet of course an individual atom, or even many individual atoms, may increase their velocity without raising the temperature, because some other neighbouring individual atoms may decrease their velocity at the same time. At constant temperature this kind of thing happens all the time. Thus we have here an example of "downward causation", of the higher level acting on the lower level. (See also section 7.)

This seems to me another important example of the general principle that a higher level may exert a dominant influence upon a lower level.

The one-sided dominance is due, in this case at least, to the random character of the heat motion of the atoms, and therefore, I suspect, to the cloudlike character of the crystal. For it seems that, were the universe *per impossibile* a perfect determinist clockwork, there would be no heat production and no layers and therefore no such dominating influence would occur.

This suggests that the emergence of hierarchical levels or layers, and of an interaction between them, depends upon a fundamental indeterminism of the physical universe. Each level is open to causal influences coming from lower *and* from higher levels.

This bears of course heavily upon the mind-body problem, upon the interaction between the physical World 1 and the mental World 2.

---

[5] The issue is whether the (probabilistic) second law of thermodynamics is completely reducible to the interaction of individual atoms or molecules. My answer is: probabilistic conclusions require probabilistic and thus non-individualistic premises for their derivation.

Chapter P2 The Worlds 1, 2 and 3

10. Interaction; The Worlds 1, 2 and 3

Whether or not biology is reducible to physics, it appears that all physical and chemical laws are binding for living things — plants and animals, and even viruses. Living things are material bodies. Like all material bodies, they are processes; and like some other material bodies (clouds, for example) they are open systems of molecules: systems that exchange some of their constituent parts with their environment. They belong to the *universe of physical entities,* or states of physical things, or physical states.

The entities of the physical world — processes, forces, fields of forces — interact among one another, and therefore with material bodies. Thus we conjecture them to be real (in the sense discussed in section 4 above) even though their reality remains conjectural.

Besides the physical objects and states, I conjecture that there are *mental states,* and that these states are real since they interact with our bodies.

A toothache is a good example of a state that is both mental *and* physical. If you have a bad toothache, it may become a strong reason for visiting your dentist; which involves a number of actions and of physical movements of your body. The caries in your tooth — a material, physico-chemical process — will thus lead to physical effects; but it does so by way of your painful sensations, and of your knowledge of existing institutions, such as dentistry. (As long as you do not feel any pain, you may be unaware of the caries, and not visit your dentist; or you may become suspicious for other reasons, and visit him without waiting for the pain: in both cases it is the intervention of some mental states — something like a conjecture, like knowledge — which explains your action, and the movements of your body.)

There are other kinds of mental states that explain human actions. A mountaineer may go on climbing, "forcing his body to go on", even though his body is exhausted: we speak of his ambition, of his wish to reach the summit, and of his determination, as mental states that may make him continue his climb. Or a motorist may press his foot on the brake because he sees the traffic lights turning red: it is his knowledge of the highway code which makes him do so.

All this is very obvious, even trivial. Nevertheless, the reality of mental states has been denied by some philosophers. Others admit that mental states are real, but deny that they interact with the world of physical states; a view which is in my opinion as unacceptable as the denial of the reality of mental states.

The question whether both physical and mental states exist, and whether they interact or whether they are otherwise related, is known as the body-mind problem, or the mind-body problem, or as the psychophysical problem.

One of the conceivable solutions of this problem is interactionism – the theory that mental and physical states interact. This leads more precisely to a description of the body-mind problem as the brain-mind problem, since it is argued that the interaction is to be located in the brain; and it has led some interactionists (notably Eccles) to formulate the body-mind problem as the problem of describing, in as much detail as possible, the "liaison" between brain and mind ("the brain-mind liaison").

It may be said that the adoption of interactionism constitutes a solution to the brain-mind problem. Of course, such a solution would have to be supported by a critical discussion of alternative views, and of the various critiques of interactionism. Interactionism can be described as a kind of research programme: it opens many detailed questions, and answers to them will demand many detailed theories.

It is sometimes said that it is the task of the solution of the brain-mind problem to make the interaction between such different things as physical states or events and mental states or events understandable.

I agree that the main task of science is to further our understanding. But I also think that complete understanding, just like complete knowledge, is unlikely ever to be achieved. Moreover, understanding can be deceptive: we had, for centuries, what appeared to be a perfect understanding of the working of clockwork mechanisms in which the cogs of the cogwheels push each other along. But this turned out to be a very superficial understanding, and the push given by a physical body to another had to be explained by the repulsion between the negatively charged electron shells of their atoms. However, this explanation and this understanding are also superficial, as is shown by the facts of adhesion and cohesion. Thus final understanding is not easy, not even in what seems the most elementary part of physical science. And when we move to the interaction between light and matter, then we get into a region of knowledge which left one of the greatest pioneers in this field, Niels Bohr, baffled; so much so that he said that in quantum theory we had to renounce the hope of understanding our subject. However, though it seems that the ideal of *complete* understanding has to be renounced, a detailed description may lead to some *partial* understanding.

Thus an understanding such as we once mistakenly believed we possessed in the case of mechanical push is not available even in physics. And we can hardly expect it in the case of brain-mind interaction, although a more detailed knowledge of the working of the brain may give us that partial understanding which, it seems, is realizable in science.

In this section, I have talked of physical states and of mental states. I think, however, that the problems with which we are dealing can be made considerably clearer if we introduce a *tripartite* division. First, there is the physical world – the universe of physical entities – to which I referred at the beginning of this section; this I will call "World 1".[1] Second, there is the world of mental states, including states of consciousness and psychological dispositions and unconscious states; this I will call "World 2". But there is also a *third* such world, the world of the contents of thought, and, indeed, of the products of the human mind; this I will call "World 3", and it will be discussed in the next few sections.

11. The Reality of World 3

I think that some increase of understanding can be obtained by studying the role of World 3.

By World 3 I mean the world of the products of the human mind, such as stories, explanatory myths, tools, scientific theories (whether true or false), scientific problems, social institutions, and works of art. World 3 objects are of our own making, although they are not always the result of planned production by individual men.

Many World 3 objects exist in the form of material bodies, and belong in a sense to both World 1 and World 3. Examples are sculptures, paintings, and books, whether devoted to a scientific subject or to literature. A book is a physical object, and it therefore belongs to World 1; but what makes it a

[1] I have adopted Sir John Eccles's [1970] suggestion to speak of "World 1", "World 2", and "World 3", instead of the "first world", "second world" and "third world", as I did prior to Eccles's publication of *Facing Reality*, in which he made this suggestion.

significant product of the human mind is its *content*: that which remains invariant in the various copies and editions. And this content belongs to World 3.

One of my main theses is that World 3 objects can be real, in the sense of section 4 above: not only in their World 1 materializations or embodiments, but also in their World 3 aspects. As World 3 objects, they may induce men to produce other World 3 objects and, thereby, to act on World 1; and interaction with World 1 – even indirect interaction – I regard as a decisive argument for calling a thing real.

Thus a sculptor may, by producing a new work, encourage other sculptors to copy it, or to produce similar sculptures. His work – not so much through its material aspects as through the new shape he has created – may influence them, by way of their World 2 experiences and, indirectly, through the new World 1 object.

An opponent of the view that World 3 objects are real may reply to this analysis by asserting that all that is involved here are World 1 objects. One man shapes such an object and thereby incites others to imitate him: nothing more is involved.

I will try to answer this by offering another and perhaps more convincing example: the production of a scientific theory; its critical discussion; its tentative acceptance; and its application which may change the face of the earth, and thus of World 1.

The productive scientist as a rule starts from a *problem*. He will try to understand the problem. This is usually a lengthy intellectual task – a World 2 attempt to grasp a World 3 object. Admittedly, in doing so he may use books (or other scientific tools in their World 1 materializations). But his *problem* may not be stated in these books; rather, he may discover an unstated difficulty in the stated *theories*. This may involve a creative effort: the effort to grasp the abstract problem situation; if at all possible, better than it was done before. Then he may produce his solution, his new theory. This may be put into linguistic form in innumerable ways. He chooses one of them. Then he will critically discuss his theory; and he may greatly modify it as a result of the discussion. It is then published and discussed by others, on logical grounds and possibly on the basis of new experiments undertaken to test it, and the theory may be rejected if it fails in the test. And only after all these intellectual efforts and these interactions with World 1 may somebody discover some far-reaching application (electronics!) that changes World 1.

To this it may be still objected that I have described nothing but the behaviour of people, including their use of books, etc.; also their social and professional behaviour, including their habitual writing of papers. I have not, so a behaviourist may allege, given any reasons for accepting theories as having an existence of their own, apart from the people whose verbal behaviour may, admittedly, be important.

However, my point is that if we do not admit problems and theories as the objects of study and of criticism, then we shall never understand the behaviour of scientists.

Admittedly, of course, theories are the products of human thought (or, if you like, of human behaviour – I will not quarrel about words). Nevertheless, they have a certain degree of *autonomy*: they may have, objectively, consequences of which nobody so far has thought, and which may be *discovered*; discovered in the same sense in which an existing but so far unknown plant or animal may be discovered. One may say that World 3 is man-made only in its origin, and that once theories exist, they begin to have a life of their own: they produce previously invisible consequences, they produce new problems.

My standard example is taken from arithmetic. A number system *may* be said to be the construction or invention of men rather than their discovery. But the difference between even and odd numbers, or divisible and prime numbers, is a discovery: these characteristic sets of numbers are there, objectively, once the number system exists, as the (unintended) consequences of constructing the system; and their properties may be discovered.

There are behaviourists who think that the truth of "$2 \times 2 = 4$" is to be explained by human convention: that this equation is true because we learned it at school. But this is not so: it is a truth, a consequence of our number system, and it is translatable into all languages, provided they are not too poor: it is a truth which is invariant with respect to convention and translation.

The situation with respect to every scientific theory is similar. It has, objectively, a huge set of important consequences, whether or not these have as yet been discovered. (In fact, it can be shown that at any time only a fraction can be discovered.[1]) It is the objective task of the scientist – an objective World 3 task which regulates his "verbal behaviour" *qua* "scientist" – to discover the relevant logical consequences of the new theory, and to discuss them in the light of existing theories.

In this way, problems may be discovered rather than invented (though some problems – not always the most interesting ones – may be described as inventions). Examples are Euclid's problem whether there is a greatest prime; the corresponding problem for twin primes; whether Goldbach's

---

[1] See for example section 7 of my autobiography [1974(b)] and [1976(g)].

conjecture that every even number greater than 2 is the sum of two primes is true; the 3-body problem (and *n*-body problem) of Newtonian dynamics; and many others.

(It is a fatal mistake to believe that there can be an adequate theory – psychological, or behavioural, or sociological, or historical – of the behaviour of scientists which does not take full account of the World 3 status of science. This is an important point which many people are not aware of.)

These considerations seem to me decisive. They establish the objectivity of World 3, and its (partial) autonomy. And since the influence of scientific theories on World 1 is obvious, they establish the reality of the objects of World 3.

12. Unembodied World 3 Objects

Many World 3 objects like books or new synthetic medicines or computers or aircraft are embodied in World 1 objects: they are material artefacts, they belong to both World 3 and World 1. Most works of art are like this. Some World 3 objects exist only in encoded form, as musical scores (perhaps never performed) or as gramophone records. Others – poems, perhaps, and theories – may also exist as World 2 objects, as memories, presumably also encoded as memory traces in certain human brains (World 1) and perishing with them.

Are there unembodied World 3 objects? World 3 objects which are not embodied like books, or gramophone records, or memory traces (nor existing as World 2 memories, nor as objects of World 2 intentions)? I think that this question is important, and that the answer to it is "yes".

This answer is implied in what I said in the preceding section about the discovery of scientific and mathematical facts, problems, and solutions. With the invention (or discovery?) of the natural numbers (cardinals) there came into existence odd and even numbers even before anybody noticed this fact, or drew attention to it. The same holds for prime numbers. There followed discoveries (discoveries are World 2 events, and may be accompanied by World 1 events) of such simple facts as that there can be no more than one even prime, namely 2, and no more than one odd triplet of primes (namely 3, 5, and 7), and that with increasing size, primes rapidly get rarer. (See also dialogue XI.) These discoveries created an objective problem situation which caused new questions to be raised such as the following: How rapidly does the rarity of the primes increase? And are there infinitely many primes (and twin primes)? It is important to realize that the objective and unembodied existence of these problems precedes their conscious discovery in the same way as the existence of Mount Everest preceded its discovery; and it is important that the consciousness of the existence of these problems leads to the suspicion that there may exist, objectively, a way to their solution, and to the conscious search for this way: the search cannot be understood without understanding the objective existence (or perhaps non-existence) of as yet undiscovered and unembodied methods and solutions.

Often we discover a new problem through our failure to reach a hoped-for solution of an older problem. For from the failure, a new problem may arise: that of proving the objective impossibility of solving the old problem (under the given conditions). Such an impossibility proof led in the time of Plato to the discovery of the irrationality of the square root of 2; that is, of the diagonal of the unit square. A similar example, which also seems to have attracted the attention of Plato, is the ancient problem of squaring the circle. Its impossibility (under the admitted conditions) was only proved by Lindemann in 1882.

Some of the most famous mathematical problems have thus been solved, if not by the originally sought for positive solution, then by an impossibility proof. "It is probably this important fact", David Hilbert writes in his lecture "Mathematical Problems" [1901], [1902], ". . . that gives rise to the conviction (shared by all mathematicians, though so far unsupported by proof) that every definite mathematical problem must be susceptible of an exact settlement, either by an answer to the question asked, or by the proof of the impossibility of its solution . . . Take any definite unsolved problem, such as the question of . . . the existence of an infinite number of prime numbers of the form $2^n + 1$ [but also of divisible numbers of the same form]. Inapproachable as these problems may seem to us . . . we have the firm conviction that their solution must follow by a finite number of purely logical steps."

Clearly, Hilbert pleads here not only for the objective existence of mathematical problems, but also for the existence of solutions, one way or another, prior to their discovery. Although his claim that his conviction is "shared by all mathematicians" goes perhaps a little too far – I have known mathematicians who think otherwise – even those who believe that mathematics itself is incomplete (and not merely its formalizations) think in terms of discovered, and thus of pre-existent, and also of undiscovered problems and solutions – of problems and solutions yet to be found.

The main reason why I consider the existence of unembodied World 3 objects so important is this. If unembodied World 3 objects exist, then it cannot be a true doctrine that our grasp or understanding of a World 3 object always depends upon our sensual contact with its material embodiment; for example, upon our reading a statement of a theory in a book. As against this doctrine I assert that the most characteristic way of grasping World 3 objects is by a method which depends little, if at all, upon their embodiment or upon the use of our senses. My thesis is that the human mind grasps World 3 objects, if not always directly, then by an indirect method (which will be discussed); a method which is independent of their embodiment, and which, in the case of those World 3 objects (such as books) that belong also to World 1, abstracts from the fact that they are embodied.

13. Grasping a World 3 Object

How do we grasp an intellectual World 3 object, such as a problem, a theory, or an argument? The problem is an old one, and I must refer here to Plato.

Plato was the first, it seems, to contemplate something analogous to our Worlds 1, 2, and 3. He sharply contrasts the world of the "visible objects" (the world of material things, corresponding closely, though perhaps not completely, to our World 1) and a world of "intelligible objects" (vaguely corresponding to our World 3). In addition, he speaks of the "affections of the soul" or "states of the soul", corresponding to our World 2.

Though Plato's world of intelligible objects corresponds in some ways to our World 3, it is in many respects very different. It consists of what he called "forms" or "ideas" or "essences" – the objects to which general concepts or notions refer. The most important essences in his world of intelligible forms or ideas are the Good, the Beautiful, and the Just. These ideas are conceived of as immutable, as timeless or eternal, and as of divine origin. By contrast, our World 3 is man-made in its origin (man-made in spite of its partial autonomy discussed in sections 11 and 12 above); a suggestion which would have shocked Plato. Moreover, while I stress the existence of World 3 objects, I do not think that essences exist; that is, I do not attribute any status to the objects or referents of our concepts or notions. Speculations as to the true nature or true definition of the good, or of justice, lead in my opinion to verbal quibbles and are to be avoided. I am an opponent of what I have called "essentialism". Thus in my opinion, Plato's ideal essences play no significant role in World 3. (That is, Plato's World 3, though clearly in some sense an anticipation of my World 3, seems to me a mistaken construction.) On the other hand, Plato would never have admitted such entities as problems or conjectures – especially false conjectures – into his world of intelligible objects; though in approaching this world, he operated with conjectures or hypotheses, to be tested by their consequences: his so-called "dialectic" is a hypothetico-deductive method.[1]

Now Plato described the grasping of the forms or ideas as a kind of vision: our mental eye (*nous*, reason), the "eye of the soul" is endowed with intellectual intuition and can *see* an idea, an essence, an object that belongs to the intelligible world. Once we have managed to see it, to grasp it, we know this essence: we can see it "in the light of truth". This intellectual intuition, once it has been achieved, is infallible.

This is a view that has been most influential among those who accept, as indeed I do, the problem "How can we understand or grasp a theory?" But while I accept the problem, I do not accept Plato's solution – or only in a greatly modified form.

First, I admit that there is something like an intellectual intuition; but I assert that it is far from infallible, and that it more often errs than not.

Secondly, I suggest that it is easier to understand how we *make* World 3 objects than it is to understand how we understand them, grasp them, or "see" them. Indeed, I will attempt to explain understanding World 3 objects in terms of making or re-making them.

Thirdly, I suggest that we do not have anything like an intellectual sense organ, although we have acquired a faculty – something like an organ – for arguing or reasoning.

According to my view, we may understand the grasping of a World 3 object as an active process. We have to explain it as the making, the re-creation, of that object. In order to understand a difficult Latin sentence, we have to construe it: to see how it is made, and to re-construct it, to re-make it. In order to understand a *problem*, we have to try at least some of the more obvious solutions, and to discover that they fail; thus we rediscover that there is a difficulty – a problem. In order to understand a *theory*, we have first to understand the problem which the theory was designed to solve, and to see whether the theory does better than do any of the more obvious solutions. In order to understand a somewhat difficult *argument* like Euclid's proof of the theorem of Pythagoras (there are simpler proofs of this theorem), we have to do the work ourselves, taking full note of what is assumed without proof. In all these cases the understanding becomes "intuitive" when we have acquired the feeling that we can do the work of reconstruction at will, at any time.

This view of grasping assumes no "eye of the mind", no mental organ of

---

[1] See my [1940(a)], now chapter 15 of my [1963(a)]. Also my [1960(d)], now the Introduction to [1963(a)]. Also section 47, below, and pp. 548ff., below.

perception. It assumes only our ability to produce certain World 3 objects, especially linguistic ones. This ability in its turn is no doubt the result of practice. A baby starts by making very simple noises. He is born with the desire to copy, to re-make, difficult linguistic utterances. The decisive thing is that we learn to do things by *doing* things, in appropriate situations, including cultural situations: we learn how to read, and how to argue.

All this looks very different from Plato's theory of the intellectual eye. However, the neurophysiology of the eye and that of the brain suggest that the process involved in physical vision is not a passive one, but consists in an active interpretation of coded inputs. It is in many ways like problem solving by way of hypotheses.[2] (Even the inputs are already partially interpreted by the receiving sense organ, and our sense organs themselves may be likened to hypotheses or theories — theories about the structure of our environment, and about the kind of information most needed and most useful to us.) Our visual perception is more like a process of painting a picture, selectively (where "making comes before matching" as Ernst Gombrich says[3]) than one of taking random photographs. Admittedly, Plato knew nothing about these aspects of vision. Yet they show that there are, after all, some important analogies between our intellectual grasp of a World 3 object and our visual perception of a World 1 object.

There are many similarities between optical vision and the understanding of World 3 objects: we can conjecture that a baby *learns* to see, by actively exploring things, and by handling things by trial and error.[4]

Nevertheless, learning to perceive through action is largely a natural process. We learn to decode the coded signals which reach us: we decode them almost completely unconsciously, automatically, in terms of real things. We *learn* to behave, and to experience, as if we were "direct realists"; that is to say, we *learn* to experience things directly, as if there was no need for any decoding. (I conjecture that this is so with all sense organs and that a bat which depends on acoustic radar "sees" the heard material obstacles as "directly" as some other mammals see them optically.)

It is similar with World 3 objects; though here the learning process is not natural but cultural and social. This holds for the most fundamental of World 3 learning processes, the process of learning a language. Decoding becomes largely unconscious for language users and for readers of books. Yet there seem to be differences. We sometimes come across complicated but correct

---

[2] See chapters E2 and E7 and the references there to Hubel's and Wiesel's work.

[3] See Sir Ernst Gombrich [1960], [1962] and later editions, and J. J. Gibson, [1966].

[4] Cp. also the experiments of R. Held and A. Hein [1963], reported by Eccles in [1970] p. 67 and in chapter E8.

sentences which we must read twice or three times before we understand them – something that happens only rarely in visual perception though it happens regularly with specially contrived optical illusions. (As a rule we are unable to decode these correctly; in fact one could say that no "correct" decoding exists.)

We have a genetically based innate curiosity and an exploring instinct which makes us active in exploring our physical and our social environment. In both fields we are active problem solvers. In the field of sense perception, this leads under normal conditions to almost faultless unconscious decoding. In the cultural field it leads us first of all to learn to speak, and later to read, and to appreciate science and art. With simple messages, language and reading becomes almost as unconscious a decoding process as optical perception. The ability to learn a descriptive and argumentative language is genetically based, and specifically human. One could say of the material genetic basis that here it transcends itself: it becomes the basis of cultural learning, of participation in a civilization and in the traditions of World 3.

14. The Reality of Unembodied World 3 Objects

Thus we learn, not by direct vision or contemplation, but by practice, by active participation, how to make World 3 objects, how to understand them, and how to "see" them. This includes the "sensing" of open problems, even of problems not yet formulated. It may incite us to think, to examine the existing theories; to discover a vaguely suspected problem; and to produce theories which we hope will solve it. In this process, published theories – embodied theories – may play a role. But the not yet explored logical relations between existing theories may also play a role. Both these theories and their logical relations are World 3 objects, and in general it makes no difference, neither to their character as World 3 objects nor to our World 2 grasp of them, whether or not these objects are embodied. Thus a not yet discovered and not yet embodied logical problem situation may prove decisive for our thought processes, and may lead to actions with repercussions in the physical World 1, for example to a publication. (An example would be the search for, and the discovery of, a suspected new proof of a mathematical theorem.)

In this way World 3 objects, including logical possibilities so far not fully explored, may act on World 2; that is to say, on our minds, on us. And we in turn may act on World 1.

This process may of course be described without mentioning what I call

World 3. Thus we may say that, incited by their knowledge about World 1, certain physicists (Szilard, Fermi, Einstein) suspected the physical possibility of making a nuclear bomb, and that these World 2 thoughts brought about the realization of their conjecture. Descriptions such as this are perfectly in order. But they hide the fact that by "their knowledge about World 1", are meant *theories* which can be objectively investigated, from a logical as well as an empirical point of view, and that these are World 3 objects rather than World 2 objects (though they can be grasped and therefore have World 2 correlates); similarly by the words "suspected the physical possibility", conjectures about *physical theories* are meant – again World 3 objects, to be investigated logically. It is perfectly true that the physicist is primarily interested in World 1. But in order to learn more about World 1 he must theorize; and this means that he must use World 3 objects as his tools. This forces him to take an interest – a secondary interest, may be – in his tools, in the World 3 objects. And only by investigating them, and working out their logical consequences, can he do "applied science"; that is, make use of his World 3 products as tools, in order to change World 1.

Thus even unembodied World 3 objects may be regarded as real, and not only the papers and books in which our physical theories are published, or the material instruments which are based on these publications.

15. World 3 and the Mind-Body Problem

It is one of the central conjectures proposed in this book that the consideration of World 3 can throw some new light on the mind-body problem. I will briefly state three arguments.

The first argument is as follows.

(1) World 3 objects are abstract (even more abstract than physical forces), but none the less real; for they are powerful tools for changing World 1. (I do not wish to imply that this is the only reason for calling them real, or that they are nothing but tools.)

(2) World 3 objects have an effect on World 1 only through human intervention, the intervention of their makers; more especially, through being grasped, which is a World 2 process, a mental process, or more precisely, a process in which World 2 and World 3 interact.

(3) We therefore have to admit that both World 3 objects and the processes of World 2 are real – even though we may not like this admission, out of deference, say, to the great tradition of materialism.

I think that this is an acceptable argument – though, of course, it is open to someone to deny any one of its assumptions. He may deny that theories are abstract, or deny that they have an effect on World 1, or claim that abstract theories can directly affect the physical world. (I think, of course, that he would have a difficult time in defending any of these views.)

The second argument partly depends upon the first. If we admit the interaction of the three worlds, and thus their reality, then the interaction between Worlds 2 and 3, which we can to some extent understand, can perhaps help us a little towards a better understanding of the interaction between Worlds 1 and 2, a problem that is part of the mind-body problem.

For we have seen that one kind of interaction between Worlds 2 and 3 ("grasping") can be interpreted as a making of World 3 objects and as a matching of them by critical selection; and something similar seems to be true for the visual perception of a World 1 object. This suggests that we should look upon World 2 as active – as productive and critical (making and matching). But we have reason to think that some unconscious neurophysiological processes achieve precisely this. This makes it perhaps a little easier to "understand" that conscious processes may act along similar lines: it is, up to a point, "understandable" that conscious processes perform tasks similar to those performed by nervous processes.

A third argument bearing on the body-mind problem is connected with the status of the human language.

The capacity to learn a language – and even a strong need to learn a language – is, it appears, part of the genetic make-up of man. By contrast, the actual learning of a particular language, though influenced by unconscious inborn needs and motives, is not a gene-regulated process and therefore not a natural process, but a cultural process, a World 3 regulated process. Thus language learning is a process in which genetically based dispositions, evolved by natural selection, somewhat overlap and interact with a conscious process of exploration and learning, based on cultural evolution. This supports the idea of an interaction between World 3 and World 1; and in view of our earlier arguments, it supports the existence of World 2.

Several eminent biologists (Huxley [1942], Medawar [1960], Dobzhansky [1962]) have discussed the relationship between genetic evolution and cultural evolution. Cultural evolution, we may say, continues genetic evolution by other means: by means of World 3 objects.

It is often stressed that man is a tool-making animal, and rightly so. If by tools material physical bodies are meant, it is, however, of considerable interest to notice that none of the human tools is genetically determined, not even the stick. The only tool that seems to have a genetic basis is language.

Language is non-material, and appears in the most varied physical shapes – that is to say, in the form of very different systems of physical sounds.

There are behaviourists who do not wish to speak of "language", but only of the "speakers" of one or the other particular language. Yet there is more to it than that. All normal men speak; and speech is of the utmost importance for them; so much so that even a deaf, dumb and blind little girl like Helen Keller acquired with enthusiasm, and speedily, a substitute for speech through which she obtained a real mastery of the English language and of literature. Physically, her language was vastly different from spoken English; but it had a one-to-one correspondence with written or printed English. There can be no doubt that she would have acquired any other language in place of English. Her urgent though unconscious need was for language – language in the abstract.

As shown by their numbers and their differences, the various languages are man-made: they are cultural World 3 objects, though they are made possible by capabilities, needs, and aims which have become genetically entrenched. Every normal child acquires a language through much active work, pleasurable and perhaps also painful. The intellectual achievement that goes with it is tremendous. This effort has, of course, a strong feedback effect on the child's personality, on his relations to other persons, and on his relations to his material environment.

Thus we can say that the child is, partly, the product of his achievement. He is himself, to some extent, a World 3 product. Just as the child's mastery and consciousness of his material environment is extended by his newly acquired ability to speak, so also is his consciousness of himself. The self, the personality, emerges in interaction with the other selves and with the artefacts and other objects of his environment. All this is deeply affected by the acquisition of speech; especially when the child becomes conscious of his name, and when he learns to name the various parts of his body; and, most important, when he learns to use personal pronouns.

Becoming a fully human being depends on a maturation process in which the acquisition of speech plays an enormous part. One learns not only to perceive, and to interpret one's perceptions, but also to be a person, and to be a self. I regard the view that our perceptions are "given" to us as a mistake: they are "made" by us, they are the result of active work. Similarly I regard it as a mistake to overlook the fact that the famous Cartesian argument "I think, therefore I am" presupposes language, and the ability to use the pronoun (to say nothing of the formulation of the highly sophisticated problem which this argument is supposed to settle). When Kant [1787] suggests that the thought "I think" must be able to accompany all our perceptions and experiences, he does not seem to have thought of a child (or of himself) in his pre-linguistic or pre-philosophical state.[1]

[1] Incidentally, I do not agree that even in an adult the idea of his self or of his ego must be able to accompany *all* his experiences. There are, definitely, mental states in which we are so absorbed in the problem before us that we forget all about our selves. For a discussion of Descartes, see section 48 below; on Kant, see section 31.

Chapter P3 Materialism Criticized

16. Four Materialist or Physicalist Positions

Three of the four views which I will classify here as "materialist" or "physicalist" (see section 3 above) admit the existence of mental processes, and especially of consciousness, but all four assert that the physical world – what I am calling "World 1" – is self-contained or *closed.* By this I mean that physical processes can be explained and understood, and must be explained and understood, entirely in terms of physical theories.

I call this the physicalist principle of the closedness of the physical World 1. It is of decisive importance, and I take it as the characteristic principle of physicalism or materialism.

I have earlier suggested that we are faced with a prima facie dualism or pluralism, with interaction between World 1 and World 2; moreover, I have suggested that by way of the mediation of World 2, World 3 can act upon World 1. By contrast, the physicalist principle of the closedness of World 1 either asserts that there is *only* a World 1 or implies that if there is anything like a World 2 or a World 3 it cannot act upon World 1: World 1 is self-contained or closed. This position is intrinsically convincing. Most physicists would be inclined to accept it without question. But is it true? And are we able, if we accept it, to provide an adequate alternative explanation of our prima facie dualism? In the present chapter, I will suggest that the theories produced by materialists to date are unsatisfactory, and that there is no reason to reject our prima facie view; a view that is inconsistent with the physicalist principle. (It might be added that, in my opinion, the openness of the physical world is needed to explain – rather than explain away – human freedom. See my [1973 (a)].)

In this introductory section I will distinguish the following four materialist or physicalist positions:

(1) Radical Materialism or Physicalism, or Radical Behaviourism. This is

the view that conscious processes and mental processes do not exist: their existence can be "repudiated" (to use a term of W. V. Quine's).

I do not think that many materialists have held this view in the past (see section 56 below), for it stands in flagrant opposition to, or tries in the end to explain away, what to most of us appear as undeniable facts, such as (subjective) pain and suffering. The great classical systems of materialism, from the early Greek materialists to Hobbes and La Mettrie, are not "radical" in the sense of denying the existence of conscious or mental processes. Nor is the "dialectical materialism" of Marx and Lenin "radical" in this sense, or the behaviourism of most behaviourist psychologists.[1]

Nevertheless, what I call radical materialism (or radical physicalism or radical behaviourism) is an important position which must not be neglected. First, because it is consistent in itself. Secondly, because it presents a very simple solution of the mind-body problem: the problem clearly disappears if there is no mind, but only body.[2] (Of course, the problem also disappears if we adopt a radical spiritualism or idealism, such as the phenomenalism of Berkeley or Mach, that denies the existence of matter.) Thirdly, because in the light of evolutionary theory, matter, and especially chemical processes, existed before mental processes existed. Current theories suggest that the evolution and the development of the body come before the evolution and the development of the mind; and they are the basis of the evolution and the development of the mind. Since this is so, it is understandable that, under the impact of contemporary science, we might perhaps become radical physicalists if we are strongly inclined towards monism and simplicity, and do not wish to accept a dualist or a pluralist view of things.

It is for reasons such as these that a radical physicalism or a radical behaviourism is accepted by some outstanding philosophers such as Quine ([1960], p.264; [1975], pp. 93ff.); and it is now often suggested by others that something very much like a radical physicalism or behaviourism will ultimately have to be accepted, perhaps because of the results of science or of philosophical analysis. Suggestions such as these, though not always unambiguous ones, can be found for example in the works of Ryle [1949], [1950] or of Wittgenstein [1953]; of Hilary Putnam [1960] or of J.J.C. Smart [1963]. Indeed one may perhaps say that, at the time of writing, radical materialism or behaviourism seems to be the view concerning the mind-body problem that is most fashionable among the younger generation of students of philosophy. Thus it has to be discussed.

---

[1] Compare, on this, the remark about Marx on p.102 of volume II of my *Open Society* [1966 (a)], and the remarks on the Stoics in footnotes 6 and 7 on p.157 of my [1972 (a)].

[2] Some radical materialists do, however, take the problem seriously. See section 25 below.

My criticism of radical materialism or radical behaviourism will be along three lines. First, I will argue that, by denying the existence of consciousness, this view of the world simplifies cosmology – but it does so by omitting rather than by solving its greatest and most interesting riddle. Further, I will argue that a principle which many adopt as "scientific", and which speaks in favour of radical behaviourism, springs from a misunderstanding of the method of the natural sciences. And lastly I will argue that this view is false, and that it is refuted by experiment (although, of course, a refutation can always be evaded).[3]

(2) All the other views which I classify here as materialistic admit the existence of mental processes and, especially, of conscious processes: they admit what I call World 2. However, they also accept the fundamental principle of physicalism – the closedness of World 1.

The oldest of these views, *panpsychism,* goes back to the earliest Pre-socratics and to Campanella. It was elaborately presented in Spinoza's *Ethics,* and in Leibniz's *Monadology.*

Panpsychism is the view that *all matter* has an inside aspect which is a soul-like or a consciousness-like "quality". Thus for panpsychism, matter and mind run *"parallel"* like the outside and the inside aspects of an eggshell (Spinozistic parallelism). In non-living matter, the inside aspect may not be conscious: the soul-like precursor of consciousness may be described as "pre-psychical" or "proto-psychical". With the integration of atoms into giant molecules and living matter, memory-like effects emerge; and with the higher animals, consciousness emerges.

Panpsychism was defended in Britain especially by the mathematician and philosopher William Kingdon Clifford [1879], [1886]. Clifford teaches (not unlike Leibniz's form of parallelism) that things in themselves are mind-stuff (pre-psychical or else psychical) but that, observed from the outside, they appear as matter.[4]

Panpsychism shares with radical materialism a certain simplicity of outlook. The universe is in both cases homogeneous and monistic. Their motto

---

[3] See my [1959 (a)], sections 19–20.

[4] Clifford mentions several German philosophers as precursors of his view. Thus, in ([1886], p.286) he refers to Kant's *Critique of Pure Reason.* Clifford refers to Rosenkranz's edition, which reprints the text of the first edition of the *Critique*; see note 1 to section 22 below. Clifford also mentions Wilhelm Wundt ([1880], volume II, pp. 460ff.) and Ernst Haeckel [1878]. Later representatives of panpsychism in Germany are Theodor Ziehen [1913], and Bernhard Rensch [1968], [1971]. The identity theory of Moritz Schlick and Herbert Feigl shows a certain similarity to panpsychism, although they do not seem to discuss the evolutionary aspects of the problem, and therefore do not say that the "things in themselves", or the "qualitites", of non-living things are pre-psychical in character. (See also section 54 below.)

could well be: "There really is no new thing under the sun", which indicates an intellectually comfortable way of living – though not an intellectually very exciting one. But everything in the universe seems to fit very nicely once the radical materialistic view, or the panpsychistic view, is adopted.

(3) Epiphenomenalism may be interpreted as a modification of panpsychism, in which the "pan" element is dropped and the "psychism" is confined to those living things that seem to have a mind. Like panpsychism it is, in its usual form, a variety of parallelism; that is to say, of the view that mental processes run parallel with certain physical processes – say, because they are the inside and the outside views of some (unknown) third entity.

However, there may be forms of epiphenomenalism which are not parallelist: what I take to be essential in epiphenomenalism is the thesis that *only* the physical processes are *causally relevant* with respect to later physical processes, while the mental processes, though existing, are causally completely irrelevant.

(4) The identity theory, or the central state theory, is at present the most influential of the theories developed in response to the mind-body problem. It may be regarded as a modification of both panpsychism and epiphenomenalism. Like epiphenomenalism, it can be seen as panpsychism without the "pan". But as opposed to epiphenomenalism it takes mental facts as important and as causally effective. It asserts that there is some kind of "identity" between mental processes and certain brain processes: not an identity in the logical sense, but still an identity such as that between "the evening star" and "the morning star" which are alternative names for one and the same planet, Venus; though they also denote different appearances of the planet Venus. In one form of the identity theory, a form due to Schlick and Feigl, the mental processes are regarded (as by Leibniz) as things in themselves, known by acquaintance, from the inside, while our theories about brain processes – processes of which we know only by theoretical description – happen to describe the same things from the outside. In contrast to an epiphenomenalist, the identity theorist can say that mental processes interact with physical processes, for the mental processes simply *are* physical processes; or more precisely, special kinds of brain processes.

In section 10 above, I discussed, briefly, the example of a visit to the dentist, to illustrate the way in which physical states (World 1), our conscious awareness (World 2), and plans and institutions (World 3) are all involved in such actions. The character of our four materialistic theories may be illustrated by the way in which they would give an account of such an incident. It might involve, for example, our damaging a tooth, our developing a toothache, our 'phoning the dentist to make an appointment, and our subsequent visit to him in order to obtain treatment.

(1) Radical materialist interpretation: there are processes in my tooth leading to processes in my nervous system. Everything that happens consists of physical processes confined to World 1 (including my verbal behaviour – my uttering words on the telephone).

(2) Panpsychistic interpretation: there are the same physical processes as in (1), but there is also another side to the story. There is a "parallel" account (which various panpsychists may explain in different ways) which tells the story as it is experienced by us. Panpsychism tells us not only that our experience in some way "corresponds" to the physical explanation as given in (1), but that the apparently purely physical objects involved (such as the telephone) have also an "inner aspect", more or less similar to our own inner awareness.

(3) Epiphenomenalist interpretation: there are the same physical processes as in (1), and the rest of the story is not unlike (2). But there are the following differences from (2): (a) only the "animate" objects have "inner" or subjective experiences; (b) whereas in (2) it was suggested that we have two different but equally valid accounts, the epiphenomenalist not only gives priority to the physical account, but emphasizes that subjective experiences are causally redundant: my felt pain plays no causal role whatever in the story; it does not motivate my action.

(4) Identity theory: the same as in (1), but this time we can distinguish between those World 1 processes which are not identical with conscious experiences (World 1_p: the subscript *p* stands for "purely physical") and those physical processes which are identical with experienced or conscious processes (World 1_m: the subscript *m* stands for "mental"). The two parts of World 1 (that is to say, the sub-worlds 1_p and 1_m) can, of course, interact. Thus my pain (World 1_m) acts upon my memory store and this makes me look up the telephone number. Everything happens as in the interactionist analysis (this is, I think, what makes this view attractive) only my World 2 (including subjective knowledge) is identified with World 1_m, that is, with a part of World 1, and World 3 is identified with other parts of World 1: with *instruments, or gadgets,* such as the telephone directory or the telephone (or perhaps with brain processes: for the identity theorist *abstract knowledge contents,* which are the heart of my World 3, do not exist).

17. Materialism and the Autonomous World 3

What does World 3 look like from a materialistic point of view? Obviously, the bare existence of aeroplanes, airports, bicycles, books, buildings, cars, computers, gramophones, lectures, manuscripts, paintings, sculptures and telephones presents no problem for any form of physicalism or materialism. While to the pluralist these are the material instances, the embodiments, of World 3 objects, to the materialist they are simply parts of World 1.

But what about the objective logical relations which hold between theories (whether written down or not), such as incompatibility, mutual deducibility, partial overlapping, etc.? The radical materialist replaces World 2 objects (subjective experiences) by brain processes. Especially important among these are dispositions for verbal behaviour: dispositions to assent or reject, to support or refute; or merely to consider — to rehearse the pros and cons. Like most of those who accept World 2 objects (the "mentalists"), materialists usually interpret World 3 contents as if they were "ideas in our minds": but the radical materialists try, further, to interpret "ideas in our minds" – and thus also World 3 objects – as brain-based dispositions to verbal behaviour.

Yet neither the mentalist nor the materialist can in this way do justice to World 3 objects, especially to the contents of theories, and to their objective logical relations.

World 3 objects just are not "ideas in our minds", nor are they dispositions of our brains to verbal behaviour. And it does not help if one adds to these dispositions the embodiments of World 3, as mentioned in the first paragraph of this section. For none of these copes adequately with the *abstract* character of World 3 objects, and especially with the *logical relations* existing between them.[1]

As an example, Frege's *Grundgesetze* was written, and partly printed, when he deduced, from a letter written by Bertrand Russell, that there was a self-contradiction involved in its foundation. This self-contradiction had been there, objectively, for years. Frege had not noticed it: it had not been "in his mind". Russell only noticed the problem (in connection with quite a different manuscript) at a time when Frege's manuscript was complete. Thus there existed for years a theory of Frege's (and a similar more recent one of Russell's) which was objectively inconsistent without anyone's having an inkling of this fact, or without anyone's brain state disposing him to agree to the suggestion "This manuscript contains an inconsistent theory".

---

[1] For a fuller discussion of this, see section 21, below.

To sum up, World 3 objects and their properties and relations cannot be reduced to World 2 objects. Nor can they be reduced to brain states or dispositions; not even if we were to admit that all mental states and processes can be reduced to brain states and processes. This is so despite the fact that we can regard World 3 as the product of human minds.

Russell did not invent or produce the inconsistency, but he *discovered* it. (He invented, or produced a way of showing or proving that the inconsistency was there.) Had Frege's theory not been objectively inconsistent, he could not have applied Russell's inconsistency proof to it, and he would not have thus convinced himself of its untenability. Thus a state of Frege's mind (and no doubt also a state of Frege's brain) was the result, partly, of the objective fact that this theory was inconsistent: he was deeply upset and shaken by his discovery of this fact. This, in turn, led to his writing (a physical World 1 event) the words, *"Die Arithmetik ist ins Schwanken geraten"* ("Arithmetic is tottering"). Thus there is interaction between (a) the physical, or partly physical, event of Frege's receiving Russell's letter; (b) the objective hitherto unnoticed fact, belonging to World 3, that there was an inconsistency in Frege's theory; and (c) the physical, or partly physical, event of Frege's writing his comment on the (World 3) status of arithmetic.

These are some of the reasons why I hold that World 1 is not causally closed, and why I assert that there is interaction (though an indirect one) between World 1 and World 3. It seems to me clear that this interaction is mediated by mental, and partly even conscious, World 2 events.

The physicalist, of course, cannot admit any of this.

I believe that the physicalist is also prevented from solving another problem: he cannot do justice to the higher functions of language.

This criticism of physicalism relates to the analysis of the functions of language that was introduced by my teacher, Karl Bühler. He distinguished three functions of language: (1) the expressive function; (2) the signal or release function; and (3) the descriptive function (see Bühler [1918]; [1934], p. 28). I have discussed Bühler's theory in various places,[2] and I have added to his three functions a fourth — (4) the argumentative function. Now I have argued elsewhere[3] that the physicalist is only able to cope with the first and the second of these functions. As a result, if faced with the descriptive and the argumentative functions of language, the physicalist will always see only the first two functions (which are also always present), with disastrous results.

---

[2] For example, my [1963 (a)], chapters 4 and 12; [1972 (a)], chapters 2 and 6.

[3] See, especially, my [1953 (a)].

In order to see what is at issue, it is necessary to discuss briefly the theory of the functions of language.

In Bühler's analysis of the act of speech he differentiates between the *speaker* (or, as Bühler also calls him, the *sender*) and the person spoken to, the *listener* (or the *receiver*). In certain special ("degenerate") cases the receiver may be missing, or he may be identical with the sender. The four functions here discussed (there are others, such as command, exhortation, advice – see also John Austin's [1962] "performative utterances") are based on relations between (*a*) the sender, (*b*) the receiver, (*c*) some other objects or states of affairs which, in degenerate cases, may be identical with *(a)* or *(b)*. I will give a table of the functions in which the lower functions are placed lower and the higher functions higher.

	functions	values	
	(4) Argumentative Function	validity/ invalidity	man
	(3) Descriptive Function	falsity truth	man
perhaps bees[4]	(2) Signal Function	efficiency/ inefficiency	man
animals, plants	(1) Expressive Function	revealing/ not revealing	man

The following comments may be made on this table:

(1) The expressive function consists in an outward expression of an inner state. Even simple instruments such as a thermometer or a traffic light "express" their states in this sense. However, not only instruments, but also animals (and sometimes plants) express their inner state in their behaviour. And so do men, of course. In fact, any action we undertake, not merely the use of a language, is a form of self-expression.

(2) The signalling function (Bühler calls it also the "release function") presupposes the expressive function, and is therefore on a higher level. The thermometer may signal to us that it is very cold. The traffic light is a signalling instrument (though it may continue to work during hours where there may not always be cars about). Animals, especially birds, give danger signals; and even plants signal (for example to insects); and when our

[4] The dancing bees *may* perhaps be said to convey factual or descriptive information. A thermograph or barograph does so in writing. It is interesting that in both cases the problem of lying does not seem to arise – although the maker of the thermograph may use it to misinform us.

self-expression (whether linguistic or otherwise) leads to a reaction, in an animal or in a man, we can say that it was taken as a signal.

(3) The descriptive function of language presupposes the two lower functions. What characterizes it, however, is that over and above expressing and communicating (which may become quite unimportant aspects of the situation), it makes statements that can be *true* or *false*: the standards of truth and falsity are introduced. (We may distinguish a lower half of the descriptive function where false descriptions are beyond the animal's (the bee's?) power of abstraction. Also a thermograph would belong here, for it tells the truth unless it breaks down.)

(4) The argumentative function adds argument to the three lower functions, with its values of *validity* and *invalidity*.

Now, functions (1) and (2) are almost always present in human language; but they are as a rule unimportant, at least when compared with the descriptive and argumentative functions.

However, when the radical physicalist and the radical behaviourist turn to the analysis of human language, they cannot get beyond the first two functions (see my [1953 (a)]). The physicalist will try to give a physical explanation — a causal explanation — of language phenomena. This is equivalent to interpreting language as expressive of the state of the speaker, and therefore as having the expressive function alone. The behaviourist, on the other hand, will concern himself also with the social aspect of language — but this will be taken, essentially, as affecting the behaviour of others; as "communication", to use a vogue word; as the way in which speakers respond to one another's "verbal behaviour". This amounts to seeing language as expression and communication.

But the consequences of this are disastrous. For if all language is seen as merely expression and communication, then one neglects all that is characteristic of human language in contradistinction to animal language: its ability to make true and false statements, and to produce valid and invalid arguments. But this must make us blind to the difference between propaganda, verbal intimidation, and rational argument.[5]

It might also be mentioned that the characteristic openness of human language — the capacity for an almost infinite variety of responses to any given situation, to which Noam Chomsky, particularly, has forcefully drawn our attention — is related to the descriptive function of language. The picture of language — and of the acquisition of language — as offered by behaviouristically inclined philosophers such as Quine seems, in fact, to be a

[5] For the theory of truth see A. Tarski [1956] and my [1963] pp. 223ff.

picture of the signalling function of language. This, characteristically, is dependent upon the prevailing situation. As Chomsky has argued [1969] the behaviourist account does not do justice to the fact that a descriptive statement can be largely independent of the situation in which it is used.

18. Radical Materialism or Radical Behaviourism

Radical materialism or radical physicalism is certainly a selfconsistent position. For it is a view of the universe which, as far as we know, was adequate once; that is, before the emergence of life and consciousness.

There is a slight awkwardness felt by most of those who hold and defend this theory now: the very fact that they propose a *theory* (*qua* theory), their own *belief,* their own *words,* their own *arguments, all* seem to contradict it. In order to get over this difficulty, the radical physicalist must adopt radical behaviourism and apply it to himself: his theory, his belief in it, is nothing; only the physical *expression* in words, and perhaps in arguments – his verbal behaviour and the dispositional states that lead to it – is something.

What speaks in favour of radical materialism or radical physicalism is, of course, that it offers us a simple vision of a simple universe, and this looks attractive just because, in science, we search for simple theories. However, I think that it is important that we note that there are *two different* ways by which we can search for simplicity. They may be called, briefly, philosophical reduction and scientific reduction.[1] The former is characterized by an attempt to simplify our view of the world; the second by an attempt to provide bold and testable theories of high explanatory power.[2] I believe that the latter is an extremely valuable and worthwhile method; while the former is of value only if we have good reasons to assume that it corresponds to the facts about the universe.

Indeed, the demand for simplicity in the sense of philosophical *rather than* scientific reduction may actually be damaging. For even in order to attempt a scientific reduction, it is necessary for us first to get a full grasp of the problem to be solved, and it is therefore vitally important that interesting problems are not "explained away" by philosophical analysis. If, say, more than one factor is responsible for some effect, it is important that we do not pre-empt the scientific judgement: there is always the danger that we might refuse to admit any ideas other than the ones we happen to have at hand; explaining away, or

---

1 See my [1972 (a)], chapter 8, where these ideas are discussed in more detail.
2 See, for example, my [1972 (a)], chapter 5.

belittling the problem. The danger is increased if we try to settle the matter in advance by philosophical reduction. Philosophical reduction also makes us blind to the significance of scientific reduction.[3]

It is in this light that I think we should consider the radical physicalist's approach to the problem of consciousness. Not only do we have, in the phenomena of consciousness, something that *seems* radically different from what, on our current view, is to be found in the physical world. We also have the dramatic and, from a physical point of view, strange changes that have taken place in the physical environment of man, due, it appears, to conscious and purposeful action. This should not be ignored, or dogmatically explained away.

I would even suggest that the greatest riddle of cosmology may well be neither the original big bang, nor the problem why there is something rather than nothing (it is quite possible that these problems may turn out to be pseudoproblems), but that the universe is, in a sense, creative: that it created life, and from it mind – our consciousness – which illuminates the universe, and which is creative in its turn. It is one of the high points in Herbert Feigl's *Postscript* [1967] to his essay *The 'Mental' and the 'Physical'* when he relates how, in a conversation, Einstein said something like this: "If there were not this internal illumination, the universe would merely be a rubbish heap."[4] This, Feigl tells us, is one of the reasons why he does not accept radical physicalism (as I call it) but the identity theory, which recognizes the reality of mental and especially of conscious processes.

It might also be worth bearing in mind that, while in science, our *quest* is for simplicity, it is a real problem whether the world is itself quite so simple as some philosophers think. The simplicity of the old theory of matter (that of Descartes or that of Newton or even that of Boscovich) is gone: it clashed with the facts. The same happened to the electrical theory of matter which, for twenty or thirty years, seemed to offer a hope of an even greater simplicity. Our present theory of matter, quantum mechanics, turns out (especially in the light of the thought experiment of Einstein, Podolsky and Rosen, and the results of J. S. Bell, and of S. J. Freedman and R. A. Holt [1975]) to be even less simple than one might have hoped. It is also clearly incomplete: in spite of Dirac's result which may be interpreted as the prediction of anti-par-

---

[3] Consider, for example, what a dogmatic philosophical reductionist of a mechanistic disposition (or even a quantum-mechanistic disposition) might have done in the face of the problem of the chemical bond. The actual reduction, so far as it goes, of the theory of the hydrogen bond to quantum mechanics is far more interesting than the philosophical assertion that such a reduction will one day be achieved.

[4] Cp. Feigl [1967], p. 138. Feigl translates a German conversation; I have slightly changed the wording of the translation (as Feigl also did, according to his report).

ticles, quantum theory cannot be said to have led to the prediction or explanation of the many new elementary particles which have been found in recent years. Thus appeals to simplicity can hardly be accepted as decisive, not even within physics. In particular, we should not deprive ourselves of interesting and challenging problems – problems that seem to indicate that our best theories are incorrect and incomplete – by persuading ourselves that the world would be simpler if they were not there. But it seems to me that modern materialists are doing just this.[5]

I may say here perhaps that I should regard radical physicalism, if it were compatible with the facts, as an intellectually satisfying theory. But it is not compatible with the facts. And the facts, difficult as they are to absorb, are intellectually challenging. So to me the decision seems to be between intellectual ease (or let us call it smugness) and unease.

Radical behaviourism, on which the radical physicalist must depend in order to explain to himself his theoretical activities as "verbal behaviour", derives most of its appeal from a misunderstanding of a problem of method. The behaviourist demands, rightly, that any scientific theory, and therefore also the theories of psychology, must be testable by reproducible experiments, or at least by intersubjectively testable observation statements: by statements about observable behaviour, which in the case of human psychology includes verbal behaviour.

But this important principle refers only to the *test statements* of a science. Just as in physics we introduce theoretical entities – electrons and other particles, or fields of forces, etc. – in order to explain our observation statements (about photographs of the events in bubble chambers, for example), so we can introduce, in psychology, conscious and unconscious mental events and processes, if these are helpful in explaining human behaviour, such as verbal behaviour. In this case, the attribution of a mind and of subjective conscious experiences to every normal human person is an explanatory theory of psychology of about the same character as the existence of relatively stable material bodies in physics. In both cases the theoretical entities are *not* introduced as something ultimate – as substances in the traditional sense; both create vast regions of unsolved problems, and so does their interaction. But in both cases our theories are well testable: in physics, by the experiments of mechanics; in psychology, by certain experiments

[5] It might be mentioned that the conflict described in the text could also be seen as the conflict between conventionalism and realism in the philosophy of science. Perhaps Charles S. Sherrington ([1947], p. xxiv) may be quoted here: "That our being should consist of *two* fundamental elements offers I suppose no greater inherent improbability than that it should rest on one only."

which lead to reproducible verbal reports (and thus to reproducible "verbal behaviour"). Since all, or almost all, experimental subjects react in these experiments with recognizably the same reports – reports about what they subjectively experience in the experimental situation – the theory of their having these subjective experiences is well tested.

I will here describe a simple experiment which every reader can carry out himself, and check with any of his friends. It is taken from the work of the great Danish experimental psychologist, Edgar Rubin ([1950], pp. 366f.).I use optical illusions because here the character of subjective experiences becomes very clear.

The following two figures are taken from Rubin, with very slight changes.

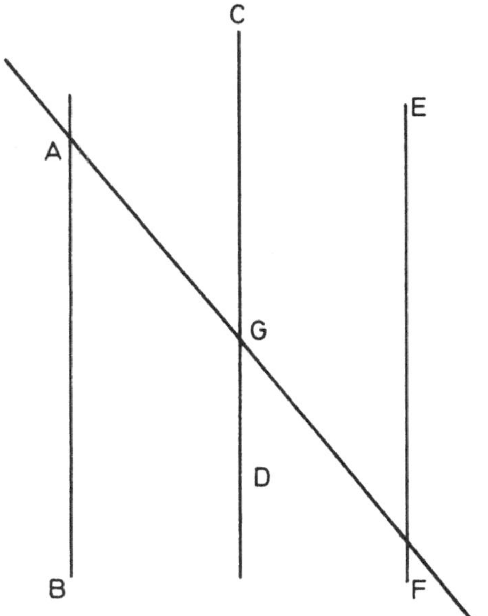

Figure 1.

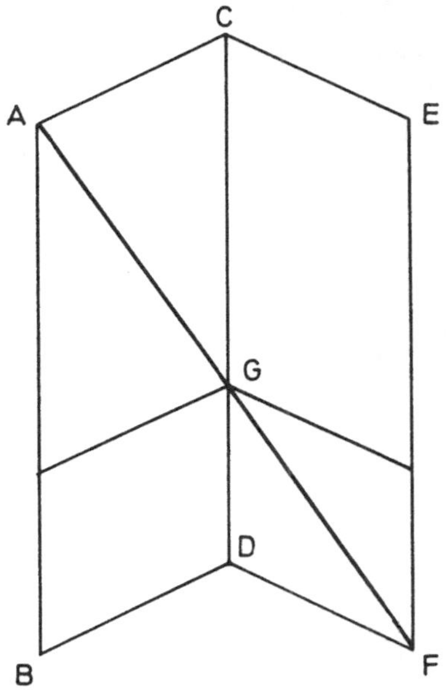

Figure 2.

It will be seen from Figure 1 that, since AB, CD, and EF are parallel and equidistant, the inclined line AF is cut in half at G; so that AG = GF.

We explain all this to our experimental subject, who thus does not need to measure the distances AG and GF in order to make sure that they are equal.

We now put to him the following questions.

(1) Look at Figure 2. You know that AG = GF, in view of the proof indicated by Figure 1. Do you agree?

We wait for the reply.

(2) Does AG *look* to you equal to GF?

We wait again for the reply.

Question (2) is the decisive question. The reply ("No") which is obtained from every (or almost every) experimental subject can be explained most directly by the conjecture that the subjective visual experience of every subject deviates systematically from what we all know (and can prove) to be objectively the case. This establishes an easily repeatable objective and behavioural test of the existence of subjective experience. (Of course, only as long as we take the reports of our experimental subjects seriously; but the radical behaviourist can still reinterpret *ad hoc* their verbal responses: every falsification can be evaded by one who is not prepared to learn from experience.)

We could have confined ourselves to Figure 3 (the so-called "Sanders Illusion"), and measured AG and GB, which is perhaps even more dramatic.

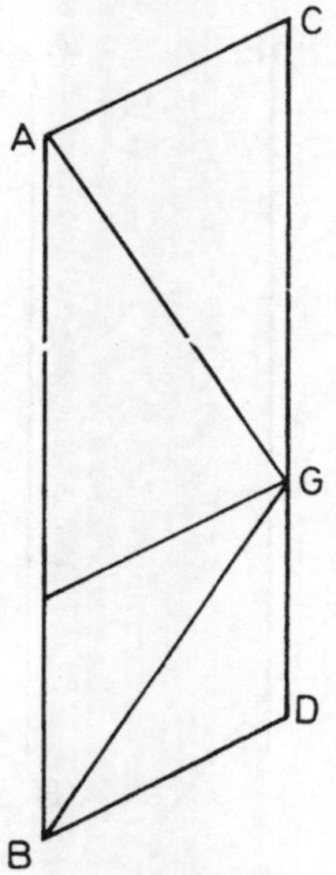

Figure 3.

Yet measurements may leave some doubt: small errors may matter and may not be easily detectable. On the other hand, it is clear that the three vertical lines in Figure 1 and Figure 2 are parallel and equi-distant. A further question is:

(3) Does your theoretical knowledge with respect to Figure 2 help you to *see* the distances AG and GF as equal?

A related but slightly different experiment may convince us that our mental processes are often *mental activities.* It operates with an ambiguous figure. (Such figures are used in Wittgenstein's *Philosophical Investigations,* yet, it seems, with very different aims or purposes.) The figure used (the "Winson Figure") is taken from a paper by Ernst Gombrich ([1973], p. 239).

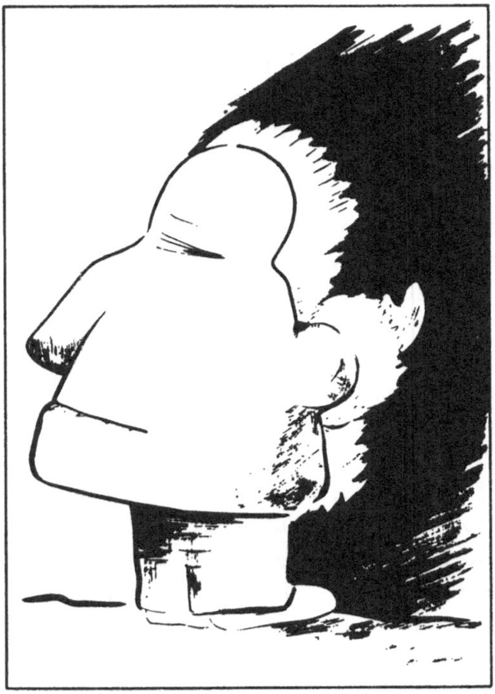

Figure 4.
Taken from R. L. Gregory and E. H. Gombrich (eds.) [1973] with the kind permission of the author, the publisher, and of Alphabet and Image.

The Figure shows ambiguously the profile of an American Indian and a view, from the back, of an Eskimo. What I wish to draw attention to is that we can voluntarily switch from the one interpretation to the other, although perhaps not easily. It seems that most people can easily see the American Indian and have difficulties in switching over to the Eskimo. (However, it is the other way round for some people.)

Now the point is that we can voluntarily and actively build up the profile of the Indian by looking at his nose, mouth, and chin, and then proceeding to his eye. As to the Eskimo, we can start to build him up from his right boot. (And of course, we can formulate experimental questions about these activities which lead to intersubjectively repeatable answers.)

There are also other sorts of intersubjectively testable experiments which are most successful and convincing tests of the theory that men have conscious experiences. For example, there are the experiments conducted by the great brain surgeon Wilder Penfield. Penfield [1955] repeatedly stimulated, with the help of an electrode, the exposed brain of patients who were being operated on while fully conscious. When certain areas of the cortex were thus stimulated, the patients reported re-living very vivid visual and auditive experiences while being, at the same time, fully aware of their actual surroundings. "A young South African patient lying on the operating table . . . was laughing with his cousins on a farm in South Africa, while he was also fully conscious of being in the operating room in Montreal." (Penfield [1975], p. 55.) Such reports, clearly reproducible, and repeated in many cases, can be only explained so far as I can see by admitting conscious subjective experiences. Penfield's experiments have sometimes been criticized for having been conducted only with epileptic patients. However, this does not affect the problem of the existence of subjective, conscious experiences.

These experiments of Penfield's may be compatible with an identity theory. They do not seem to be compatible with radical physicalism – with the denial of the existence of subjective states of consciousness. There are many similar experiments.[6] They test and establish, by behaviourist methods, the conjecture – if it is to be called a conjecture rather than a fact – that we have subjective experiences; conscious processes. Admittedly, there is every reason to think that these go hand in hand with brain processes. It is, it appears, the brain rather than the self which "insists", as it were, on the inequality of distances we know to be equal. (A corresponding remark holds for the *Gestalt* switch.) Yet my main point here is merely that we can establish empirically, by behaviourist methods, that subjective, conscious experience exists.

A word may be added on the unusual or paradoxical character of both types of experiment here mentioned – optical illusion and Penfield's stimulation of the cortex. Our mechanism of perception is normally not reflexively directed onto itself, but directed towards the outside world. Thus we can forget about ourselves in normal perception. In order to become quite clear about our subjective experience it is therefore useful to choose experiments in which something is out of the ordinary and clashes with the normal perceptual mechanism.

[6] One important type of experiment is due to modern sleep research: rapid eye movements have been shown to indicate dreaming; and dreaming is clearly a (low-level) conscious experience. (The radical behaviourist or materialist would have to say, in order to avoid refutation, that rapid eye movements signify a manifestation of a disposition which would lead people if woken up to say that they had been dreaming, while in reality no such things as dreams exist. But this would obviously be an *ad hoc* way of evading refutation.)

19. Panpsychism

Panpsychism is a very ancient theory. Traces of it can be found in the earliest Greek philosophers (who are often described as "hylozoists", that is, as holding that all things are animate). Aristotle reports of Thales (*De anima* 411a7; cp. Plato, *Laws* 899 b) that he taught "Everything is full of gods". This may, Aristotle suggests, be a way of saying that "soul is mingled with everything in the whole universe", including what we usually regard as inanimate matter. This is the doctrine of panpsychism.

Among the Presocratic philosophers down to Democritus, panpsychism has a materialist or at least semi-materialist character in so far as the psyche, or mind, was regarded as a very special kind of matter. This attitude changes with the moral or ethical theory of the soul developed by Democritus, by Socrates, and by Plato. Yet even Plato (*Timaeus* 30 b/c) calls the universe "a living body endowed with a soul".

Panpsychism, like pantheism, is widespread among Renaissance thinkers (for example Telesius, Campanella, Bruno). It is fully developed in Spinoza's treatment of the mind-body relationship, his doctrine of psycho-physical parallelism: ". . . all things are animate in various degrees". (*Ethics* II, XIII, Scholium.) According to Spinoza, matter and soul are the outside and inside aspects, or attributes, of one and the same *thing in itself* (or *things in themselves*); that is to say, of "Nature, which is the same as God".

A very similar yet atomist version of the theory is the monadology of Leibniz. The world consists of monads (= points), of unextended intensities. Being unextended, these intensities are souls. They are, as in Spinoza, animate in various degrees. The main difference from Spinoza's theory is this: while in Spinoza, the thing in itself is the (inscrutable) Nature, or God, of which body and soul are outside and inside aspects, Leibniz teaches that his monads – which are the things in themselves – are souls, or spirits, and that extended bodies (which are spatial integrals over the monads) are their outside appearances. Leibniz is therefore a metaphysical spiritualist: bodies are accumulations of spirits, seen from the outside.

Kant teaches, by contrast, that the things in themselves are unknowable. Yet there is a strong suggestion that, as moral characters, we ourselves are things in themselves; though there is also a suggestion that the other things in themselves (those which are not human) are not of a mental or spiritual character: Kant is not a panpsychist.

Schopenhauer takes up Kant's suggestion that as moral characters – as moral wills – we are things in themselves; and he generalizes this: the thing in itself (Spinoza's God) is will, and will manifests itself in all things. Will is the essence, the thing in itself, the reality of everything, and will is what, from outside, for the observer, appears as body or matter. One can say that Schopenhauer is a Kantian who has turned panpsychist. In order to carry out this idea, Schopenhauer emphasizes the unconscious: although his will is mental, or psychical, it is largely unconscious – completely so in inanimate matter, but largely so even in animals and in man. Schopenhauer is thus a spiritualist; but his spirit is mainly unconscious will, drive, and appetite, rather than conscious reason. This theory[1] exerted a great influence upon German, English and American panpsychists who, partly under the influence of Schopenhauer, interpret the chemical affinities, the binding forces of atoms, and other physical forces such as gravity, as the outward manifestations of the drive-like or will-like properties of the things in themselves which, seen from outside, appear to us as matter.

This may serve as a sketch of the idea of panpsychism.[2] (An excellent historical and critical introduction by Paul Edwards may be found in his [1967 (a)].) Panpsychism has many varieties, and it offers what appears to its defenders a comfortable solution of the problem of the emergence of mind in the universe: mind was always there, as the inside aspect of matter. This seems to be the reason why panpsychism is accepted by several well-known contemporary biologists, such as C. H. Waddington [1961] in England or Bernhard Rensch [1968], [1971] in Germany.

It is obvious that panpsychism is, from a metaphysical (or ontological) point of view, nearer to spiritualism than to materialism. However, many panpsychists, from Spinoza and Leibniz to Waddington, Theodor Ziehen, and Rensch, accept what I called in section 16 above the physicalist principle of *the closedness of the physical world.* They believe,[3] like Spinoza and Leibniz, that psychological or mental processes and physical or material processes run parallel, without interacting; that mental (World 2) processes can act only upon other mental processes, and that physical (World 1) processes can act only upon other physical processes, so that World 1 is closed, self-contained.

---

[1] It seems to have been influenced by Goethe's novel *Elective Affinities* (*Die Wahlverwandtschaften = The Chosen [Chemical] Affinities*) in which sympathy, and attraction, were interpreted as akin to chemical affinity. Schopenhauer, who knew Goethe personally, was greatly influenced by him.

[2] For a fuller discussion of the history of the mind-body problem, see chapter P5, below.

[3] (Added in proofs.) Professor Rensch has kindly informed me that he disagrees with the view stated in the first part of this sentence, since he is not a parallelist, but an identity theorist. (But in my view the identity theory is a special case – a degenerate case – of parallelism; see also sections 22 to 24, below.)

I will here present three arguments against panpsychism.

(1) My first criticism of panpsychism is that the assumption that there must be a pre-psychical precursor of psychical processes is either trivial and completely verbal, or grossly misleading. That there is something in evolutionary history which preceded, in some sense, the mental processes, is trivial as well as vague. But to insist that this something must be mind-like *and* that it can be attributed even to atoms is a misleading way of arguing. For we know that crystals and other solids have the property of solidity *without* solidity (or pre-solidity) being present in the liquid before crystallization (though the presence of a crystal or some other solid in the liquid may help in the crystallization process).

Thus we know of processes in nature which are "emergent" in the sense that they lead, not gradually but by something like a leap, to a property which was not there before. Although the mind of a baby develops, gradually, from a pre-mental state to full consciousness of self, we do not need to postulate that the food which the baby eats (and which in the end may form its brain) has qualities which can be, with informative success, described as pre-mental or as in any way even distantly similar to mind. Thus the *pan*-element in *pan*psychism seems to me gratuitous and also fantastic. (But I should not say that the idea shows much imagination.)

(2) Panpsychism accepts, of course, that what we usually call inanimate or inorganic matter has a very much poorer mental life than any organism. Thus to the great step from non-living to living matter will correspond a great step from pre-psychical processes to psychical processes. It is therefore not very clear how much panpsychism gains for a better undertstanding of the evolution of the mind by assuming pre-psychical states or processes: even on the panpsychistic account, something totally new enters the world with life, and with heredity, if only in several steps. Yet the main motive of post-Darwinian panpsychism was to avoid the need to admit the emergence of something totally novel.

To say this is not, of course, to deny the fact that there exist not only unconscious mental states, but also many different degrees of consciousness. There can be little doubt that dreaming is conscious, but on a low level of consciousness: it is a far cry from a dream to a critical evaluation and revision of a difficult argument. Similarly, a newborn child has clearly a low level of consciousness. It probably takes years, and the acquiring of language, and perhaps even of critical thinking, before the full consciousness of self is achieved.

(3) Although there exists, no doubt, something that may be described as unconscious memory — that is, memory of which we are not aware — there

cannot be, I propose, consciousness or awareness without memory.

This may be explained with the help of a thought experiment.

It is well known that, as a consequence of an injury, or an electric shock, or a drug, a person may lose consciousness (and that a period of time prior to the event may be extinguished from his memory).

Now let us assume that, by taking a drug, or by some other treatment, we may extinguish the recording of memory for several minutes or seconds.

Let us further assume that we are treated in this way *repeatedly* – say, after every p seconds – every time extinguishing our memory for a short blacked out span of q seconds. (We assume $p > q$.)

(a) We see at once that if the periods p were made equal to the extinguished periods q, no recorded memory would be left of the whole period of the experiment.

(b) Since the periods p are somewhat longer than the periods q, there will be a sequence of recordings left, each of the length $p-q$.

(c) Now assume (b); and further, that $p-q$ becomes very short. I suggest that in this case we should lose consciousness for the whole period of the experiment. For after every memory loss (even upon waking up from deep sleep) it takes some little time before we can, as it were, re-assemble ourselves and become fully conscious. If this time needed to become fully conscious (say 0.5 seconds) exceeds $p-q$ then, I suggest, there will not be any brief moments of consciousness or awareness whose memory is extinguished; rather, there will be no moment of consciousness or awareness at all.

To put my thesis in a different way, a certain minimum span of continuity of memory is needed for consciousness or awareness to arise. Thus the atomization of memory must destroy conscious experience and, indeed, any form of conscious awareness.

Consciousness, and every kind of awareness, *relates* certain of its constituents to earlier constituents. Thus it cannot be conceived of as consisting of arbitrarily short events. There is no consciousness without a memory that links its constituting "acts of awareness"; and these, in their turn, cannot exist unless they are linked to many other such acts.

These results of a purely speculative thought experiment are corroborated, as far as this is possible, by some of the results of brain physiology. I am told that some drugs used as total anaesthetics – that is, for producing unconsciousness – act in the manner described, that is, as more or less radical atomizers of memory connections, and thus of awareness. Some forms of epilepsy also seem to work in a similar way. In all these cases parts of the long term memory are kept intact, in the sense that upon the recovery of consciousness the patient can remember events of his earlier life or events up to losing consciousness; and it is this past memory (or so it seems) which makes it possible for the patient to preserve his self-identity.[4]

Now this thought experiment speaks strongly against the theory of panpsychism according to which atoms, or elementary particles, have something like an inside view; an inside view that constitutes the unit, as it were, out of which the consciousness of animals and men is formed. For according to modern physics, atoms or elementary particles have emphatically no memory: two atoms of the same isotope are physically completely identical, *whatever their past history*. For example, if they are radioactive, their probability or propensity to decay is exactly the same, whatever the difference in their past radioactive history may be. But this means that they have, physically, no memory. If psycho-physical parallelism is assumed, their "inside state" must also be one without memory. But then, this cannot be anything like an inside state: it cannot be a state of consciousness, or even of consciousness-like pre-consciousness.

Memory-like states do occur in inanimate matter; for example, in crystals. Steel "remembers" that it has been magnetized. A growing crystal "remembers" a fault in its structure. But this is something new, something emergent: atoms and elementary particles do not "remember", if present physical theory is correct.

Thus we should not assign inside states, or mental states, or conscious states to atoms: the emergence of consciousness is a problem that cannot be avoided, or mitigated, by a panpsychist theory. Panpsychism is baseless, and Leibniz's monadology must be rejected.

It might be added that it now looks as if the beginning of human or animal memory is to be found in the genetic mechanism; that memory in the conscious sense is a late product of genetic memory. The physical basis of genetic memory seems to be within the reach of science, and the explanations that we have of it seem to make it totally unrelated to any panpsychistic effect. That is to say, instead of a straight progression from memory-lacking atoms to the memory of magnetized iron, and further to the memory of plants and to conscious memory, there appears to be a huge detour via genetic memory. Thus the results of modern genetics speak strongly against the view that there is any value in panpsychism — that is, against its explanatory power or explanatory prospects, although panpsychism as such is so metaphysical (in a bad sense) and has so little content that we can hardly talk about its explanatory value.

---

[4] See especially the remarks on the patient H.M. in Brenda Milner [1966].

20. Epiphenomenalism

William Kingdon Clifford was a panpsychist. His friend, Thomas Huxley, was an epiphenomenalist. Both agreed in adopting the physicalist principle of the closedness of the physical world (World 1). In Clifford's words ([1886], p. 260): "all the evidence that we have goes to show that the physical world gets along entirely by itself . . .".

The difference between epiphenomenalism and panpsychism is mainly this.

(1) Epiphenomenalism does *not* assert that *all* material processes have a psychical aspect, and

(2) Epiphenomenalism is very far from regarding conscious states or processes as the things in themselves, as at least some of the post-Leibnizean and post-Kantian panpsychists do.

(3) Epiphenomenalism *may* be linked with a parallelist view (like a partial panpsychism) or it *may* allow for a one sided causal action of the body upon the mind. (The latter view is liable to clash with Newton's third law – the equality of action and reaction.[1]) I will criticize here a parallelist epiphenomenalism; but nothing in my criticism depends on this choice.

Huxley ([1898], p. 240; cp. pp. 243 f.) puts his epiphenomenalism very well: "Consciousness . . . would appear to be related to the mechanism of [the] body, simply as a . . . [side] product of its working, and to be as completely without any power of modifying that working as the [sound of a] steam-whistle which accompanies the work of a locomotive . . . is without influence upon its machinery."

Thomas Huxley was a Darwinian – in fact, the first of all Darwinians. But I think that his epiphenomenalism clashes with the Darwinian point of view. For from a Darwinian point of view, we are led to speculate about the survival value of mental processes. For example we might regard pain as a warning signal. More generally, Darwinists ought to regard "the mind", that is to say mental processes and dispositions for mental actions and reactions, as analogous to a bodily organ (closely linked with the brain, presumably) which has evolved under the pressure of natural selection. It functions by helping the adaptation of the organism (cp. the discussion of organic evolution in section 6, above). The Darwinian view must be this: consciousness and more generally the mental processes are to be regarded (and, if possible, to be explained) as the product of evolution by natural selection.

[1] The principle is re-affirmed by Einstein ([1922]; [1956], chapter 3, p. 54) when he says: ". . . it is contrary to the mode of thinking in science to conceive of a thing . . . which acts itself, but which cannot be acted upon."

The Darwinian view is needed, especially, for understanding intellectual mental processes. Intelligent actions are actions adapted to foreseeable events. They are based upon foresight, upon expectation; as a rule, upon short term *and* long term expectation, and upon the comparison of the expected results of several possible moves and countermoves. Here *preference* comes in, and with it, the making of decisions, many of which have an instinctual basis. This may be the way in which emotions enter the World 2 of mental processes and experiences; and why they sometimes "become conscious", and sometimes not.

The Darwinian view also explains at least partly the first emergence of a World 3 of products of the human mind: the world of tools, of instruments, of languages, of myths, and of theories. (This much can be of course also admitted by those who are reluctant, or hesitant, to ascribe "reality" to entities such as problems and theories, and also by those who regard World 3 as a part of World 1 and/or World 2.) The existence of the cultural World 3 and of cultural evolution may draw our attention to the fact that there is a great deal of systematic coherence within both World 2 and World 3; and that this can be explained – partly – as the systematic result of selection pressures. For example, the evolution of language can be explained, it seems, only if we assume that even a primitive language can be helpful in the struggle for life, and that the emergence of language has a feedback effect: linguistic capabilities are competing; they are being selected for their biological effects; which leads to higher levels in the evolution of language.

We can summarize this in the form of the following four principles of which the first two, it seems to me, must be accepted especially by those who are inclined towards physicalism or materialism.

(1) The theory of natural selection is the only theory known at present which can explain the emergence of purposeful processes in the world and, especially, the evolution of higher forms of life.

(2) Natural selection is concerned with *physical survival* (with the frequency distribution of competing genes in a population). It is therefore concerned, essentially, with the explanation of World 1 effects.

(3) If natural selection is to account for the emergence of the World 2 of subjective or mental experiences, the theory must explain the manner in which the evolution of World 2 (and of World 3) systematically provides us with instruments for survival.

(4) Any explanation in terms of natural selection is partial and incomplete. For it must always assume the existence of many (and of partly unknown) competing mutations, and of a variety of (partly unknown) selection pressures.

These four principles may be briefly referred to as the Darwinian point of view. I shall try to show here that the Darwinian point of view clashes with the doctrine usually called "epiphenomenalism".

Epiphenomenalism admits the existence of mental events or experiences – that is, of a World 2 – but asserts that these mental or subjective experiences are causally ineffective byproducts of physiological processes, which alone are causally effective. In this way the epiphenomenalist can accept the physicalistic principle of the closedness of World 1, together with the existence of a World 2. Now the epiphenomenalist must insist that World 2 is indeed irrelevant; that only physical processes matter: If a man reads a book, the decisive thing is not that it influences his opinions, and provides him with information. These are all irrelevant epiphenomena. What matters is solely the change in his brain structure that affects his disposition to act. These dispositions are indeed, the epiphenomenalist will say, of the greatest importance for survival: it is only here that Darwinism comes in. The subjective experiences of reading and thinking exist, but they do not play the role we usually attribute to them. Rather, this mistaken attribution is the result of our failure to distinguish between our experiences and the crucially important impact of our reading upon the dispositional properties of the brain structure. The subjective experiential aspects of our perceptions while reading do not matter; nor do the emotional aspects. All this is fortuitous, casual rather than causal.

It is clear that this epiphenomenalist view is unsatisfactory. It admits the existence of a World 2, but denies it any biological function. It therefore cannot explain, in Darwinian terms, the evolution of World 2. And it is forced to deny what is plainly a most important fact – the tremendous impact of this evolution (and of the evolution of World 3) upon World 1.

I think that this argument is decisive.

To put the matter in biological terms, there are several closely related systems of controls in higher organisms: the immune system, the endocrinal system, the central nervous system, and what we may call the "mental system". There is little doubt that the last two of these are closely linked. But so are the others, if perhaps less closely. The mental system has, clearly, its evolutionary and functional history, and its functions have increased with the evolution from lower to higher organisms. It thus has to be linked with the Darwinian point of view. But epiphenomenalism cannot do this.

An important but separate criticism is this. If applied to arguments, and our weighing of reasons, the epiphenomenalist view is suicidal. For the epiphenomenalist is committed to arguing that arguments or reasons do not really matter. They cannot really influence our dispositions to act – for example, to speak or to write – nor the actions themselves. These are all due to mechanical, physico-chemical, acoustical, optical and electrical effects.

Thus the epiphenomenalist argument leads to the recognition of its own irrelevance. This does not refute epiphenomenalism. It merely means that if epiphenomenalism is true, we cannot take seriously as a reason or argument whatever is said in its support.

The problem of the validity of this argument was raised by, among others, J. B. S. Haldane. It will be discussed in the next section.

21. A Revised Form of J. B. S. Haldane's Refutation of Materialism

The argument against materialism mentioned at the end of the previous section was concisely formulated by J. B. S. Haldane. Haldane [1932] puts it thus: ". . . if materialism is true, it seems to me that we cannot know that it is true. If my opinions are the result of the chemical processes going on in my brain, they are determined by the laws of chemistry, not of logic."[1]

The argument (retracted by Haldane in a paper "I Repent an Error" [1954][2]) has a long history. It can be traced back at least to Epicurus: "He who says that all things happen of necessity cannot criticize another who says that not all things happen of necessity. For he has to admit that the assertion also happens of necessity."[3] In this form, it was an argument against determinism rather than against materialism. But the close relationship between the arguments of Haldane and Epicurus is striking. Both indicate that if our opinions are the result of something other than the free judgement of reason,[4] or the weighing of reasons, of the pros and cons, then our opinions are not worth taking seriously. Thus an argument that leads to the conclusion that our arguments and opinions are not arrived at in this way defeats itself.

Haldane's argument (or more precisely, the second of the two sentences

---

[1] See J. B. S. Haldane [1932], reprinted in Penguin Books ([1937], p. 157); see also Haldane [1930], p. 209.

[2] J. B. S. Haldane [1954]. See also Antony Flew [1955]. A more recent rejection of what I call Haldane's argument, due to Keith Campbell, can be found in Paul Edwards, ed. [1967 (b)] vol. 5, p. 186. See also J. J. C. Smart [1963], pp. 126f. (and Antony Flew [1965], pp. 114–15) where further references will be found, and section 85 of my (unpublished) *Postscript*.

[3] Epicurus, Aphorism 40 of the Vatican Collection. See Cyril Bailey [1926] pp. 112–113. This may well have been Epicurus's central argument against determinism, and the motive of his theory of the "swerve" of the atoms (if this was his theory rather than that of Lucretius).

[4] Cp. Descartes, *Meditation* IV; *Principles* I, 32–44.

quoted above) cannot be upheld in the form here stated. For a computing machine may be said to be determined in its working by the laws of physics; but it may nevertheless work in full accordance with the laws of logic. This simple fact invalidates (as I pointed out in section 85 of my unpublished *Postscript*) the second sentence of Haldane's argument as it stands.

However, I believe that Haldane's argument (as I will call it in spite of its antiquity) can be so revised as to become unexceptionable. Although it does not show that materialism destroys itself, I suggest that it shows that materialism is self-defeating: it cannot seriously claim to be supported by rational argument. The revised argument of Haldane could be put more concisely, but I think it is clearer if developed at length.

I will represent the revised argument in the form of a dialogue between an interactionist and a physicalist.

Interactionist I am quite prepared to accept your refutation of Haldane's argument: the computer constitutes a counter-example to this argument as it stands. However, it seems to me important to remember that the computer, which admittedly works on physical principles and, at the same time, also according to logical princples, has been *designed by us* – by human *minds* – to work like this. In fact, a great amount of logical and mathematical theory is being used in the making of a computer. This explains why it works according to the laws of logic. It is far from easy to construct a piece of physical apparatus that works (according to the laws of physics and, at the same time) according to the laws of logic. Both the computer and the laws of logic belong emphatically to what is here called World 3.

Physicalist I agree, although I admit only the existence of a *physical* World 3 to which, for example, books on logic and mathematics belong, and, of course, also computers: this World 3 of yours is in fact part of World 1. Books and computers are products of men and women – they are designed; they are products of human *brains*. Our brains in turn are not really designed – they are largely the products of natural selection. They are so selected as to adapt themselves to their environment; and their dispositional capacities for reasoning are the result of this adaptation. Reasoning consists in a certain kind of verbal behaviour and in acquiring dispositions to act and to speak. Apart from natural selection, positive and negative conditioning through the success and failure of our actions and reactions also play their role. So does schooling; that is to say, conditioning through a teacher who works upon us – somewhat like a designer who works on a computer. In this way we become conditioned to speak and to act and to reason rationally or intelligently.

Interactionist It seems that you and I agree on a number of points. We agree that natural selection *and* individual learning play their role in the evolution of logical thinking. And we agree that a reasonable or a reasoning materialism is bound to assert that a well trained brain, like a reliable computer, is built in such a way that it works in accordance with the principles of logic *and* with those of physics and electro-chemistry.

Physicalist Precisely. I am even prepared to admit that if this view cannot be upheld, then Haldane's argument would actually upset materialism: I would have to admit that materialism undermines its own rationality.

Interactionist Do computers or brains never make mistakes?

Physicalist Of course computers are not perfect. Nor are human brains. This goes without saying.

Interactionist But if so, you need World 3 objects, such as standards of validity, which are *not* embodied or incarnated in World 1 objects: you need them to be able to appeal to the *validity of an inference*; yet you deny the existence of such objects.

Physicalist I do deny the existence of non-corporeal World 3 objects; but I do not quite see your point yet.

Interactionist My point is quite simple. If computers or brains may fail, what do they fall short of?

Physicalist Of other computers or brains or of the contents of books on logic and mathematics.

Interactionist Are these books infallible?

Physicalist Of course not. But mistakes are rare.

Interactionist I doubt that, but let it be so. I still ask: if there is a mistake – mind you, a logical mistake – by what standard is it a mistake?

Physicalist By the standards of logic.

Interactionist I fully agree. But these are abstract, non-corporeal World 3 standards.

Physicalist I do not agree. They are not abstract standards. but the standards or principles which the great majority of logicians – in fact, all except a lunatic fringe – are disposed to accept as such.

Interactionist Are they so disposed because the principles are valid, or are the principles valid because logicians are disposed to accept them?

Physicalist A tricky question. The obvious answer to it, and at any rate your answer, would seem to be "logicians are disposed to accept logical standards because these standards are valid". But this would admit the existence of non-corporeal and thus of abstract standards or principles whose existence I deny. No, I have to give a different reply to your question: the standards exist, so far as they exist, as states or dispositions of the brains of people: states, or dispositions, which make people accept the proper standards. You may now, of course, ask me "What else are the *proper* standards but the *valid* standards?" My answer is "certain ways of verbal behaviour, or of connecting some beliefs with others; ways which have proved useful in the struggle for life, and which therefore have been selected by natural selection, or learned by conditioning, perhaps in school, or otherwise".

These inherited or learned dispositions are what some people would call "our logical intuitions". I admit that they exist (as opposed to abstract World 3 objects). I also admit that they are not always reliable: logical errors exist. But these mistaken inferences may be criticized, and eliminated.[5]

Interactionist I do not think that we have made much progress. I have long admitted the role of natural selection and of learning (which I, incidentally, should certainly not describe as "conditioning"; but never mind the terminology). I also would insist, as you seem to do now, on the importance of the fact that we often approach truth by way of the elimination and correction of error; and like yourself, I am inclined to say that the same holds with mistaken inferences as opposed to valid inferences: we learn of an inference, or a certain way of drawing inferences, that it is invalid if we find a counter-example; that is to say, an inference of the same logical form, with true premises and a false conclusion. In other words: *an inference is valid if and only if no counter-example to this inference exists*. But this statement (which I have italicized) is a *characteristic example of a World 3 principle*. And although the emergence of World 3 can be, partly, explained by natural selection, that is to say, but its usefulness, the principles of valid inference, and their applications, which belong to World 3, cannot all be explained in this way. They are partly the unintended autonomous results of the making of World 3.

Physicalist But I stick to my point that only the physiological dispositions (more precisely, dispositional states[6]) exist. Why should not dispositions evolve or develop which I may describe as dispositions to act in accordance with a routine? For example, in accordance with what you call the logical standards of truth and validity? The main point is that the dispositions are useful in the struggle for survival.

Interactionist That may *sound* all right, but it seems to me to avoid the real issue. For dispositions must be dispositions to do something. If we ask what this something is, you seem to indicate that your answer would be "to act in

---

[5] My physicalist seems to me to do somewhat better here than those materialists for whom truth is ensured by direct causation rather than by the elimination of error, e.g. by selection (partly by natural selection). See also section 23 below.

[6] See Armstrong [1968], pp. 85–8.

accordance with a routine". But can we not then ask "*What* routine?" – and this, I think, would lead us back to World 3 principles.

But let us look at the matter from another angle. The property of a brain mechanism or a computer mechanism which makes it work according to the standards of logic is not a purely physical property, although I am very ready to admit that it is in some sense connected with, or based upon, physical properties. For two computers may physically differ as much as you like, yet they may both operate according to the same standards of logic. And *vice versa*; they may differ physically as little as you may specify, yet this difference may be so amplified that the one may operate according to the standards of logic, but not the other. This seems to show that the standards of logic are not physical properties. (The same holds, incidentally, for practically all relevant properties of a computer *qua* computer.) Yet the standards of logic are, according to you and me, useful for survival.

Physicalist But you say yourself that the property of a computer which makes it work according to the standards of logic is based upon physical properties. I do not see why you deny that this property *is* a physical property. Surely, it can be defined in purely physical terms. We simply build a logical computer, which is a physical object. Then we define the relations between its input and its output as the standards of logic. In this way we have defined a standard of logic in purely physical terms.

Interactionist No. Your computer may break down. This may happen to any computer. Incidentally, you could just as well choose as your standard a particular copy of a logical text book. However, it may have mistakes in it, either printing mistakes or others. No, standards belong to World 3, but they are useful for survival; which means that they have causal effects in the physical world, in World 1. Thus the abstract World 3 property of a computer which we can describe by saying "its operations conform to logical standards" has physical effects: it is "real" (in the sense of section 4 above). This causal action upon World 1 is precisely the reason why I call World 3, including its abstract objects, "real". If you admit that conformity with logical standards is useful for survival, you admit the usefulness of logical standards, and so their reality. If you deny their reality, why is the similarity between useful computers and the differences between a useful computer and a useless one not to be found in their physical similarity or dissimilarity but in their ability or disability to work in accordance with logical standards?

Physicalist I am still unconvinced. Is usefulness for survival purposes according to you a property belonging to World 1, as I think, or do you count it as belonging to World 3?

Interactionist It depends. The usefulness of a natural organ I am inclined to count as a property belonging to World 1 objects, while that of man-made tools may be a property belonging to World 3 objects.

Physicalist But the brain, and its states and processes, are World 1 objects; and so are verbal expressions such as statements or theories. Could we not simply accept a suggestion of William James's and call a theory true if it is useful? And could we not similarly call an inference valid if it is useful?

Interactionist You can, of course, but you do not gain anything. Admittedly, truth is useful in many contexts; it is so especially if one adopts the World 3 aims and purposes of a scientist, a theoretician; that is, to explain things. From this point of view, valid inference is particularly valuable or "useful", because we can look at explanation as a certain kind of (usually abbreviated) valid inference. But although we can say that in this sense truth is useful, it leads to great trouble if we try (with William James) to identify truth and usefulness.

Physicalist How does it lead to trouble?

Interactionist If one thinks of a true theory as useful, then one does so mainly because of the usefulness of its true informative content. But a theory may be true even if its informative content is negligible, or nil: a tautology like "All tables are tables" or perhaps "1 = 1" is true; but it has no useful informative content. This has its repercussions on the usefulness of validity.

A valid inference always transmits truth from the premises to the conclusion and retransmits falsity from the conclusion to at least one of the premises. Is this perhaps enough to show its instrumental value? It is not, for the premises may be true and useful but the conclusion may be true and useless, as I have just shown. The point is that the *informative content* of a validly derived conclusion can never exceed that of the premises. (If it does a counterexample can be found.) But the informative content can deteriorate in a valid inference. In fact, it may be zero. For example, a valid conclusion drawn from some highly informative and useful theory may be just a tautology like "1 = 1", which is not informative and therefore no longer useful.

Thus a valid inference always transmits truth, but not always usefulness. It cannot therefore be shown that every valid inference is a useful instrument, or that the routine of drawing valid inferences is as such always useful.

You might wonder why you as a physicalist could not say that it is not so much every particular valid inference that is useful but the whole system of valid inferences; that is to say, logic as such. Now, it is indeed true enough that it is the system – logic – which is useful. *But the problem for the physicalist is that it is just this that he cannot admit; for the point at issue between him and the interactionist is precisely whether such things as logic (which is an abstract system) exist (over and above particular ways of linguistic behaviour).* The interactionist here takes the commonsensical view that valid inference is useful — and this, indeed, is one of the reasons why he admits its reality. The physicalist is prevented from accepting this position.

So far the dialogue. In it I have tried in brief to state some of the reasons why a materialist theory of logic and with it of World 3 does not work.

Logic, the theory of valid inference, is indeed a valuable instrument; but this cannot be made clear by an instrumentalist interpretation of valid inference. Nor can, I think, such ideas as that of the *informative content of a theory* (an idea that depends on that of deducibility or valid inference) be made clear as long as we do not transcend the materialist point of view — the point of view that admits only the physical aspects of World 3.

I do not claim that I have refuted materialism. But I think that I have shown that materialism has no right to claim that it can be supported by rational argument — argument that is rational by logical principles. Materialism may be true, but it is incompatible with rationalism, with the acceptance of the standards of critical argument; for these standards appear from the materialist point of view as an illusion, or at least as an ideology.

I think that the argument of this section concerning validity can be generalized.

Some people assert[7] that all argument is ideological and that science is just another ideology. This is clearly a self-defeating relativism. It is sometimes connected with the thesis that there is no such thing as a pure standard of validity, or a pure theory, but that all knowledge works in the interest of human interests — such as socialism and capitalism. Reply: are computers in a socialist Utopia to be constructed differently from those in a capitalist society? (Of course, they may be differently programmed; but this is trivial, as they will always be differently programmed if used to solve different problems.)

22. The So-Called Identity Theory

I always try to avoid discussing the meaning of words, and as a consequence, I also try to avoid criticizing a theory for using the wrong words or words with a wrong meaning or with no meaning at all. My standard policy in these cases is

---

[7] Perhaps under the influence of Thomas Kuhn's *The Structure of Scientific Revolutions* [1962].

to see whether the theory under discussion cannot be so reformulated or interpreted that objections based on the meaning of words disappear.

This applies to the identity theory. (The identity theory often occurs linked with panpsychism, for example in its founder, Spinoza, or in our own time in the work of Rensch. However, it needs to be clearly distinguished from panpsychism as a theory.) I very much doubt whether a formulation like "mental processes are identical with a certain kind of (physico-chemical) brain processes" can be taken at its face value, in view of the fact that we understand, since Leibniz, "*a* is identical with *b*" to imply that any property of the object *a* is also a property of the object *b*. Some identity theorists certainly seem to assert identity in this sense; but it seems to me more than doubtful whether they really can mean it. (Two very powerful though very different criticisms of the identity claim in this sense can be found in Judith Jarvis Thomson [1969] and in Saul A. Kripke [1971]; each of them appears to me pretty conclusive.) In view of this situation I will adopt here the following policy. I will criticize the identity theory by criticizing a logically weaker consequence of it, the Spinozistic theory that mental processes are physical processes experienced "from the inside"; that is, I shall criticize a form of parallelism. (A parallelist theory is weaker than an identity theory because the identity of two lines or two surfaces is a limiting case of their being parallel: they are parallel with the distance zero.) In this way I can avoid criticizing the identity claim and still criticize the identity theory, and some weaker theories at the same time. Moreover, in adopting this policy, I am not prevented from presenting the identity theory in as reasonable and convincing a form as I can.

The identity theory in some of its versions is very old. It is reformulated in Diogenes of Appolonia (DK B5). Democritus no doubt regarded psychical processes as identical with atomic processes, and Epicurus (Letter I, to Herodotus, 63 ff.) indicates clearly that he regards sensations and passions (or feelings) as mental or psychical, and the soul or mind as a body of fine particles; and these ideas are no doubt even older. Descartes stresses the different character of the mental (unextended; intensive) and the physical (extended); but the Cartesian Spinoza stresses that "the order and the connection of [mental] ideas is the same as [or identical with] the order and the connection of [physical] things" (*Ethics* Part II, proposition VII; Part V, proposition I, demonstration); and he explains this by the theory that mind and matter are two different ways of comprehending, or aspects of, one and the same substance (or thing in itself) which he also called "Nature" or "God". This theory – a parallelism between mind and matter, explained by their being two aspects of a thing in itself – is, I suppose, the beginning of the modern physicalistic identity theory which replaces "Nature" by either "mental process" or by "physical process" and which restricts the identity thesis to a small subclass of material processes: to a subclass of the brain processes, which it identifies with mental processes.

It is interesting that the Spinozistic theory of two aspects was often described as an identity theory. Thus the great nineteenth century neurologist John Hughlings Jackson ([1887] = [1931], volume ii, p. 84) distinguished the following three doctrines of the relation between consciousness and "the highest nervous centres" of the nervous system. [The remarks in square brackets have been added by me.]

(1) The "mind acts through the nervous system". [Interactionism.]

(2) The "activities of the highest centres and mental states are one and the same thing, or are different sides of one and the same thing". [Identity theory; and Spinozism.]

(3) The two things, though "utterly different", "occur together . . . in parallelism", there being "no interference of one with the other". [Parallelism.]

It is clear that (2) comprises the identity theory and Spinozism, while (3) distinguishes a non-Spinozistic (Leibnizean?) parallelism from (2). (Jackson himself opted for (3).) I too shall regard here the identity theory as a more radical form of Spinozistic parallelism.

The theory called by Herbert Feigl "the psychophysical identity theory" aims at avoiding the implausibilities and the difficulties of epiphenomenalism. It does so by stressing that the mental phenomena – or the mental processes – are *real.* (Feigl, following Schlick, goes so far as to say that they are *the* real things or, in Kantian terminology, the things in themselves.[1]) Thus mental processes do not play here the objectionable role of redundant epiphenomena. They are conjectured, however, to be "identical" with a certain subclass of the *physical processes* that occur in our brains. This is the central conjecture of the theory. It does not mean that the mental experiences or processes as known by acquaintance must be *logically* identi-

[1] Feigl ([1967], pp. 84, 86, 90.) In a footnote on p. 84 Feigl refers to Kant's *Critique of Pure Reason* (see *Kritik der reinen Vernunft, first* edition, p. 361; transcendentale Dialektik, zweites Buch, dritter Paralogism = Kants *Werke,* Akademieausgabe, Band 4, 1911, p. 227; Cassirer's edition, Band 3, 1913, p. 643), where indeed the theory is mentioned that the thing in itself may be of a mindlike character. Thus we get the following parentage of this form of the identity theory: Kant – Schopenhauer (the thing in itself = will) – Clifford (whose identity theory is a kind of parallelism) – Schlick – Feigl – Russell (Russell's "Mind and Matter" [1956] is discussed in H. Feigl and A. E. Blumberg [1974], pp. XXIIff., and Feigl [1975]). For Clifford, see note 4 to section 16, above; for some additional remarks on the history of the identity theory, see section 54 below.

cal with physical processes as described by physical theory. On the contrary, as Schlick emphasizes, the mental processes of which we have a *knowledge by acquaintance* are conjectured, according to his theory, to be "identical" with a kind of physical process of which we may obtain only a *knowledge by description*; "identical" in the sense that the objects the brain physiologist tries to describe in theoretical terms turn out empirically to be, in part, our subjective experiences. This knowledge is *theoretical* knowledge (and thus, incidentally, conjectural knowledge). Or as Feigl likes to put it; the mental processes of which we have knowledge by acquaintance turn out, if we want to obtain of them knowledge by description, to be physical brain processes. Thus according to Feigl's theory a type of mental process may, regarded as a type of brain process, consist of the fact that a sufficiently large number of neurons are all doing microchemically the same thing – say, synthesizing certain transmitter molecules in a peculiar rhythm.

The identity theory (or the "central state theory") can be formulated thus. Let us call "World 1" the class of processes in the physical world. Then let World 1 (or the class of objects belonging to it) be divided (as in section 16) into two exclusive subworlds or subclasses, in such a manner that World 1_m (*m* for mental) consists of the *description* in physical·terms of the class of all the *mental* or psychological processes that will ever be *known by acquaintance,* while the vastly larger class, World 1_p (*p* for purely physical) consists of all those physical processes (described in physical terms) which are not mental processes as well.

In other words, we have

(1) World 1 = World 1_p + World 1_m

(2) World $1_p \cdot$ World $1_m = 0$ (that is, the two classes are exclusive of each other)

(3) World 1_m = World 2

The identity theory stresses the following points:

(4) Since World 1_p and World 1_m are parts of the same World 1, there is no problem raised by their interacting. *They can clearly interact according to the laws of physics.*

(5) Since World 1_m = World 2, mental processes are real. They interact with World 1_p processes, exactly as interactionism asserts. So we have interactionism (without tears).

(6) Accordingly, World 2 is not epiphenomenal, but real (also in the sense of section 4, above). Therefore the clash between the Darwinian point of view and the epiphenomenal view of World 2 described in section 20 does not occur (or so it might seem – but see the next section).

(7) The "identity" of World 1_m and World 2 can be made intuitively acceptable by considering a cloud. It consists, physically speaking, of an accumulation of water vapour, that is, a region of physical space in which water drops of a certain average size are distributed with a certain density. This is a physical structure. It looks from the outside like a white reflecting surface; it is experienced, from the inside, as a dull, only partially translucent, fog. The thing as experienced is, in theoretical or physical description, identical with a structure of water drops.

According to U. T. Place [1956], we can compare the inside view and the outside view of the cloud with the inside or subjective experience of a brain process and the outside observation of the brain. Moreover, the theoretical description in terms of water vapour, or of a structure of water drops, can be compared to the not yet fully known theoretical physical description of the relevant physico-chemical brain processes involved.

(8) If we say that fog was the cause of a car accident, then this can be analysed, in physical terms, by pointing out how the water drops absorbed light, so that light quanta which otherwise would have stimulated the driver's retina never reached the retina.

(9) The upholders of the central state theory or identity theory point out that the fate of the theory will depend on empirical corroboration which can be expected to come from the progress of brain research.

I have presented what I regard as the essentials of the theory. The following points I regard as inessential.

(a) Herbert Feigl's suggestion ([1967], p. 22) that the theory does not assume the hypothesis of emergent evolution. (This is even a crucially important point for Smart.) I think that the theory does assume it: there was no World 1_m before it emerged from World 1_p. Nor could its peculiar mental properties be predicted. However, I regard this emergent character of World 1_m as perfectly in order, and not as a point of weakness of the theory.[2]

(b) It will be remembered that in my presentation of the theory I have tried to avoid any purely verbal argument connected with the term "identical" or with the question what it may mean to say that mental or experienced processes (World 2 = World 1_m) are "identical" with objects of our physical descriptions. This "identity" certainly has its difficulties. But in my view it

[2] The point is far from crucial; but it is not merely verbal. Smart, more especially, has a different attitude towards scientific knowledge from mine: while I am impressed by our immense ignorance on all levels, he holds that we can assert that our knowledge of physics will one day suffice to explain everything — even (to quote Peter Medawar) our foreign exchange deficit; see section 7 above.

need not be taken as crucial for the theory or for some version of it; just as it may not be essential for our metaphor of the cloud to decide in which sense the three aspects – the outside view, the inside view, and the description in physical terms – are all aspects of *one and the same* object. What I regard as crucial is that the identity theory adheres to the physicalist principle of the closedness of World 1. Thus in my view a theory which gives up the term "identity" and replaces it by "very close association" (say) would be just as mistaken if it adhered to this physicalist principle.

(c) Feigl rightly stresses the "reality" of the mental processes, and this point seems to me essential. But he also stresses the character of the mental processes as things in themselves. This seems to me to make him a spiritualist rather than a physicalist, but it invites discussions which may easily become quite verbal. Take again our cloud metaphor. It seems to me (but I should be loth to argue the point) that the physical description – that of the cloud as a space in which water drops of a certain kind are distributed – comes in a way perhaps nearer to describing the thing in itself than either the outside description as a cloud or as a bulky surface reflecting light, or the inside experience as a fog. But does it matter? What does matter is that all the descriptions are descriptions of the same real thing – a thing that can interact with a physical body (for example, by condensing on it and thus making it wet).

I think that we may assume that there is no problem here; we can still criticize the theory on non-verbal grounds. In the next section I will criticize the identity theory as a physicalist theory. In a later section (54) I will point out that as a spiritualist theory, bordering on panpsychism, it accords badly with modern cosmology.

23. Does the Identity Theory Escape the Fate of Epiphenomenalism?

Before starting to criticize the identity theory, let me make it quite clear that I regard it as a perfectly consistent theory of the relation of mind and body. In my opinion the theory *may* therefore be true.

What I regard as inconsistent is a wider and stronger theory: the materialist view of the world, which involves Darwinism, and which together with the identity theory leads to a contradiction – the same as in the case of epiphenomenalism. My thesis is that the identity theory combined with Darwinism faces the same difficulties as epiphenomenalism.

Admittedly, the identity theory is somewhat different from epiphenomenalism; especially from an intuitive point of view. From this point of view it seems not so much a form of psychophysical parallelism;[1] rather, it seems close to dualistic interactionism.

For in view of

(3) World 1_m = World 2

we have, by (4), that World 1 interacts with World 2. Moreover, the reality of World 1_m (= World 2) and its efficacy could not be stressed more strongly. All this takes World 1_m (= World 2) far away from epiphenomenalism.

Moreover, the identity theory has the great advantage over epiphenomenalism that it gives a kind of explanation – and an intuitively satisfying explanation – of the nature of the link between World 1_m and World 2. In parallelistic epiphenomenalism, this link has just to be accepted as one of the ultimate inexplicables of the world – as a Leibnizian pre-established harmony. In the identity theory (whether we take or do not take the term "identity" quite seriously) the link is satisfying. (It is at least as satisfying as that between the inside view and the outside view of reality in Spinozism.)

All this seems to distinguish the identity theory sharply from epiphenomenalism. Nevertheless, the identity theory is as unsatisfactory as epiphenomenalism from a Darwinian point of view. But we (and especially the materialists among us) *need Darwinism* as the only known explanation of the emergence of purposeful behaviour in a purely material or physical world, or even in a world which at some stage of its evolution was confined to World 1_p (so that at this stage World 1_m = World 2 = 0).

Thus it is my thesis that my critical remarks about epiphenomenalism apply here too, *mutatis mutandis,* though admittedly with less intuitive force.

For the identity theory is, by intention, a purely physicalistic theory. Its fundamental principle is still the principle of the closedness of World 1; which leads to the lemma that (causal) explanation, so far as it is knowledge by description, must be in terms of strictly physical theory. This allows us (perhaps) to accept the emergence of a new World 1_m; *but it does not allow us to explain that the characterizing feature of this World 1_m is that it consists of mental processes, or that it is closely linked with mental processes.*

On the other hand, we must demand that all major novelties emerging under the pressure of natural selection must be explained entirely within World 1.

To put it in another way, the World 2 of the identity theory remains with respect to the Darwinian point of view logically in exactly the same situation as the epiphenomenal World 2. For although it is causally effective, this fact is

---

[1] The idea that World 1 and World 2 run parallel, without interacting, is suggested by epiphenomenalism if we remember that it accepts the physicalistic principle that World 1 is causally closed.

irrelevant when it comes to *explaining* any causal action of World 2 upon World 1. This has to be done entirely in terms of the closed World 1.

The real thing, the thing in itself, and causality known by acquaintance — all this remains, from the point of view of the physicalistic principle and of knowledge by description, outside of the physical explanation, and, indeed, of what is physically explicable.

The principle of the closedness of World 1 demands that we still *explain,* truthfully, my going to the dentist in purely physical terms. But if so, the fact that World 1_m is identical with World 2 — the world of my pains, my aim to get rid of them, and my knowledge about the dentist — remains causally redundant. And this is not changed by the assertion that another causal explanation, a World 2 one, is also true: it is not needed; the world works without it. But Darwinism explains the emergence of things or processes only if they make a difference. The identity theory adds a new aspect to the closed physical world, but it cannot explain that this aspect is of advantage in the struggles and pressures of World 1.[2] For it can explain this only if the purely physical World 1 contains these advantages. But if so, then World 2 is redundant.

Thus the identity theory, contrary to its intuitive character, is logically in the same boat as a parallelist theory that employs the physicalist principle of the closedness of World 1.

24. A Critical Note on Parallelism. The Identity Theory as a Form of Parallelism

In this section I am going to discuss what one may describe as the empirical background of psycho-physical parallelism. By way of an afterthought, I shall suggest that whatever may appear as a piece of supporting evidence in favour of the identity theory is also one of the cases which seem to support parallelism; an additional reason for interpreting the identity theory as a special case (a "degenerate case") of parallelism.

I shall start from the relation of perception to the other contents of our consciousness, and I shall try to throw some light on certain characteristics of perceptions by discussing the biological function of perception.

Under the influence of Descartes and also of British empiricism, a kind of *atomistic theory of mental events or processes* became widely established. In

[2] Jeremy Shearmur has drawn my attention to a very similar argument in Beloff [1965].

its simplest form, this theory interpreted consciousness as a *sequence of elementary ideas*. It does not matter for our purposes whether the ideas were regarded as unanalysable atoms, or as molecular (and consisting, say, of atomic sensations or of sense data or what not). What is important is the doctrine that there are elementary mental events ("ideas") and that the stream of consciousness consists of an ordered sequence of such events.

Some of the Cartesians then assumed that to each elementary mental event there corresponds a definite brain event. This correspondence was assumed to be of the one-to-one kind. The result is mind-body parallelism, or psycho-physical parallelism.

Now it is to be admitted that there is a kernel of truth in this theory. When I look at a red flower, then (keeping still) close my eyes for a second, and then open them and look again, the two perceptions will be so similar that I recognize the second perception as a repetition of the first. We all assume that this repetition is to be explained by the similarity of the two temporally distinct irritations of my retina, and of the two corresponding brain processes. If we generalize from such considerations (a generalization which to a Humean, particularly, may appear valid, since for Hume all consciousness consists only of such experiences) we arrive at psycho-physical parallelism. (The *Gestalt* switch of a Necker cube[1] which, no doubt, is due to changing functioning of the brain would seem to add further confirmation.)

It is therefore understandable why psycho-physical parallelism appears so convincing, indeed obvious, to many. Nevertheless I shall try to combat it here. My fundamental objection will be that the examples of repeated perceptions have been misinterpreted, and that our states of consciousness

[1] The following seems to work with most people: if we stare for long enough at a diagram of a Necker cube, then it switches on its own into the opposite interpretation (that is, with that side

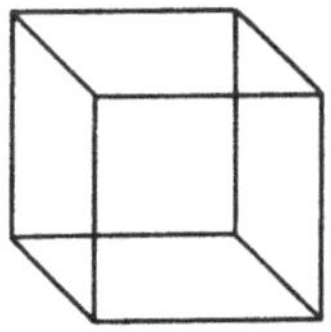

Necker Cube

which previously looked at the front now appearing to be at the back). The effect may be related to the tendency for anything to disappear if we have stared at it for long enough. This tendency, and perhaps with it the former effect, can be explained biologically. It is well known that a not too loud noise disappears subjectively after a time, unless we draw our attention to it consciously. See also note 2, below.

are not to be thought of as sequences of elements – neither of atoms nor of molecules.

True: I did look twice, with attention, at the same object; and since my mind has learned how to inform me about my environment, it informed me of this fact. It did so by producing the hypothesis, or the conjecture: "This is the same flower as before (and the same aspect of it, since neither the flower nor I have moved)."

But it is precisely because I was thus informed when I allegedly "identified the two experiences" that the second experience or state of consciousness was different from the first. The identification was one of *objects,* and of their aspects. The subjective experience (the "judgement" formed, the conjecture formed) was different: I experienced a repetition, which with the first I did not. If this is so, then the theory of consciousness as a sequence of (often repetitive) elementary or atomic perceptions is mistaken. And in consequence, the theory of a one-to-one correspondence between elementary conscious events and brain events will have to be given up as baseless (though certainly not as empirically refuted). For if our states of consciousness are not sequences of elements, then it is no longer clear what is supposed to correspond to what, in a one-to-one manner.

A parallelist might try to avoid this conclusion, insisting that our perceptions (and the corresponding brain events) are not atomic but molecular: in this case, the (postulated) experiential atoms and elements of the objective brain events may still be in one-to-one correspondence, although there may perhaps in fact never be two molecular experiences (and their corresponding brain events) which are identical.

It seems to me that two points may be made against such a view.

First, while the original theory which we were discussing was straightforward and informative, describing, as it did, actual experiences as elementary or atomic perceptions, and suggesting that there was some elementary brain event in one-to-one correspondence with each of these, we are now offered an atomistic ghost as a replacement. For the replacement theory is completely speculative, merely alleging that all actual experiences are *composed* in some unspecified way of atomic components, to which there are supposed to be brain correlates: it transfers atomism dogmatically from physics to psychology. Such things may exist – we cannot rule them out – but such a theory cannot claim any empirical support.

Second, considered as a theory of perception, I think that it is on the wrong track. I shall suggest below that we should take a biological approach to consciousness, and that one of the functions of consciousness is to allow us to recognize physical objects when we meet them again. This is arbitrarily interpreted by the theory we have been discussing as the recurrence of a psychological event and a corresponding brain event.

(The theory of perception which I am criticizing is, incidentally, a part of the very popular but nevertheless mistaken theory of a one-to-one correspondence between stimulus and response, or between input and output; and this theory, in its turn, is part of the theory, apparently upheld by Sherrington in [1906], but rejected by him in [1947], that there is one elementary kind of atomic or molecular brain function – the "reflexes" and the so-called "conditioned reflexes" – of which all the others are complexes or integrations. See Roger James [1977].[2])

What, then, of the status of perception? I suggest that we proceed in a different way. Instead of starting from the assumption of a one-to-one stimulus response mechanism (though such mechanisms may perhaps exist and may perhaps even play an important role), I suggest that we start from the fact that consciousness or awareness has a number of biologically useful functions.

If we regain consciousness after a spell of unconsciousness, a typical problem arises: "Where am I?". I take this as an indication that it is an important function of consciousness to keep track of our whereabouts in the world by constructing a kind of schematic model (as Kenneth J. W. Craik [1943] suggested) or a schematic map; detailed as far as our momentary immediate environment is concerned, but very sketchy as far as more distant regions are concerned. This model or map, I suggest, with our own position marked on it, is part of our ordinary consciousness of self. It normally exists in the form of vague dispositions or programmes; but we can focus our attention upon it whenever we wish, whereupon it may become more elaborate and precise. This map or model is one of a great number of conjectural *theories* about the world which we hold and which we almost constantly call to our aid, as we go along and as we develop, specify, and realize, the programme and the timetable of the actions in which we are engaged.

If we now look at the function of perception with this in mind then, I suggest, our sense organs should be regarded as auxiliaries to our brain. The brain in turn is programmed to select a fitting and relevant model (or theory or hypothesis) of our environment, as we move along, to be interpreted by the mind. This I should call the original or primary function of our brain and of our sense organs – in fact, of the central nervous system: in its most

[2] See also section 40. In this context, reference should be made to the experiments which show that stabilized images, stabilized noises, and stabilized touches (for example from our clothes) show a tendency to fade. For clearly the fading effect depends upon something like physical or stimulational similarity. But as this leads to fading, there is a dissimilarity of response.

primitive form it developed as a steering system; as an *aid to movement.* (The primitive central nervous system, in worms, is an aid to movement; and so are the far more primitive senses of fungi. See Max Delbrück [1974] for a report of his fascinating investigations into the beginning of sense organs and of problem solving in phycomycetes.)

The frog is programmed for the highly specialized task of catching moving flies. The frog's eye does not even signal to its brain a fly within reach if it does not move.[3]

Many years ago I quoted David Katz (*Animals and Men,* chapter VI; see my [1963 (a)], pp. 46f.) in a similar context: "A hungry animal divides the environment into edible and inedible things. An animal in flight sees roads to escape and hiding places." In general, an animal will perceive what is relevant according to its problem situation; and its problem situation, in turn, will depend not only on its external situation, but upon its inner state: its programme, as given by its genetic constitution, and its many sub-programmes – its preferences and choices. In the case of man, this involves personal aims and personal, conscious decisions.

Looking back from here to our experiment which led to a sequence of two practically identical perceptions, I do not deny that the two perceptions were extremely similar *qua* perceptions: our brain, supported by our eyes, would not have done its biological duty had it not informed us that *our environment* did not change from the first instant of time to the second. This explains why in the field of perception there will be a consciousness of repetition if the objects perceived do not change, *and if our programme does not change.* But this does not mean that the content of our consciousness was repeated, as I have already hinted. Nor does it mean that the two brain states were very similar. In fact, our programme (which was, in this special case, "compare your response to a stimulus repeated in two consecutive instants of time") did not change between the first instant and the second. But the two instants of time played decidedly different roles in that programme, just because of the repetition; and this alone ensured that they were experienced in different ways.

We now see that, even as far as the consciousness of perceptions is concerned (which represents only a part of our subjective experiences) there is no one-to-one correspondence of stimulus and response, as indicated by David Katz's remark about possible changes in our interest and in our

[3] See Lettvin & others [1959].

attention. Nevertheless, perceptions would not fulfil their task unless, *in cases when interest and attention did not change,* there was there something approaching to a one-to-one correspondence. But this is *a very special case.* And the usual procedure of generalizing from this special case, and of looking at stimulus and response as a simple one-to-one mechanism, and of confining the contents of our conscious experiences to this, is grossly mistaken.

But if we discard the idea of two one-to-one correlated sequences of events, the idea of psycho-physical parallelism loses its main prop. This does not *refute* the idea of parallelism, but it dissolves, I think, its apparently empirical basis.

Incidentally, the theory of brain-mind identity turns out, in the light of the present considerations, to be a special case of the idea of parallelism; for it too is based on the idea of a one-to-one correlation: it is an attempt rationally to *explain* this one-to-one correlation which it takes, uncritically, for granted.

25. Additional Remarks on some Recent Materialist Theories

Armstrong's book *A Materialist Theory of the Mind* [1968] is in many respects excellent. Yet as opposed to Feigl's identity theory or central state theory – a theory which emphatically accepts the existence of a world of conscious experience – Armstrong minimizes the significance of what Feigl ([1967], p. 138) describes as "the internal illumination" of our world through our consciousness. First, he stresses, not unfairly, the significance of subconscious or unconscious states. Next, he gives a most interesting theory of perception as an unconscious or conscious process of acquiring dispositional states. Thirdly, he suggests (without saying so explicitly) that consciousness is nothing but inner perception, perception of a second order, or perception (scanning) of an activity of the brain by other parts of the brain. But he skips and skims over the problem why this scanning should produce consciousness or awareness, in the sense in which all of us are well acquainted with consciousness or awareness; for example with the conscious, critical assessment of a solution to a problem. And he never goes into the problem of the difference between conscious awareness and physical reality.

Armstrong's book is divided into three parts: Part I is an introductory survey of theories of the mind; Part II, "The Concept of Mind", is a general theory of mental states and processes, and it has in my opinion some excellent things to say; though it can be, I gather, criticized on neurophysiological grounds. Part III, which is very sketchy, contains hardly more than the bare thesis that the mental states as described in Part II can be identified with states of the brain.

Why do I regard Part II in the main as excellent? The reason is this. Part II gives a description of states and processes of the mind seen from a *biological point of view*; that is, as if the mind could be regarded as an *organ*.

This attitude is due, of course, to the fact that Armstrong wishes later (in Part III) to *identify* the mind with an organ: with the brain. I need not stress that I do not agree with this identification, though I feel inclined to regard the identification of *unconscious* mental states and processes with brain states and brain processes as a very important conjecture. And although I am inclined to assume that even conscious processes somehow go "hand in hand" with brain processes, it seems to me that an *identification* of conscious processes with brain processes is liable to lead to panpsychism.

However mistaken Armstrong's metaphysical motives may be, his method of considering the mind as an organ with Darwinian functions seems to me excellent, and Part II of his book proves, in my opinion, the fruitfulness of this biological approach.

To turn to criticism. Armstrong's theory may either be classified as a radical materialism with a denial of consciousness, and criticized as such, or it may be classified as a not quite outspoken form of epiphenomenalism, *as far as the world of consciousness is concerned,* whose significance it tries to minimize. In this case my criticism of epiphenomenalism as incompatible with the Darwinian point of view applies.

I do not think that this theory of Armstrong's should be classified as an identity theory in the sense of Feigl, that is, in the sense that conscious processes are not merely linked with brain processes, but actually identical with them. For Armstrong nowhere discusses, or suggests, that conscious processes may be the things in themselves of which certain brain processes may be the appearances: he is very far from Leibniz's animism. However, if Armstrong should move nearer to Feigl, then my criticisms in section 23 would apply. In any case, my criticism in section 20 seems to me applicable.

I think that many (though not all) of the analyses of Armstrong's in his Part II are lasting contributions to biological psychology. But his treatment of the problem of consciousness is ambiguous and weak.

The reason for this weakness is to be found not so much in the fact that Armstrong, though not denying consciousness or awareness, minimizes and fails to discuss its significance, but rather in the fact that Armstrong ignores, and fails to discuss (in whatever terminology), what I call World 3 objects: he considers only World 2 and its reduction to World 1. But the main biological function of World 2, and especially of consciousness, is the grasping and the critical evaluation of World 3 objects. Even language is hardly mentioned.

Following a suggestion by Armstrong, it has become fashionable to refer to the identification of

gene = DNA

as an analogue of the suggested identification of

mental state = brain state

But the analogy is a bad one, because the identification of genes with DNA molecules, while a most important empirical discovery, did not add anything to the metaphysical (or ontological) status of the gene or DNA. Indeed, even before the gene theory was developed there was Weismann's theory of the "germ plasm" *(Keimplasma)* in which the instructions for development were assumed to be given in the form of a material (chemical) structure. Later it was suggested (on the basis of Mendel's discovery) that there were "particles" in the germ plasm representing "characters". Genes themselves were, from the beginning, introduced as such "particles": as material structures; or more precisely as substructures of the chromosomes. More than thirty years before the DNA theory of genes, detailed maps of chromosomes were proposed that showed the relative positions of the genes (cp. T. H. Morgan and C. B. Bridges [1916]); maps whose principle was confirmed in detail by recent results of molecular biology. In other words, something like the identity *gene = DNA* was expected, if not taken for granted, from the beginning of the gene theory. What was unexpected to some people was that the gene turned out to be a nucleic acid rather than a protein; so also, of course, was the structure and function of the double helix.

The identification of the mind with the brain would be analogous to this only if it was assumed, to start with, that the mind is one of the physical organs, and then found empirically that it was not (say) the heart, or the liver, but rather the brain. While the dependence (or interdependence) of thought, intelligence, subjective experiences, and brain states was expected since Hippocrates's *On the Sacred Disease,* only materialists asserted an identity – in the face of considerable factual and conceptual difficulties.

This analysis shows that there is no analogy between the two identifications. The claim that they are analogous is not only unwarranted, but misleading.

An even stronger criticism can be directed against the claim that the identification of mental processes with brain processes is analogous to that of a flash of lightning with an electrical discharge.

The conjecture that a flash of lightning is an electrical discharge was suggested by observing that electrical discharges were like miniature flashes of lightning. And then came Franklin's experiments which strongly supported this conjecture.

Very interesting critical remarks on these identifications are made by Judith Jarvis Thomson [1969].

Armstrong has recently published a very clearly and compactly reasoned book *Belief, Truth and Knowledge* [1973]. The book is essentially a traditional empiricist theory of knowledge, translated into materialist terms. None of the problems of the dynamics of the growth of knowledge, of the correction of knowledge, or of the growth of scientific theories are even mentioned, which is disappointing.

Quinton in *The Nature of Things* [1973] proposes an identity theory which, like Feigl's and unlike Armstrong's, stresses the importance of consciousness, but which does not appeal to the relationship between the thing in itself and its appearance.

How is this identification to be conceived? Quinton refers to Armstrong's example of the flash of lightning and the electric discharge. Like Feigl, Smart, and Armstrong, he regards the identification as empirical. So far so good. But he does not say how we proceed empirically to test conjectural identifications. And like his predecessors, he does not suggest the kind of test which could possibly be regarded as a test of the identity thesis of mind and brain, as distinct from an interactionist thesis (especially from one which does not operate with a mental substance).

There are also those who simply say that the mind is an activity of the brain, and who leave it at that. Not much can be said against this, as far as it goes. But it does not go far enough: the question arises whether the mental activities of the brain are just part of its many physical activities or whether there is an important difference; and if so, what we can say about the difference.

26. The New Promissory Materialism

A somewhat half-hearted retreat from the identity theory has become fashionable lately. It is a retreat into what may be described as a "promissory materialism". The popularity of promissory materialism is perhaps a reaction to some striking criticisms which have been advanced against the identity theory in recent years. These criticisms show that the identity theory is hardly compatible with ordinary language or with common sense. At any rate, it seems that the new promissory materialism accepts that, at the present time, materialism is not tenable. But it offers us the promise of a better world, a world in which mental terms will have disappeared from our language, and in which materialism will be victorious.

The victory is to come about as follows. With the progress of brain research, the language of the physiologists is likely to penetrate more and more into ordinary language and to change our picture of the universe, including that of common sense. So we shall be talking less and less about experiences, perceptions, thoughts, beliefs, purposes and aims; and more and more about brain processes, about dispositions to behave, and about overt behaviour. In this way, mentalist language will go out of fashion and be used only in historical reports, or metaphorically, or ironically. When this stage has been reached, mentalism will be stone dead, and the problem of mind and its relation to the body will have solved itself.

In support of promissory materialism it is pointed out that this is exactly what has happened in the case of the problem of witches and their relation to the devil. If at all, we now speak of witches either to characterize an archaic superstition, or we speak metaphorically or ironically. The same will happen with mind language, we are promised: perhaps not so *very* soon – perhaps not even during the life span of the present generation – but soon enough.

Promissory materialism is a peculiar theory. It consists, essentially, of a historical (or historicist) prophecy about the future results of brain research and of their impact. This prophecy is baseless. No attempt is made to base it upon a survey of recent brain research. The opinion of researchers who, like Wilder Penfield, started as identity theorists, but ended as dualists (see Penfield [1975], pp. 104f.) is ignored. No attempt is made to resolve the difficulties of materialism by argument. No alternatives to materialism are even considered.

Thus it appears that there is, rationally, not more of interest to be found in the thesis of promissory materialism than, let us say, in the thesis that one day we shall abolish cats or elephants by ceasing to talk about them; or in the thesis that one day we shall abolish death by ceasing to talk about it. (Indeed, did we not get rid of bedbugs simply by refusing to talk about them?)

Promissory materialists like, it seems, to state their prophecy in the at present still fashionable jargon of linguistic philosophy. But I suggest that this is inessential; and a physicalist might drop the jargon of linguistic philosophy and reply to what I have said here along the following lines.

Physicalist: "You claim, as a critic of physicalism, that reports about subjective experience, and empirically testable theories about subjective experience, constitute evidence against our thesis. However, as you yourself [1934 (b)] always emphasize, all observation statements are theory-impregnated; and as suggested by yourself ([1957 (i)] = [1972 (a)], chapter 5), it has happened in the history of science that statements about facts, and well-tested theories, have been *corrected* when they have been explained by later theories. Thus it is certainly not impossible that what we now regard as statements about subjective experience will, in the future, be explained and corrected by physicalist theories. If this happens, subjective experience will be left in much the same position as, say, demons or witches are now: it will be part of a theory which was once accepted, but which has now been discarded; and the old evidence for it will have been reinterpreted and corrected."

While I do not wish to suggest that it is *impossible* that things may happen as the physicalist says here (see my [1974 (c)], p. 1054), I do not think that this argument can be taken seriously. For it says no more than that no observational evidence is final, beyond the possibility of correction, and that all our knowledge is fallible. This is true, of course; but it is not enough to be used, on its own, as a defence of a theory against empirical criticism. The argument, as it stands, is too weak. As mentioned before, it could be applied to argue against the existence of cats or of elephants just as well as it has been applied to argue against the existence of subjective experience. While there is always a risk involved in accepting evidence and arguments like those here used by me, it seems to me reasonable to take the risk. For all the physicalist offers is, as it were, a cheque drawn against his future prospects, and based on the hope that a theory will be developed one day which solves his problems for him; the hope, in short, that something will turn up.

27. Results and Conclusion

It appears then from our analysis that, in the present Darwinian climate, a consistent materialist view of the world is only possible if it is combined with a denial of the existence of consciousness.

However, as John Beloff says at the end of his excellent book ([1962], p. 258), "A doctrine which can sustain itself only by elaborate evasions is little better than humbug."[1]

[1] Where I do not follow Beloff is in his attitude towards "the paranormal" as he calls it. I believe that radical physicalism can be regarded as refuted, quite independently of the paranormal.

It appears, further, that if we adopt a Darwinian point of view (see section 20) and admit the existence of an evolved consciousness, we are led to interactionism.

What I call the Darwinian point of view appears to be part of our present scientific outlook, and also an integral part of any materialist or physicalist creed.

On the other hand, if separated from the Darwinian point of view, the identity theory seems to me consistent. Yet apart from its incompatibility with Darwinian principles, it does not seem to me to be empirically testable, as Feigl ([1967], p. 160 and *passim*) suggests, by any prospective results of neurophysiology. Such results can, at best, show a close parallelism between brain processes and mental processes. But this would not support the identity theory any more than parallelism (for example, epiphenomenalism) or even interactionism.

I may perhaps show this in a little more detail for interactionism.

According to interactionism, an intense brain activity is the necessary condition for mental processes. Thus brain processes will go on contemporaneously with any mental processes, and being necessary conditions, may be said to "cause" them, or to "act" upon them. Take a simple example, like looking at a tree and closing and opening your eyes. The causal effect of the nervous changes upon your experiences is obvious. Or look at one of the figures illustrating *Gestalt* switch – either initiated by yourself or by your nervous system. This illustrates the action of the nervous system on consciousness *and* the – voluntary – effect of "concentration".[2] Owing to the constant goings on of brain processes on all levels it does not seem possible to distinguish interaction from, say, the alleged identity *empirically*; nor have any serious suggestions been made how this could be done, although it has often been asserted that it can be done (as we have seen).

To sum up, it appears that Darwinian theory, together with the fact that conscious processes exist, lead beyond physicalism; another example of the self-transcendence of materialism, and one quite independent of World 3.

---

[2] A good example is the following well-known figure, called "double cross" by Wittgenstein [1953], p. 207. One can operate it by "concentrating" either on the white cross or on the black cross; either voluntarily, or withholding our volition.

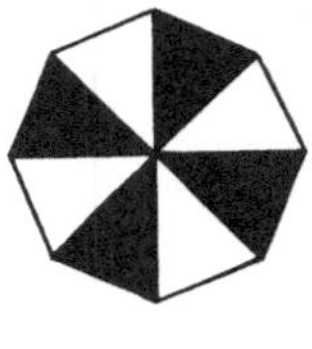

Chapter P4 Some Remarks on the Self

28. Introduction

The present chapter is difficult; not (I hope) so much for the reader as for the writer. The trouble is that although the self has a peculiar unity, my somewhat scattered remarks on the self do not pretend to have any such unity or system (except perhaps in stressing the dependence of the self upon World 3). A discussion of the self, of persons and of personalities, of consciousness and of the mind, is only too liable to lead to questions like "What is the self?" or "What is consciousness?". But as I have often pointed out,[1] "what is" questions are never fruitful, although they have been much discussed by philosophers. They are connected with the idea of *essences* – "What is the self essentially?" – and so with the very influential philosophy which I have called "essentialism" and which I regard as mistaken.[2] "What is" questions are liable to degenerate into verbalism – into a discussion of the meaning of words or concepts, or into a discussion of definitions. But, contrary to what is still widely believed, such discussions and definitions are useless.

It is of course to be admitted that the words "self", "person", "mind", "soul" and similar words are not synonyms, but have somewhat different meanings in sensitive English usage. For example, "soul" is often used, in contemporary English, with the implication that it is a substance which can survive death. (In German, the word "*Seele*" is used differently, more like the English word "mind".)

I have no intention here of discussing the question of the immortality of the soul. (But see the discussion between Eccles and myself in dialogue XI.) I will however quote here a brief statement about this question with which I agree closely. It is due to John Beloff ([1962], p. 190).

---

[1] Cp. my [1974 (z_7)]; [1974 (z_8)]; [1974 (z_4)]; [1975 (r)] and [1976 (g)].

[2] See my [1975 (r)] and [1976 (g)]. Cp. also note 2 to section 30.

"I have no craving for personal immortality; indeed I would think the poorer of a world in which my ego was to be a permanent fixture."

I shall for this reason try to avoid using the word "soul"; though if I were writing in German, I might perhaps not feel that I should avoid the word "*Seele*". I will not, however, continue to discuss words, but rather use them, as well as I can, to discuss not verbal issues, but real ones.

Having stated my attitude to the problem of the survival of the soul, I want to state briefly, before entering into arguments and controversies, my attitude to the main questions.

I agree with the great biologist Theodosius Dobzhansky who wrote, shortly before his death in December 1975:[3]

"I am not only alive but aware of being alive. Moreover, I know that I shall not remain alive for ever, that death is inevitable. I possess the attributes of self-awareness and death awareness."

We are not only aware of being alive, but each of us is aware of being a self; aware of his identity through considerable periods of time, and through breaks in his self-awareness due to periods of sleep, or to periods of unconsciousness; and each of us is aware of his moral responsibility for his actions.[4]

This self-identity is no doubt closely related to the self-identity of our body (which changes greatly during its life, and which constantly changes its constituent material particles). Both in the case of the identity of our selves and in the case of the identity of our bodies, we should always be clear that this numerical identity is not a strictly logical identity. (It is, rather, what Kurt Lewin [1922] called "genidentity": the numerical sameness of some thing that changes in time.) This kind of identity constitutes a problem even with changing inanimate bodies, and more so with living bodies; and it is an even greater problem with selves, or minds, or self-conscious minds.

29. Selves

Before starting my remarks about the self, I wish to state clearly and unambiguously that I am convinced that *selves exist.*

This statement might seem somewhat superfluous in a world in which

[3] Dobzhansky [1975], p. 411.

[4] I should perhaps mention, at the outset, that in my discussion of the self I am not going to discuss issues from the field of abnormal psychology or the related problems posed by results obtained concerning brains split by commissurotomy. For a discussion of the split brain, see Eccles, chapter E5.

overpopulation is one of the great social and moral problems. Obviously, people exist; and each of them is an individual self, with feelings, hopes and fears, sorrows and joys, dreads and dreams, which we can only guess since they are known only to the person himself or herself.

All this is almost too obvious to be written down. But it must be said. For some great philosophers have denied it. David Hume was one of the first who was led to doubt the existence of his own self; and he had many followers.

Hume was led to his somewhat strange position by his empiricist theory of knowledge. He adopted the commonsense view (a view which I regard as mistaken; see my [1972 (a)], chapter 2) that all our knowledge is the result of sense experience. (This overlooks the tremendous amount of knowledge which we inherit and which is built into our sense organs and our nervous system; our knowledge how to react, how to develop, and how to mature. See my [1957 (a)] = [1963 (a)], chapter 1, p. 47.) Hume's empiricism led him to the doctrine that we can know nothing but our sense impressions and the "ideas" derived from sense impressions. On this basis he argued that *we cannot have anything like an idea of self*; and that, therefore, there cannot be such a thing as the self.

Thus in the section *"Of Personal Identity"* of his *Treatise*,[1] he argues against "some philosophers who imagine that we are every moment intimately conscious of what we call our SELF"; and he says of these philosophers that "Unluckily all these positive assertions are contrary to that very experience, which is pleaded for them, nor have we any idea of *self*. . . For from what impression cou'd this idea be deriv'd? This question 'tis impossible to answer without manifest contradiction and absurdity . . .".

These are strong words, and they have made a strong impression on philosophers: from Hume to our own time the existence of a self has been regarded as highly problematical.

Yet Hume himself, in a slightly different context, asserts the existence of selves just as emphatically as he here denies it. Thus he writes, in Book II of the *Treatise*:[2]

"'Tis evident, that the idea, or rather impression of ourselves is always intimately present with us, and that our consciousness gives us so lively a

---

[1] [1739], Book I, Part IV, Section VI (Selby-Bigge edition [1888], p. 251). In Book III [1740], Appendix ([1888], p. 634) Hume slightly mitigates his tone; yet he seems in this Appendix to have completely forgotten about his own "positive assertions" such as those in [1739], Book II, referred to in the next note.

[2] [1739], Book II, Part I, Section XI ([1888], p. 317). A similar passage is [1739], Book II, Part II, Section II, Sixth Experiment ([1888], p. 339) where we read: "'Tis evident that . . . we are at all times intimately conscious of ourselves, our sentiments and passions . . .".

conception of our own person, that 'tis not possible to imagine, that anything can in this particular go beyond it."

This positive assertion of Hume's amounts to the same position that he attributes in the more famous negative passage quoted before to "some philosophers", and that he there emphatically declares to be manifestly contradictory and absurd.

But there are lots of other passages in Hume supporting the idea of selves, especially under the name of "character". Thus we read:[3]

"There are also characters peculiar to different . . . persons . . . The knowledge of these characters is founded on the observation of an uniformity in the actions, that flow from them . . ."

Hume's official theory (if I may call it so) is that the self is no more than the sum total (the bundle) of its experiences.[4] He argues – in my opinion, rightly – that talk of a "substantial" self does not help us much. Yet he again and again describes actions as "flowing" from a person's character. In my opinion we do not need more in order to be able to speak of a self.

Hume, and others, take it that if we speak of the self as a substance, then the properties (and the experiences) of the self may be said to "inhere" in it. I agree with those who say that this way of speaking is not illuminating. We may, however, speak of "our" experiences, using the possessive pronoun. This seems to me perfectly natural; and it need not give rise to speculations about an ownership relation. I may say of my cat that it "has" a strong character without thinking that this way of talking expresses an ownership relation (in the reverse direction to the one when I speak of "my" body). Some theories – such as the ownership theory – are incorporated in our language. We do not, however, have to accept as true the theories that are incorporated in our language, even though this fact may make it difficult to criticize them. If we decide that they are seriously misleading, we may be led to change the aspect of our language in question; otherwise, we may continue to use it, and simply bear in mind the fact that it should not be taken too literally (for example the "new" moon). All this, however, should not prevent us from always trying to use the plainest language we can.

Memory is obviously important for self-awareness: those states of which I have lost my memory *completely* can hardly be said to be states of myself;

---

[3] [1739], Book II, Part III, Section I ([1888], p. 403; see also p. 411). Elsewhere, Hume attributes to us as agents "motives and character" from which "a spectator can commonly infer our actions". See, for example, [1739], Book II, Part III, Section II ([1888], p. 408). See also the Appendix ([1888], pp. 633 ff.).

[4] See also the text to note 1 to section 37 for a criticism of this theory.

except in the sense that I *may* recover the memory of those states. Nevertheless, I think that there is more to self-awareness than memory, in spite of Quinton's excellent reply to F. H. Bradley [1883] who wrote: "Mr. Bain thinks the mind is a collection [= what Hume called a bundle]. Has Mr. Bain reflected: who collects Mr. Bain?". Quinton ([1973], p. 99) comments: "The answer is that the later Mr. Bain collects the earlier Mr. Bain by recollecting him."

Recollecting is important, but it is not everything. The capacity for recollection is perhaps more important than the actual recollection. We obviously are not all the time "recollecting" our earlier selves. And we live more for the future – acting, preparing for the future – than in the past.

30. The Ghost in the Machine

It may perhaps be helpful to comment here a little more fully on the question of self-knowledge and self-observation, and on Gilbert Ryle's views in his most remarkable book, *The Concept of Mind* [1949].

Materialists have welcomed this book as expounding their creed; and Ryle himself writes in the book that its "general trend . . . will undoubtedly, and harmlessly, be stigmatized as 'behaviourist' " (p. 327). He also explicitly declares (p. 328) "that the two-worlds story is a myth". (Presumably, the three-worlds story is even worse.)

Yet Ryle is decidedly not a materialist (in the sense of the principle of physicalism). Of course he is no dualist; but he is definitely not a physicalist or a monist. This becomes very clear from the section entitled "The Bogy of Mechanism". There he writes (p. 76): "Whenever a new science [he is alluding to mechanics] achieves its first big successes, its enthusiastic acolytes always fancy that all questions are now soluble"; and in this and the next paragraph he makes it quite clear that he does not take seriously the hope, or the fear, of a "reduction" of biological, psychological and sociological laws to what he calls "mechanical laws"; and although he does not distinguish between classical (mechanical) materialism and modern physicalism, there can be no doubt that he would reject a physicalistic monism as strongly as he rejects a mechanistic monism.

It is in this light that we have to read the following statement of Ryle's which certainly shows his humanistic tendencies: "Man need not be degraded to a machine by being denied to be a ghost in a machine . . . There has yet to be ventured the hazardous leap to the hypothesis that perhaps he is a man." (p. 328).

The question arises, what does Ryle wish to deny when he says that man is not a "ghost in a machine"? If it is his intention to deny the view of Homer according to whom the *psyche* – a shade resembling the body – survives the body, one could not object. But it was Descartes who most clearly rejected this semi-materialist view of human consciousness; and Ryle calls the myth which he rejects the "Cartesian myth".[1] This looks as if Ryle wishes to deny the existence of consciousness. From some of his arguments one might indeed think that this is his point; but this impression would be mistaken. (See p. 206: "observation entails having sensations"; or see p. 240: "sensation is now returning to my numbed leg"; or see pp. 37–8 where an excellent discussion of imagined noises can be found; and many other places.) So what does Ryle wish to deny? He certainly wishes to deny that there is a Cartesian thinking "substance"; something I also wish to deny, because I suggest that the very idea of substance is based on a mistake. However, he also wishes no doubt to deny the (Socratic and Platonic) idea of the mind as the pilot of a ship – the body; a simile which I regard as in many ways excellent and adequate; so much so that I can say of myself "I believe in the ghost in the machine".[2]

(The adequacy of the simile may be seen from the neurologist's description of "automatism" (or "*petit mal* automatism") a state of loss of the full

---

[1] The myth, as others have also remarked, is hardly to be ascribed to Descartes. It is, if anything, a popular ancient legend, rather than a philosophical and "fairly new fangled legend", as Ryle ([1950], p. 77) calls it (see section 44, below).

[2] See dialogue IV. The theory of the pilot will be discussed later; see, for example, sections 33 and 37. I may perhaps say here that while I remain opposed to "essentialism", to the raising of and to attempts to answer, "what is" questions, I nevertheless believe in something that may be called the quasi-essential (or quasi-substantial) nature of the self. The self is linked with what is usually called character or personality. It changes: it depends in part on a person's physical type, and also on his intellectual initiative and inventiveness, and on his development. Nevertheless, I think that we are psycho-physical processes rather than substances.

The point here is that the idea of an essence is indeed taken from our idea of the self (or the soul, or the mind); we experience that there is a responsible, controlling, centre of ourselves, of our persons; and we speak about essences (the essence of vanilla) or spirits (the spirit of wine) by analogy with these selves. These extensions may be rejected as anthropomorphisms. But there is no objection to being anthropomorphic in discussing man (as Hayek has reminded us).

Aristotelian essentialism strangely enough fits very well biological organisms that have an essence in the sense of a genetic programme. It also fits man-made tools whose essence is their purpose: it is the essence of a watch to measure time. (A tool is an exosomatic organ.) These comments contain no concession to essentialism – to the asking of "what is" questions – although in biology and with respect to tools it is fruitful to ask teleological " what is it for" questions.

consciousness of self, and of memory, sometimes observed in epileptic patients: the pilot has left the ship.[3])

Taking Ryle's book as a whole, there seems to be a general tendency to deny the existence of most subjective conscious experiences, and a suggestion that they should be replaced by sheer physical states – by dispositional states, by dispositions to behave. However, there are many places in Ryle's book in which it is admitted that we may genuinely *feel* these states. Thus Ryle says (p. 102) that there is a difference between a sham avowal of a feeling and a sincere avowal of a feeling. I am sure Ryle would also distinguish between the sincere avowal "I am bored" (pp. 102 f.) and the suppression of this sincere avowal out of politeness. And he not only admits (p. 105) that we may feel pain but he points out, interestingly, what many neurologists (including Descartes) have found: that we may be mistaken in locating the pain. To say I have a pain in my leg may be a mistaken "causal hypothesis", a "wrong diagnosis" even though I may feel the pain which I wrongly judge to originate in an amputated leg.

It seems, however, that there is at least one important question of fact where Ryle and I differ. It is the question of self-knowledge, and the somewhat different question of self-observation. (The questions are different, because knowledge is not always based on observation.)

Thus the section entitled "Introspection", in chapter VI of *The Concept of Mind,* seems to me open to criticism. For there exists an introspective psychology of considerable interest and capable of yielding objectively testable results. I have in mind especially the schools of psychology related to the Würzburg School; particularly Otto Selz, and his pupils Julius Bahle and Adriaan D. de Groot. I myself studied psychology under Karl Bühler who was a prominent member of the Würzburg School, and I well remember something about these matters. And although I gave up psychology because I was dissatisfied with its methods and its results, and although I am inclined to approach the psychological World 2 mainly from the point of view of its (biological) function in relating World 3 to World 1, I do not find that what Ryle writes in his section on Introspection (pp. 163 ff.) about introspective psychology resembles the real thing, even as it existed in my youth. What

[3] Wilder Penfield ([1975], p. 39) tells us: "In an attack of [epileptic] automatism the patient becomes suddenly unconscious, but, since other mechanisms in the brain continue to function, he changes into an automaton. He may . . . continue to carry out whatever purpose his mind was in the act of handing on to his automatic sensory-motor mechanism when the highest brain-mechanism went out of action. Or he follows a stereotyped, habitual pattern of behaviour. In every case, however, the automaton can make few, if any, decisions for which there has been no precedent. If Patient C was driving a car . . . he might discover later that he had driven through one or more red lights."

Ryle says is perhaps a valid if somewhat exaggerated criticism of introspective psychology before the Würzburg School, before Wolfgang Köhler and the *Gestalt* school, before David Katz and Edgar Rubin and Edgar Tranekjaer Rasmussen; before Albert Michotte or, more recently, J. J. Gibson. But it has no similarity with what these people did and still do. I can only say that reproducible and very interesting results (for example, about optical illusions) have been unearthed by partly introspective methods.

Now one of the interesting things in this connection is that Ryle seems to have tried to observe himself, but apparently he did not succeed in making any interesting self-observations. The reason may be that he did not utilize the main principle of the Würzburg School: to be presented with an interesting and absorbing task, and *afterwards* (immediately afterwards) to try to remember, and describe, the mental operations that went into the solution of the problem. (There are of course more recent methods; see for example A. D. de Groot's [1965], [1966], or R. L. Gregory [1966].) It is clear that we cannot concentrate on a problem and observe ourselves *at the same time*. But from various remarks in Ryle's book it seems that this is precisely what he tried to do. Of course he found the "I" (which he somehow linked with the "now") elusive. This is very well described by him. Had he tried to follow the Würzburg precepts, he might have got better results. Indeed, with a little training, some very interesting results can be obtained.[4] For example, Julius Bahle ([1936] and especially [1939]) discovered that a group of outstanding composers of music, Richard Strauss among them, were all adopting a method of problem finding and of problem solving which was unexpectedly similar to that described by Otto Selz [1913], [1922], [1924] in his work on purely intellectual tasks.

There are also many introspective reports on scientific discoveries. Famous is Kekulé's report of the way he arrived at the ring model of the benzene molecule. Half asleep he saw chains of carbon atoms, in the symbolic representation invented by himself, which seemed to come alive, and one of the chains coiled itself up like a snake, to form a ring. It was the end of a long search. (The introspective observation came, of course, after the event.) A very similar report is given by Otto Loewi ([1940]; see also F. Lembeck and W. Giere [1968], and dialogue VI) about his idea of how to test the hypothesis of chemical nervous transmission.

A number of interesting reports of a similar kind are contained in a

[4] It is interesting that Ryle's arguments against introspection are closely similar to those of Auguste Comte, and that John Stuart Mill's answer to Comte anticipated the Würzburg School. See A. Comte [1830–42] volume I, pp. 34–8, and J. S. Mill [1865(a)] (third edition, 1882, p. 64). See William James [1890] volume I, pp. 188 f.

famous book, *The Psychology of Invention in the Mathematical Field,* by Jacques Hadamard [1945], [1954]. In these reports, the solution is often arrived at intuitively, suddenly; but it must not be overlooked that it is usually reached only after hard and laborious work, and after repeated rejections of earlier trials and after severe criticism of unsatisfactory results.

It is clear that these critical methods, even where the final solution was intuitive, are necessary stages, and are made possible by the existence of language, and of other forms of symbolism. For as long as we carry an intuitive belief with us, without a symbolic representation, we are one with it, and cannot criticize it. But once we have formulated it, or written it down in symbolic form, we can look at it objectively, as a World 3 object, and criticize it, and learn from it, even from its rejection; see also section 34, below.

In the cases referred to, the self is very active indeed. Cases in which the self is comparatively passive, and no doubt almost completely dependent upon what the central nervous system delivers, are well known. One of the simplest cases known to me of a comparatively passive self shown by self-observation is due to Aristotle.[5] It is the experiment of softly pressing one of one's eyes, while looking at some object. The object *seems* to move with the increasing pressure, but we are so well *aware* of the causal connection that we are not deceived; and we realize the *subjective character* of the experience.

In section 18, when discussing illusions, we noted in connection with the Winson figure (the Eskimo/Red Indian picture) that we could actively try to achieve one of the two interpretations rather than the other. Cases such as these – and those in which we are conscious of having an illusion and of being unable to prevent it – illustrate the fact that we can sometimes distinguish between what is delivered to us, as it were, by the brain, and our active efforts at interpretation.

The activity of the self, or of the consciousness of self, leads us to the question of *what it does*; of *what function it performs,* and so to a biological approach to the self. This will be the topic of some of my later sections in this chapter. Before this, however, I will touch upon one of the other topics of this chapter: the relation of the self to World 3.

31. Learning to be a Self

In this section my thesis is that we – that is to say our personalities, our selves – are anchored in all the three worlds, and especially in World 3.

[5] See section 46 below, text to note 11.

It seems to me of considerable importance that we are not born as selves, but that we have to learn that we are selves; in fact we have to learn to be selves. This learning process is one in which we learn about World 1, World 2, and especially about World 3.

Much has been written (by Hume, by Kant, by Ryle, and many others) about the question whether one can observe one's self. I regard the question as badly formulated. We can – and this is important – know quite a bit about our selves; but, as I have indicated before, knowledge is not always (as so many people believe) based on observation. Both pre-scientific knowledge and scientific knowledge are largely based on action and on thought: on problem solving. Admittedly, observations do play a role, but this role is that of posing problems to us, and of helping us to try out, and weed out, our conjectures.

Moreover, our powers of observing are primarily directed to our environment. Even in the experiments with optical illusions referred to in section 18, what we observe is an environmental object, and to our surprise we find that it *seems* to have certain properties while we *know* that it does not have them. We know this in a World 3 sense of "know": we have well-tested World 3 theories which tell us, for example, that a printed picture does not change, physically, while being looked at. We can say that the background knowledge which we possess, dispositionally, plays an important role in the way in which we interpret our observational experience. It has also been shown by experiments (see Jan B. Deregowski [1973]) that some of this background knowledge is culturally acquired.

This is why, when we try to live up to the command "observe yourself!", the outcome is usually so meagre. The reason is not, in the first instance, a special elusiveness of the ego (even though there is, as we have seen, something in Ryle's [1949] contention[1] that it is almost impossible to observe oneself as one is "now"). For if you are told "observe the room you are sitting in" or "observe your body", the result is also likely to be pretty meagre.

How do we obtain self-knowledge? Not by self-observation, I suggest, but by becoming selves, and by developing theories about ourselves. Long before we attain consciousness and knowledge of ourselves, we have, normally, become aware of other persons, usually our parents. There seems to be an inborn interest in the human face: experiments by R. L. Fanz [1961][2] have

---

[1] Gilbert Ryle [1949], chapter VI, (7): The Systematic Elusiveness of the "I".

[2] R. L. Fanz [1961], p. 66. See also Charlotte Bühler, H. Hetzer and B. H. Tudor-Hart [1927] and Charlotte Bühler [1927]; these older studies obtained (with less sophisticated methods) positive results only at an age of more than one month. Fanz obtained positive results at an age of five days.

shown that even very young babies fixate a schematic representation of a face for longer periods than a similar yet "meaningless" arrangement. These and other results suggest that very young children develop an interest in and a kind of understanding of other persons. I suggest that a consciousness of self begins to develop through the medium of other persons: just as we learn to see ourselves in a mirror, so the child becomes conscious of himself by sensing his reflection in the mirror of other people's consciousness of himself. (I am very critical of psycho-analysis, but it seems to me that Freud's emphasis upon the formative influence of social experiences in early childhood was correct.) For example, I am inclined to suggest that when the child tries actively "to draw attention to himself" it is part of this learning process. It seems that children, and perhaps primitive people, live through an "animistic" or "hylozoistic" stage in which they are inclined to assume of a physical body that it is animate – that it is a person[3] – until this theory is refuted by the passivity of the thing.

To put it slightly differently, the child learns to know his environment; but persons are the most important objects within his environment; and through their interest in him – and through learning about his own body – he learns in time that he is a person himself.

This is a process whose later stages depend much upon language. But even before the child acquires a mastery of language, the child learns to be called by his name, and to be approved or disapproved of. And since approval and disapproval are largely of a cultural or World 3 character, one may even say that the very early and apparently inborn response of the child to a smile already contains the primitive pre-linguistic beginning of his anchorage in World 3.

In order to be a self, much has to be learned; especially a sense of time, with oneself extending into the past (at least into "yesterday") and into the future (at least into "tomorrow"). But this involves *theory*; at least in its rudimentary form as an expectation:[4] there is no self without theoretical orientation, both in some primitive space and some primitive time. So the self is, partly, the result of the active exploration of the environment, and of the

[3] It seems to me that Peter Strawson ([1959], p. 136) is right when he suggests that the general idea of a person must be had prior to learning the use of the word "I". (I doubt however whether this priority can be described as "logical".) He is also right, I think, when he suggests that this helps to dissolve the so-called "problem of other minds". However, it is well to remember that the early tendency to interpret all things as persons (called animism or hylozoism) needs correction, from a realistic point of view: a dualistic attitude is nearer to the truth. See William Kneale's excellent lecture *On Having a Mind* ([1962], top of p. 41), and also my discussion of Strawson's ideas in section 33.

[4] See my [1963 (a)], chapter 1, especially p. 47.

grasp of a temporal routine, based upon the cycle of day and night. (This will no doubt be different with Eskimo children.)[5]

The upshot of all this is that I do not agree with the theory of the "pure self". The philosophical term "pure" is due to Kant and suggests something like "prior to experience" or "free from (the contamination of) experience"; and so the term "pure self" suggests a theory which I think is mistaken: that the ego was there prior to experience, so that all experiences were, from the beginning, accompanied by the Cartesian and Kantian "I think" (or perhaps by "I am thinking"; at any rate by a Kantian "pure apperception"). Against this, I suggest that being a self is partly the result of inborn dispositions and partly the result of experience, especially social experience. The newborn child has many inborn ways of acting and of responding, and many inborn tendencies to develop new responses and new activities. Among these tendencies is a tendency to develop into a person conscious of himself. But in order to achieve this, much must happen. A human child growing up in social isolation will fail to attain a full consciousness of self.[6, 7]

Thus I suggest that not only perception and language have to be learned – actively – but even the task of being a person; and I further suggest that this involves not merely a close contact with the World 2 of other persons, but also a close contact with the World 3 of language and of theories such as a theory of time (or something equivalent[8]).

What would happen to a human child growing up without *active* participation in social contacts, without other people, and without language? There are some such tragic cases known.[6] As an indirect answer to our question, I

---

[5] The baby smiles; no doubt unconsciously. Yet it is a kind of (mental?) *action*: it is quasi-teleological, and it suggests that the baby operates with the psychologically *a priori* expectation of being surrounded by *persons*; persons who have the power of being friendly or hostile – friends or strangers. This, I would suggest, comes prior to the consciousness of self. I would suggest the following as a conjectural schema of development: first, the category of persons; then the distinction between persons and things; then the discovery of one's own body; the learning that it is one's own; and only then the awakening to the fact of being a self.

[6] See the case of Genie, discussed in chapter E4, and the reference there to Curtiss & others [1974].

[7] Since I wrote this section, Jeremy Shearmur has drawn my attention to the fact that Adam Smith [1759] puts forward the idea that society is a "mirror" which enables the individual to see and to "think of his own character, of the propriety or demerit of his own sentiments and conduct, of the beauty or deformity of his own mind", which suggests that if it were "possible that a human creature could grow up to manhood in some solitary place, without any communication with his own species" then he could not develop a self. (See Smith [1759] Part III, Section II; Part III, Chapter I in the sixth and later editions.) Shearmur has also suggested that there are certain similarities between my ideas here and the "social theory of the self" of Hegel, Marx and Engels, Bradley and the American pragmatist G. H. Mead.

[8] I have added the words "or something equivalent" in view of what Whorf [1956] says about time and the Hopi Indians.

will refer to a report by Eccles [1970][9] of a very important experiment comparing the experiences of an active and a non-active kitten, designed by R. Held and A. Hein [1963]; it is fully described in chapter E8.

The non-active kitten learns nothing. I think that the same must happen to a child deprived of active experience in the social world.

There is a most interesting recent report which bears on this issue. Scientists at Berkeley operated with two groups of rats, one living in an enriched environment and one living in an impoverished environment. The first were kept in a large cage, in social groups of twelve, with an assortment of playthings that were changed daily. The others were living alone in standard laboratory cages. The main result was that the animals living in the enriched environment had a heavier cerebral cortex than the impoverished ones. It appears that the brain grows through activity, through having to solve problems actively.[10] (The increment resulted from a proliferation of dendritic spines on cortical cells and of glial cells.)

32. Individuation

In his discussion of individual and personal identity – identity during change – John Locke ([1690], [1694], book II, chapter XXVII, sections 4–26) starts from biological considerations: he starts from a discussion of the identity of individual plants and animals. An oak may be said to be the same individual, from its beginning as an acorn to its death; and similarly an animal. And Locke points out that the individual identity of a man consists essentially "in nothing but a participation . . . [in] the same continued life, by constantly fleeting particles of matter" (section 6).

I think that Locke is right in his biological approach, and that in this he has done better than some of the succeeding philosophers who often tried to establish by *a priori* arguments such questions as whether every experience must belong to, or inhere in, one individual spiritual "substance". Instead of raising these questions we rather should raise the question of the individuation of living matter.

Higher animals are, clearly, individuals; that is to say, individual organ-

---

[9] J.C. Eccles [1970], pp. 66f. See also Figure E8–8.

[10] See Mark R. Rosenzweig & others [1972(a)]; P. A. Ferchmin & others [1975]; see also section 41, below.

isms (processes, open systems; see below). They may be part of a family, a herd, or of some other animal society, such as a swarm, or a state. Now these individual organisms illustrate what appears to be a very important tendency of life as we know it on earth: that it tends to be individualized. Important as this tendency is, it has exceptions: forms of life which deviate from the principle of individuation do exist. There are animals, such as earthworms, which are individuals but can be, contrary to most animals, subdivided into two or more individuals. There are animals such as sea urchins which do not have a fully centralized nervous system (see section 37) and which therefore do not act in the way we expect individuals to act. There are also the sponges which have no nervous system, and no individualized character as we know it from unicellular and most multicellular animals and even from viruses. And there are such animal colonies as the Portuguese man of war whose specialized members act like organs.

Thus although it may seem at first sight that the biological principle of individuation is founded on the fundamental structures and mechanisms of molecular biology, this is not true. For when it comes to multicellular life, deviations from the principle occur: multicellular structures and animal colonies or states exist which are not wholly centralized by one nervous system or not wholly individualized. But it seems that these evolutionary experiments, although clearly not unsuccessful, are not quite as successful as individual multicellular organisms with highly centralized nervous systems. This seems intuitively understandable, considering the mechanisms of natural selection. Individuation seems to represent one of the best ways of establishing an instinct for defence and survival; and it seems fundamental for the evolution of a self.

I suggest that we look upon the existence of human individual persons, and of human selves, or human minds, against this contingent and not even universal biological background of the principle of individuation. We may conjecture, somewhat trivially, that without biological individuation, mind and consciousness would not have emerged; not, at least, in the way we know them from our own experience.

Let us look a little more closely at the individuality of an organism. It is, clearly, not quite the same as the individuality of (say) a diamond or a piece of hard metal. These pieces of solid matter are crystals. They are systems of oscillating atoms, atoms which in the main are neither leaving nor joining the system within fairly long periods of time: they are *closed systems* – closed with respect to the material particles of which they consist (though they are open with respect to energy flow). By contrast, organisms are open systems – like flames. They exchange material particles (and also, of course, energy) with the environment: they have a metabolism. Nevertheless, they are identifiable individuals. They are, as indicated by Locke, identifiable even during growth: they are identifiable dynamic processes; or perhaps better, material systems undergoing exchange of matter. When we speak of an organism, we often forget this, because *during a sufficiently short time span an organism is approximately closed,* almost like a crystal.

Thus the changing self which yet remains itself appears to be based on the changing individual organism which yet retains its individual identity.

But we may conjecture perhaps more than this. While we do not in general ascribe *activity* or *agency* to material bodies (even if they are in motion, or attract other bodies, as the sun attracts the planets) we do ascribe something like activity to a flame, to a fire, and to a chemical process, especially if it gets beyond our control; and we ascribe activity even more decidedly to an organism, to a plant, and, more especially, to a higher animal. (Incidentally, the distinction between movement and activity was not clearly made by the Presocratic Greek philosophers who were inclined to say that the *psyche* is the cause of movement in general rather than of an active way of behaving or moving; see Aristotle, *De anima* 403b26–407b11, *etc.*)

In ascribing activity to an inanimate process, and more especially in ascribing activity to an organism, we regard the process or the organism as a centre of control and (unless it gets out of control) as self-controlling. Even an inanimate process such as a gas flame may indeed be said to be a self-controlling (homeostatic) system. Organisms certainly are; and at least some of them establish centres of control which keep them in a kind of dynamic equilibrium. In those animals to which we conjecturally ascribe a mind or consciousness, the biological function of the mind is clearly closely related to the mechanisms of control (self-control) of the individual organism.

What is usually described as the unity of the self, or the unity of conscious experience, is most likely a partial consequence of biological individuation — of the evolution of organisms with inbuilt instincts for the survival of the individual organism. It seems that consciousness, and even reason, have evolved very largely owing to their survival value for the individual organism. (See also section 37, below.)

In this section I have suggested that we should look at the problem of self-identity from the biological point of view. This shows that self-identity is, at least partly, of a surprisingly contingent character. Further aspects of this problem will be discussed in subsequent sections. In the next section I will look briefly at Peter Strawson's view of self-identity, and at the way in which self-identity depends upon the brain.

33. Self-Identity: The Self and Its Brain

Is a new born baby a self? Yes and no. It feels: it is capable of feeling pain and pleasure. But it is not yet a person in the sense of Kant's two statements:[1] "A person is a subject that is responsible for his actions", and "A person is something that is conscious, at different times, of the numerical identity of its self." Thus a baby is a body — a developing human body — *before* it becomes a person, a unity of body and mind.

Temporally, the body is there before the mind. The mind is a later achievement; and it is more valuable. Juvenal tells us to pray that we are given a sound mind in a sound body. Yet in order to save our life, we all would be prepared to have a leg cut off. And we would all, I think, refuse an operation which would prevent us from being responsible for our actions, or which would destroy the consciousness of our numerical identity at different times: an operation that would save the life of the body, but not the integrity of the mind.

It is fairly clear that the identity and integrity of the self have a physical basis. This seems to be centred in our brain. Yet we can lose considerable portions of our brain without interference with our personality. On the other hand, damage to our mental integrity seems to be always due to brain damage or some other physical disorder of the brain.

Recently it has been often suggested, especially by Strawson, that it is a mistake to assume a distinction between body and mind to start with; we should start, rather, from the integrated person. We can then distinguish various aspects or kinds of properties: those which are clearly physical, and those which are partly or wholly personal or mental. (P. F. Strawson [1959] gives examples like "weighs ten stone" for a physical property of a person, and "is smiling" or "is thinking hard" for two different personal properties. A similar suggestion — that we use "person" as fundamental — was made in 1948 or thereabouts by J. H. Woodger in a lecture he gave in one of my seminars.) Persons, it is rightly said, can be *identified*, in the same way in which we identify physical bodies. And this, it is said, solves the problem of the identity of selves. I think it a very attractive suggestion that we take the person as primary, and its analysis into body and mind as a secondary

---

[1] The first quotation is from *Die Metaphysik der Sitten* [1797], Einleitung in die Metaphysik der Sitten, 4: Vorbegriffe zur Metaphysik der Sitten *(philosophia practica universalis)* = *Kants Werke,* Akademieausgabe, Band 6, 1914, p. 223 = Cassirer edition, Band 7, p. 24. The second is from *Kritik der reinen Vernunft,* first edition [1781], p. 361, transcendentale Dialektik, zweites Buch, dritter Paralogism = *Kants Werke,* Akademieausgabe, Band 4, 1911, p. 227; Cassirer edition, Band 3, p. 643.

abstraction. Unfortunately, I shall have to raise, a little later, some objections to it.

But first I want to say several things in favour of this suggestion. It seems to me, especially, that it agrees with our mental development. As mentioned in section 31, I think that much speaks for the conjecture that the child is born with a "knowledge" of persons – an inborn attitude towards persons: it smiles at a very early age, and it is attracted by the human face and by a face-like imitative contraption or dummy.[2] In time, *things* are differentiated from *persons*. And in time, the child discovers that he is a person himself, like others. Thus I conjecture that, genetically and psychologically, the idea of a person is indeed prior to that of the self or of the mind.

I therefore do not agree with John Beloff's criticism of Peter Strawson. Beloff writes in his excellent book *The Existence of Mind* ([1962], p. 193): "All we can ever know about other persons must . . . come . . ., ultimately, from our own sense experience. If pressed to justify our belief that other persons have minds like ours we are still driven back on analogical arguments . . . [Thus] to maintain, as Strawson does, that our own personal identity somehow depends upon our recognition of the identity of others appears an unwarranted reversal of the traditional position".

Beloff is quite right to speak here of "the traditional position". Indeed, the position is all but universally accepted.[3] It is, I suggest, just one of the "dogmas of empiricism", as Quine calls them.

The young baby is actively interested in his surroundings. He shows by his behaviour a knowledge of the existence of the external world which he cannot have "inferred" from his own sense experience: he is guided by what is best described as his innate knowledge – a knowledge that partly guides him in his explorations, and that he develops and expands through his active adventures. (Compare the active kitten in Held and Hein's experiment, referred to in section 31; see chapter E8.)

In addition to the baby's innate knowledge of persons, especially his mother, there is also little doubt that the baby has to learn what belongs to his body and what does not, and that this knowledge antedates and forms the basis of his discovery of being a self. The resistance which the external world offers to his intentions and to his actions also contributes to this discovery.

I now turn to consider some objections to Strawson's and similar theories.

We learn to distinguish between bodies and minds. (This is not, as has been argued especially by Gilbert Ryle, a philosopher's invention. It is as old

---

[2] See note 2 to section 31. R. L. Fanz [1961] compares the baby's reaction with that of a young bird; see also my [1963(a)], p. 381.

[3] But see note 7 to section 31.

as the memory of mankind. See my section 45.) We learn to distinguish between parts of our body that are sensate and others (nails, hair) that are not. This is still part of what we may describe as the "naturally" developed world view. But then we learn about surgical operations: we learn that we can do without appendix, gall bladder, parts of our stomach; without limbs, without eyes; that we can do without our own kidneys, and even without our own heart. All this teaches us that our bodies are, to a surprising and even shocking extent, expendable. And this teaches us that we cannot simply identify our personal selves with our bodies.

Theories of the seat of the mind, or of consciousness, in the body are very old. Even the theory of the brain as the seat of the mind is at least 2,500 years old. It goes back to the Greek physicians and philosophers Alcmaeon (DK A 10)[4] and Hippocrates (*On the Sacred Disease*) and to Plato (*Timaeus* 44d, 73 d). The present view may be formulated sharply and somewhat shockingly by the conjecture that the flawless transplantation of a brain, were it possible, would amount to a transference of the mind, of the self. I think that physicalists and most non-physicalists would agree with this.[5]

(Objections to this close liaison of brain and mind would be raised, I suppose, from believers in parapsychology, and from those impressed by reports of people who have been possessed by departed spirits. See for example William James [1890], vol. i, pp. 397f. I do not intend to discuss parapsychology at any length here, simply because I am not competent to do so: it seems that one can easily spend twenty years on the subject without becoming competent. This is due to the fact that the results – or the alleged results – are not reproducible, nor claimed to be reproducible. To my knowledge there is only one theory of any promise available in the subject, though it is not testable so far – that due to Robert Henry Thouless and Berthold Paul Wiesner.[6])

Now if we accept the conjecture of the transplantability of the self and its brain, then we must give up Strawson's theory that the *person,* with its physical properties (of the whole human body) and its personal properties

---

[4] DK = Diels & Kranz [1951–2].

[5] Cp. Anthony Quinton [1973], p. 93.

[6] In this theory (see Thouless & Wiesner [1947]) it is suggested that there is a mind-body dualism, and that acts of will (mind acting on body) and perception (body acting on mind) are the two typical cases of interaction. Moving our limbs at will and ordinary perception are special cases in which the body and the mind involved belong to the same person. It is suggested that phenomena such as clairvoyance (or extra sensory perception) and telekinesis are more general cases of the same types of interaction. Here bodies affect minds without involving the senses, and minds affect bodies without involving muscular innervation. I will not say more about the theory here, because of our decision, announced in our Preface, not to discuss parapsychology. See also Beloff [1962], pp. 239ff.

(those with a mental component) must be taken as *logically* primitive. (We may however say that it is *psychologically* primitive.) No such simple and natural theory will do; for a person's body no longer provides the unfailing basis of his personal identity. Nor can we identify the brain with the mind, as I have tried to show at length in chapter P3. (Indeed, this would hardly do even for an identity theorist, for he would not wish to identify the brain with the mind, but rather certain processes and states of *parts* of the brain with mental processes and states of the mind.)

And if we are asked why, in the case of a successful brain transplantation, we should expect the personality or the personal character to be transplanted, and so the personal identity of the body to be changed, then we can hardly answer this question without speaking of the mind or the self; nor without speaking of its conjectured liaison with the brain. Also, we should have to say that the mind is essential to the person; and we should have to predict (it would be a prediction testable in principle) that, after the transplantation, the person will claim identity with the donor of the brain, and that he will be able to "prove" this identity (by means like those used by Odysseus to prove his identity to Penelope).

All this shows that we regard the mind and its self-identity as crucial for personal identity; for, were we to think with Aristotle that the heart is the seat of the mind, we would expect personal identity to go with the heart rather than with the brain. (If I have understood Strawson [1959] aright, this view of mine contradicts his view, and he would say that it takes us back to Cartesianism.)

Thus in *ordinary* circumstances we can regard the identity of the body as a criterion of the identity of the person, and of the self. But our thought experiment, the transplantation (which I hope will never be carried out on a human being), shows that the identity of the body is a criterion only as long as it entails the identity of the brain; and the brain plays this role in its turn only because we conjecture its liaison with the mind, because we conjecture that due to this liaison the brain is the carrier of the self-identity of the person.

This also explains why, in a case of pathological loss of memory, we should regard the identity of the body as sufficient for identifying the person. But this does not imply that we accept the identity of the body as an ultimate criterion.

The liaison between the self and its brain is conjectured to be extremely close. But there are a number of very important facts to be remembered which speak against too close and too mechanical a relationship.

Much work has been done on finding out the functions played by the various areas of the human brain. One of the results is that there are what Wilder Penfield calls *"committed areas"* of the cortex as well as large *"uncommitted areas"*. The sensory and the motor areas, for example, are committed to these functions from birth. The speech centre, for example, is not fully committed: up to five or six years, the right hemisphere cooperates with the left in controlling the function of speech. (See chapter E4.) This explains the recovery of speech when the main centre in the left hemisphere is damaged. If the child is too old when the speech centre is damaged, the loss of speech will be permanent.

The uncommittedness of large areas of the cortex is seen also in other ways. Considerable parts of the non-committed cortex may be removed without noticeable damage to any mental function. Operative removal of parts of the brain in order to treat attacks of epilepsy has even led in some cases to improved intellectual performances.

All this is not, of course, sufficient to refute the physicalist view that the physical structure of the brain, including this plasticity of its functioning, can explain everything about the mind: I have argued against physicalism in chapter P3, and I shall not continue the argument here. Yet at least some outstanding brain scientists have pointed out that the development of a new speech centre in the undamaged hemisphere reminds them of the reprogramming of a computer. The analogy between brain and computer may be admitted; and it may be pointed out that the computer is helpless without the programmer.

There seem to be some brain functions which are in a one-to-one relationship with experience; for example, a *Gestalt* switch (see section 18). But there must be many cases for which this kind of relationship cannot be empirically supported. Think of the typical fact that there are sentences which we use once, and never again. There could be a one-to-one relationship between the words and certain brain processes. But the experience of understanding the sentence is something beyond understanding the sequence of the words (as we find out whenever we have to read a difficult sentence twice in order to understand it); and since this experience may be one of those many experiences which are essentially *unique,* we should not arbitrarily assume that a brain process is one-to-one related to it (one can speak of a one-to-one relation only if there is some *universal* law or rule correlating the two processes, and this is here not assumed to exist; see also section 24 above). Of course few interactionists would doubt that there is a brain process, perhaps also unique, going on at the same time, and interacting with the experience. (Similar considerations pertain to creative experiences; in fact, we might describe the forming of any new sentence as creative – which would render most of us creative most of time.)

Another point, stressed by Eccles, is that there is not only the problem of the identity of the self (linked to that of the brain), but also the problem of the unity of the self. Our experiences are often complex, and sometimes even our attention is divided; yet each of us knows — obviously from introspective experience — that he or she is *one.* But there does not seem to be a definite part of the brain which corresponds to this one self; on the contrary, it seems that the whole brain must be in high activity to be linked with consciousness — a teaming process of unimaginable complexity.

I have called this section "The Self and Its Brain", because I intend here to suggest that the brain is owned by the self, rather than the other way round. The self is almost always active. The activity of selves is, I suggest, the only genuine activity we know. The active, psycho-physical self is the active programmer to the brain (which is the computer), it is the executant whose instrument is the brain. The mind is, as Plato said, the pilot. It is not, as David Hume and William James suggested, the sum total, or the bundle, or the stream of its experiences: this suggests passivity. It is, I suppose, a view that results from passively trying to observe oneself, instead of thinking back and reviewing one's past actions.

I suggest that these considerations show that the self is not a "pure ego" (cp. section 31 above, text following note 5); that is, a mere subject. Rather, it is incredibly rich. Like a pilot, it observes and takes action at the same time. It is acting and suffering, recalling the past and planning and programming the future; expecting and disposing. It contains, in quick succession, or all at once, wishes, plans, hopes, decisions to act, and a vivid consciousness of being an acting self, a centre of action. And it owes this selfhood largely to interaction with other persons, other selves, and with World 3.

And all this closely interacts with the tremendous "activity" going on in its brain.

34. The Biological Approach to Human Knowledge and Intelligence

By the biological approach to knowledge I mean an approach that regards knowledge, whether animal or human, as the evolutionary result of adaptation to the environment — to an external world.

We can here introduce several important distinctions.

(1) Inherited adaptations *versus* learned adaptations, acquired by the

individual organism. The latter will be, especially, adaptations to newly emerged aspects of the environment, or to the aspects of a newly chosen environment, or to aspects which are unstable. Note however that all learned adaptation has a genetic basis in the sense that the heredity of the organism (its "genome") must provide for the aptitude of acquiring new adaptations.

(2) Conscious *versus* unconscious knowledge; a distinction of importance on the human level. This raises the problem of the biological function of consciousness.

(3) Knowledge in the subjective sense (World 2 knowledge) *versus* knowledge in the objective sense (World 3 knowledge). This distinction (see my [1972(a)]) arises only on the human level.

Both inherited and acquired knowledge can be of extreme complexity. (Its informative content can be very great.) Without the background of inherited knowledge, which is almost all unconscious, and which is incorporated in our genes (or so it seems), we would not, of course, be able to acquire any new knowledge. Classical empiricist philosophy sees the human mind as a *tabula rasa,* an empty blackboard, or an empty sheet, empty until sense perception makes an entry ("there is nothing in our intellect which has not entered it through our senses"). This idea is not merely mistaken, but grotesquely mistaken: we have only to remember the ten thousand million neurons of our cerebral cortex, some of them (the cortical pyramidal cells) each with "an estimated total of ten thousand" synaptic links (Eccles [1966], p. 54). These may be said to represent the material (World 1) traces of our inherited and almost entirely unconscious knowledge, selected by evolution. Although there is really no method of comparing the two (this is so in general with the nature *versus* nurture problem) I should be intuitively inclined to say that the huge amount of information we can acquire in a lifetime through our senses is small compared with the amount of this inherited background of potentialities. At any rate, there are two great sources of our information: that which is acquired through genetic inheritance and that which is acquired throughout our life. Moreover all knowledge, whether inherited or acquired, is historically a modification of earlier knowledge; and all acquired knowledge can be traced back, step by step, to modifications of inborn or instinctive knowledge. The importance of acquired information lies almost entirely in our inborn ability to use it in connection with or in correction of our unconscious hereditary knowledge.

Of course, most of the acquired information received through our senses is also unconscious. What is, largely, consciously acquired knowledge, and what may remain conscious for a time, is the theoretical World 3 knowledge which results from theory construction and especially from the critical correction of our theories. This is a process in which World 2 and World 3 interact. (See section 13 above.) We are thus led to the conjecture that *fully conscious intelligent work largely depends upon this interaction between World 2 and World 3.*

In the discovery of new World 3 problems, and in the invention of new World 3 theories, unconscious knowledge (perhaps becoming conscious as "intuition") seems to play a highly important role. The main function of World 3 objectification is, however, to make our theories accessible to conscious fault finding: to criticism. And although what may be called our "critical acumen" may largely be unconscious knowledge, the theory to be criticized (and perhaps also our critical arguments) must be conscious, and capable of being formulated in language: we expose our World 3 conjectures to selection by *conscious* criticism.

There is an important distinction between "knowledge" in the subjective or personal sense, or in the World 2 sense, and "knowledge" in the objective or World 3 sense, in the sense of "that which is known", or the contents or results of tradition and of research. This distinction, I should perhaps emphasize, concerns facts or, if you like, things, rather than usage. My aim in making it is to draw attention to some important differences between these two sorts of "knowledge" (see my [1972(a)]).

However, some philosophers have taken me up on a point of usage; and I have been criticized by some people who deny that "knowledge" can, in ordinary English, have the meaning of what I call knowledge in the objective sense. This criticism is wrong on two counts. First, it is irrelevant to my point whether or not the distinction that I am proposing to make exists in English usage – or, indeed, in any other language. Second, I believe that the criticism is in fact wrong about usage. Admittedly, the English verb "I know" is used with a personal pronoun almost exclusively in the personal sense; but a phrase like "It is known that . . ." or "All that is known is that . . ." is often used to refer to the *contents* of some tradition or of research. Admittedly, Archbishop Whately correctly described the basic subjective usage when he wrote "Knowledge implies . . . firm belief, . . . of what is true, . . . on sufficient grounds." But the *Oxford English Dictionary*, from which this quotation supporting the World 2 sense is taken, considers *two* senses of the word "knowledge" derived from the verb "know"; the first, "the fact or condition of knowing", is my World 2 sense; but there is also a second: "The object of knowing; that which is known or made known"; and this is my World 3 sense. (I would, however, add that the main category given under this heading "The sum of what is known" seems to me not to do full justice to the objective or World 3 usage, for we can also use the term "knowledge" in speaking about single items of knowledge; say about results of current research on nerve deafness, announced in learned books and journals.)

What is important is that there is no self-contradiction whatever in describing *scientific knowledge* or, say, *historical knowledge*, as consisting largely or wholly of hypotheses or conjectures, rather than as a body of known and well-established truths (see my Autobiography [1974(b)], p. 87, and [1976(g)], p. 110). Nor does my emphasis on the objective and conjectural character of scientific knowledge in any sense amount to a denial of the significance of the personal or World 2 experiences of those who produce the scientific conjectures. On the contrary; my emphasis upon the importance of the World 3 of the objective products of the human mind may well lead to increased respect for the subjective minds who are the creators of that World 3.

A word may be said in this connection about differences in intelligence.

It seems likely that there are innate differences of intelligence. But it seems almost impossible that a matter so many-sided and complex as human inborn knowledge and intelligence (quickness of grasp, depth of understanding, creativity, clarity of exposition, *etc.*) can be measured by a one-dimensional function like the "Intelligence Quotient" (I. Q.). As Peter Medawar [1974(b)] writes:

"One doesn't have to be a physicist or even a gardener to realize that the quality of an entity as diverse and complex as soil depends upon . . . [a] large number of variables . . . [Yet] it is only in recent years that the hunt for single-value characterizations of soil properties has been virtually abandoned."[1]

The single-valued I. Q. is still far from being abandoned, even though this kind of criticism is leading, slowly and belatedly, to attempts to investigate such things as "creativity". However, the success of these attempts is very doubtful:[2] creativity is also many-sided and complex.

We must be clear that it is perfectly possible that an intellectual giant like Einstein may have a comparatively low I. Q. and that among people with an unusually high I. Q. talents of the kind that lead to creative World 3 achievements may be quite rare, just as it may happen that an otherwise highly gifted child may suffer from dyslexia. (I have myself known an I. Q. genius who was a blockhead.)

Moreover, it is quite possible that, among most normal people, inborn differences in talent are comparatively negligible; compared, that is, with the

---

[1] Peter Medawar [1974(b)], p. 179; see also his [1977].

[2] Cp. John Beloff [1973], pp. 186–97 and 207–9 and the references that he gives there.

tremendous intellectual achievement of almost all children in being able, by their active efforts, to acquire a human dialect with all its intricacies at an early age.

35. Consciousness and Perception

According to psychological sensualism or empiricism, it is the sensory input of information on which our knowledge and perhaps even our intelligence depend. This theory is in my opinion refuted by a case like that of Helen Keller whose sensory input of information — she was blind and deaf — was certainly far below normal, but whose intellectual powers developed marvellously from the moment she was offered the opportunity of acquiring a symbolic language. She even seems to have learned, to some extent, to "see" and "hear" through the eyes and ears of her teacher with whom she was in close tactile (and symbolic) contact.

Her linguistic achievements were connected for her with a strong and unforgettable experience of happiness and gratitude. These were powerful conscious experiences, but they had nothing to do with sense perception. It was not the touch of her teacher's hand that made her happy, but her sudden realization that a certain sequence of touches was a *name*: the name for water. (Another powerful conscious experience of hers came later when she was accused — wrongly — of plagiarism.)

I think it is a bad philosophical habit, established under the influence of traditional commonsense empiricism (see chapter 2 of my [1972(a)]), to take sense perceptions, and especially visual sense perceptions, as a standard example of conscious experience. (See section 24 above.) The tradition is understandable enough. I *know* that I am conscious; but *how can I establish it to myself*? The problem is solved, very simply, by just looking at some nearby object and by doing so *consciously*. It is all so easy. Indeed, it is too easy. It is liable to make me overlook that I have not only *experienced a sensation*, but that I have consciously *solved a problem*; that I was probably having visual sensations all the time (but perhaps only unconscious ones, or at any rate not fully conscious ones) until I was faced with the *problem* of how to establish to myself that I was conscious. It is the intellectual grasp of the problem and its conscious solution which has really exemplified to myself the fact of being conscious; and the conscious visual experience was only a handy means, used as part of the procedure.

However, British empiricism — Locke, Berkeley, Hume — established the tradition of taking sense perception as the main or even the only paradigm of a conscious experience, and of an experience of knowing. As a consequence, Hume could deny that he was conscious of anything like a self, over and above being conscious of perceptions or memories of perception.[1] I suggest that we should try to teach ourselves to take as examples of conscious experience such things as our admiration and pleasure due to some striking formulation ("This happy breed of men"), or our experience of helpless irritation when being faced with a great problem (How to end the armaments race? How to stop population increase?) or our effort, our trials and rejections, when reading, re-reading, interpreting and re-interpreting a difficult passage of some ancient book.

36. The Biological Function of Conscious and of Intelligent Activity

I propose that the evolution of consciousness, and of conscious intelligent effort, and later that of language and of reasoning – and of World 3 – should be considered teleologically, as we consider the evolution of bodily organs: as serving certain purposes, and as having evolved under certain selection pressures. (Compare section 25 above.)

The problem can be put as follows. Much of our purposeful behaviour (and presumably of the purposeful behaviour of animals) happens without the intervention of consciousness.[1] What, then, are the biological achievements that are helped by consciousness?

I suggest as a first reply: the solution of *problems of a non-routine kind*. Problems that can be solved by routine do not need consciousness. This may explain why intelligent speech (or still better, writing) is such a good example of a conscious achievement (of course, it has its unconscious roots). As has been often stressed, it is one of the characteristics of human language that we constantly produce new *sentences* – sentences never before formulated – and understand them. As opposed to this major achievement, we constantly make use of *words* (and, of course, of phonemes) which are used routinely, again and again, though in a most varied context. A fluent speaker produces most of these words unconsciously, without paying attention to them, except where the choice of the best word may create a problem – a new problem,

[1] See section 29, above.

[1] Thus John Beloff [1962] says somewhere: " . . . all those reflex processes on which successful vision depends: lens accommodation, pupillary contraction, binocular convergence, eye movement, etc., all take place at an unconscious level."

not solved by routine. " . . . new situations and the new responses they prompt are kept in the light of consciousness", Erwin Schrödinger ([1958], p. 7; [1967], p. 103) writes; "old and well practised ones are no longer so [kept]."[2]

A closely related idea concerning the function of consciousness is the following. Consciousness is needed to select, critically, new expectations or theories — at least on a certain level of abstraction. If any one expectation or theory is invariably successful, under certain conditions, its application will after a time turn into a matter of routine, and become unconscious. But an unexpected event will attract attention, and thus consciousness. We may be unconscious of the ticking of a clock, but "hear" that it has stopped ticking.

We cannot know, of course, how far animals are conscious. But novelty can excite their attention; or more precisely, it can excite behaviour which, because of its similarity to human behaviour, many observers will describe as "attention", and interpret as conscious.

But the role of consciousness is perhaps clearest where an aim or purpose (perhaps even an unconscious or instinctive aim or purpose) can be achieved by *alternative means*, and when two or more means are tried out, after deliberation. It is the case of making a new decision. (Of course, the classical case is Köhler's chimpanzee Sultan who fitted a bamboo stick into another, after many attempts to solve the problem of obtaining fruit out of his reach: a detour strategy in problem solving.) A similar situation is the choice of a non-routine programme, or of a new aim, such as the decision whether or not to accept an invitation to lecture, in addition to much work in hand. The acceptance letter, and the entry into the engagement calendar, are World 3 objects, anchoring our action programme; and the general principles we may have developed for accepting or rejecting such invitations are also programmes, also belonging to World 3, though perhaps on a higher hierarchical level.

---

[2] Schrödinger actually went further than this: he suggested that whenever, in any organism, a new problem arises, it will give rise to consciously attempted solutions. This theory is too strong, as was shown by Peter Medawar [1959] in a review of Schrödinger's [1958]. Medawar pointed out that the immune system is constantly faced with new problems, but it solves them unconsciously. Medawar has shown me some correspondence between Schrödinger and himself, in which Schrödinger agrees that Medawar has produced a counter-example to his thesis. See also note 1 to section 38 and text.

37. The Integrative Unity of Consciousness

From the biological point of view it is, especially in the case of the higher animals, the individual organism that is fighting for its existence; that is relaxing; that is acquiring new experiences and skills; that is suffering; and that is ultimately dying. In the case of the higher animals it is the central nervous system which "integrates" (to use Sherrington's [1906], [1947] phrase) all the activities of the individual animal (and, if I may say so, all its "passivities" which will include *some* "reflexes"). Sherrington's famous idea of "the integrative action of the nervous system" is perhaps best illustrated by the innumerable nervous actions which have to co-operate in order to keep a man standing quietly upright, at rest.

A great many of these integrative actions are automatic and unconscious. But some are not. To these belong, especially, the selection of means to certain (often unconscious) ends; that is to say, the making of decisions, the selection of programmes.

Decision making or programming is clearly a biologically important function of whatever the entity is that rules, or controls, the behaviour of animals or men. It is essentially an integrative action, in Sherrington's sense: it relates the behaviour at different instants of time to expectations; or in other words, it relates present behaviour to impending or future behaviour. And it directs *attention*, by selecting what are relevant objects, and what is to be ignored.

As a wild conjecture I suggest that it is out of four biological functions that consciousness emerges: pain, pleasure, expectation and attention. Perhaps attention emerges out of primitive experiences of pain and pleasure. But attention is, as a phenomenon, almost identical with consciousness: even pain may sometimes disappear if attention is distracted and focussed elsewhere.

The question arises: how far can we explain the individual unity of our consciousness, or our selfhood, by an appeal to the biological situation? I mean by an appeal to the fact that we are animals, animals in whom the instinct for individual survival has developed, as well as, of course, an instinct for racial survival.

Konrad Lorenz ([1976], pp. 46f.) writes of the sea-urchin that its "non-centralized nervous system . . . makes it impossible for such animals to inhibit completely one of a number of potentially possible ways of behaviour, and thus to 'decide' in favour of an alternative way. But such a decision (as shown so convincingly by Erich von Holst in the case of the earthworm) is the most fundamental and the most important achievement of a brainlike central nervous organ". In order to achieve this, the relevant situation must be signalled to the central organ in an adequate manner (that is to say, both in a realistic manner and, by suppressing the irrelevant aspects of the situation, in an idealizing manner). Thus a unified centre must inhibit some of the possible ways of behaviour and only allow one single way at a time to proceed: a way, Lorenz says, "which in the situation just existing can contribute to survival . . . The greater the number of possible ways of behaviour, the higher the achievement which is required from the central organ."

Thus (1) the individual organism – the animal – is a unit; (2) each of the various ways of behaving – the items of the behavioural repertoire – is a unit, the whole repertoire forming a set of mutually exclusive alternatives; (3) the central organ of control must act as a unit (or rather, it will be more successful if it does).

Together these three points, (1), (2), and (3), make even of the animal an active, problem solving *agent*: the animal is always actively attempting to control its environment, in either a positive sense, or, when it is "passive", in a negative sense. In the latter case it is undergoing or suffering the actions of an (often hostile) environment that is largely beyond its control. Yet even if it is merely contemplating, it is actively contemplating: it is never merely the sum of its impressions, or of its experiences. Our mind (and, I venture to suggest, even the animal mind) is never a mere "stream of consciousness", a stream of experiences. Rather, our active attention is focussed at every moment on just the relevant aspects of the situation, selected and abstracted by our perceiving apparatus, into which a selection programme is incorporated; a programme which is adjusted to our available repertoire of behavioural responses.

When discussing Hume, we considered the view that there is no self beyond the stream of our experiences; so that the self is nothing but a bundle of the experiences. This doctrine,[1] which has been so often reasserted, seems to me not only untrue but actually refuted by the experiments of Penfield's, briefly referred to in section 18 above. Penfield stimulated what he called the "interpretative cortex" of the exposed brain in his patients and thereby managed to make them re-experience most vividly some of their past experiences. Nevertheless, the patients fully retained their awareness that they were lying on the operating table in Montreal. Their consciousness of self was not affected by their perceptual experiences, but was based on their knowledge of the localization of their bodies.

The importance of this localization (of the question "Where am I?" on recovering from a fit) is that we cannot act coherently without it. It is part of

[1] See section 29, above.

our self-identity that we try to know where we are, in space and time: that we relate ourselves to our past and the immediate future, with its aims and purposes; and that we try to orientate ourselves in space.

All this is well understandable from a biological point of view. The central nervous system had from its beginning the main function of *steering* or *piloting* the moving organism. A knowledge of its location (the location of one's body image) relative to the biologically most relevant aspects of the environment is a crucial prerequisite of this piloting function of the central nervous system. Another such prerequisite is the centralized unity of the steering organ, of the decision maker who will, wherever possible, devolve some of his task upon a hierarchically lower authority, upon one of the many unconscious integrative mechanisms. To these devolved tasks belong not only executive tasks (such as keeping the body's balance) but even the acquisition of information: information is selectively filtered before it is admitted to consciousness. (See chapter E2.) An example of this is the selectivity of perception; another is the selectivity of memory.

I do not think that what I have said here or in the preceding sections clears up any mystery; but I do think that we need not regard as mysterious either the individuality, or the unity, or the uniqueness of the self, or our personal identity; at any rate not as more mysterious than the existence of consciousness, and ultimately that of life, and of individualized organisms. The emergence of full consciousness, capable of self-reflection, which seems to be linked to the human brain and to the descriptive function of language, is indeed one of the greatest of miracles. But if we look at the long evolution of individuation and of individuality, at the evolution of a central nervous system, and at the uniqueness of individuals (due partly to genetic uniqueness and partly to the uniqueness of their experience), then the fact that consciousness and intelligence and unity are linked to the biological individual organism (rather than, say, to the germ plasm) does not seem so surprising. For it is in the individual organism that the germ plasm – the genome, the programme for life – has to stand up to tests.

38. The Continuity of the Self

We may say of the self that, like any living organism, it extends through a stretch of time, roughly from birth to death. While consciousness is interrupted by periods of sleep, we take our selves to be continuous. This means that we do not necessarily identify the self with consciousness: there are unconscious "parts" of the self. The existence of such "parts" does not, however, normally disturb what we (I suggest) all know as the unity and continuity of the self.

The self, or the ego, has often been compared to an iceberg, with the unconscious self as the vast submerged part and the conscious self as the tip projecting from the water. Although there is little basis for estimating magnitudes here, it nevertheless appears that at any given moment what is selected, filtered, and admitted to full consciousness, is only a small fraction of all that which we act upon and which acts upon us. Most of what we "learn", what we acquire and integrate into our personality, our self, what we make use of in action or in contemplation, remains unconscious or subconscious. This has been confirmed by interesting psychological experiments. They show that we are always ready to learn – in some cases quite unconsciously – new skills, such as the skill of avoiding something unpleasant (an electric shock, for example[1]). It may be conjectured that such unconscious skills of avoidance play a considerable role in the process of acquiring almost any skill, including the ability to speak a language.

I think that the views of Gilbert Ryle and of D. M. Armstrong can throw much light on the unconscious self which is indeed largely dispositional, and at least partly physical. It consists of dispositions to act, and of dispositions to expect: of unconscious expectations. Our unconscious knowledge can well be described as a set of dispositions to act, or to behave, or to expect. It is very interesting that these unconscious and dispositional states may, somehow, become retrospectively conscious, if our expectation is disappointed; remember that we may hear that the clock has just stopped ticking. It may mean that a new, *unexpected problem* arises which demands our attention. This illustrates one of the functions of *consciousness.*

Our unconscious dispositions are certainly very important for our selves. Much that contributes to the unity of the self, and, more especially, to its temporal continuity, seems to be unconscious. There is a kind of memory – the ability to recall what has happened to us in the immediate past – which is, like all latent memory, unconscious, but can be recalled into consciousness. We usually "know" in considerable detail what we have done and experi-

[1] Michael Polanyi [1966], [1967] gives in the first three notes of his book ([1967], pp. 95–97) some interesting references on this subject. See especially: R. S. Lazarus & R. A. McCleary [1949], [1951]; C. W. Eriksen [1960]; R. F. Hefferline & T. B. Perera [1963]. Most of these adopt a conditioned reflex theory, as criticized here in section 40, below. The question which kinds of skills are acquired by conscious attention (see text to note 2, section 36) and which may be acquired unconsciously ought to be made the subject of a more systematic theoretical and experimental investigation.

enced a minute ago, in the sense that we know how to recall it into consciousness, *if we so wish.* It is this unconscious disposition which gives a self its continuity from moment to moment, in its normal states of wakefulness.

I have to stress here, in contradistinction to radical materialism or radical behaviourism, that these unconscious dispositions to recall, if wanted, the immediate past, are not dispositions to *behave*, not dispositions to any observable behaviour, but rather dispositions to relive an experience. This does not hold for all kinds of memory: learning a skill like walking or bicycling or playing the piano consists in the acquiring of a disposition to behave, *at will*; at the same time, many behavioural details may remain completely unconscious.

All this suggests that there are at least two kinds of unconscious dispositional states, which may or may not be the result of a learning process:

(1) Dispositions to recall to consciousness (which may or may not lead to conscious action).

(2) Dispositions to behave unconsciously.

It seems that both of these bear heavily on the self. The first kind is most important in what we may describe as the memory which produces the potential continuity of the self, or the continuity-producing memory.

The continuity-producing memory may be conjectured to be a kind of reverberation, probably reverberating nervous circuits, or something of the kind. However, it has to be understood in its biological function. It is always interpreted *theoretically*, in the light of a theory of our position in the environment, represented by a "feeling" of our body and its place in a kind of model or map. This theory too is unconsciously and dispositionally held, as a disposition to recall our relation or orientation towards objects of the environment which may be significant or problematic in connection with any of our actions or expectations.

Thus the active self is orientated and anchored in space by means of World 3 theories or models which we have a disposition to make conscious and explicit at will. Similarly, we are anchored in time by our disposition to recall our past, and by our theoretical expectations and our action programmes for the future.

Within the model of our environment, interpreted and highlighted by our action programmes, the continuity-producing memory draws, unconsciously, a spatio-temporal track of our immediate past, like the trail of an aeroplane in the sky, or like the track of a skier in the snow; a track that with the passing of time becomes somewhat indistinct.

The continuity-producing memory is to be distinguished from memory in the sense of what one has acquired by some method of *learning*. This is, essentially, theory formation or skill formation by *action and selection*, leading to unconscious dispositions to expect and to act.

I have stressed, in this section, the unconscious and dispositional character of certain aspects of the self, especially of memory. This should not be misunderstood. I regard as decisively important the conscious self, and especially its relationship to World 3, to the world of our theories about ourselves and our environment, including our expectations and our programmes for action. All this can take the form of dispositions; and these dispositions represent our "knowledge" in the subjective sense, or World 2 sense. This dispositional knowledge is part of ourselves; but it consists, at least in part, in dispositions to "grasp" World 3 objects; that is to say, "knowledge" in the objective sense.

39. Learning from Experience: The Natural Selection of Theories

The self changes. We start as children, we grow up, we grow old. Yet the continuity of the self ensures that the self remains identical, in a sense. (The sense is Kurt Lewin's [1922] "genidentity".) And it remains more truly identical than its changing body (which also remains "genidentical" in Lewin's sense). The self changes slowly due to ageing, and due to forgetting; and much faster due to learning from experience. According to the theory here defended, we learn from experience *by action and selection*. We act with certain aims or preferences, and with certain expectations or theories, especially expectations of realizing or approaching these aims: we act on the basis of action programmes. According to this view, learning by experience consists in modifying our expectations and theories and our action programmes. It is a process of modification and of selection, especially by the refutation of our expectations. Organisms can learn from experience, according to this view, only if they are active; if they have aims or preferences; and if they produce expectations. Since we can speak instead of the holding of expectations of the holding of theories or action programmes, all this can also be stated by saying that we learn by modifying our theories or our action programmes by selection, that is to say, by trial and by the elimination of error. (Of course, our aims or preferences may also change in the learning process, but as a rule such changes are rare and slow, although they are sometimes of the nature of a conversion.)

The theory of the learning process which I have sketched applies equally to adaptive learning on the level of animal behaviour (where my theory clashes with the old theory of the conditioned reflex, to be criticized in the next section), and on the level of the formation of objective knowledge, for example scientific theories. And it corresponds closely to adaptation by natural selection on the most basic level, the level of genetic adaptation.

On all three levels of adaptation (the genetic level, the behavioural level, the level of scientific theory formation) adaptive changes always start from some *given structures*: on the genetic level, the structure is the genome (the DNA structure). On the level of animal and of human behaviour, the structure consists of the genetically inherited repertoire of possible forms of behaviour and, in addition, of the rules of behaviour handed on by tradition. (On the human level, some of these belong to World 3.) On the scientific level, the structure consists of the dominant scientific theories, handed on by tradition, and of open problems. These structures or starting points are always transmitted by *instruction*: the genome is replicated *qua* template, and thus by instruction; the tradition is handed on by direct instruction, including imitation. But the new adaptive changes in the inherited structure happen on all three levels by way of natural *selection*: by way of competition, and of the elimination of unfit tentative trials. More or less accidental mutations or variations come under the selection pressure of mutual competition, or under external selection pressure which eliminates the less successful variations. Thus the conservative power is *instruction*; the evolutionary or revolutionary power is *selection.*[1]

On each of the levels, adaptation starts from a highly complex structure which may be described (somewhat metaphorically if we have the genetic level in mind) as the transmitted structure of highly complex *theories* about the environment, or as a structure of *expectations.* And adaptation (or adaptive learning) consists in a modification of this highly complex structure, by trial mutations, and by selection.

These trial mutations seem to be, on the genetic level, completely random, or blind. On the behavioural level they are not completely blind, because they are influenced by the (momentarily constant) background knowledge, which includes the internal structure of the organism, and by the (relatively constant) aim structure and preference structure of the organism. On the level of World 3 theory formation they are of the character of planned gropings into the unknown.

Adaptation on the behavioural and on the scientific level is usually *an intensely active process.* I may refer to the young animal at play, and to the

---

[1] For a more detailed analysis see my [1975(p)].

behaviour called by Pavlov ([1927], pp. 11–12) "exploratory behaviour" and "freedom behaviour". (I think that Pavlov failed to see the significance of these forms of behaviour; see also the next section.) These activities are largely genetically programmed, but they can be repressed by environmental constraints. (Recall the experiments of R. Held and A. Hein, and the experimental results of Mark R. Rosenzweig and his collaborators, referred to in section 31.) In the case of such constraints, the animal fails to learn; and its brain fails to grow, and to mature. The immensely complex new growth of glial cells and dendritic spines and of synaptic junctions, reported by Rosenzweig and others [1972(a)], depends on the activity of the subjects, and on their active contact with an enriched environment (Ferchmin and others [1975]; see also chapter E8).

On the scientific level, discoveries are revolutionary and creative, and they are also usually the result of much activity: of a new way of looking at problems, of new theories, new experimental ideas, new criticism, and new critical tests. On all three levels there is an interaction and a co-operation of conservative and revolutionary tendencies. The conservative tendencies preserve and protect an immensely complex structural achievement; and the revolutionary tendencies add new variations to these complex structures.

In none of these adaptive procedures of learning new things, or making adaptive discoveries, do we find anything like inductive procedures, or anything like discovery by induction or repetition. Repetition *does* play a role in behavioural adaptation, but it does not contribute to discoveries. Rather, it helps, after the discovery is made, to make of it an unproblematic routine and therefore to make it unconscious. (This is so with the skills mentioned before, like walking, or bicycling, or piano playing.) Repetition, or practising, is no way of acquiring new adaptations: it is a way of turning new adaptations into old ones, into unproblematic background knowledge; into unconscious dispositions.

I have written much against the myth of induction by repetition – the myth according to which we discover a regularity by deriving it from repeated observations or experiments – and I shall repeat here only one of my arguments. It is this.

All observations (and even more all experiments) are *theory impregnated*: they are interpretations in the light of theories. We observe only what our problems, our biological situation, our interests, our expectations, and our action programmes, make relevant. Just as our observational instruments are based upon theories, so are our very sense organs, without which we cannot observe. *There is no sense organ in which anticipatory theories are not genetically incorporated.* An example (compare section 24 above) is the inability of the frog to see a nearby fly that does not move: it is not recognized as possible prey. Thus our sense organs are products of adaptation – they can be said to be theories, or to incorporate theories: theories come before observation and so they cannot be the results of repeated observations.

The theory of induction by repetition has thus to be replaced by the theory of the tentative variation of theories or action programmes and their critical testing, by using them in our actions.[2]

The fact that our organs are adaptations and therefore "assume" regularities, like theories, will be used in criticizing the theory of the reflex, especially of the conditioned reflex.

40. Criticism of the Theory of Unconditioned and Conditioned Reflexes

A very different theory of adaptive learning – the reflex theory and the closely connected association theory – has been dominant from Descartes, Locke, and Hume to Jacques Loeb, Bechterev and Pavlov; to the founder of behaviourism, J. B. Watson, and his followers, and even the first edition [1906] of Sherrington's *Integrative Action of the Nervous System,* though Sherrington repudiated it in the preface of the second edition [1947].

The reflex theory is an explanatory theory of behaviour. Somewhat simplified and idealized, it can be briefly put as follows.

Animal behaviour consists of muscular responses to stimuli. The *stimulus* is in the simplest case an irritation or excitation of a sense organ; that is, of a centripetal nerve. The signal is carried by the centripetal nerve to the central nervous system (spinal cord and brain), and is there *reflected*; that is to say, it excites (possibly after having been processed in the central nervous system) a centrifugal nerve which in turn is responsible for the excitation and contraction of a muscle. This causes a physical movement of some part of the body: a *behavioural response.*

The nervous connection, from the irritated centripetal nerve to the excitation of the muscle, is the reflex arc. In the simplest conceivable case the reflex arc would consist of two neurons, the centripetal and the centrifugal, and their junction, called by Sherrington the "synapse". It is clear that in general some interneurons will intervene that belong neither to the centripetal nor to the centrifugal system but to the central nervous system.

[2] See my [1934(b)], [1959(a)], [1963(a)] and [1972(a)].

The reflex theory (Bechterev calls it "reflexology") is the thesis that in principle all behaviour is explicable as due to the co-operation of more or less complicated reflex arcs.

The reflex theory distinguishes between unconditioned or innate reflexes and conditioned or acquired reflexes. All learning, especially all adaptive learning, is explained with the help of conditioned reflexes or conditioning. The fundamental process of conditioning ("Pavlov's dog") is as follows. Let there be an unconditioned reflex like the response of saliva flow in a dog to the visual stimulus of something edible. If an auditory stimulus like the ringing of a bell is arranged to accompany the visual stimulus several times, then the new auditory stimulus alone will be able to lead to the response of saliva flow.

The new conditioned reflex (bell – saliva flow) can be "positively reinforced" by rewarding the dog with food when or after it has responded to the ringing of the bell.

There is also a method of "negative reinforcement". It consists in punishing the dog (for example by an electric shock) whenever it does not respond in the desired way. Negative reinforcement is effective especially if the conditioned response is an *avoiding response.* Example: a bell is rung just before the dog receives a shock in his right foreleg. If it lifts the paw when the bell is rung, no shock is administered. Lifting the right foreleg when the bell rings is then the new or conditioned reflex; the electric shock is the negative reinforcement.

To proceed to criticism, let us first see how the reflex theory of learning looks from the point of view here developed in the preceding section.

As seen from our point of view, neither the conditioned reflex, nor the unconditioned reflex exist.

From our point of view, Pavlov's dog, actively interested in the environment, *invents a theory* either consciously or unconsciously, and then tries it out. It invents the true and obvious theory, or expectation, that the food will arrive when the bell rings. This expectation makes its saliva flow – exactly as the expectation raised by the visual perception or the smell of food.

What is the difference between the two interpretations of Pavlov's experiment? At first sight one might perhaps be inclined to think that Pavlov's and my interpretations differ only verbally; moreover, one may feel that Pavlov's interpretation is simple, mine complicated; and that my interpretation, but not Pavlov's, is anthropomorphic.

But the two interpretations differ not only verbally. Pavlov's interpretation sees the dog as a passive mechanism, while my interpretation attributes to the dog an active (though no doubt unconscious) interest in its environment, an exploratory instinct. Pavlov indeed noticed exploratory behaviour in the dog. But he did not see that this was not a "reflex" in his sense: not a response to a stimulus, but a general attitude towards the environment, a general curiosity and activity, something like a Bergsonian *élan vital*, yet perhaps explicable in Darwinian terms, since it clearly can contribute much to the survival of the organism if it takes an active exploratory interest in the structure of its environment. As opposed to this, Pavlov has to assume that all biologically important regularities to which the organism can adapt itself consist in coincidences, like that of the bell and the arrival of the food. But the structure of our environment to which we must adapt ourselves, and dogs must adapt themselves, has no similarity with Hume's constantly conjoined impressions. Animals and men have to find their way, and have to fend for themselves, in a world of partial changes and partial invariants. A cat sitting in the grass near a mouse hole and waiting patiently does not mechanically "respond" to a "stimulus", but it carries out an action programme. Rain, hail and snow change the world radically for birds and for mammals, yet quite a few manage to adapt themselves. Rats, as we have seen, adapt themselves to an "enriched environment"; and it is important that they do so not by passive laziness but by increased activity. It is this activity that makes their brains grow: clearly a case of the exploratory drive.

I should also perhaps emphasize that from my point of view for something to be a stimulus, it must relate to the action programme of the animal concerned, and to its active relation to the environment. The fact that something is or is not a stimulus, and the kind of stimulus that it is, depends on the animal, and on its momentary state. (Compare section 24 above.)

Admittedly, the learning mechanism postulated by Pavlov is very simple. It is far simpler than any explanation of the formation of theories or of expectations could possibly be. But living organisms are not so very simple; nor are their adaptations to the environment.

I propose that organisms do not wait, passively, for repetitions of an event (or two) to impress or impose upon their memory the existence of a regularity, or of a regular connection. Rather, organisms actively try to impose guessed regularities (and, with them, similarities) upon the world.

Thus we try to discover similarities in our world; similarities in the light of the laws, the regularities, which we have ourselves tentatively invented. Without waiting for repetitions, we produce guesses, conjectures; without waiting for premises, we jump to conclusions. These may have to be discarded; or if we do not discard them in time, we may be eliminated with them.

It is this theory of actively proffered conjectures and their refutation (by a kind of natural selection) which I propose to put in the place of the theory of the conditioned reflex and of the theory that there are naturally repeatable stimuli which the organism cannot fail to recognize as being the same. (Two sparrows look to us extremely similar, but hardly to sparrows.[1])

How does the theory of World 3 affect all this? The guessed regularities through which we try to introduce an order into our world, an order to which we may adapt ourselves, and the similarities that depend on them, may perhaps be conscious. But even so, they will be dispositional in character, and for most of the time they will be part of our physiology. It is only by formulating them in language, by making them World 3 objects, that they can become objects of inspection, of consideration, and of rational criticism. As long as our conjectures are part of ourselves, there is a great likelihood that, if they are not well adapted, we shall die with them. It is one of the main biological functions of World 2 to produce theories and conscious anticipations of impending events; and it is the main biological function of World 3 to make it possible for these theories to be rejected – to let our theories die in our stead.

Let us now look at the unconditioned reflex; say the famous pupillary reflex which makes our pupils contract when the amount of light increases, and which makes them expand when the amount of light decreases.

This, it seems, is a genuine example of a reflex in the sense of the reflex theory. And it cannot be denied that it may be consistently so regarded. Yet from my point of view it is part of the genetically determined functioning of an organ – the eye – which can be understood only from the point of view that it solves, like a theory, certain problems, problems of adaptation to a changing environment. The pupillary reflex solves the problem of keeping the amount of light that reaches the retina between certain definite bounds. It thereby allows the retina to be more sensitive to light than if it were unprotected, and so to be useful even in very dim light. Our organs are problem solvers. In fact, all organisms are highly active problem solvers. That we use, sometimes, a reflex arc in order to solve our problems is not surprising. But the reflex theory according to which all behaviour is of the stimulus-response character is mistaken and should be abandoned.[2] Organisms are problem solvers and explorers of their world.

---

[1] With all this compare chapter 1 of my [1963(a)], especially pp. 46–48; see also my [1959(a)], pp. 420–422.

[2] An interesting criticism of the theory will be found in Robert Efron [1966]. (His paper criticizes mainly the meaning of the concepts of the theory, while I prefer to criticize the *truth of its assertions*.) Another excellent recent discussion is R. James [1977].

41. Kinds of Memory

As will be seen from the previous section, I am an opponent of associationist psychology, and the associationist theory of learning. I attribute comparatively little significance to repetition, especially to passive repetition (except that it may lead to some actions becoming automatic), and much significance to action, and to interpretation in the light of aims, purposes, and explanatory theories.

When I was about ten years old I discovered that I could best learn long poems by heart by trying to *reconstruct* them. I was greatly surprised by the results of this method. The method consisted in an attempt to understand the structure and the ideas of the poem, and then of trying to reconstruct it without looking at the text, noting those passages which were dubious. Only after the whole was reconstructed and the dubious passages reduced to a minimum did I look them up, once. This was as a rule enough, even though I did not, before I invented this method, memorize easily; nor was the method of reconstruction easy. The whole point was to replace mechanical repetition by construction, and thus by problem solving.

One aspect of this experience was that I felt very strongly that the method of reconstruction appealed to faculties which were totally different from those underlying the more mechanical method of repetition. It appealed to the understanding rather than to the "mechanical" memory. It was active rather than passive, and the activity was almost akin to that of solving an equation.

Ever since I have felt that there may be any number of very different structures deserving to be subsumed under the term "memory".

The oldest theory of a mechanism of memory is, I suppose, that of Descartes. It is interesting because it can be "translated" into a quite modern theory of long term memory; in the following sense: when we speak of an (electric) nerve impulse, Descartes speaks of the flow of animal spirits. When we speak of a synapse or a synaptic knob, Descartes speaks of pores through which the animal spirits can flow. When we conjecture that long term memory traces or engrams consist of sets of synaptic knobs which are enlarged owing to use, leading to an increase in synaptic efficacy, Descartes ([1649], Article XLII = Haldane & Ross [1931], volume i., p. 350) says that "these traces [engrams] are nothing but the fact that those pores of the brain through which the spirits have formerly flown . . . have in that way acquired a greater facility than the others for being once more opened by the animal spirits that move towards them . . ."

More recently this Cartesian theory has been (1) extended and (2) modified; and a considerable amount of empirical evidence ("on synaptic plasticity") in support of the modified theory has been collected. (See Eccles's chapter E8; also Eccles's [1973].)

(1) The synaptic growth theory of learning, as we may call it, has been extended by a theory that solves the following two problems: (a) What is the mechanism of the growth of the synapses? (b) What was the mechanism of the memory before the synapses had time to grow? The answer to these two questions lies in the distinction between short term memory and long term memory (see Eccles [1973]) or in an even more elaborate distinction between short term, intermediate, and long term memory, discussed in chapter E8. (See especially Fig. E8−7.) The fundamental idea is this. Any experience leads to reverberating circuits in the brain (a dynamic engram, one might say), involving a large number of synapses. These reverberating circuits constitute the short term and/or the intermediate memory. But the reverberating circuits not only explain the short term and the intermediate memory; they also explain the growth of the synapses which constitute the long term memory (the anatomic or histological engram). For the reverberating circuits make use of a certain set of synapses; and it can be shown experimentally (see Fig. E8−3) that the efficacy of synapses increases with their use; and there is also evidence that the synapses grow with use (Fig. E8−4).

(2) The main recent modifications of the synaptic growth theory of memory are these: there is not only growth of some synapses, but others are weakened or eliminated. (See Mark K. Rosenzweig and others, [1972(b)].) Moreover, there also seem to be other changes, perhaps subsidiary: chemical changes (Holger Hydén [1959], [1964]) must be involved in synaptic growth (Eccles [1966 (b)], p. 340), and there is experimental work indicating growth of glial cells.

These results are most interesting. Yet I am dissatisfied.

I am unconvinced that it is sufficient to distinguish between two or three mechanisms of memory according to the period of duration of the memory; that is to say, according to their short term, intermediate, and long term character. I believe that there must be also other mechanisms and other structures at work. I conjecture that problem solving and mere passive repetition of an experience are not likely to work in the same way, as far as their memory aspect is concerned.

This conjecture is supported by various experimental results; for example by the role of activity in the experiments with kittens of Held and Hein [1963], discussed by Eccles in chapter E8, and the results of Rosenzweig and Ferchmin mentioned in section 39.

I suggest that it is useful to list the phenomena which may be comprised under the term "memory" in its widest sense, in order to obtain a general view of the problems involved.

We could begin with pre-organic "memory", such as shown by a bar of iron with respect to the "experience" of magnetization; or of a growing crystal with respect to a "fault". However, the list of such pre-organic effects would be long, and not very enlightening.

(1) The first memory-like effect in organisms is, most likely, the retention of the programme for protein (enzyme) synthesis encoded in the gene (DNA or perhaps RNA). It shows, among other things, the occurrence of mistakes of memory (mutation), and a tendency for such mistakes to persist.

(2) The inborn nervous pathways are likely to constitute a kind of memory consisting of instincts, ways of action, and skills.

(3) In addition to this structural or anatomic engram (2), there is an additional innate memory of functional character; this includes, it seems, the innate capacity for various functions to mature (such as in learning to walk or in learning to speak).

Immunological memory may also be mentioned here.

(4) Other innate capacities for learning which are not closely linked with maturation; such as for learning how to swim, or to paint, or to teach.

(5) Memory acquired through some learning process
- (5.1) Actively acquired (a) consciously (b) unconsciously
- (5.2) Passively acquired (a) consciously (b) unconsciously

(6) Further distinctions, partly combinable with the foregoing:
- (6.1) Recallable at will
- (6.2) Not recallable at will (but, say, turning up, uncalled, as "expectancy waves")
- (6.3) Manual skills and other physical skills (swimming, skiing)
- (6.4) Linguistically formulated theories
- (6.5) Learning of speeches, vocabularies, poems.

There does not seem to be any reason to assume that the processes of acquiring these various memories are all based on the same simple mechanism such as the growth of synapses by repeated use. Moreover, the kind of memory which I have called in section 38 "the continuity-producing memory" is likely to be based on a mechanism very different from dispositional knowledge, or from the memory gained by active problem solving (or by action and selection).

(7) The continuity-producing memory. In connection with this there exist several interesting theories. It is, or so it seems to me, related to what Henri Bergson [1896], [1911] calls "pure memory" (as opposed to "habits"),

a record of all our experiences in their proper temporal order. This record, however, is not according to Bergson recorded in the brain, or in any matter: it exists as a purely spiritual entity. (The function of the brain is to act as a filter for the pure memory, to prevent it from intruding on our attention.) It is interesting to compare this theory with the experimental results obtained by Penfield and Perot [1963] by stimulating selected regions of the exposed brains of conscious patients, described by Eccles in chapter E8: Bergson might perhaps have claimed that these experiments support his theory, since they prove the existence of a perfect record of (at least some) past experiences. However, as Eccles points out, we have no such reports from non-epileptic patients; besides, Penfield was stimulating the brain, rather than preventing it from acting as a Bergsonian filter. It still seems the most likely conjecture that the continuity-producing memory is not perfectly stored; neither in the mind nor in the brain, and that Penfield's amazing discoveries show only that certain splinters of it may be perfectly stored in some people – perhaps only in epileptics. The normal memory of past situations does not, of course, have the character of immediate re-experience, but rather of a dim "I remember that" or "I remember how".

(8) As to the process of actively learning by trial and error, or by problem solving, or by action and selection, I suggest that we have to distinguish at least between the following different stages:

(8.1) The active exploration, guided by inborn and acquired "knowledge how", and by (background) "knowledge that".
(8.2) The production of a new conjecture, a new theory.
(8.3) The criticism and testing of the new conjecture or theory.
(8.4) The rejection of the conjecture, and the recording of the fact that it does not work. ("Not this way.")
(8.5) Repetition of this process (8.2) to (8.4) with modifications of the original conjecture or with new conjectures.
(8.6) The discovery that a new conjecture seems to work.
(8.7) The application of the new conjecture involving additional tests.
(8.8) The practical and standardized use of the new conjecture (its adoption).

I conjecture that only in (8.8) does the process take on, in stages, the character of a repetition.

There does not seem to be any reason to assume that any of these procedures are very similar in character or that the various underlying activities of the brain are very similar. Let us assume that all a neuron can do is to fire. (This is not true: it appears that it can grow, or wither away, or form new synapses, etc.) But the complexity of the brain is immense; and learning in the sense of theory production, and the other forms of establishing memory traces, need not happen on the level of the firing of neurons or on the level of anatomic structures, though these levels undoubtedly play a role: such learning could well consist in the hierarchical organization of structures of structures. (A non-dynamic example of such structures of structures would be a hologram, as discovered by Dennis Gabor.)

Among the reasons that speak against the purely repetitive theory of reverberating currents and synaptic growth induced by them are the following: the role played in learning by such partly emotional elements as interest or attention or the expected significance of the event cannot be neglected (see chapter E8); nor the tendency to forget certain events which are unflattering to our idea of ourselves; nor the tendency to modify these in our memory. Such things cannot be explained, I think, by a mere repetitive mechanism, but only, I feel inclined to conjecture, by the action which a discerning mind exerts upon memory contents — contents which are related to the World 3 of theories and of action programmes.

One of the major controversial problems in the theory of memory is the difference of opinion between the defenders of the classical electrophysiological (or synaptic) theory of memory storage and the defenders of a chemical theory (for example Holger Hydén; see Georges Ungar [1974] and the references cited there). The latter group has submitted evidence which seems to indicate that learned habits can be transferred from animal to animal by way of injecting certain chemicals (which are possibly related to "transmitter substances"; see Eccles [1973], chapter 3, and chapter E1).

Although I am only a layman in this field, I cannot help feeling that a theory which combines the electrophysiological with the chemical theory is the most promising one, for the following reasons. (a) An electrophysiological theory seems needed for all animals with a central nervous system. (b) A chemical theory seems the only possible one for plants (in which, it appears, a kind of "memory" exists) and lower animals without a nervous system. It appears that something approaching memory exists on this level, and if so, it would seem unlikely that this chemical "memory" completely disappears on the higher rungs of the evolutionary ladder. It seems more likely that it plays a role in combination with the action of the nervous system.

42. The Self Anchored in World 3

In most of what has been said so far I have co-ordinated the self with the living individual organism, and I have tried to glean from this biological approach some facts that explain the unity, individuality, and continuity of the self, as well as some facts that may perhaps throw some light upon the biological function of that greatest of miracles: the human consciousness of self.

But the human consciousness of self transcends, I suggest, all purely biological thought. I may put it like this: I have little doubt that animals are conscious, and especially that they feel pain and that a dog can be full of joy when his master returns. But I conjecture that only a human being capable of speech can reflect upon himself. I think that every organism has a programme. But I also think that only a human being can be conscious of parts of this programme, and revise them critically.

Most organisms, if not all, are programmed to explore their environment, taking risks in doing so. But they do not take these risks consciously. Though they have an instinct for self preservation, they are not aware of death. It is only man who may consciously face death in his search for knowledge.

A higher animal may have a character: it may have what we may call virtues or vices. A dog may be brave, affable, and loyal; or it may be vicious and treacherous. But I think that only a man can make an effort to become a better man: to master his fears, his laziness, his selfishness; to get over his lack of self control.

In all these matters it is the anchorage of the self in World 3 that makes the difference. The basis of it is human language which makes it possible for us to be not only subjects, centres of action, but also objects of our own critical thought, of our own critical judgement. This is made possible by the social character of language; by the fact that we can speak about other people, and that we can understand them when they speak about themselves.

The social character of language together with the fact that we owe our status as selves – our humanity, our rationality – to language, and thus to others, seems to me important. As selves, as human beings, we are all products of World 3 which, in its turn, is a product of countless human minds.

I have described World 3 as consisting of the products of the human mind. But human minds react, in their turn, to these products: there is a feedback. The mind of a painter, for example, or of an engineer, is greatly influenced by the very objects on which he is working. And he is also influenced by the work of others, predecessors as well as contemporaries. This influence is both conscious and unconscious. It bears upon expectations, upon preferences, upon programmes. In so far as we are the products of other minds, and of our own minds, we ourselves may be said to belong to World 3.

I have (in section 33) quoted Kant as saying: "A person is a subject that is responsible for his actions." In so far as a person is responsible or answerable for his actions to others and to himself, he may be said to be acting rationally; and he may be described as a moral agent, or as a moral self.

Of course, to call somebody a "moral agent" in this sense does not involve a positive judgement that he is a responsible or a rational person; it does not mean that he is in fact acting rightly or justly or morally: a moral agent may be acting in a morally blameable or even in a culpable way. How his actions are to be regarded from a moral point of view will depend on the intended aims of his actions; more especially on the way in which he has taken other people and their interests into consideration.

In his in many ways very important book *A Theory of Justice* [1971], John Rawls introduces the idea of a *plan of life* (taken over from Josiah Royce;see note 10 on p. 408) to characterize the purposes or aims which make of a man "a conscious, unified moral person". I suggest that this idea of a man-made World 3 plan of life may be somewhat modified: it is not the unity of one unified and perhaps unchanging plan of life which is needed to establish the unity of the self, but rather the fact that there is, behind every action taken, a plan, a set of expectations (or of theories), aims and preferences, which may develop and mature, and which at times, though infrequently, may even change radically, for example under the impact of a new theoretical insight. It is this developing plan which – following Rawls – gives unity to the person, and which largely determines our moral character. The idea is closely similar to my idea that our selves are anchored in World 3; only that I should lay much stress, in addition to the aims and preferences, on the expectations and theories of the universe (of Worlds 1, 2, and 3) which are held by a person at a certain time. It is the possession of such a (changing) plan, or set of theories and preferences, which makes us transcend ourselves – that is to say, transcend our instinctive desires and inclinations ("*Neigungen*", as Kant called them).

The most widespread aim in such a plan of life is the personal task of providing for oneself and for one's dependants. It may be described as the most democratic of aims: remove it, and you make life meaningless for many. This does not mean that there is no need for a Welfare State to help those who do not succeed in this. But even more important is that the Welfare State should not create unreasonable or insurmountable difficulties for those who try to make this most natural and democratic of tasks a major part of their aims in life.

There is much heroism in human life: actions which are rational, but undertaken for aims which clash with our fears, our instincts for safety and security.

Climbing high mountains, climbing Everest for example, always seemed to me a striking refutation of the physicalist view of man. To overcome difficulties, just for the sake of doing so; to face grave dangers, just for the sake of doing so; to go on at the point of utter exhaustion: how can these ways of fighting all our natural inclinations be explained by physicalism or behaviourism? Perhaps, in a few cases, by the ambition of achieving great distinction: some mountaineers have become famous. But there were, and there are, many mountaineers that scorn notoriety and fame: they love mountains, and they love the overcoming of difficulties for their own sake: it is part of their plan of life.

And is not something like this part of the plan of life of many great artists and scientists? Whatever the explanation – even if it is ambition – the explanation cannot be physical; or so it seems to me. Somehow the mind, the conscious self, has taken over.

If I should be asked to expose the bare bones of this chapter, I should say that there seems to me no reason to believe in an immortal soul, or in a psychical substance which can exist independently of the body. (I leave open the possibility, which I regard as far-fetched, that the results of psychical research may change my judgement on this point.) Yet it has to be recognized that the talk about a substantial self is far from being a bad metaphor; especially if we remember that "substances" are, it seems, to be replaced, or to be explained, by processes, as was foreseen by Heraclitus. We certainly experience ourselves as an "essence": the very idea of an essence seems to be derived from this experience, which explains why it is so closely akin to the idea of a spirit. Perhaps the worst of this metaphor is that it does not stress the intensely active character of the self. If one rejects essentialism, one may still describe the self as a "quasi essence", as that which seems essential to the unity and continuity of the responsible person.

What characterizes the self (as opposed to the electrochemical processes of the brain on which the self largely depends – a dependence which seems far from one-sided) is that all our experiences are closely related and integrated; not only with past experiences but also with our changing *programmes for action*, our *expectations*, and our *theories* – with our models of the physical and the cultural environment, past, present, and future, including the *problems* which they raise for our evaluations, and for our programmes for action. But all these belong, at least in part, to World 3.

This relational idea of the self is not quite sufficient because of the essentially active and integrative character of the self. Even so far as sense perception and memory is concerned, the model of "inflow" (and perhaps "output") is quite insufficient, since everything depends upon a constantly changing programme: there is active selection, and partially active digestion, and active assimilation; and all of these depend upon active evaluations.

Chapter P5 Historical Comments on the Mind-Body Problem

43. The History of Our Picture of the Universe

Human thought in general, and science in particular, are products of human history. They are, therefore, dependent on many accidents: had our history been different, our present thinking and our present science (if any) would be different also.

Arguments like these have led many people to relativistic or to sceptical conclusions. Yet these are far from inevitable. We may accept it as a fact that there are accidental (and of course irrational) elements in our thought; yet we may reject relativistic conclusions as self-defeating and as defeatist. For we may point out that we can, and sometimes do, learn from our mistakes, and that this is the way science progresses. However mistaken our starting points, they can be corrected and thus transcended; especially if we consciously seek to pin down our mistakes by criticism, as we do in the sciences. Thus scientific thought can be progressive (from a rational point of view), irrespective of its more or less accidental starting points. And we can actively help it along by criticism, and so get nearer to the truth. The scientific theories of the moment are the common product of our more or less accidental (or perhaps historically determined) prejudices, *and* of critical error elimination. Under the stimulus of criticism and of error elimination their truthlikeness tends to increase.

Perhaps I should not say "tends"; for it is not an inherent tendency of our theories or hypotheses to become more truthlike: it is rather the result of our own critical attitude, which admits a new hypothesis only if it looks like an improvement over its predecessors. What we demand of a new hypothesis before allowing it to replace an earlier one is this.

(1) It must solve the problems which its predecessor solved at least as well as did its predecessor.

(2) It should allow the deduction of predictions which do not follow from

the older theory; preferably predictions which contradict the old theory; that is to say, crucial experiments. If a new theory satisfies (1) and (2), then it represents possible progress. The progress will be actual if the crucial experiment decides in favour of the new theory.

Point (1) is a necessary demand, and a conservative demand. It prevents regression. Point (2) is optional and desirable. It is revolutionary. Not all progress in science has a revolutionary character, although every important breakthrough in science is revolutionary. The two demands together ensure the rationality of scientific progress; that is, an increase in verisimilitude.

This view of scientific progress seems to me to be strictly opposed to relativism and even to most forms of scepticism. It is a view that allows us to distinguish science from ideology, and to take science seriously without overrating or dogmatizing its often dazzling results.

Some of the results of science are not only dazzling but unfamiliar and quite unexpected. They seem to tell us that we live in a vast universe, consisting almost wholly of space empty of matter and filled by radiation. It only contains a little matter, most of it in violent agitation; also a vanishingly small amount of living matter; and a still smaller amount of living matter endowed with consciousness.

Not only are vast amounts of space empty of any living matter, according to present scientific views, but also vast periods of time. We can learn from molecular biology that the origin of life from lifeless matter must be an event of extreme improbability: even under very favourable conditions – themselves improbable – life, it seems, could originate only after innumerable and long sequences of events, each of them nearly but not wholly successful in producing life.

One cannot say that this picture of the universe, as it is painted by contemporary science, strikes us as familiar or as intuitively quite satisfactory (though it is certainly intellectually and intuitively exciting). But why should it? It may well be true, or near to the truth: we should have learned by now that the truth is often strange. Or else it might be far from the truth – we may in an unexpected way have misread the whole story, or rather, what we regard as the evidence supporting our story. Still, it is improbable[1] that there has been no increase of verisimilitude in the critical evolution of the story. There is, it appears, inanimate matter; life; and consciousness. It is our task to think about these three, and their interrelations; and especially also about the place of man in the universe, and of human knowledge.

I may mention in passing that the strangeness of the scientific picture of

[1] "Improbable" in the sense of my [1972 (a)], pp. 101–3.

the universe seems to me to refute the subjectivist (and the fideist) theory of probability, and also the subjectivist theory of induction or, more precisely, of "probable belief". For according to this theory, the familiar thing, the thing to which we are accustomed, should also be the rationally and scientifically acceptable thing; while in fact the evolution of science corrects and replaces the familiar by the unfamiliar.

According to our latest theories, these cosmological matters could hardly look more unfamiliar; a fact that shows, incidentally, how far science has moved away, under the pressure of criticism, from its beginnings in anthropomorphic myths. The physical universe bears – or so it seems – several independent and consistent traces of having originated in a violent explosion, the "first big bang". Moreover, what seem to be the best of our contemporary theories predict its ultimate collapse. These two terminal events have even been interpreted as the beginning and the end of space *and time* – though obviously when we say such things we hardly understand what we are saying.

The strangeness of scientific theory, as compared with a more naive view, was discussed by Aristotle who said, alluding to the proof of the incommensurability of the diagonal with the side of the square: "The acquisition of knowledge must establish a state of mind right opposite to that from which we originally started our search . . . For to those who have not yet grasped the reason it must seem a marvel that there should be something [that is, the diagonal of the square] that cannot be measured, not even by the smallest unit." (*Metaphysics* 983a11.) What Aristotle appears not to have seen was that the "acquisition of knowledge" may be an unending process, and that we may *continue* to be surprised by the progress of knowledge.

There could hardly be a more dramatic example of this than the story of the development of the theory of matter. From the Greek *"hulē"* which we translate by "matter" and which often means firewood in Homer, we have progressed to what I described in section 3 above as the self-transcendence of materialism. And some leading physicists have gone even further in their dissolution of the idea of matter. (Not that I am prepared to follow them in this.) Under the influence of Mach, a physicist who believed neither in matter nor in atoms, and who proposed a theory of knowledge reminiscent of Berkeley's subjective idealism, and under that of Einstein – who was a Machian when young – idealistic and even solipsistic interpretations of quantum mechanics have been put forward by some of the great pioneers of quantum mechanics, especially by Heisenberg and by Wigner. "Objective reality has evaporated", wrote Heisenberg [1958]. As Bertrand Russell ([1956], p. 145) puts it: "It has begun to seem that matter, like the Cheshire

Cat, is becoming gradually diaphanous until nothing of it is left but the grin, caused, presumably, by amusement at those who still think it is there."

My remarks on the history of thought will be very sketchy. This would be unavoidable even if telling the story were my main purpose; but it is not. My main purpose is to make the present problem situation concerning the relation of mind and body better understandable by showing how it arose out of earlier attempts to solve problems — and not only the mind-body problem. Incidentally, it should illustrate my thesis (see especially [1972(a)], chapter 4) that history ought to be written as a history of problem situations.

44. A Problem to be Solved by What Follows

One of my main aims in writing on the ancient history of the mind-body problem is to show the baselessness of the doctrine that this problem is nothing but part of a modern ideology and that it was unknown in antiquity. This doctrine has a propagandist bias. It is suggested that a man who has not been brainwashed by a dualist religion or philosophy would naturally accept materialism. It is asserted that ancient philosophy was materialist — an assertion which, though misleading, contains a grain of truth; and it is suggested that those of us who are interested in the mind, and in the mind-body problem, have been brainwashed by Descartes and his followers.

Something on these lines is suggested in the brilliant and valuable *Concept of Mind* by Gilbert Ryle [1949]; and it is even more strongly suggested in a broadcast in which Ryle [1950] speaks of "the legend of the two theatres" (p. 77) which he describes as a "fairly new-fangled legend". He also says that "For the general terms in which the scientists [the allusion is to Sherrington and Lord Adrian] have set their problems of mind and body, we philosophers have been chiefly to blame" (p. 76). For "we philosophers" one must read here "Descartes and the post-Cartesian philosophers".

Views like this are not only to be found in an outstanding philosopher (and a student of Plato and Aristotle) such as Ryle, but they are widespread. William F. R. Hardie, author of *A Study in Plato* [1936] and *Aristotle's Ethical Theory* [1968], examines in a recent article [1976] in *Mind* two books and eight articles on Aristotle, of which he says: "In most of these articles [and books] what is being said or suggested in different ways is that Aristotle, for better or worse, had no concept of consciousness or not one corresponding closely to ours." Hardie examines with great care the best of the articles, and concludes — not totally unexpectedly — that Aristotle was not a Cartesian. Yet Hardie makes it clear that, if "being 'conscious' or having a 'mind' [is] what distinguished animals from plants or what distinguished men from other animals", then Aristotle, "who gave us the terminology ('psychology', 'psychical', 'psychophysical', 'psychosomatic') which we use to mark" this distinction, cannot be said to have "neglected" the distinction. In other words, even though Aristotle may not have had a term corresponding precisely to our "consciousness" in its very wide and somewhat vague sense, he had no difficulty in speaking of the various kinds of conscious events.

Nor did Aristotle have any doubt that body and mind interact – though his theory of this interaction was different from the ingenious but inconsistent (and thus untenable) detailed elaboration which Descartes gave to interactionism.

In the brief historical sketch that constitutes this chapter I shall try to argue in favour of the following views.

(1) Dualism in the form of the story of the ghost in the machine (or, better, of the ghost in the body) is as old as any historical or archaeological evidence reaches, though it is unlikely that prior to the atomists the body was regarded as a machine.

(2) All thinkers of whom we know enough to say anything definite on their position, up to and including Descartes, were dualist interactionists.

(3) This dualism is very marked, in spite of the fact that certain tendencies inherent in human language (which originally was, apparently, appropriate only for the description of material things and their properties) seem to make us inclined to speak of minds or souls or spirits as if they were a peculiar (gas-like) kind of body.

(4) The discovery of the moral world leads to the realization of the special character of the mind. This is so in Homer (see *Iliad* 24 that recounts, as the climax of the whole poem, the visit of Priam to Achilles in which moral and humane considerations play a decisive role); in Democritus; and in Socrates.

(5) In the thought of the atomists, one finds materialism, interactionism, and also the recognition of the special moral character of the mind; but they did not, I think, draw the consequences of their own moral contrast between mind and matter.

(6) The Pythagoreans, Socrates, Plato and Aristotle tried to transcend the "materialist" way of talking about the mind: they recognized the *non-material character of the psyche* and tried to make sense of this new conception. An important speech attributed to Socrates by Plato in the *Phaedo* (see section 46 below) deals explicitly with the moral explanation of human action in terms of ends, and decisions, and contrasts this with the explanation of human behaviour in terms of physiological causes.

(7) Alternatives to interactionism arose only after Descartes. They arose because of the special difficulties of Descartes's elaborate interactionism and its clash with his theory of causation in physics.

These seven points obviously indicate a very different view from the one which seems so widespread at present. To these seven points I shall add an eighth:

(8) We know that, but we do not know *how,* mind and body interact; but this is not surprising since we have really no definite idea how physical things interact. Nor do we know how mental events interact, unless we believe in a theory of mental events and their interaction which is almost certainly false: in associationism. The theory of the association of ideas is a theory which treats mental events or processes like things (ideas, pictures) and their interaction as due to something like an attractive force. Associationism is therefore probably just one of those materialist metaphors which we almost always use when trying to speak about mental events.

45. The Prehistoric Discovery of the Self and of World 2

The history of the theories of the self or of the mind is very different from the history of the theories of matter. One gets the impression that the greatest discoveries were made in prehistoric times, and by the schools of Pythagoras and of Hippocrates. More recently, there has been much critical activity, but it has hardly led to great revolutionary ideas.

The greatest achievements of humanity lie in the past. They include the invention of language and of the use of artificial tools for making other artefacts; the use of fire as a tool; the discovery of the consciousness of self and of other selves, and the knowledge that we all have to die.

The last two of these discoveries seem to depend on the invention of language, and so perhaps may the others. Language certainly looks the oldest of these achievements, and it is the one most deeply rooted in our genetic make-up (although of course a specific language has to be acquired from tradition).

The discovery of death, and the sense of loss, of bereavement, must also be very old. From the old customs of burial, reaching back to Neanderthal man, one is led to the conjecture that these people were not only conscious of death, but that they also believed in survival. For they buried their dead with gifts – most likely gifts they thought useful for the journey to another world and to another life. Moreover, R. S. Solecki [1971] reports that he found in the Shanidar cave in northern Iraq the grave of a Neanderthal man (perhaps of several) who apparently had been buried on a bed of twigs, decorated with flowers.[1] He also reports that he found the skeletons of two old men, one of them "a very handicapped individual" the other "a rehabilitation case" (Solecki [1971], p. 268). It appears that they were not only tolerated, but helped by their family or group. It seems that the humane idea of helping the weak is very old, and that we must revise our ideas of the primitivity of Neanderthal man, supposed to have lived in the period from 60,000 to 35,000 years ago.

Much speaks, it seems, for the conjecture that the idea of surviving death entails some kind of dualism of body and mind. No doubt the dualism was not Cartesian. Everything speaks for the idea that the soul was regarded as extended: as a ghost or a spectre – as a shade with a physical shape resembling the body. This, at any rate, is the idea which we find in our oldest literary sources, especially in Homer, in sagas and in fairy tales (and also in Shakespeare).

It is, in a sense, a form of materialism, especially if we accept the Cartesian idea that matter is characterized by (three dimensional) extension. Nevertheless its dualistic character is clear: the ghostlike soul is *different* from the body, it is *less* material than the body, it is finer; more like air, like vapour, like breath.

In Homer, we have a plurality of words for the mind or the soul, and for its functions, the "processes of consciousness", as R. B. Onians [1954] calls them: feeling, perceiving, thinking, scorning, anger, and so on.

I shall refer here to only three of these words.[2] (Their use in Hesiod is similar.)

Of the foremost importance in Homer is *thymos,* the stuff of life, the vaporous breath soul, the active, energetic, feeling and thinking material related to blood.[3] It leaves us when we faint or, with our last breath, when we die. Later this term is often restricted in meaning, so as to mean courage, energy, spirit, vigour. By contrast, *psyche* in Homer (although sometimes used as a synonym of *thymos*) is hardly a principle of life, as it is in later authors (Parmenides, Empedocles, Democritus, Plato, Aristotle). It is, in Homer, rather the sad remainder which is left over when we die, the poor unintelligent shade, the ghost that survives the body: it is "not concerned in ordinary consciousness"; it is that which "persists, still without ordinary

---

[1] Samples of the soil were analysed eight years after the discovery by a French paleobotanist, a specialist in pollen analysis, Mme Arlette Leroi-Gourhan, who made this staggering discovery.

[2] For two further words *(phrēn* or *phrēnes* and *eidōlon)* see notes 5 and 8 below, and note 1 to section 47.

[3] Onians ([1954]; p. 48).

consciousness [or ordinary life] in the house of Hades, . . . the visible but impalpable semblance of the once living" body.[4] Thus when Odysseus in the eleventh book of the *Odyssey* visits the underworld, the dark and gloomy house of Hades, he finds that the shades of the dead are almost completely lifeless until he has fed them with blood, the stuff which has the power of restoring a semblance of life to the shade, the *psyche*. The scene is one of utmost sadness, of despairing pity for the state in which the dead survive. For Homer, only the living body is a fully conscious self.

The third term, *noos* (or *nous*, in the decisively important passage *Odyssey* 10, 240 to be discussed presently), is usually quite well translated into English as "mind" or "understanding". Usually it is mind with an intention, a purpose (in German *"Absicht"*; see *Odyssey* 24, 474). Onians ([1954], p. 83) characterizes it well as "purposing consciousness". It involves, as a rule, an understanding of a situation, and it sometimes means, in Homer, conscious intelligence, or even intelligent consciousness of self.

In view of the fact that it has been sometimes denied, by implication, that a (dualistic) idea of mind occurs before Descartes, which would make my ascription of this idea to Homer grossly unhistorical, I wish to refer to a passage (*Odyssey* 10, 240) which to me appears as absolutely crucial for the pre-history and the early history of the mind-body problem.

It is the story of a magical transformation of the body, a metamorphosis which leaves the mind unchanged, one of the oldest and most widespread topics of fairy tales and folklore. In this, almost the oldest extant literary document of our Western civilization, it is explicitly stated that the magical transformation of the body leaves the self-identity of the mind, of consciousness, intact.

The passage, in the tenth book of the *Odyssey*, describes how Circe smote some of the companions of Odysseus with her wand: "They had the head, and voice, and bristles, and the body (*demas*[5]) of swine; but their mind (*nous*) remained unchanged, as before. So they were penned there, weeping . . .". Clearly, they understood their frightful situation, and remained conscious of their self-identity.

[4] Op. cit., p. 94.

[5] In Homer *demas* (in later writers, from Hesiod and Pindar on, often *soma*) the body, the frame or stature of men, is often opposed to the mind, for which various terms are used, for example *phrenes;* see note 8 below, and *Iliad* 1, 113–115; cp. also *Odyssey* 5, 211–213. See further *Iliad* 24, 376–377, with the contrast of body (*demas*) and mind (*noos*); *Odyssey* 18, 219f., with the contrast of bodily size (*megethos*, here used as a synonym for *demas*, as can be seen from 251) and mind (*phrenes*); *Odyssey* 17, 454, where bodily shape (*eidos*) is contrasted with mind (*phrenes*). In *Odyssey* 4, 796, a *phantom* (*eidōlon*, similar to the Homeric *psyche*) is clad by the goddess into a body (*demas*). Cp. the opposition of phantom or mind (*eidōlon*) and body (*sōma*) in Pindar quoted in note 1 to section 46, below; and my [1974 (z_4)], pp. 409f.

This, I think, is clear enough; and we have every reason to interpret the many magical metamorphoses of classical antiquity and of other fairy tales accordingly. Thus the conscious self is not an artefact of Cartesian ideology. It is the universal experience of mankind, whatever contemporary anti-Cartesians may say.

Once this is seen, it is also seen that mind-body dualism is in evidence everywhere in Homer,[6] and of course in later Greek authors. This dualism is typical of the very ancient tendency to think in polar opposites, such as the antithesis "mortal-immortal".[7] For example, Agamemnon says of Chryseis (*Iliad* 1, 113–115): "Know you, I prefer her to Clytemnestra, my wedded wife, as she is no whit inferior to her, neither in body or its bearing, nor in her mind[8] or in its accomplishments." The opposition, or dualism, of body and mind is quite characteristic of Homer (see note 5 to the present section); and since the mind is usually conceived as material, there is no obstacle whatever to the obvious doctrine of mind-body interaction.

Concerning dualism, it should be made clear that the opposition or polarity of body and mind must not be exaggerated: "my mind" and "my body" may well occur as synonyms of "my person", although they are rarely synonyms of each other. An example may be found in Sophocles, when Oedipus says "My mind (*psyche*) bears the weight of my and your sorrows" and, at another place, "He [Creon] has been cunningly plotting against my body (*soma*)". In both cases, "my person" (or simply "I") would do as well in English, or even better; but in the Greek as well as in English we could not replace in either case the one expression (*psyche*) by the other (*soma*).[9] That we cannot always do this holds for Homer or for Sophocles as well as for ourselves.

Concerning what I have just said about interactionism — the interaction of a material soul with a material body — I do not wish to imply that the interaction was conceived in a mechanistic way. Consistent mechanistic

---

[6] Interesting Homeric passages from the *Iliad* indicating dualism (of course, a materialistic dualism) are, for example, the golden girl robots (see note 1 to section 2 above) who are clearly described as *conscious* robots: they have understanding or mind (*nous*) in their hearts (cp. *Iliad* 18, 419). See also *Iliad* 19, 302; 19, 339; and 24, 167; passages in which overt speech is contrasted with concealed thought; and also 24, 674, where Priam and the herald are going to sleep in the forecourt of Achilles's hut, "their minds heavy with cares". (E. V. Rieu, in the Penguin Classics edition, translates very freely but very well "with much to occupy their busy minds".)

[7] Cf. G. E. R. Lloyd [1966].

[8] Here the term *phrenes* (according to Onians originally in Homer the lungs and the heart) is used for "mind"; see Onians ([1954] chapter 2).

[9] See Sophocles, *King Oedipus,* lines 64 and 643; cp. E. R. Dodds [1951], p. 159, note 17.

thinking becomes prominent only very much later, with the atomists, Leucippus and Democritus, although there were of course plenty of skilled users of mechanics before. There was much that was not well understood, neither in mechanical nor in other terms, in Homeric times and for a long time after, and that was interpreted in a crudely "animistic" way, such as the thunderbolt of Zeus. Causation *was* a problem, and animistic causation was something bordering the divine. And there was divine action on both bodies and minds. Infatuation, such as Helen's, and blind anger and pigheadedness, such as Agamemnon's, were attributed to the gods. It was "an abnormal state which [demanded] a supernormal explanation", as E. R. Dodds ([1951], p. 9) puts it.

There is an abundance of important evidence that supports the hypothesis that dualistic and interactionist beliefs concerning body and mind are very old – prehistoric and of course historic. Apart from folklore and fairy tales, it is supported by all we know about primitive religion, myth, and magical beliefs. There is, for example, shamanism, with its characteristic doctrine that the soul of the shaman may leave the body and may go on a journey; in the case of the Eskimos, even to the moon. The body is meanwhile left in a state of deep sleep or coma, and survives without food. "In that condition he is not thought, like the Pythia or like a modern medium to be possessed by an alien spirit; but his own soul is thought to leave its body . . ." (Dodds [1951], p. 140). Dodds gives a long list of prehistoric and historic Greek shamans;[10] of the prehistoric ones, only legends are left, but they are sufficient evidence for dualism. The story of the Seven Sleepers of Ephesus probably belongs to this tradition, also perhaps the theory of metempsychosis or reincarnation. (Among the shamans of historical times, Dodds counts Pythagoras and Empedocles.)

Interesting from our point of view is the distinction, due to the social anthropologist E. E. Evans-Pritchard [1937], between witches (male or female) and sorcerers. His analysis of the ideas of the Azande led him to distinguish witches from sorcerers according to whether or not conscious intention plays a part. According to Zande views, witches have inherited special innate supernatural powers to harm others, but they are completely unconscious of their dangerous potentialities. (An evil eye may be an example of such a potentiality.) By contrast, sorcerers have acquired the techniques of handling substances and charms by which they can intentionally harm others. This distinction appears to be applicable to numerous, though not all,

---

[10] See also K. Meuli [1935].

primitive African cultures.[11] The applicability shows the existence of a widespread primitive distinction between conscious intentional actions and unconscious and unintended effects.

Myths and religious beliefs are attempts to explain to ourselves theoretically the world we live in – including of course the social world – and how this world affects us and our ways of living. It seems clear that the old distinction between soul and body is an example of such a theoretical explanation. But what it explains is the experience of consciousness – of intelligence, of will, of planning and of carrying out our plans; of using our hands and feet as tools; and of using artificial, material tools, and of being affected by them. These experiences are not philosophical ideologies. The doctrine of a substantial (or even a material) soul to which they lead us may well be a myth; indeed, I conjecture that the substance theory as such is a myth. But if it is a myth, it may be understood as the result of grasping the reality and effectiveness of consciousness and of our will; and grasping its reality leads us first to conceive of the soul as material, as the finest matter, and later to conceive of it as a non-material "substance".

I may perhaps finally summarize the major discoveries in this field which, it appears, were made by primitive man and prehistoric man (and partly by Neanderthal man who is generally classified as prior and distinct from our own species, and more recently conjectured to have mixed his blood with *homo sapiens*).

Death and its inevitability are discovered; the theory is accepted that the states of sleep and of unconsciousness are related to death and that it is consciousness or spirit or mind (*thymos*) which "leaves" us at death. The doctrine of the reality and therefore the materiality and substantiality of consciousness – of the soul (or mind) – is developed, and further, the doctrine of the complexity of the soul or mind: desire, fear, anger, intellect, reason or insight (*nous*) are distinguished. Dream-experience and states of divine inspiration and possession and other abnormal states are recognized, also involuntary and unconscious mental states (such as those of "witches"). The soul is regarded as the "mover" of the living body, or as the principle of life. Also, the problem of our lack of responsibility for unintentional acts or acts committed in abnormal states (of frenzy) is grasped. The problem of the position of the soul in the body is raised, and usually answered by the theory that it pervades the body, yet is centred in the heart and the lungs. (See Dodds [1951], chapter 1, p. 3, on Agamemnon's apology (*Iliad* 19, 86ff.); and compare Sophocles, *Oedipus at Colonus,* 960ff.).

---

[11] S.F. Nadel [1952].

Some of these doctrines are no doubt hypostatizations, and they have been, or may have to be, modified by criticism. Others are mistaken. Yet they are nearer to modern views and modern problems than the pre-Ionian and even the Ionian theories of matter,[12] though admittedly this may be due to the primitive character of our modern views about consciousness.

46. The Mind-Body Problem in Greek Philosophy

It is sometimes asserted that the Greeks were aware of a soul-body problem, but not of a mind-body problem. This assertion seems to me either mistaken or a verbal quibble. In Greek philosophy, the soul played a role very similar to that of the mind in post-Cartesian philosophy. It was an entity, a substance, which sums up the conscious experience of the self. (It may be said to be a hypostatization – almost unavoidable and possibly justified – of conscious experience.) Moreover, we find as early as in fifth century Pythagoreanism a doctrine of the incorporeality of the soul; and several concepts (for example *nous* and *psyche*) in several authors sometimes correspond very closely to the modern concept of mind. (Remember also that the English concept "mind" has often to be translated into German as *"Seele"*, which is also the translation of "soul"; a symptom of the fact that "mind" and "soul" are not so different as the assertion at the beginning of this section indicates.) Although the use of certain terms may often be indicative of the theories held, and of the views taken for granted, this is not always so: theories which are closely similar or even identical are sometimes formulated in very different terminologies. Indeed, some of the main changes after Homer regarding mind and body are terminological; and they do not run parallel with changes in theory.[1]

In what follows, I will briefly sketch the history (I) of the material soul

---

[12] See my [1963(a)], chapter 5.

[1] For Homer *psyche* (or *eidōlon*) meant phantom or shade; later *psyche* assumes a meaning near to Homer's *thymos*: the active conscious self, the living and breathing self. In this way, the *psyche* or the *eidōlon* becomes the principle of life, while in Homer (and later sometimes in Pindar) it seems to have been asleep when the person was alive and awake, and awake when the person was asleep or unconscious or dead. (Not that these rules of usage were ever quite consistently adhered to by any author.) Thus we read in Pindar (Fragment 116 Bowra = 131 Sandys (Loeb)): "The body of every man follows the call of mighty death; yet there is left alive a phantom or image (*eidolon*) from his time of life, which alone stems from the gods. It sleeps while his limbs are active; but while he sleeps it often announces in dreams their [the gods] decision of coming joy or sorrow." We see that Homer's phantom *psyche*, which was a projection of all the terrors of extreme old age far beyond the grave, has lost some of its ghastly and ghostlike character, although there are some traces left of the Homeric usage.

from Anaximenes to Democritus and Epicurus (including that of the location of the mind); (II) of the dematerialization or spiritualization of the mind, from the Pythagoreans and Xenophanes to Plato and Aristotle; (III) of the moral conception of the soul or mind, from Pythagoras to Democritus, Socrates, and Plato.

I

In Homer the material soul of the living body was a vaporous breath. (It is not quite clear how this breath-soul was related to intelligence or understanding or mind.) In the Ionian philosophic tradition from Anaximenes down to Diogenes of Appolonia it remains very nearly the same: the soul consists of air. (Aristotle tells us that "the poems known as Orphic say that the soul, borne by the winds, enters from the all into the animals when they breathe".[2])

As Guthrie ([1962], p. 355) points out, *"psyche"* meant for a Greek thinker of the fifth century B. C. "not only *a* soul but soul; that is, the world was permeated by a kind of soul-stuff which is better indicated by the omission of the article". This certainly is true of the materialist thinkers of the time: they regarded soul as air (and the soul as a portion of air) because air is the finest and lightest of the known forms of matter.

As Anaxagoras, who perhaps no longer believed in a material mind, puts it (DK 59 B12), "Mind (*nous*) . . . is the most rarefied of things and the purest; it has all the knowledge with respect to everything, and it has the greatest power. And all that has life (*psyche*), the biggest [organisms] and the smallest, all these mind rules." Whether or not Anaxagoras believed in a material mind, he certainly distinguished sharply between mind and all other existing (material) substances. For Anaxagoras, mind is the principle of motion and order, and therefore the principle of life.

Even before Anaxagoras a more exciting though still a materialist interpretation of the doctrine of soul – of the soul stuff – was given by Heraclitus, the thinker who of all materialists was perhaps furthest removed from mechanical materialism, for he interpreted all material substances and especially the soul as material *processes.* The soul was *fire.* That we are flames, that our selves are processes, was a marvellous and a revolutionary idea. It was part of Heraclitus's cosmology: all material things were in flux: they were all processes, including the whole universe. And all were ruled by law (*logos*). "The limits of the soul you will not discover, not even if you travel every road: so deep is its *logos.*" (DK B45.) The soul, like fire, is killed by water: "It is death for souls to become water" (DK B36). Fire is for

---

[2] DK 1 B 11 = *De anima* 410b28. (DK = Diels & Kranz [1951–2].)

Heraclitus the best and the most powerful and the purest (and no doubt also the finest) of material processes.

All these materialist theories were dualist in so far as they gave the soul a very special and exceptional status within the universe.

The schools of medical thinkers were also certainly materialist *and* dualist in the sense here described. Alcmaeon of Croton, who is usually regarded as Pythagorean, seems to have been the first Greek thinker to locate sensation and thought (which he seems to have sharply distinguished) in the brain. Theophrastus reports "that he spoke of passages (*poroi*) leading from sense organs to the brain" (Guthrie [1962], p. 349; DK A5, p. 212, l. 8). He thereby created a tradition to which the school of Hippocrates adhered, and Plato; but not Aristotle who, adhering to an older tradition, regarded the heart as the common sensorium, and thus as the seat of consciousness.

The Hippocratic medical treatise *On the Sacred Disease* is of the greatest interest. Not only does it assert with great emphasis that the brain "tells the limbs how to act", but also that the brain "is the messenger to consciousness (*sunesis*) and tells it what is happening". The brain is also described as the interpreter (*hermeneuos*) of consciousness. Of course, the word "*sunesis*", here translated by "consciousness", can also be translated as "intelligence" or "sagacity" or "understanding". Yet the meaning is clear – and so is the fact that the author of the treatise discussed at length what we should call the mind-body problem, and mind-body interaction. (See especially chapters XIX and XX.) He explains the influence of the brain by the fact that "it is the air that gives it intelligence" (chapter XIX); thus the air is interpreted as soul, as with the Ionic philosophers. The explanation is that "when a man draws breath into himself, the air first reaches the brain". (It may be worth mentioning that Aristotle, who was greatly influenced by the medical tradition yet gave up the connection between air and soul, retained the connection between air and the brain, and regarded the brain as a mechanism for cooling by means of air – as a kind of air-cooled radiator.)

The greatest and most consistent of the materialist thinkers was Democritus. He explained all natural and psychological processes mechanically, by the movement and the collision of atoms and by their joining or separating, their composition or dissociation.

In a brilliant essay "Ethics and Physics in Democritus", first published in 1945–46, Gregory Vlastos [1975] discusses in considerable detail the mind-body problem in Democritus's philosophy. He points out that Democritus, himself a writer of medical treatises, was arguing against the professional tendency to make "the body the key to the well-being of both body and soul". He points out that a famous fragment of Democritus' (DK B187) should be interpreted in this sense. The fragment says: "It is fitting for men that they should make a *logos* [= law, or theory] more about the soul than about the body. For the perfection of the soul puts right the faults of the body. But bodily strength without reasoning does not improve the soul."

Vlastos points out that "the first axiom of this *logos* of the soul" is the principle of responsibility: the soul, not the body, is the responsible agent. This follows from the principle of physics "that the soul moves the body".

In Democritean atomic physics, soul consists of the smallest atoms. They are (according to Aristotle *De anima* 403b31) the same atoms as those of fire. (Clearly, Democritus was influenced by Heraclitus.) They are round and "best able to slip through anything and to move other things by their own movement".

The small soul atoms are distributed throughout the body in such a way that atoms of soul and body alternate (see Lucretius *De rerum natura* III, 371–73). More precisely, "the soul has two parts; the one, which is rational (*logicos*) is located in the heart, while the unreasoning part is dispersed throughout the whole body" (DK A105). This is no doubt an attempt to solve certain aspects of the mind-body problem.

Like Socrates who taught (cp. the *Apology*) "Care for your souls", so did the mechanical materialist Democritus: "Men don't get happiness from bodies or from money, but by acting right and thinking wide." (DK B40.) Another ethical fragment is "Who chooses the goods of the soul, chooses the more divine; who chooses those of the body chooses the more human." (DK B37; cp. Vlastos [1975], pp. 382f.) Like Socrates, his contemporary, he teaches: "He who commits an act of injustice is more unhappy than he who suffers it". (DK B45.)

One can describe Democritus not only as a materialist but as a monistic atomist. But owing to his moral teaching he was also a kind of dualist. For although he plays a major part in the history of the materialist theory of the soul, he also plays an important part in the history of the moral conception of the soul and its contrast with the body, to be treated below under (III). Here I will only briefly mention Democritus's, Epicurus's and Lucretius's theory of dreams (*De rerum natura* IV), from which we see that the materialist theory of the soul did not neglect conscious experience: dreams are not given by the gods but consist of memories of our own perceptions.

II

We have just seen that the Homeric idea of the soul as breath – as air, or as fire: as a very fine corporeal substance – survived for a long time. So Aristotle was not quite correct when he said of his predecessors (*De anima*

405b11): "Almost all of them characterize the soul by three of its attributes: [the power of] movement; sensation; and incorporeality." The last term should be weakened to "comparative incorporeality" to make this quite correct; for some of his predecessors thought that the soul was a fine body.

However, Aristotle's slip is excusable. Even the materialists, I suggest, were dualists who habitually contrasted the soul with the body. I suggest that they all saw in the soul or in the mind the *essence* of the body.

There are, obviously, two ideas of essence: a corporeal essence and an incorporeal one. The materialists, down to and beyond Democritus, regarded the soul or spirit of man as analogous to the spirit of wine – or the spirit of wine as analogous to the soul. (See note 2 to section 30 above.) Thus we come to a (material) soul substance like air. But another idea, due I suspect to Pythagoras, or to the Pythagorean Philolaus, was that the essence of a thing is something abstract (like number or the ratio of numbers).

Perhaps transitory, or already within the tradition of incorporeality, is Xenophane's monotheism. Xenophanes, who brought the Ionian tradition to Italy, emphasizes that the mind or the thought of God is the divine essence; though his God is not conceived in the likeness of man (DK B23–26):

> One god, alone among gods and alone among men, is the greatest,
> Neither in body does he nor in mind resemble the mortals.
> Always in one place he abides: he never is moving;
> Nor is it fitting for him to change now hereto, now thereto.
> Effortless he moves the world by thought and intention.
> All of him is sight; all is knowing; and all is hearing.[3]

Mind is here identified with perception, with thought, with the power of will, and with the power of acting.

In the Pythagorean theory of immaterial hidden essences, numbers, and relations between numbers such as "ratios" or "harmonies", take the place of the substantial "principles" of Ionian philosophy: the water of Thales, the unlimited of Anaximander, the air of Anaximenes, the fire of Heraclitus. This is a very striking change, and it is best explained by the assumption that it was Pythagoras himself who discovered the numerical ratios which underlie the concordant musical intervals:[4] on the monochord, an instrument of one string which can be stopped with the help of a moveable bridge, one can show that the octave corresponds to the ratio of 1 : 2, the fifth to the ratio of 2 : 3, and the fourth to the ratio of 3 : 4 of the length of the string.

---

[3] Cp. Epicharmus, DK B12: "Only mind sees, only mind hears: all else is deaf and blind."

[4] Plato's *Republic* 530c–531c may be taken as evidence that the discovery was made by some Pythagorean. For the discovery and its ascription to Pythagoras himself see Guthrie ([1962], pp. 221 ff.). See also Diogenes Laertius viii, 12.

Thus the hidden essence of melodic or harmonic concords is the ratio of certain simple numbers 1:2:3:4 – even though a concord or harmony as experienced is clearly not a quantitative but a qualitative affair. This was a surprising discovery. But it must have been even more impressive when Pythagoras discovered that a right angle (clearly another qualitative affair) was connected with the ratios 3:4:5. Any triangle with sides of these ratios was rectangular.[5] If, as it seems, it was Pythagoras himself who made this discovery, then the report is likely to be true that "Pythagoras spent most of his time upon the arithmetical aspects of geometry" (Diogenes Laertius viii, 11f.).

These reports explain the background of the Pythagorean theory that the hidden essences of all things are abstract. They are numbers; numerical ratios of numbers; and "harmonies". Guthrie ([1962], p. 301) puts it as follows: "To the Pythagoreans *everything* was an embodiment of number. They included what we should call abstractions like justice, mixture, opportunity . . .". It is perhaps interesting that Guthrie writes here "embodiment". Indeed, we feel still that the relation of the essence to that of which it is the essence is like the relation of the soul or the mind to the body.

Guthrie has suggested ([1962]; see also the brilliant article by Charles H. Kahn [1974]) that there were in fact two theories of the soul which went under the name "Pythagorean". The first, the original theory, probably due to Pythagoras himself, or perhaps to Philolaus the Pythagorean, was that the immortal soul of man was a harmony or attunement of abstract numbers. These numbers and their harmonious relations precede and survive the body. The second theory, put by Plato in the mouth of Simmias, a pupil of Philolaus, was that the soul is a harmony or attunement of the body, like the harmony or attunement of a lyre (it should be noted that the lyre is not just a World 1 object but also a World 3 object; and so is its proper attunement or harmony). It must perish with the body, as the harmony of the lyre must perish with the lyre. The second theory became popular, and was extensively discussed by Plato and Aristotle.[6] Its popularity was clearly due to the fact that it offered an easily grasped model of mind-body interaction.

We have here two related but subtly different theories; two theories which may be interpreted as describing "two kinds of soul" (Guthrie [1962], p. 317), an immortal and higher kind of soul, and a perishable and lower kind

---

[5] For the generalization of this problem see chapter 2, section IV, of my [1963(a)].

[6] See Plato, *Phaedo* 85e ff., especially 88c-d; Aristotle, *De anima* 407b27 ". . . many regard it as the most credible of all . . . theories"; and p. 21 of volume XII (*Select Fragments)* of the Oxford edition of *The Works of Aristotle* edited and translated by Sir David Ross, 1952, where Themistius describes the theory as very popular.

of soul; both are harmonies. There is historical evidence for the existence of both theories, of Pythagoras's theory and of Simmias's theory. But to my knowledge, they have not been clearly distinguished before Guthrie's searching and brillant discussion of Pythagoras and the Pythagoreans.

The question should be raised of how the theory which we may with Guthrie describe as Pythagoras's theory (in contradistinction to Simmias's theory) envisages the relation of soul (harmony, ratio of numbers) to body.[7] We may conjecture that the answer to this question could have been similar to a theory — a Pythagorean theory — that can be found in Plato's *Timaeus*. There the formed or shaped body is the result of a pre-existing form that impresses itself on unformed or indefinite space (corresponding to Aristotle's first matter).[8] This form would be of the nature of a number (or a numerical ratio, or of a triangle). From this we might conclude that the organized body would be organized by a pre-existing harmony of numbers which therefore could also outlast the body.

The philosophers who followed the Pythagoreans (including "Simmias") in proposing a theory of the soul and/or of the mind which interpreted them as incorporeal essences were (possibly) Socrates and (certainly) Plato and Aristotle. They were later followed by the Neo-Platonists, by St. Augustine and other Christian thinkers, and by Descartes.

Plato proposed, at different times, somewhat different theories of the mind, but they were always related to his theory of forms or ideas in a way similar to that in which Pythagoras's theory of the mind was related to his theory of numbers or ratios. The Pythagorean theory of numbers and their ratios can be interpreted as a theory of the true nature or essence of things in general, and so can Plato's theory of forms or ideas. And while, for Pythagoras, the soul is a ratio of numbers, for Plato, the soul, though it is not a form or idea, is "akin" to the forms or ideas. The kinship is very close: the soul is, very nearly, the essence of the living body. Aristotle's theory is again similar. He describes the soul as the "first entelechy" of the living body; and the first entelechy is, more or less, its form or its essence. The main difference between Plato's and Aristotle's theory of the soul is, I think, that Aristotle is a cosmological optimist, but Plato rather a pessimist. Aristotle's world is essentially teleological: everything progresses towards perfection. Plato's world is created by God, and it is, when created, the best world: it does not

---

[7] I owe this question to Jeremy Shearmur, who also suggested that the relation might be like that of the Platonic ideas to matter.

[8] See my [1963(a)], chapter 3, page 26 and note 15.

progress towards something better. Similarly, Plato's soul is not progressive; if anything it is conservative. But Aristotle's entelechy is progressive: it strives towards an end, an aim.

It seems to me probable that this teleological theory – the striving of the soul towards an end, the good – goes back to Socrates who taught that acting for the best purpose, and with the best aim, follows with necessity upon knowing what is best, and that the mind, or the soul, was always trying to act so as to bring about what is best. (See also Socrates's autobiographical remarks in the *Phaedo,* 96aff., especially 97d which I am inclined, following Guthrie [1969] vol. iii, pp. 421ff., to regard as historical.[9])

Plato's doctrine of the world of essences – his theory of forms or ideas – is the first doctrine of what I call World 3. But (as I have explained in section 13, above) there are considerable differences between my theory of World 3, the world of products of the human mind, and Plato's theory of forms. However, Plato was one of the first (together, perhaps, with Protagoras and Democritus) to appreciate the importance of ideas – of "culture", to use a modern term – for the forming of our minds.

As to the mind-body problem, Plato regards this problem mainly from an ethical point of view. Like the Orphic-Pythagorean tradition, he regards the body as a prison of the soul (it is perhaps not quite clear how we can escape from it through transmigration). But according to Socrates and Plato the soul, or mind, or reason *ought* to be the ruler of the body (and of the lower parts of the soul: the appetites, which are akin to the body, and liable to be ruled by it). Plato often points out parallelisms between mind and body, but he accepts an interactionism of mind and body as a matter of course: like Freud he upholds the theory that the mind has three parts: (1) reason; (2) activity or energy or liveliness (*thymos,* often translated by spirit, or by courage); and (3) the (lower) appetites. Like Freud he assumes a kind of class struggle between the lower and the higher parts of the soul. In dreams, the lower parts may get out of control; for example, our appetites may make a man dream (*Republic,* beginning of book ix, 571dff.) of marrying his mother,

---

[9] Reading Guthrie ([1969], vol. iii), whose book contains the best presentation of Socrates known to me, has convinced me that Socrates's autobiographical remarks in Plato's *Phaedo,* 96aff., are likely to be historical. I first accepted Guthrie's criticism (p. 423, n. 1) of my *Open Society* (vol. i, p. 308) without re-reading what I had written. In preparing the present passage I looked up my *Open Society* vol. i, again, and I found that I did not, on p. 308, argue against the historicity of the autobiographical passage (*Phaedo* 96aff.), but against the historicity of the *Phaedo* in general, and of *Phaedo* 108dff. in particular, with its somewhat authoritative and dogmatic exposition of the nature of the cosmos, especially of the earth. This exposition still seems to me incompatible with the *Apology*.

or of "any foul deed of blood" (such as parricide, James Adam adds). It is clearly implied that such dreams arise from the action of our bodies on "the beastly and savage part" of the soul; and that it is the task of reason to tame these parts, thereby ruling the body. The interaction between mind and body is due to forces which Plato regards here, and in some other places, as similar to *political* forces rather than to *mechanical* forces: certainly an interesting contribution to the mind-body problem. He also describes the mind as the pilot of the body.

Aristotle too has a theory of lower (irrational) and higher (rational) parts of the soul; but his theory is biologically rather than politically or ethically inspired. (But he says, in the *Nicomachean Ethics* 1102b6ff., probably alluding to the dream passage in Plato, that "the dreams of good men are better than those of ordinary people".)

Aristotle's ideas anticipate, in several respects, biological evolution. He distinguishes the nutritive soul (found in all organisms including plants) from the sensory soul and the soul which is the source of motion (only found in animals) and the rational soul (*nous*), which is to be found only in man, and which is immortal. He frequently stresses that these various souls are "forms" or "essences". But Aristotle's theory of essence is different from Plato's. His essences do not like Plato's belong to a separate world of forms or ideas. Rather they are inherent in the physical things. (In the case of organisms, they may be said to live in the organism, as its principle of life.) The irrational souls or essences of Aristotle may be said to be anticipations of modern gene theory: like DNA they plan the actions of the organism and steer it to its *telos,* to its perfection.

The irrational parts or potentialities of Aristotle's sensory and moving souls have much in common with Rylean dispositions to behave. They are, of course, perishable, and they are altogether similar to Simmias's "harmony of the body" (though Aristotle has much to say in criticism of the harmony theory). But the rational part, the immortal part of the soul, is different.

Aristotle's rational soul is, of course, conscious of its self, like Plato's. (See for example the *Posterior Analytics* 99b20 to the end, with the discussion of *nous* which here means intellectual intuition.) Even Charles Kahn [1966] who is prepared to stress the differences between the Aristotelian notion of soul and the Cartesian notion of consciousness arrives, after a brilliant and most careful investigation, at the conclusion (which I regard as almost obvious) that Aristotle's psychology *does* possess the notion of the consciousness of self.[10]

---

[10] See also the remarks on W. F. R. Hardie [1976] in section 44 above.

In this context I will refer only to one important passage which at the same time shows Aristotle's realization of the interaction between our physical sense organs and our subjective awareness. In Aristotle *On Dreams,* 461b31, we read: "If a man is unaware that a finger is being pressed below his eye, not only will one thing *seem* to be two, but he may think that it is two; whereas, if he is not unaware [of the finger being pressed below his eye], it will still appear to be two, but he will not think that it is two." This is a classical experiment to demonstrate the reality of conscious awareness, and of the fact that sensation is *not* a disposition to believe.[11]

III

In the development of the theory of the soul or the mind or the self, the development of ethical ideas plays a major role. It is, in the main, the changes in the theory of the survival of the soul which are most striking and important.

It must be admitted that in Homer and in some other myths of Hades the problem of the reward and punishment of the soul for its unusual excellence or for its moral failures is not always avoided. But in Homer, the status of the surviving soul of ordinary people who have never done much evil is terrible and depressing. Odysseus's mother is just one of them. She is not punished for any crime. She suffers merely as part of the condition of being dead.

The mystery cult of Eleusis (and perhaps what is called "the Orphic religion") led to a change in this belief. Here was a promise of a better world to come – if the right religion with the right rituals was adopted.

For us post-Kantians, this kind of promise of a reward does not seem to be a moral motivation. But there can be little doubt that it was the first step on the way to the Socratic and the Kantian point of view in which the moral action is done for its own sake; in which it is its own reward, rather than a good investment, a price paid for a promised reward in the life to come.

The steps in this development can be seen clearly; and the developing idea of a soul, a self, which is the responsible acting person, plays a most important part in this development.

Possibly under the influence of the Eleusian mysteries and of "Orphism", Pythagoras taught the survival and the reincarnation of the soul, or metempsychosis: the soul is rewarded or punished for its action by the quality – the *moral* quality – of its next life. This is the first step towards the idea that goodness is its own reward.

Democritus, who in many respects was influenced by the tenets of the Pythagoreans, taught like Socrates (as we have seen earlier in this section)

---

[11] Cp. section 30 above, text to note 5.

that it is worse to commit an act of injustice than to suffer it.[11a] Democritus, the materialist, did not of course believe in survival; and Socrates seems to have been an agnostic with respect to survival (according to Plato's *Apology* though not according to the *Phaedo*[12]). Both argued in terms of reward and punishment – terms unacceptable to moral rigorism of a Kantian kind. But both far transcended the primitive idea of hedonism – of the "pleasure principle". (Cp. *Phaedo* 68e–69a.) Both taught that to commit an act of injustice was to debase one's soul; in fact, to punish one's self. Both would have accepted Schopenhauer's simple maxim "Do not hurt anybody; but help everybody as well as you can!" (*Neminem lede; imo omnes, ut potes, juva!*) And both would have defended this principle by what, in essence, was an appeal to self respect, and the respect of other individuals.

Like many materialists and determinists Democritus did not seem to see that materialism and determinism are, in fact, incompatible with their enlightened and humanitarian moral teaching. They did not see that, even if we look upon morality not as being God-given, but as being man made, it is part of World 3: that it is a partly autonomous product of the human mind. It was Socrates who first realized this clearly.

Most important for the mind-body problem are two comments, probably genuinely Socratic, which are reported in the *Phaedo*, the dialogue in which Plato describes the last hours in prison and the death of Socrates. The two comments to which I am alluding occur in the passage in the *Phaedo* (96a – 100d) that is famous for containing some autobiographical remarks by Socrates.[13] The first comment (96b) is one of the crispest formulations of the mind-body problem in the whole history of philosophy. Socrates reports that when he was young he was interested in questions such as these. "Does the hot or the cold bring about the organization of animals by a process of fermentation, as some say? Do we think with our blood, or with air, or with fire? Or is it none of these but, rather, the brain that produces the sensations – hearing, sight, and smell; and do memory and opinion arise from these? And does demonstrative knowledge (*episteme*) derive from firmly established memory and opinion?" Socrates makes it clear that he soon rejected all such physicalist speculations. Mind, or thought, or reason, he decided,

---

11a See Diels & Kranz [1951–2] 68 B45. Cp. also 68 B187.

12 Concerning the incompatibility of certain parts of the *Phaedo* (especially *Phaedo* 108d ff.) with Plato's *Apology*, see note 9 to this section above, and p. 308 of my [1966(a)], volume i.

13 The historicity of this autobiographical passage is defended convincingly by Guthrie [1969] vol. iii, pp. 421–3; see also note 9 above.

always pursued an aim, or an end: it always pursued a purpose, doing what was best. Upon hearing that Anaxagoras had written a book in which he taught that the mind (*nous*) "orders and causes all things", Socrates was most eager to read the book; but he was severely disappointed. For the book did not explain the *purposes* or the *reasons* underlying the world order, but it tried to explain the world as a machine driven by purely mechanical *causes*. "It was (Socrates says in the second of the two comments, *Phaedo* 98c–99a) . . . as if somebody would first say that Socrates acts with reason or intelligence; and then, in trying to explain the causes of what I am doing now, should assert that I am now sitting here because my body is composed of bones and sinews; . . . and that the sinews, by relaxing and contracting, make me bend my limbs now, and that this is the cause of my sitting here with my legs bent . . . Yet the real causes of my sitting here in prison are that the Athenians have decided to condemn me, and that I have decided that . . . it is more just if I stay here and undergo the penalty they have imposed on me. For, by the Dog, . . . these bones of mine would have been in Megara or Boetia long ago . . . had I not thought it better and nobler to endure any penalty my city may inflict on me, rather than to escape, and to run away."

John Beloff ([1962], p. 141) rightly calls this passage a "superb affirmation of moral freedom in the face of death". But it is meant as a statement distinguishing sharply between an explanation in terms of physical causes (a World 1 causal explanation) and an explanation in terms of intentions, aims, ends, motives, reasons and values to be realized (a World 2 explanation that also involves considerations of World 3: Socrates's wish not to violate the legal order of Athens). And it makes clear that both kinds of explanation may be true, but that so far as the explanation of a responsible and purposeful action is concerned the first kind (the World 1 causal explanation) would be absurdly irrelevant.

In the light of some modern developments we can well say that Socrates considers here certain parallelist and identity theories; and that he rejects the claim that a causal physicalist explanation or a behaviourist explanation of a human action could possibly be equivalent to an explanation in terms of ends, purposes, and decisions (or to an explanation in terms of the logic of his situation). He rejects a physicalist explanation not as untrue, but as incomplete and as lacking any explanatory value. It omits all that is relevant: the conscious choice of ends and means.

Here we have a second and very different comment on the mind-body problem, even more important than the previous one. It is a statement in terms of responsible human actions: a statement within an essentially ethical context. It makes it clear that the ethical idea of a responsible moral self has played a decisive part in the ancient[14] discussions connected with the mind-body problem, and the consciousness of self.

The position here taken by Socrates is one that any interactionist must subscribe to: for any interactionist, even a full explanation of human bodily movements, *taken purely as physical movements,* cannot be provided in purely physical terms: the physical World 1 is not self-contained, but causally open to World 2 (and through it, to World 3).[15]

47. Conjectural versus Ultimate Explanation

Even for those who are not interested in history but mainly in understanding the contemporary problem situation, it is necessary to go back to two opposed views on science and on scientific explanation which can be shown to be part of the tradition of the Platonic and the Aristotelian Schools.

The Platonic and the Aristotelian traditions can be described as objectivist and rationalist (in contrast to the subjectivist sensualism or empiricism which takes as its starting point sense impressions and tries to "construct" the physical world out of these). Almost[1] all the forerunners of Plato and Aristotle were rationalists in this sense: they tried to explain the surface phenomena of the world by postulating a hidden world, a world of hidden realities, behind the phenomenal world. And they were right.

Of course, the most successful of these forerunners were the atomists, Leucippus and Democritus, who explained many properties of matter, such as compressibility, porousness, and the changes from the liquid state to the gaseous state, and to the solid state.

Their method can be called *the method of conjecture or hypothesis,* or that of *conjectural explanation.* It is analysed in some detail in Plato's *Republic*

---

[14] In modern times this second passage from Plato's *Phaedo* was repeatedly referred to by Leibniz in his various discussions of the mind-body problem. See section 50 below.

[15] If one does not insist on this point – if, say, one says that the physical movements of our bodies can be in principle completely explained in World 1 terms alone, and that this explanation may merely be complemented by one in terms of meanings – then, it seems to me, one has unwittingly adopted a form of parallelism, in which human aims, purposes and freedom become merely a subjective epiphenomenon.

[1] The only exceptions were some of the Sophists, especially Protagoras. Subjective empiricism became important again with Berkeley, Hume, Mach, Avenarius, and with the early Wittgenstein and the logical positivists. I regard it as mistaken and I shall not devote much space to it. I regard as its characteristic doctrine the saying of Otto Neurath, "Everything is surface: the world has no depth"; or the saying of Wittgenstein: "*The riddle* does not exist." (*Tractatus* [1921], 6.5.)

(e. g. 510b–511e), in the *Meno* (86e–87c) and in the *Phaedo* (85c–d). It consists, essentially, in making some assumption (we *may* have nothing to say in its favour) *and seeing what follows.* That is to say, *we test our assumption or our conjecture by exploring its consequences*; aware of the fact that in doing so, we can never establish the assumption. The assumption may or may not appeal to us intuitively: intuition is important, but (within this method) never decisive. One of the main functions of the method is to explain the phenomena, or "to save the phenomena".[2]

A second method which in my opinion ought to be sharply distinguished from the method of conjecture or hypothesis is *the method of the intuitive grasp of the essence*; that is to say, *the method of essentialist explanation* (the intuition of the essence is called, in German, "*Wesensschau*"; this is Husserl's term[3]). Here "intuition" (*nous,* intellectual intuition) implies infallible insight: it guarantees truth. What we see or grasp intuitively is (in this sense of intuition) the essence itself. (See for example Plato's *Phaedo,* 100c; and Aristotle's *Posterior Analytics,* esp. 100b.) The essentialist explanation allows us to answer a "what is" question, and (according to Aristotle) to state the answer in a *definition of the essence,* a formula of the essence. (Essentialist definition, real definition.) Using this definition as a premise we can then try, again, to explain the phenomena deductively – to save the phenomena. However, if we do not succeed, then it cannot be the fault of our premise: the premise must be true, if we have properly grasped the essence. Moreover, an explanation by the intuition of the essence is an *ultimate explanation*: it is neither in need nor capable of any further explanation. By contrast, any conjectural explanation can give rise to a new problem, to a new demand for an explanation: the "why?" question can always be reiterated, as even small children know. (Why did daddy not come home for lunch? He had to go to the dentist. Why does he have to go to the dentist? He has a bad tooth. Why does he have a bad tooth?) It is different with "what is" questions. Here an answer may be ultimate.

I hope I have made clear the difference between conjectural explanation – which, even if guided by intuition, always remains tentative – and, on the other hand, essentialist or ultimate explanation – which, if guided by intuition (in another sense) is infallible.

---

[2] This method must be clearly distinguished from the theory of instrumentalism with which it was conflated by Duhem. (See my [1963(a)], chapter 3, note 6, p. 99, where references to Aristotelian passages discussing this method can be found, e. g. *De caelo* 293a25.) The difference between this method and instrumentalism is that we put the truth of our tentative explanations to the test mainly because we are *interested* in their truth (like an essentialist, see below) though we do not think that we can *establish* their truth.

[3] See my *Open Society,* ii, p. 16.

There are, incidentally, two corresponding methods of criticizing an assertion. The first method ("scientific criticism") criticizes an assertion by drawing logical *consequences* from it (perhaps from it in conjunction with other, unproblematic assertions), and by trying to find *consequences which are unacceptable*. The second method ("philosophical criticism") tries to show that the assertion is *not really demonstrable*: that it cannot be derived from intuitively certain premises, and that it is itself not intuitively certain.

Almost all scientists criticize assertions by the first method; almost all philosophical criticism I know proceeds by the second method.

Now the interesting thing is that the distinction between the two methods of explanation can be found in the works of Plato and of Aristotle: both the theoretical description of the two methods is there, and also their use, in practical examples. But what is missing, from Plato right down to our own day, is a full consciousness that the methods are two: that they differ fundamentally; and, even more important, that only the first method, conjectural explanation, is valid, and feasible, while the second is just a will-o'-the-wisp.

The difference between the two methods is more radical than a difference between two methods that lead to what has been termed "knowledge claims"; for only the second method leads to knowledge claims. The first method leads to *conjectures* or *hypotheses*. Although these may be described as belonging to "knowledge" in an objective or World 3 sense, they are not *claimed* to be known or to be true. They may be *conjectured* to be true; but this is an entirely different thing.

Admittedly, there exists an old traditional movement against essentialist explanation, starting from ancient scepticism; a movement that influenced Hume, Kirchhoff, Mach, and many others. But the members of this movement do not distinguish the two kinds of explanation; rather, they identify "explanation" with what I call "essentialist explanation" and they therefore reject explanation altogether. (They recommend instead that we take "description" to be the real task of science.)

Oversimplifying things (as we always have to in history) we can say that, in spite of the existence of the two kinds of explanation, clearly recognized at some places by Plato and Aristotle, there is an almost universal conviction, even among the sceptics, that only the essentialist type of explanation is really an explanation, and that it alone is to be taken seriously.

I suggest that this attitude is almost unavoidable in the absence of a clear distinction between World 2 and World 3. Unless this distinction is clearly made, there is no "knowledge" except in the subjective or World 2 sense. There are no conjectures or hypotheses, no tentative and competing theories. There is only subjective doubt, subjective uncertainty, which is almost the opposite of "knowledge". We cannot say of two theories that the one is better than the other — we can only believe in the one and doubt the other. There can be, of course, different degrees of subjective belief (or of subjective probability). But as long as we do not recognize the existence of an objective World 3 (and of objective reasons which may make one of the competing theories objectively preferable or objectively stronger than another though none of them may be known to be true), there cannot be different theories or hypotheses of different degrees of objective merit or preferability (short of outright truth or falsity). As a consequence, while from the point of view of World 3, theories *are* conjectural hypotheses, for those who interpret theories and hypotheses in terms of World 2 beliefs there is a sharp division between theories and hypotheses: theories are known to be true, while hypotheses are provisional and at any rate not yet known to be true. (Even the great William Whewell — who in some ways comes near to the point of view here advocated — believed in the essential difference between a hypothesis and a finally established theory: a point of agreement between Whewell and Mill.)

It is interesting that Plato almost always stresses, when he comes to relate a myth, that the myth has only verisimilitude, not truth. But this does not affect his belief that what we seek is certainty, and that certainty is to be found in the intellectual intuition of essences. He agrees with the sceptics that this may not (or not always) be available. But the method of conjecture is, it seems, regarded by all parties not only as tentative but as a provisional *stop-gap for something better.*

One of the most interesting incidents in the history of science is due to the fact that this view is held even by Newton. His *Principia* may be described, I believe, as the most important of all works of conjectural or hypothetical explanation in history, and Newton clearly realized that his own theories in the *Principia* were not essentialist explanations. Yet he never rejected, and implicitly accepted, the philosophy of essentialism. Not only did he say "I do not feign hypotheses" (this particular remark may well have been meant "I do not offer *speculations* about possible ultimate explanations, as does Descartes"), but he agreed that essentialist explanations are to be searched for and that they would, if found, be final, and superior to his attraction at a distance. It never occurred to him to give up his belief in the superiority of an essentialist explanation to his own type of explanation (which he wrongly believed to be based on induction from the phenomena rather than on hypotheses). In contradistinction to some of his followers, he admitted that his theory was not an explanation; and he merely claimed that it was "the best and safest method first diligently to investigate the properties of things . . .

and [only] then to seek hypotheses to explain them".[4] In the third edition of the *Principia* [1726], Newton added to the beginning of Book III at the end of the Rules of Reasoning in Philosophy, "Not that I affirm gravity to be essential to bodies", thus disclaiming that the force of gravity could be taken as an essentialist explanation.[5]

To sum up, Newton, probably the greatest master ever of the method of conjectural explanations which "saved the phenomena", was of course right in appealing to the phenomena. He wrongly believed himself to have avoided hypotheses and to have used (Baconian) induction. He rightly believed that his theory might be explained by a deeper theory, but he wrongly believed that this would be an essentialist explanation. He also wrongly believed that inertia was essential to matter — an inherent *vis insita* of matter. (A further and complementary discussion of Newton's theory and its relation to essentialism will be found in section 51 below.)

Before proceeding to Descartes and his essentialist explanation of matter and of mind, I will only briefly state my belief that most of our difficulties are due to the fact that we still are inclined to ask "what is" questions: that we hope to find out one day what mind really is. Against this, I wish to point out that we do not know what matter is, though we now know quite a bit about the physical structure of matter. Thus we do not know (for example) whether the "elementary particles" which enter this structure are, or are not, "elementary" in any relevant sense of the term.

In a similar way, though we know nothing about its essence, we know quite a bit about the structure of mind. We know something about waking and sleeping. We know much about its purposeful activity; about its problem solving activity; about this activity of the mind going on even during sleep, and unconsciously; about virtues, heroism, forgetfulness of self, and the readiness to make sacrifices; about vices, and egoism, and self-centredness; and altogether about the richness and variousness of human personality. And we know much, though far too little, about the social and cultural traditions of man, and about the way in which our minds are anchored in World 3. These are the "phenomena" (in Newton's sense); and somehow we look, like Newton, for an ultimate explanation. No doubt, wrongly. We may not even

---

[4] Newton, letter to Oldenburg, 2 June 1672. (Cp. Newton's *Opera*, ed. S. Horsley, vol. IV, pp. 314f.)

[5] Cp. also the letters to Richard Bentley, 17th January and 25th February 1692–3. See my [1963(a)] notes 20 and 21 to chapter 3 (and text), and Newton's *Opticks*, query 31, where Newton mentions the possibility that attraction "may be performed by impulse, or by some other means unknown to me".

get very far with conjectural explanation. But this is only to be expected. For the mind is a process, or a phenomenon, of life – of the life of higher organisms; and although we know very much about organisms, and especially about one great unifying fact – the genetic code – almost all we know is even less unified than our typically pluralistic knowledge about matter. Though we must try for as much unification as possible, we must not expect an essentialist or a similarly unified answer to our problems.

48. Descartes: A Shift in the Mind-Body Problem

> Soul and body, I suggest, react sympathetically upon each other: a change in the state of the soul produces a change in the shape of the body, and conversely: a change in the shape of the body produces a change in the state of the soul.
> ARISTOTLE

Whether this programmatic statement from the beginning of chapter IV of the *Physiognomics (Minor Works,* 808b11) is due to Aristotle himself, under whose name it is transmitted, or whether it is due to one of his pupils (perhaps Theophrastus) is irrelevant for my purpose, which is to show that the mind-body problem, and its interactionist solution, were common possessions of the school of Aristotle. The members of this school, who accepted the doctrine that the mind was incorporeal, also accepted, tacitly but none the less clearly, that the mind-body relation was based on an *interaction* which was as a matter of course *non-mechanical.* The mind-body problem was solved in this way, as I have already suggested, by all thinkers of the time, except by the atomists who believed in a mechanical interaction.

My thesis in the present section is simple. First, I wish to stress that there was common ground between Aristotle and Descartes in respect of the doctrines of the incorporeality of the soul and of interactionism, and also in respect of their acceptance of the idea of essentialist explanation. Descartes, however, got into particular difficulties with the problem of interaction. It became for him the problem of how a non-material soul could act upon a physical world of clockwork mechanisms, in which all physical causation was, essentially and necessarily, based on mechanical push. My thesis is that, in trying to combine the doctrine of the incorporeality of the soul, and of interaction, with a mechanistic and monistic principle of physical causation, Descartes created an entirely new and unnecessary difficulty. This difficulty led to a new shift in the mind-body problem (and, with the successors of Descartes, to mind-body parallelism and later to the identity thesis).

Descartes, as I have said, was an essentialist, and his physical ideas rested upon an intuitive idea as to the essence of body.[1] The reliability of this intuition was supposed to be guaranteed by God. Descartes tried to show, by arguments starting from his "I think, therefore I am", that God existed, and that, as He was perfect, He could not allow us to be deceived when we had a clear and distinct intuition or perception. Thus clarity and distinctness of our perceptions (and of some other subjective thoughts) are for Descartes reliable *criteria of truth.*

Descartes defined a body as something which was (three-dimensionally) spatially extended. Thus *extension was the essence of bodyhood or materiality.* (This was not very different from Plato's theory of space in the *Timaeus,* or from Aristotle's theory of the first matter.) Descartes shared with many previous thinkers (Plato, Aristotle, St. Augustine[2]) the view that mind and the consciousness of self are non-corporeal. Accepting the view that extension was the essence of matter, he was forced to say that the incorporeal substance, soul, was "unextended". (This led Leibniz to identify souls with unextended Euclidean points; that is, with "monads".) The essence of the soul-substance was, according to Descartes, that it was a "thinking" substance.[3] "Thinking" is here, clearly, meant as synonymous with "conscious". The definition of matter or body as *extended* led Descartes direct to his peculiar form of a mechanistic theory of causality — to the theory that all causation in World 1 is by push.

This was, in a way, an old theory. It is the theory of the warrior who wields a sword or a spear and who defends himself with a shield and a helmet; and it is the theory of the craftsman, the potter, the shipbuilder, the smith. (It is hardly the theory of the smelter of bronze or iron, for the application of heat uses a causal factor different from mere push; nor is it the theory of the alchemist or chemist; nor is it the theory of the shaman or the soothsayer, or

---

[1] By "essence" Descartes means the essential or unchanging properties of a substance (for Descartes's idea of substance, see note 1 to section 49, below) — very much like Aristotle, or like Newton (who said that gravity cannot be essential to matter because it diminishes with distance).

[2] It is interesting that Descartes's famous argument, "I think, therefore I am.", was anticipated by St. Augustine, in his *De libero arbitrio,* as was pointed out by Arnauld to Descartes. (See Haldane & Ross [1931], vol. ii, pp. 80 and 97.) It was also (according to Bertrand Russell [1945], p. 374) anticipated in St. Augustine's *Soliloquia.* On the relation of mind to body, much can be found in Augustine's *Confessions* (e. g. X, 8) and his *De quantitate animae.*

[3] For Descartes's idea of substance see note 1 to section 49.

the astrologist; but of course, push is almost universal, and within everyone's experience from childhood on.)

The first philosopher who made push the (almost) universal causal agent was Democritus; even the combination of atoms was (partly) due to push, when the hooks of atoms got entangled. In this way, he "reduced" pull to push.

By contrast, Descartes did not accept atomism. His identification of geometrical extension and bodyhood or materiality prevented him from accepting it. This identification led him to two arguments against atomism: there could be no void, no empty space; for geometrical space was extension and thus the very essence of body or matter. And there could be no finite limit to divisibility; for geometrical space was infinitely divisible. Nevertheless, Descartes accepted, apart from the theory of push, many of the cosmological ideas of the atomists (as had Plato and Aristotle); first of all the theory of vortices. He was forced to accept this theory by his definition of the essence of matter. Since this definition forced him to accept that space is full, every movement had to be, in principle, of the character of a vortex, like the movement of tea leaves in a tea cup.

In Descartes's cosmology, like in that of the atomists, the world was a huge mechanical clockwork, with cogwheels: vortices geared to each other and pushing each other along. All animals were part of this huge clockwork mechanism. Each animal was a sub-clockwork, like the automatic puppets driven by water which at his time were fashionable show pieces in some noblemen's gardens.

The human body was no exception. It was an automaton — *except for its voluntary movement.* Here was the *only* exception in the universe: the immaterial human mind could cause movements in the human body. It could also become conscious of some of the mechanical impressions made by physical light, sound, and touch, on the human body.

It is clear that this theory of mind-body interaction does not fit well into an otherwise completely mechanical cosmology.

To see this we have only to compare Descartes's cosmology with that of Aristotle.

The immaterial and immortal human soul in the philosophy of Descartes corresponds very closely to the rational soul or mind (*nous*) in the philosophy of Aristotle. Both are, clearly, endowed with consciousness of self. Both are immaterial and immortal. Both can consciously pursue an aim, and use the body as an instrument, an organ, to achieve their ends.

Aristotle's vegetative soul and his sentient soul (and the appetitive and locomotive soul) correspond to what Descartes calls the "animal spirits". Contrary to the first impressions conveyed by the term "spirit", the animal spirits of Descartes are part of the purely mechanical apparatus of the body. They are fluids – very rare fluids – which in all animals and in man do a lot of the mechanical work of the brain, and which connect the brain with the sense organs and with the muscles of the limbs. They are conducted in the nerves (and are thus anticipations of nervous electric signals).

So far there is little difference between the theories of Aristotle and of Descartes. The discrepancy is very great, however, if we look at the cosmological picture as a whole. Aristotle sees man as an elevated animal, as a rational animal. But all animals and plants, and even the whole inanimate cosmos, are striving for aims or ends; and the plants and animals are steps (possibly even evolutionary steps) leading from inanimate nature to man. Aristotle is a teleologist.

Descartes's world is totally different. It consists almost exclusively of lifeless mechanical contrivances. All plants or animals are such contrivances, and only man is truly animate, truly alive. This picture of the universe was felt by many to be unacceptable and even shocking. It led to doubts as to the sincerity of Descartes – whether he was not, perhaps, a camouflaged materialist who introduced the soul into his system merely because he was afraid of the Roman Church. (That he was afraid of the Church is known from the fact that he gave up the plan to publish his first book *On the World* when he heard of the trial and condemnation of Galileo.)

This suspicion is probably unfounded. Yet there are difficulties in dismissing it. Descartes accepted the Copernican system, and the infinite universe of Giordano Bruno (because Euclidean space is infinite). Within a pre-Copernican cosmology, the unique exception made for man might have been understandable. But it fits badly into the Copernican cosmology.

The Cartesian soul is unextended; but it is localized. It is, therefore, located in an unextended Euclidean point in space. Descartes does not seem (like Leibniz) to have drawn this conclusion from his premises. But Descartes did locate the soul "mainly" within a very small organ – the pineal gland. The pineal gland was the organ immediately moved by the human soul. In its turn, it acted on the animal spirits like a valve in an electrical amplifier: it steered the movements of the animal spirits, and through them, the movement of the body.

Now this theory led to two grave difficulties. The graver of the two was this. The animal spirits (which are extended) moved the body by push, and they, in their turn, were also moved by push: this was a necessary consequence of Descartes's theory of causality. But how could the unextended soul exert anything like a push on an extended body? Here was an inconsistency.

This particular inconsistency was the main motive of the evolution of Cartesianism. It was ultimately removed by Leibniz, as I will show; and in this solution of the problem, Leibniz was influenced and partly anticipated by Thomas Hobbes.[4]

The second difficulty is less serious. Descartes believed that the action of the soul on the animal spirits was to deflect the direction of their motion; and he believed that this could be done without violating any law of physics, as long as the "amount of motion", mass multiplied by velocity, was conserved. Leibniz showed that this was a mistake. He discovered the law of conservation of momentum (mass multiplied by *motion in any given direction*), and he emphasized repeatedly that the law of conservation of momentum demands that momentum, and therefore *the direction* of motion, must be conserved.

While this is a telling point against Descartes's specific suggestion, I do not think that physical conservation laws pose any serious problem for the interactionist. This may be shown by the fact that a vessel or a vehicle *can* be steered from the inside without violating any physical law. (And this can be done by such weak forces as wireless signals.) All that is necessary is (1) that the vehicle carries with it a source of energy and (2) that, in order to change its direction, it can compensate for the change by pushing some mass – for example the earth, or some amount of water – in the opposite direction. (One could also say: if there were a serious difficulty here then we could never change our own direction; as it is, when we get up from a chair, we push the whole earth in the opposite direction, if ever so lightly: thus the law of the conservation of momentum is preserved.)

If, in addition, we interpret Descartes's mechanical "animal spirits" not mechanically, but physicalistically as electrical phenomena, then this particular difficulty becomes altogether negligible since the mass of the deflected electrical current is almost equal to zero so that there is no problem in compensating for a switch which changes the direction of the current.

To sum up. The great difficulty of the Cartesian theory of mind-body interaction lies in the Cartesian theory of physical causality according to which all physical action must be by mechanical push.

---

[4] See the reference to John W. N. Watkins in note 1 to section 50.

49. From Interactionism to Parallelism: The Occasionalists and Spinoza

Most of the important thinkers who followed Descartes rejected interactionism. To understand why this happened, we need to glance briefly back at Descartes.

Descartes, as we have seen, was an essentialist; and critics of his ideas raised against him the objection that, if soul and body are substances of entirely different natures, then there could be no interaction between them. Descartes himself protested against this: "I declare . . . [that it is] a false supposition that can by no manner of means be proved . . . that if the soul and the body are two substances of diverse nature, that prevents them from being capable of acting on one another."[1] I agree that the mere diversity of nature or essence does not create a difficulty. However, *if* one accepts Descartes's essentialist theory of physical causation, in addition to Descartes's essentialist view of soul and body, then it would, indeed, seem difficult to understand how this interaction could take place. This explains the widespread rejection of interaction in the Cartesian school.

As a historical point, this is all understandable enough. But what is perhaps surprising is that the distrust of interactionism, on the grounds of the dissimilarity of the two substances, still exists. The argument against interactionism based on the dissimilarity of body and soul is taken quite seriously even by contemporary philosophers of outstanding merit.[2]

But I suggest that it is *only* the Cartesian idea of physical causation (admittedly, derived by Descartes from the essential property of physical substance) that creates a serious problem, and not the idea of an essential difference of the substances. Even if we were to presuppose the idea of *ultimate explanation based on ultimate essentialist substances,* even then the dissimilarity of substances would not necessarily create an argument against

[1] See Haldane and Ross [1931], vol. ii, p. 132. The prehistory of the concept of substance goes far back to the early Ionian "principles": water, or the indefinite (*apeiron*), or air, or fire. It may be said to denote whatever remains identical with itself when a thing *changes*; or to denote the thing that it the carrier of its properties (which may change). In the *Meditations,* Descartes uses "substance" frequently as a synonym of "thing". But in the *Principles,* he says first (i, 51), as he also does in *Meditation* III, that a substance is a thing that depends upon nothing else for its existence, adding that only God is truly a substance (the view later adopted by Spinoza); yet immediately afterwards (i, 52–54) he says that we may also call soul and body substances, namely created substances: having been created by God they can be destroyed only by God. Locke obviously had Descartes in mind when complaining about the confused idea of substance (*Essay* ii, xxiii). By and large, the popular usage of "substance" is at least as clear as the Cartesian usage. (See also Quinton [1973], Pt. i.)

[2] Cp. John Passmore [1961], p. 55.

the possibility of their interaction; but from the point of view of *conjectural explanation,* this difficulty simply does not arise.

And indeed, in the present state of physics (which operates with conjectural explanations) we are faced, not with a plurality of substances, but with a plurality of different kinds of forces, and thus with a pluralism of different interacting explanatory principles.[3]

(Perhaps the clearest physical example against the thesis that only like things can act upon each other is this. In modern physics, the action of bodies upon bodies is *mediated* by fields – by gravitational and electrical fields. Thus like does not act upon like, but bodies act first upon fields which they modify, and then the (modified) field acts upon another body.[4])

Thus the difficulty of mind-body interaction arises only as a necessary consequence of Descartes's essentialist theory of causation.

The first proposed solution of this difficulty is due to some Cartesians (Clauberg, Cordemoy, De la Forge, Geulincx, Malebranche) who were also "occasionalists".

Occasionalism is the theory that every instance of causation is a miracle: God intervenes on the occasion of every particular case of causal action or interaction. The Cartesian occasionalists applied this view especially to actions of mind on body and of body on mind.

Their theory that God intervened at such occasions had some backing in an important part of Descartes's own theory. For Descartes had appealed to the truthfulness of God, who could not deceive us, when he argued that clear and distinct ideas must be true. This implied (a) that clear and distinct sense-perceptions are true, (b) that God intervened, and was at least co-responsible, in putting these perceptions into our minds on the proper occasions; that is to say, on all occasions when the perceived physical objects acted on our bodily sense organs.

This shows that the occasionalists were good Cartesians: they made use of an essential part of Descartes's philosophical system in order to amend another part which had turned out to be untenable and, indeed, inconsistent with Descartes's own essentialist definitions of mind and body.

---

[3] J. O. Wisdom [1952] discussed electromagnetism, and suggested that the interdependence between electrical and magnetic forces may serve as a model of mind-body interaction. See also Watkins ([1974], pp. 394–5). Jeremy Shearmur has also drawn my attention to a report in Beloff ([1962], p. 231) that Sir Cyril Burt has argued "that physicists ought to be more tolerant . . . towards . . . dualism inasmuch as physics itself, as currently understood, is pluralistic." On causality, see also my [1972(a)], *Appendix*; [1959(a)], section 12; [1972(a)], chapter 5; [1967(k)]; and [1974(c)], pp. 1125–39.

[4] See Watkins ([1974], p. 395).

Thus it was the occasionalists who first rejected the psychophysical *interactionism* which until then had ruled supreme and unquestioned. They replaced it by a psychophysical *parallelism*: there was no interaction between mind and body. Rather, there was a parallelism which created the appearance of interaction: on every occasion when the mind, the will, wished consciously to move a limb, the limb moved, as if caused by the will; and *vice versa,* on every occasion when a bodily sense organ was stimulated, the mind experienced a perception, as if caused by the sense organ. But in reality, there was no causation. The parallelism was miraculous: it was due to the intervention of God, it was due to God's veracity and goodness.

This kind of miracle was, however, not really satisfactory; neither for the orthodox believer in miracles and in Christianity, nor for the sober rationalist – to say nothing of the sceptic. (If we live in a world of constant miracles, miracles that happen on the most trivial occasions, then the miracles which are essential to the Christian faith are robbed of part of their character as miraculous, and of part of their value.)

It is understandable that Cartesian philosophers searched for a version of parallelism which retained the advantages of occasionalism without its manifest disadvantages.

The first version of such a parallelistic theory was due to Spinoza, who regarded himself as a Cartesian. The second and, in my opinion, more important version was due to Leibniz.

Spinoza's theory, like the theory of occasionalism, appealed to a remark of Descartes's. Descartes had described mind and body as "substances". But he had also said that only God deserved, strictly speaking, to be described as a substance; for a substance should, Descartes said (in *Meditation* III), be defined as "a thing which exists without depending for its existence upon any other thing"; and this, strictly speaking, can hold only of God.

This idea was taken up by Spinoza. God alone is the substance of everything, of the universe. He is identical with the Essence of the universe, with its Nature. There cannot be more than one substance; that is, God.

This one *substance,* God, has an infinity of *attributes.* (The term "attribute" had also been used in a similar sense by Descartes (*Principles* I, 56).) Of this infinity of attributes, the human intellect can grasp only two: *cogitatio,* thought, consciousness, mind; and *extensio,* extension, bodyhood. Since both are merely attributes of God, their parallelism can be explained without the appeal to occasional miracles. They run parallel because they are different aspects of one and the same underlying entity, of the one substance: God.

One sees that, and why, Spinoza must be a pantheist: since there is no other essence or substance in the universe than God, God must be identical with the essence or substance of the universe, with nature.

One also sees that, and why, Spinoza must be a panpsychist: mind is an attribute and an aspect of the one substance; so there are mental aspects running everywhere parallel to all material aspects.

50. Leibniz's Theory of Mind and Matter: From Parallelism to Identity

Leibniz, I believe, can be best understood as a Cartesian who, following in the footsteps of the other great Cartesians, was critical of Descartes. He was a critical ecletic, much influenced by Plato, Aristotle and St. Augustine, as well as by all the great productive philosophers of his time: by Descartes; by Hobbes[1] and Gassendi; by Geulincx and Malebranche; by Spinoza and by Arnauld. (He read and criticized Locke; but he seems never to have read Newton's *Principia.*) He was a parallelist, like Spinoza, and he frequently criticized Spinoza and the occasionalists, especially Malebranche. Yet his own theory of mind-body parallelism is strikingly similar to both occasionalism and Spinozism. Like the occasionalists, he gave up mind-body interaction, and replaced it by the action of God. Like Spinoza, he avoided the appeal to a divine miracle on every single occasion. But he also avoided Spinoza's pantheism and his form of monism. Leibniz's explanation of mind-body parallelism is his famous doctrine of the pre-established harmony: when God created the world, he foresaw and pre-established everything; and in doing so, he pre-established, for every soul, that its ideas (its perceptions, its subjective experiences) would correctly (if often only vaguely) mirror the physical events of the universe, from its particular point of view: from the point in the universe which it occupied. Accordingly, our perceptions (so far as they are clear and distinct) are truthful, and this does not require the special intervention of God on every particular occasion; and similarly, when we decide to move a limb, this is followed by both the perception of the motion of the limb and, of course, the physical motion of the limb.

Like Spinoza, Leibniz was a kind of panpsychist: there was an inner aspect, a soul-like experience, of all matter. However, he differed from Spinoza in at least two important ways concerning the mind-body relation. While Spinoza was a monist — there was one substance only, that is, God —

[1] Leibniz's dependence upon Hobbes and his theory of *conatus* (= endeavour or appetite or striving or will) has been generally noticed, though its full significance has, to my knowledge, been observed only by John W. N. Watkins [1965], [1973].

Leibniz was a pluralist and an individualist: there were infinitely many substances, each of them corresponding to a point in space; and each of them was soul-like, though only comparatively few of them — the animal souls — were endowed with perception and memory, and still fewer — the human souls or minds — were endowed also with reason. Since each of these souls or soul-like substances, differing in the degree of clarity of consciousness, corresponded to a point in space, Leibniz called them "monads" (*monas,* in Euclid, is a unit or point).

Another important difference between Leibniz's cosmology and that of Spinoza is this. While in Spinoza's theory soul and body were merely two *attributes* of the one substance, God, Leibniz taught that the *many* monads were each real substances. In Kantian terminology, each was a *real thing in itself*; while matter was, merely, the well-founded *appearance,* from outside, of the accumulations and extensions of these substantial things in themselves. ("Well-founded" in the sense that though the unity of a body was an illusion, its spatial continuity and its extension were not illusions.) God, more particularly, did not appear as matter, as He did in Spinoza's system; but He was a soul, a monad, a thing in itself, though of course different from all the monads in His omniscience and omnipotence. He was the creator of the other monads — created in His likeness, and endowed with different degrees of knowledge and power. (He was *not* the creator of matter since this was merely the outside appearance of accumulations of monads.)

Leibniz's theory of mind (of monads) and of matter takes literally the Cartesian definition of mind as essentially unextended and of matter as essentially extended: mind, being unextended must be, regarded from outside, an *unextended point in space.* (Descartes, as mentioned above, does not say exactly the same; but his unextended mind is concentrated *mainly* in the pineal gland; and being unextended *and* having position together seem to imply the Leibnizean doctrine that the soul is contained in a point in space.) Every piece of matter, on the other hand, being *extended* in space, must consist of an infinity of points, and thus of an infinity of monads; "inanimate" matter consisting of monads without clear and distinct ideas and without memory; "animate" matter or organisms consisting of monads with more or less clear and distinct ideas (perceptions) and more or less memory; mind consisting of monads with very clear and distinct ideas and memory.

Thus Leibniz accepts here some basic Cartesian ideas. But he differs from Descartes in stressing that matter is not a substance (or a thing in itself), but a mere appearance. Also, he postulates a continuity of steps from mindless or inanimate monads to animals and further to human rational souls.

Leibniz obtains this result by way of a criticism of Descartes.

Extension – geometrical extension – implies, as in Descartes, *divisibility*. Thus there can be no indivisible extended atoms. (Descartes taught the same.) Yet every extended thing consists of an infinity of unextended substances. Thus each unextended substance must be an *intensity located in a point.*

Leibniz had met such intensities located in a point in his differential calculus. For example, a force was an unextended intensity located in a point. Since a force was an unextended intensity, the Cartesian dichotomy (*mind* = *unextended* and *matter* = *extended*) showed that force must be something *mental.* This was in passable agreement with the very wide usage of the Cartesian conception of a thinking substance: thinking meant for Descartes anything from perceiving and doubting to planning, intending, and willing; to experiencing appetites and drives. All these are intensities, and appetites and drives are not unlike forces.

Descartes's mechanics consisted of matter (extension) in motion. It did not operate with the idea of force. Leibniz criticized this at an early date. He showed that extension, though characteristic of matter, was not satisfactory (as Descartes thought) as an explanation of matter, and of causation by push. For it could not establish the important *impenetrability* of matter (its *"antitypy"*[2] or repellent power). What distinguished matter from a phantasma, or from a shade, was this impenetrability or *antitypy.* But this was a power of resistance – for example, of resistance to touch – and therefore a force. Thus matter was extension filled by forces, by intensities.

This is Leibniz's argument which led him to the conclusion, all-important for his theory of the mind-body problem, that *matter was extension, filled by mindlike substances.*

The idea of identifying the mental concept of striving (*conatus,* endeavour, will) with the idea of a localizable but unextended physical force goes back to Hobbes (see note 1 above). Leibniz must have been greatly encouraged when he found that the differential calculus strongly supported this idea: force was equal to acceleration times mass, and acceleration was a second differential of the motion of a point: obviously *a localized intensity,* and obviously *unextended*; and therefore, according to Descartes, *mental.*

---

[2] See Leibniz's letter to Thomasius, April 20/30, 1669. (Gerhardt IV [1880], pp. 162ff., especially pp. 171, 173; Loemker i [1956], pp. 144ff., especially pp. 148–160.)

This is the background of Leibniz's cosmology, his theory of the universe of mental substances or monads – his monadology. Later[3] he added the doctrine of the pre-established harmony. This was, in the first instance, a harmony, established at their creation, between the intensities (the experienced perceptions and strivings) of the various individual mental substances, the monads. *As a consequence* of this, there had to be also a harmony between the individual substances and the appearances (which were accumulations of substances as seen from outside).

A consequence of the doctrine of pre-established harmony was this. Since all experience, especially also will and perception (also apperception; that is, consciousness, reflection; see Gerhardt IV, p. 600) was pre-established in the monads, the monads did not need any "windows" or sensoria to observe the world: they just mirrored the changing world (the outside view of the physical accumulations of monads) because that faculty was built into them by God in the beginning.

Thus there was no interaction between the monads. *But the physical world behaved as if there was mechanical interaction by push.*

From this follows an important further consequence: a parallelism between the world of mental experience – of purposes, of ends, of will – and the physical world of appearances, the world of mechanical causation, the world of matter. Leibniz stresses repeatedly that his theory of pre-established harmony solves the second formulation of the Socratic mind-body problem as stated in the autobiographical passage of the *Phaedo* (see the end of section 46, above). It shows that there is an explanation in terms of *reasons* or *purposes,* in addition to an explanation in terms of *mechanical causes or of push.* And it shows that the former explanation is, wherever applicable, more relevant, since it pertains to the substances, the teleological world of minds which are things in themselves; while the explanation in terms of push pertains to physical appearances only.

Another important consequence of the theory is the doctrine of the *absolute individuality* of the monads, the mental substances, with their intrinsic properties, their ideas (for example, perceptions). Since each monad was created intrinsically to mirror the universe from a different point of view, no two substances could be intrinsically equal. This leads to Leibniz's doctrine of the identity of indiscernibles: any two substances that were *intrinsically indiscernible* could not really be two, but were identically the same. (This

---

[3] In "A New System of the Nature and Communication of Substances", 1695. (Gerhardt IV, 477 ff.; Loemker ii, 740 ff.)

clashes with the modern theory of elementary particles which are of course extrinsically or positionally different but intrinsically indiscernible in a most important way. One can say that Newton foresaw this, and that Leibniz did not.[4])

It is important to remember that Leibniz's theory is pluralistic, as compared to Spinoza's monism: it contains infinitely many intrinsically different individual substances. But it is also in a certain sense dualistic: it distinguishes sharply between minds (real substances) and bodies (appearances). And in another sense it is even monistic: the only substances, the only realities, the only things in themselves, are mindlike. And the minds or souls differ in their ideas, not accidentally, but essentially. For the carrying of ideas is their essence, which God has implanted into them, and which distinguishes them individually.

It is interesting to compare Leibniz's theory with the ancient theories of Pythagoras and Simmias (see section 46, above) and with the modern identity theories of Schlick, Russell, and Feigl (see sections 22 and 23 above, and section 54, below).

Pythagoras's theory of the immaterial soul described the soul as a harmony – a harmony of numerical relations. Leibniz describes the *relations between* his souls as a harmony: what is harmonious are the ideas, the divinely implanted contents, of the different individual souls. Thus "soul" in general – the universe of souls as distinct from the individual souls – is harmonious.

Simmias (Plato in the *Phaedo*) describes the soul as a harmony of the body (of a living organism). According to Leibniz, the body of a living organism consists of an accumulation of souls which are in harmony, with one of them dominant, and ruling the organism.

Obviously, this dominant soul is in harmony with the body – that is, with the infinity of souls constituting the body.

The modern identity theories of Schlick, Russell, and Feigl describe "the mental" as an inside view (knowledge by acquaintance) of some brain processes. As in Leibniz's theory, this inside view is *real*; it is a view of a *thing in itself*. The corresponding brain process is an outside *appearance* of the same thing ("knowledge by description"). Schlick, Russell, and Feigl are not, in intention, panpsychist, and still less spiritualist monists. It is arguable, however, that they are committed to a theory which differs only verbally from Leibniz's monadology. (Of course, in Leibniz's theory the "mental" is not

---

[4] See *A Collection of Papers which passed between the Late Learned Mr. Leibniz and Dr. Clarke in the Years 1715 and 1716* (London 1717); Loemker ii, pp. 1095ff.

identical with anything "physical" or "extended"; but it is identical with an indivisible element of something "physical" or "extended".)

It should be noted, finally, that Leibniz's idea of the *monad as a force* comes sometimes very close to an idea of the *monad as a process* – an idea stressed, in a somewhat different way, by Whitehead.

51. Newton, Boscovich, Maxwell: The End of Ultimate Explanation

Were the history of human thought more fully under the control of reason, then the idea of ultimate explanation (for example, of explanation by an appeal to self-evident axioms, or to clear and distinct ideas; see section 47 above) would have been discarded after the publication of the first edition of Newton's *Principia,* 1687, or at least after the more or less general acceptance of Newton's theory – say fifty years later. For Newton's *Principia,* as Newton, Leibniz, Berkeley, and almost everybody saw, clashed with the idea of essentialist or ultimate explanation. Ultimate explanations in physics ought to have been based on the essence of matter, on its intrinsic or essential property – extension – which explains push, impulse, *repulsion.* But Newton operated with gravitational *attraction.*

This problem situation led to four possible positions.

(1) Dismissing the Newtonian theory. This was the position of Leibniz.

(2) Interpreting Newton's attraction as a new inherent or essential property of matter (claiming for it, *ad hoc,* intuitive self-evidence). This was half-heartedly suggested by Cotes and, as will be shown below, also by Newton, though he almost at once withdrew the suggestion.

(3) Dismissing essentialism, and interpreting Newton's theory as a conjectural explanation. This, in my opinion, is the correct position. At first sight, it may seem to have been the position of Berkeley, who denied the existence of a real world of physical essences behind the world of appearances. However, not only did Berkeley remain an essentialist (especially with respect to mind or spirit and God), but his views are more accurately described as a fourth position:

(4) Adopting an instrumentalist interpretation of Newton's theory.

This should be clearly distinguished from (3): while (3) looks upon Newton's theory as a conjecture which may *possibly be true,* (4) looks upon it as a *mere instrument for prediction* (Berkeley also said a [mere] "mathematical hypothesis") which cannot be true, though it may be useful, for example for prediction.[1]

[1] For this position see chapters 6 (on Berkeley) and 3 of my [1963(a)].

Newton's own position was, I suppose, somewhat unsettled. Not only did he never give up essentialism, but he never quite gave up his objections to considering gravity as an acceptable essential cause. Nor did he ever quite give up hope that he or a successor of his may find the essential cause of gravity, and so may be able to give an ultimate explanation of the inverse square law of gravitational attraction. It is only in the fourth edition of his *Opticks*, published three years after his death, that he argues, in the form of queries (query 31) for what in my opinion can be interpreted as the suggestion that attraction may be, after all, like repulsion ("a repulsive Virtue"), a "Virtue" or inherent property of bodies, and thus an ultimate explanation. However, even after making this suggestion, he protects himself by repeating his often made statements against the use of "hypotheses" or "occult Qualities" which "put a stop to the Improvement of natural Philosophy". But (as he said before) "to derive two or three Principles of Motion from Phaenomena" is "a very great step in Philosophy, though the [essential] Causes of those Principles were not discovered".

Thus the position of Newton whose *Principia* clearly offered what I have called "conjectural explanations" is here again of great interest. (a) He believed that his laws of motion were obtained by induction from the phenomena. (b) He admitted that induction was not a valid proof. (c) He believed that in this special case of the laws of motion, he was entitled to claim their factual truth, although he was not entitled to claim their character as "causes" or as explanations. (That the law of gravity *may* after all be acceptable as an essential cause he hardly dared to suggest in this final query in the *Opticks*.) I suggest that all this was due to a deep-seated belief in essentialism; a belief which he tried to replace, unsuccessfully, by appeals to the phenomena, and to induction from the phenomena.

If I am more or less right in this analysis, then it makes Newton's achievements even more admirable: they were achieved against the odds of false methodological beliefs. Wrongly believing, and modestly believing, that what he offered was not the best but only the second best, he unerringly achieved the best theory that could possibly have been achieved at the time, and in the best possible way. (Who can say that his attacks of depression were not due, or partly due, to his inherited essentialism?)

Newton was an atomist, and an admirer of the ancient atomists, but not with respect to the mind-body problem: here he followed Descartes, and the Platonic and Aristotelian immaterialist traditions. (*Opticks*, queries 28 and 31.)

Roger Joseph Boscovich, the great Yugoslav physicist and philosopher, may be said to be one of the greatest, if not the greatest, of Newtonians. He combined, in a most original way, one of Leibniz's ideas with many of the ideas of Newton, especially with Newton's atomism. The idea that Boscovich took from Leibniz was the unextendedness of the atoms: like Leibniz's monads, Boscovich's atoms were unextended monads, geometrical points in space, and centres of force. However, in every other respect Boscovich's monads (and also Kant's monads, developed contemporaneously with, and independently of, Boscovich) were utterly different from those of Leibniz.

Leibniz's monads were densely, or more precisely continuously, packed in space: to every point in three-dimensional space there corresponded a monad, which was non-material since it was unextended. On the other hand, any three-dimensionally extended accumulation in space appeared as matter, as body: it *appeared,* because in reality it consisted of non-extended and non-material substance; it appeared as matter or as body because it was extended, because it filled an extended part of three-dimensional space. Thus there was no vacuum, no empty space between the closely packed monads.

Boscovich's (and also Kant's) theory was different.[2] They were atomists; that is to say, they believed in *atoms and the void.* Their atoms were points, monads. But they were not closely packed. On the contrary, no two of their atomic monads could touch each other: they were prevented from doing this by *repulsive forces* which increased with diminishing distances and approached infinity when the two monads approached each other indefinitely. Thus the monads are spaced; and as Kant makes particularly clear, the forces radiating from the monads fill the void, with varying intensity or density.

According to Boscovich, the forces radiating from the monads change with the distance, as follows. For *very* short distances, the force is highly repulsive. With increasing distances the repulsion quickly decreases to zero; then the force becomes attractive. This explains cohesion between particles (or perhaps chemical forces between atoms, forming molecules). Then they become again zero, then repulsive. Owing to the repulsive forces, the atoms take up space. Thus matter is expanded, but it remains always compressible, even though, owing to the repulsive forces, further compression may only be possible if the compressive forces are very great.

This theory is in a sense purely speculative, or purely rational — the result of rational, critical model building and of criticism of earlier models (like those of Leibniz and of the earlier atomists). It is of course purely conjectural: it is a paradigm of conjectural explanation. It is interesting to note that,

---

[2] Kant published his *Monadologica Physica* in 1756, two years before the first edition of Boscovich's great book *Theoria Philosophiae Naturalis,* Vienna, 1758. But Boscovich had earlier published some of his main ideas in a dissertation, *De Viribus Vivis,* in 1745, and in *De Lege Virium in Natura existentium* in 1755.

apart from the assumption that the basic atoms are unextended points, the theory of changing repulsive and attractive forces was anticipated by Newton who wrote, in the *Opticks* (query 31) of attractive chemical forces: "And as in Algebra where affirmative Quantities vanish and cease, there negative ones begin; so in Mechanicks, where Attraction ceases, there a repulsive Virtue ought to succeed." This is, essentially, Boscovich's theory. (Boscovich refers to several passages of query 31.)

From our point of view it is interesting that Boscovich is, like Descartes and Newton, a believer in essentialist or ultimate explanation; and he makes explicit use of it in order to establish interaction of mind and body. Concerning his own physical theory, Boscovich's position is almost the same as Newton's, although he is, clearly, less disturbed by the methodological problem than is Newton.

Since Boscovich proposes a dynamic theory of matter, like that of Leibniz, he has, as an interactionist, to make clear that his monads are not Leibnizian spirits, and that his matter interacts with spirit or mind, and does not run parallel in a pre-established harmony: ". . . this theory of mine", Boscovich writes ([1763], article 157), "can be conjoined in an excellent manner with the immateriality of spirits. The theory ascribes to matter the properties inertia, impenetrability, sensibility [this is a consequence of impenetrability to touch] and incapacity for thinking; and to spirits it ascribes an incapacity for affecting our senses by impenetrability, and the faculties of thinking and willing. Indeed, I assume the incapacity for thinking and willing in the very definition [the essentialist definition] of matter itself and of corporeal substance . . . If this definition is accepted, it is clear that matter cannot think. And this is a sort of metaphysical conclusion that follows with absolute certainty from accepting the definition." One sees the danger of essentialist definitions even for a man as great as Boscovich. However, he is right in defending himself against the suspicion that the acceptance of unextended dynamic intensities such as Leibniz's monads commits him to accepting a Leibnizian attitude towards the mind-body problem.

Thus essentialism was not superseded, neither as a result of Newton's theory, nor of Boscovich's. It was superseded, however, as a result of Maxwell's field theory of electromagnetism. Maxwell tried first to base his theory on a mechanical model of the ether. (This was still essentialism.) At first this mechanical model was a great help for the formulation and interpretation of his equations (which described the interdependence of electrical and magnetic forces). But the *mechanical* essentialist model became very clumsy, and in the end it became inconsistent: it broke down. The equations, on the other hand, were consistent, and testable. They were tested by Heinrich Hertz.

Thus here was a most successful and important physical theory whose mechanical substance and essence had evaporated. It was the end of essentialism. Nobody could ask any longer what self-evident intuition lay "behind" the equations: the equations simply stated the laws of electromagnetic interaction, and thereby explained the phenomena in question: just as Newton's equations had stated the laws of mechanics, and thereby explained the phenomena – as he had always insisted.

Thus with Newton, and now, plainly, with Maxwell, the idea that there must be intuitively self-evident ultimate principles (such as, allegedly, those of a clockwork mechanism) behind explanation, had been exploded. Successive "self-evident" intuitions as to the "true nature" of matter had been shattered. So it became possible to ask of any suggested explanation the question "Can this be further explained?", or, more simply, "Why?". (Since this is always possible, no ultimate explanation can be attained.) What there was of value in essentialism – the desire to discover *structures behind appearances*, and the search for *simple* theories – was fully accommodated by the method of conjectural explanation.

The success of Maxwell's theory led for a time to a turning of the tables: instead of a mechanical explanation of electromagnetism, an electromagnetic theory of matter and of mechanics was for a time (especially after H.A. Lorentz[3]) generally accepted. In fact, quantum mechanics started its career as part of this electromagnetic theory of matter. But this theory also broke down (with Yukawa's theory of non-electrical nuclear forces).

In this way, modern physics became non-essentialistic and pluralistic. Almost certainly, this pluralism is not the last word. There is the (generalized) law of the conservation of energy and momentum; and this makes a monistic simplification hopeful. Such a monistic simplification of the theories of matter and the various kinds of forces would be a tremendous success, and it is being tried. But I conjecture that the essentialist "what is" question will in time disappear for ever.

For a long time, essentialism had been identified by all parties, including its positivist opponents, with the view that the task of science (and of philosophy) was to reveal the ultimate hidden reality behind the appearances. It has turned out that although there are such hidden realities, none of them is ultimate; although some are on a deeper level than others.[4]

---

3 Additional remarks on these developments can be found in the text following note 3 to section 3, above.

4 See also my [1963(a)], chapter 3, pp. 114–17, and [1972(a)], chapter 5, pp. 196–204.

52. The Association of Ideas as an Ultimate Explanation

Descartes was an interactionist, but he was also a dualist, and questions connected with the extended substance, matter or body, may suggest similar questions concerning the unextended substance, mind. Mind and matter interact; but from a cosmic point of view, it is even more important that matter (bodily events, bodily movements) may interact with matter; for Descartes, as we know, by push. Thus the question arises: What about mind interacting with mind, that is, mental events with mental events?

An answer to this question which has been very influential is a theory which in its intuitive simplicity and persuasiveness may be compared to the theory that bodies push each other mechanically. It is the theory that ideas (regarded as elements of the mental substance) pull each other mechanically (into the focus of consciousness). This theory of a mechanism of the mind had a tremendous influence. It starts, I believe, with Aristotle; it is important in Descartes and Spinoza,[1] and even more so in the school of British empiricists, Locke, Berkeley, Hume (and especially his younger contemporary Hartley whose main work [1749] was published ten years after Hume's *Treatise*); it achieved something like dominance with Bentham and James Mill, and with Herbart; and it remained a powerful element in Freud's psychoanalysis, and even in the *Gestalt* school (although it was highly critical of associationism). But it was John Stuart Mill ([1865 (b)], p. 190) who was, I suppose, the first to say explicitly what had been at least since Spinoza implicit in the claims of the associationists: that the "laws of association" represented a mechanism of the mind analogous to, and of equal importance with, the laws of motion (and of gravity in Newton's mechanics) of physical bodies. The "ideas" – simple or complex – were the atoms and molecules of the mind, subject to a mechanics of association, and their complexes, bound by association, were subject to a "mental chemistry".

(All this, I suggest, is the most terribly misleading doctrine which has emerged from Cartesian dualism under the influence of later parallelistic ideas. Nothing, I suggest, can be further from the truth. The doctrine of ideas as particles of mind, and of mental mechanisms – all this is far removed from reality; as far as can be. Organisms love and hate, solve problems, try out valuations. World 2 is indeed very different from World 1.)

---

[1] Descartes himself tried to explain memory and association physiologically (see section 41 above). Spinoza has no such theory. In his *Ethics* II, prop. 7, he establishes the parallelist principle "The order and connection of the ideas is the same as the order and connection of the [physical] things" and in II, prop. 18, he formulates the principle of association by the coincidence of events.

It is interesting that, just as the theory of push is intended as an ultimate explanation in terms of the essence of bodies (push is due to extension), the theory of the association of ideas can be presented as an ultimate explanation in terms of the essence of mind: *thinking;* which is connecting ideas.[2]

Locke may be said to be sceptical of ultimate explanation and of essentialism (*Essay* III, vi, 3) in general and especially of the Cartesian theory of extension and push (II, xiii, 11). Yet in spite of this, his theory of thinking – of knowing, of judging – can be understood as *an ultimate and essentialist theory of thinking by association.* (II, xxxiii, 5ff.) Thought is, essentially, a joining or separating of ideas (IV, v, 2; IV, i, 2 and 5; etc.) As in categorical Aristotelian subject-predicate propositions, two ideas (say, man and mortal) are joined or separated by a copula (man is mortal; man is not mortal). The copula is a sign of the positive or negative *association.* (Cp. IV, v, 5.) Thus the laws of thinking (or of thinking according to Aristotle) are laws of the association of ideas; where *ideas* are Aristotelian *terms.* Locke turned Aristotelian subject-predicate logic into a psychological theory.

Let us look briefly at the prehistory of associationism.

In Plato, forms or ideas are of course not mental objects (or World 2 objects) but World 3 objects existing independently of anybody's grasping them; the grasping of an idea is not, in its turn, called "idea". Similarly in Aristotle, forms or ideas or essences are inherent in things: a stone sculpture consists of matter *and* form; and the inherent form or idea is its essence.

But in Descartes, in Spinoza, and in Locke, ideas are in the mind, and are the atoms or elements of thought processes: they are the mental conceptions or notions which we use in thinking of the essential properties of things; they are the elements of thinking. Thus the historical problem arises: how did the transition take place which leads to the theory of *the association of ideas*? (I consciously neglect, among other things, the history of the theory of recollection by similarity – of knowledge = recognition = recollection – which of course is due to Plato's *Meno* and *Phaedo.*)

Aristotle (*On Memory* 451b12-452b7) has an associationist theory of recollection. He does not speak there of the association of "ideas", yet I think that it was Aristotle who first placed ideas (forms, essences), which according to him normally inhere in World 1 objects, into our minds (though not as its atoms or elements or elementary experiences). If I am not mistaken it happened as follows.

---

[2] As I have mentioned in dialogue VIII, the adoption of causation by push in the physical world, and causation by association in the mental world, reinforced the theory of psychophysical parallelism.

According to Aristotle (*De anima* 430a20), "Actual knowledge is identical with its object". (Cp. my [1966] vol. i, p. 314; also Theophrastus *De sensu* 1 = DK 28 A46.) He explains more fully (*Metaphysics* 1075a1) that knowledge is identical with the form or essence of its object, omitting the matter. Or as he puts it (*De anima* 431b26-432a1): "The contents of the sensorium and of the scientific grasp of the soul . . . must either be identical with the objects themselves or with their forms or essences. But they are not identical with the objects; for the stone does not exist in the soul but only its form or essence or idea". In this way, we find that the Platonic ideas which for Plato exist only in a World 3, and which for Aristotle are inherent in World 1, also come to exist, for Aristotle, in World 2. I suspect that is the step which turns the term "idea" into a mental or psychological term. It explains its psychological usage in Descartes, Spinoza, Locke, and the moderns (a use against which Schopenhauer protested – I think wrongly, in view of Aristotle's use). Once the important term "idea" had become a term for something contained in the mind, it is not surprising that ideas became the mind's main or even the only elements, and that a theory of the mind resulted such as Hume's, according to which there were no minds but only ideas, and bundles of ideas.

53. Neutral Monism

While the psycho-physical parallelism of the occasionalists, but also of Spinoza and of Leibniz may be described as a metaphysical parallelism, that of the so-called neutral monists, whose classical representatives are Hume, Mach, and Russell (in one of his phases), may be described as an epistemological parallelism. I shall present this view without following very closely the actual historical forms in which it was presented by David Hume and by Ernst Mach. As in the case of metaphysical parallelism, its proponents offer us a painless, non-interactionist theory of the relation of mind and body.

According to neutral monism, there is no body or mind in the sense in which the metaphysical philosophers conceived them. There is hardly a physical world, or a mental world. What there really is is a physical ordering of (neutral) things or events and a mental ordering of *the same* things or events. That is to say, the things or events are considered to be "physical" or to be "mental" according to the context in which we conceive them. This, the neutral monist could argue, must be so, because "physical" means somehow or other something that comes within the scope of physical theory; "physical" is something that can be grasped or explained or dealt with by physical theory with its concepts of physical action, physical interaction, and so on. Similarly, "mental" is that which can be explained with the help of theories which we hold about the mind – theories of psychology and about human action. So we have two realms of theories – physical theories and psychological theories – or two systems for ordering things. The physical theories order things in what we may call a physical order or a physical interpretation, and the mental theories order the same things in a mental order or a mental interpretation. Whether we call something physical or mental will therefore depend on the order in which we conceive it. Certain simplexes, or elements, more especially, may be interpreted as belonging to physical complexes or to mental complexes. But the elements themselves are supposed to be neutral, just because they may, alternatively, become parts of either physical complexes or mental complexes.

In putting things this way we have given no indication at all of what these supposedly neutral elements really are. However, neutral monists have usually taken the elements to be something like impressions or ideas or sensations. Mach's term *"Empfindungen"* – which is his term for these elements – can be perhaps translated by "sensations" (or perhaps by "feelings"). The best way to describe neutral monism (if we wish to start from the elements rather than from the theories) is this.

The elements may be taken as "data" or as "given". These data may be bundled together or lumped together in two different ways, as will be shown by means of a two-dimensional diagram. Let us represent the elements as points on a plane (represented by crosses); the two ways of bundling them together can then be represented by drawing vertical and horizontal columns through the plane; various minds are represented by various vertical columns, and various material objects by various horizontal columns. This may be seen from the diagram on the top of the next page.

In this diagram, every element belongs to both orderings, but this is, of course, an oversimplification; for an element, although belonging to a mind, may not belong to a body – for example, if this element is something like a feeling of relaxation or a feeling of joy. On the other hand, an element, although belonging to a physical body, may perhaps not belong to any mind. (Although this possibility is difficult for the neutral monist to admit.) Or it may belong to some physical event which is not necessarily a body; for example, a flash of lightning. The main point of the theory is that the physical world and the mental world are both *theoretical constructions* out of a given material, and that the various entities belonging to these worlds are also theoretical constructions out of this given material.

	Jack's self	Karl's self	Tom's self	Jeremy's self	Freddy's self
This table	×		×	× ×	×
This book	× ×	×		×	
Jack's body	×	× ×			××
Jack's pen	× ×		×	×	
Karl's body	×	×	×		
Tom's body			×× ×		×
Tom's pipe	×	×	×		×
Jeremy's body		× ×× ×		×	
Freddy's body			×		× ×
Freddy's pencil			× ×		×

Now how does the mind-body problem appear in this view? As with Spinozism, we have here a view which is fundamentally monistic: it knows only one really fundamental kind of reality. But while in Spinoza's theory this fundamental reality is God, in neutral monism it is "the given". Furthermore, while Spinoza says that body and mind are two attributes of his fundamental reality, in neutral monism body and mind are two constructs made from the given. In Spinoza we have actual causation, causal interaction of bodies with bodies and of mind with mind, but no interaction between mind and body. In neutral monism we have physical theories, that is to say, theories which explain how the physical constructs interact with other physical constructs; and we have mental theories, that is to say, theories which explain how mental constructs interact with other mental constructs. But the question of an interaction between the mental constructs and the physical constructs does not arise, because action and interaction are theoretical concepts, and the two theories — the physical theory and the mental theory — are each self-contained. No interaction between them arises unless we introduce a new (unnecessary) theory. Such a theory would mean, from the neutral monist point of view, that there would not be only the two theories but also another one: a theory of a higher type, relating the two theories rather than the elements, the given.

But in neutral monism there is no place for such an interactionist theory: interaction can be, and therefore is to be, avoided. Thus the relation between the mental and the physical becomes parallelistic. We can describe it as an epistemological parallelism, as opposed to the metaphysical parallelism of Spinoza or of Leibniz, in so far as the reality with which it starts is supposed to be something which is epistemologically ultimate or "given".

The view that physical objects are constructs was first proposed by sensationalist or phenomenalist epistemology, which tried to reduce all our empirical knowledge to sensations or "impressions". From the point of view of this epistemology, neutral monism is not merely a painless theory of the mind-body relation but an ingenious as well as natural way of looking at it.

What speaks in favour of neutral monism? It is, I believe, true that nearly all the things which a naive view would consider as simply existing are in a sense theoretical interpretations or constructions. However, while neutral monism might seem attractive, especially to a thoroughgoing empiricist, I do not think that it is a satisfactory theory. Its allegedly neutral elements are only called "neutral": they are, unavoidably, *mental*; and so is, clearly, the procedure of the "construction" of physical objects. Thus "neutral" monism is so only in name. In fact, it is a subjective idealism, very much in the Berkeleyan manner.

54. The Identity Theory After Leibniz: From Kant to Feigl

In Leibniz's theory the things in themselves are monads; and monads are essentially, though not all to the same degree, minds or spirits. They are thinking substances whose thought may be more or less clear and distinct, more or less conscious. According to the degree of clarity and distinctness of their state of consciousness, the substances are ordered in a hierarchy. Organisms each have one ruling or dominant monad — their soul. Lower things such as stones may not have even a dominant monad. This theory is clearly a form of panpsychism, with all its difficulties. It is also a theory that takes things in themselves to be of a mental or of a spiritual character (and *vice versa*). And it regards matter as the (well founded) outside appearance of collections or accumulations of mind-like things in themselves. If we take Leibniz's view of the physical world as modified and clarified by Boscovich and Kant (see section 51 above), together with Leibniz's view that the monads (the atoms) are mind-like, then we reach a position which is very similar to, if not identical with, the modern form of the identity theory. This theory can be found in many German philosophers, from Kant, Herbart and Fechner to Moritz Schlick; and in the work of Bertrand Russell, Bernhard Rensch and, I believe, Herbert Feigl. It has been discussed and criticized in sections 22 and 23, above.

Regarded as a modification of Leibniz's view, the identity theory is, in brief, that the monads, the mind-like entities – or perhaps the experiences, the sensations, the thoughts – are the things in themselves. We know either our selves, or our experiences ("raw feels" as Feigl, following Tolman, calls them) immediately "by acquaintance". Seen from outside – or perhaps taken as the basis of logical constructions – these experiences are the objects of the theoretical physical world: the world of physical objects which we do not know immediately or by acquaintance, but rather "by description", through our theoretical constructions. This world of physical particles, atoms, and molecules is clearly our construction, our theoretical invention. This also holds for organisms and their parts, such as the brain.

The identity theory as here sketched must, for obvious reasons, accept and incorporate a physical theory – the physical theory of the day; for it is this theory which constructs the physical world, according to the identity theory. In this sense, the identity theory may be described as "physicalistic". However, it may be equally well, or even more properly, described as a form of spiritualism or mentalism since it regards as real, or as things in themselves, the mind and other mind-like entities.

The mature philosophy of Kant was strangely divided into two parts: theoretical or speculative philosophy and practical or moral philosophy. The first, theoretical philosophy, implied that we could say nothing about things in themselves: we could neither assert nor deny their spiritual character. The second, moral or practical philosophy, asserted that morality makes us believe in God and in an immortal soul; and it makes us believe that souls are things in themselves. (It leaves it open whether or not all things in themselves are souls.) Thus although Kant's epistemology is very different from Leibniz's, his physics as well as his (morally based) theory of the soul comes very close to that of Leibniz – closer perhaps than he himself realized.

However this may be, several post-Kantian philosophers in Germany gave up the Kantian thesis that knowledge (that is, theoretical knowledge) of things in themselves was impossible; and most of them made the things in themselves soul-like. They claimed, as against what Kant said, that we can obtain some knowledge (knowledge by acquaintance) of a thing in itself — that is, of our ego — by immediate self-experience (by way of "raw feels").

The outcome of all this was, broadly speaking, two theories, a monistic one that we could say goes back to Spinoza, and a pluralistic and individualistic one that we could say goes back to Leibniz. The first assumes that individuality is a matter of appearance rather than of reality. Its main representative among the followers of Kant was Schopenhauer.[1] The second assumes that individuality is real, and that things in themselves are individuals. It seems that this was Kant's own view. It was the view of Fechner, and also of Lotze. It was essentially the view of Schlick, and of Russell. All these were greatly influenced by Leibniz. (It is interesting that Schlick [1925], p. 209; [1974], p. 227, draws attention to the influence of Leibniz on Russell.)

In our own time, the theory was renewed, and thoroughly and fairly discussed, by Herbert Feigl, who had been a student and a close friend of Schlick's. Feigl brought the theory up to date, and combined it with a physicalist position. He has done much in the way of supporting it by new arguments. He is aware of its similarities with the views of Leibniz and of Kant, although he seems to think that these similarities are partly accidental (a view in which I cannot follow him). This is connected with the fact that he thinks of himself more as a materialist than a spiritualist.

Some detailed criticism of the identity theory as a physicalistic theory has been given in section 23 above. My objection to it, as a mentalistic theory, may be briefly summarized as follows. The theory does not agree with what our present cosmology presents as a fact: a world in which there was, for eons, no trace of life or mind, in which first life and later mind emerged, and even a World 3. I admit that all this can be explained away; but I feel that it has to be taken as a starting point for the mind-body problem. I admit the intellectual attractiveness of monism. I also admit that some form of monism may become acceptable one day; but I do not think it probable that this situation will arise.

[1] Schopenhauer, in section 18 of volume 1 of *The World as Will and Representation* not only proposed an identity theory ("The act of will and the action of the body . . . are one and the same thing, though given [to us] in two totally different ways"), but he used the term "identity": he speaks of "the identity of body and will".

55. Linguistic Parallelism

Another theory that avoids interaction, and that may be regarded as a psycho-physical parallelism, is the two-language theory. According to this theory there is only one world; only one reality. But there are two ways of speaking about this one reality: one way of speaking about it is to treat it as physical and another is to treat it as mental. This is a view which is very closely related to neutral monism. In the place of the two theories or the two ways of bundling elements together of neutral monism, it puts two languages or language systems or two ways of talking about reality. *Theories* and *language systems* are of course very closely related, and this indicates the close relation between linguistic parallelism and epistemological parallelism. Linguistic parallelism can take on different forms according to what is meant by saying that there are two languages in which we speak about the same reality. I will distinguish three versions of linguistic parallelism.

According to the first version, by two languages we mean simply two different kinds of vocabularies. Both vocabularies may be used in the same language, but we can nevertheless clearly distinguish two classes of words, that is to say, mental words and physical words.

According to the second version, we have two vocabularies because we have two theories, and within these two theories we have two sets of concepts which are meaningful only within their respective theoretical contexts.

According to the third version, the situation is a little different. In this interpretation, the talk about the two languages is taken as a kind of metaphor to indicate that if one man speaks about bodies, and another man speaks about minds, then these two men can never really communicate with one another. They are like a Chinese man and an Englishman who have never learned one another's language. Thus the impossibility of cross-communication between a mentalist and a physicalist language is here the main point: this theory amounts to the view that there are here two languages between which no communication is possible. But why, one could ask, is no communication possible? After all, some Englishmen have learned to speak Chinese, and many more Chinese have learned to speak and to write English. If these two languages refer to the same world – if the two persons speak different languages but live in the same world – then it should be possible for them to establish some sort of basic communication, some sort of translation from one language to the other language, however different their interpretations of the world may be to start with.

These are the three main versions known to me of the two-language view or of linguistic parallelism. The attitude of linguistic parallelism towards the mind-body problem is again of course that interaction is impossible. It is impossible because causal action must be described in a language, and we have only either a physical or a mental language available. The tendency of this view, as of neutral monism, is to solve the mind-body problem by explaining away what up to and including Descartes was an obvious fact — the fact of interaction — by showing that this obvious fact is not a fact but a misinterpretation. According to this view, it is a misinterpretation of language.

Why is linguistic parallelism attractive? First of all, because it presents some sort of solution of a very intractable problem, by showing that the problem really does not arise or that it arises out of linguistic misunderstandings. Thus this view is particularly attractive to the linguistic school of philosophy, especially to those language analysts who still say that philosophical problems in general arise out of linguistic misunderstandings. A second reason why this view is attractive is that there is undoubtedly an element of truth in it. Linguistic parallelism emphasizes the view that all ideas of interaction arise out of an inadmissible mixing of two languages. If you mix two languages, this view suggests, you may not get just another language, but, rather, something like meaningless pseudo-statements. Thus Socrates might be said to have suggested (see section 46, above) that it is inadmissible to say that he stayed in prison because his legs did not take him away.

I now come to my criticism of linguistic parallelism, and I will start with the first and second versions; that is to say, with the versions in which the two languages are two vocabularies, or two sets of concepts, connected by theories, or meaningful within the context of certain theories. My comment here is that this may be so. But, I would ask, how is it that these theories are supposed to be unrelated? Take, for example, the characteristic concepts or the characteristic vocabulary of three theories like optics, acoustics and mechanics. You have here three different theories, each with its own peculiar vocabulary and with its own peculiar language. But this does not prevent physicists from trying to unify these theories. They may try, for example, to explain acoustics mechanically, or to develop a theory of radiation (an optical theory) which is connected with the mechanics of the atom. What is more, optics has been linked with mechanical effects, such as light pressure. And acoustics, of course, also has mechanical effects (for example, resonance), and we can produce acoustic effects by mechanical means. And we can also produce radiant heat, and therefore something within the province of optics, by mechanical means.

All this shows that we have every reason to try to develop connections between theories which at first may have arisen independently, and which use different languages. And it shows that the use of different languages does not establish that there may be no interaction or interconnection between the entities treated by these different theories.

I will now discuss the third version of linguistic parallelism. Here the point was that the two languages are supposed to be (more or less) untranslatable. I have already indicated that I have certain criticisms of this thesis – particularly if the two languages refer to the same world or the same reality, and if the speakers of the languages have certain aims or problems in common. But let us put these reservations aside, and work with the assumption that the two languages are not intertranslatable.

It is clear what this means for the mind-body problem. Statements in the one language like "I feel cold" and in the other like "My brain is in a certain state", are not, it is assumed, inter-translatable. No dualist, I think, would disagree.

But it may be possible for us to establish connections between these two different sorts of statements. We may discover, for example, that there is a universal connection between a certain brain state – or certain sorts of brain states – and certain sorts of pain. Nobody (except possibly a materialist) would wish to suggest that in so doing we have inter-translated the two statements. What we have done, rather, is that we have produced a rudimentary theory about psycho-physical interaction. We have done exactly what linguistic parallelism was trying to avoid.

To put this point another way, if two languages are not translatable, and especially if we are told (as we are by linguistic parallelists) that they both refer to the same reality, then it will clearly be interesting to ask what the relations are – if any – between the "facts" of the different languages. This, in turn, will lead us to try to develop a language in which we can talk about facts of both kinds, and pose problems about their possible interrelations.

To repudiate all of this, and to insist on the maintenance of a parallelism, appears to me as obscurantist. Consider an example. Take the case of someone who is accidentally poisoned, as a result of eating two different types of food that happen to contain preservatives which react together to produce some toxic substance. If, say, the coroner wants to investigate the case he will talk in terms both of chemical theory (a theory of World 1) and of the human aspects of it (World 2) and the legal aspects of it (World 3), and about their *interrelations*. The mixture of these languages, far from creating some sort of confusion, will itself provide a statement about the event in question. But even the purely chemical account could be given only if we allow it to start from, and to be constantly guided by, the "human" and legal aspects of the problem. For, from a strictly scientific point of view, there is nothing to tell the chemist *which* of all the many different chemical reactions going on in the region of space and time in question are here *relevant* to the problem — the fatal issue — and which are not.

It will be remembered that we said that linguistic parallelism is attractive because there are some cases in which pseudo-problems may arise because of a mixing of languages. This fact is perfectly explicable, however, even if we turn down the two-language interpretation. For such cases arise out of a confusion of *theories*, or from asking confused questions. It is better to sort out such problems *ad hoc* when the need arises than to construct a philosophical system with the dubious aim of preventing them from arising.

56. A Final Look at Materialism

My discussion of linguistic parallelism brings us quite naturally to the ideas that I have earlier called "radical materialism" and "promissory materialism". For it is a fairly simple step, from the two-language theory, to suggest the following:

There are two languages, a "mental" language and a "physical" language. However, we may be able to *eliminate* the mental language, by philosophical and scientific analysis, either now ("radical materialism") or at some unspecified time in the future ("promissory materialism"). (Alternatively, of course, a mentalist or spiritualist might suggest an analogous programme for the elimination of the physical language.)

I am not very impressed with such suggestions, for reasons that I have explained in chapter P3, even though I am in favour of the idea that we should attempt scientific reductions.

However, let us have a brief, final look at materialism, and its post-Cartesian history.

Descartes was a mechanist and a materialist as far as the world without man was concerned. Man alone was not just a machine, for he consisted of body and soul.

Those who felt that this kind of reasoning exaggerated the gulf between man and the animals had two ways of reacting. They could say, as Arnauld suggests in his *Objections to Descartes's Meditations*, that animals are more than machines, and have souls; that is, some kind of consciousness.[1] Or they

[1] See Haldane and Ross [1931], vol. ii, p. 85. (Descartes's reply is on pp. 103f.) It is interesting that in the *Port-Royal Logic* (Pt iii, end of chapter xiii) Arnauld gives a syllogism (in

could be more radical than Descartes, and say that man is a machine since he is an animal.

One would not, however, expect anybody who believes in the superiority of man over other animals to hold both that *animals are more than machines* and that *man is a machine.* This, however, was the position taken up tentatively by Pierre Bayle, and after him by Julien Offray de la Mettrie, the famous author of *Man a Machine* [1747]. It is less well known that La Mettrie published, two years later, a book under the title *Animals More than Machines (Les animaux plus que machines).*

It is thus necessary to look a little more closely at the materialism of this most famous of materialists. It turns out that he certainly taught that the soul depended on the body. But he did not deny consciousness (as Descartes had denied it to animals); neither to animals nor to men. In fact he proposed something like an empirical and naturalistic view, involving evolutionary emergence. (His view may perhaps he described as bordering on epiphenomenalism.) He allowed purposive activity to animals and men. His main thesis was that the state of the soul depends upon that of the body.[2]

Although La Mettrie's influence upon the development of a materialist man-machine theory was certainly very great, he was not himself a radical materialist, for he did not deny the existence of subjective experience. It is interesting to note that many of those who call themselves materialists or physicalists are not radical materialists – neither Haeckel nor Schlick nor Anthony Quinton nor Herbert Feigl, nor, indeed, the "dialectical materialists". Nor are, I think, those who merely deny (as I am also inclined to do) the existence of disembodied minds, nor those who emphasize that mind is the product of the brain, or of evolution; nor those who suggest that matter, if highly organized, can think. It is not that I regard all these views as acceptable (as I have explained in chapter P3). Rather, I think that it is important to remember that the proponents of such views, while sometimes calling themselves materialists, accept the existence of consciousness, even though they belittle its importance.

Whether the theories of Democritus and Epicurus are properly described

---

Celarent) establishing that the soul of an animal does not think. Thus he did not commit himself to the soulless animal, but only to an unthinking animal soul, making perhaps allowance for perception. (See Leonora C. Rosenfield [1941], p. 281.)

[2] One can well interpret La Mettrie as an interactionist (in contradistinction, for example, to Malebranche) and as a vitalist with respect to animal physiology (in contradistinction to Descartes). La Mettrie himself refers to Claude Perrault and Thomas Willis as his predecessors. (See the [1960] edition of *L'Homme Machine,* p. 188.) But these two were animists, in different ways.

as radical materialism is difficult to say. They are, it seems, radical materialists in their programme, but are hardly so in its execution. They believed in the existence of the soul, which they tried, as did many before them, to explain as very subtle matter, but (as I have indicated in sections 44 and 46, above) I think that they ascribed to mind a moral status different from that of the body.

In fact, there are only three types of materialism known to me which do deny the existence of consciousness: the theories of such thinkers as Quine, who explicitly adopt a form of radical behaviourism; the theory of Armstrong and Smart (described above in section 25); and what I have called "promissory materialism" (see section 28). The last of these seems to me not to merit further discussion. As to the first two, Schopenhauer described such radical materialism as "the philosophy of the subject who forgot to take account of himself". Although this is a good remark, it does not go far enough; for (as we have seen in section 18) there are perfectly objective regularities testable by intersubjective behaviour which the radical materialist and the radical behaviourist tend to forget — or to explain away in a somewhat far-fetched manner.

The main motives of all materialistic theories are intuitive. One such intuitive motive I have briefly mentioned and criticized in section 7. It is the reductionist belief that there can be no "downward causation". The other is the intuition of the causal closedness of the physical World 1 — an intuitively most compelling view which, I suggest, is clearly refuted by the technical, scientific, and artistic achievements of mankind; in other words, by the existence of World 3. Even those who think that mind is "just" the causal product of self-organizing matter should feel that it is difficult to regard the Ninth Symphony in this way, or *Othello,* or the theory of gravitation.

I have said nothing so far about a question which has been debated quite a lot: whether we shall one day build a machine that can think. It has been much discussed under the title "Can Computers Think?". I would say without hesitation that they can not, in spite of my unbounded respect for A. M. Turing who thought the opposite. We *may* perhaps be able to teach a chimpanzee to speak — in a very rudimentary way; and if mankind survives long enough we may even speed up natural selection and breed by artificial selection some species which may compete with us. We also may perhaps be able in time to create an artificial micro-organism capable of reproducing itself in a well-prepared environment of enzymes. So much that is incredible has happened that it would be rash to assert this to be impossible. But I predict that we shall not be able to build electronic computers with conscious subjective experience.

As I wrote many years ago [1950 (b) & (c)] at the very beginning of the debate about computers, a computer is just a glorified pencil. Einstein once said "my pencil is cleverer than I". What he meant could perhaps be put thus: armed with a pencil, we can be more than twice as clever as we are without. Armed with a computer (a typical World 3 object[3]), we can perhaps be more than a hundred times as clever as we are without; and with improving computers there need not be an upper limit to this.

Turing [1950] said something like this: specify the way in which you believe that a man is superior to a computer and I shall build a computer which refutes your belief. Turing's challenge should not be taken up; for any sufficiently precise specification could be used in principle to programme a computer. Also, the challenge was about behaviour – admittedly including verbal behaviour – rather than about subjective experience. (For example, it would be easy to programme a computer in such a way that it responds with any desired statement to the stimulus of my figures 1, 2 and 3 in section 18 which show optical illusions.)

I do not really believe that we shall succeed in creating life artificially; but after having reached the moon and landed a spaceship or two on Mars, I realize that this disbelief of mine means very little. But computers are totally different from brains, whose function is not primarily to compute but to guide and balance an organism and help it to stay alive. It is for this reason that the first step of nature towards an intelligent mind was the creation of life, and I think that should we artificially create an intelligent mind, we would have to follow the same path.

[3] The "reason" that the programmer and the artificial intelligence worker discern in the computer was put there by us; that the computer can do *more* than we can is due to the fact that we put into the computer powerful operating principles; in fact, autonomous World 3 principles. (See section 21 above and also my [1953(a)].)

Chapter P6 Summary

To sum up the main results of my contribution, the following points seem to me of interest.

(1) The criticism of materialism, especially section 21.

(2) The criticisms of parallelism and the identity theory. (Sections 20, 23, 24.)

(3) The defence of interaction and the thesis that parallelism is the result of Descartes's mistaken theory of causation. (Sections 48–9.)

(4) The rejection of the view that the theory of the existence of mind is just another ideology. (Section 44.)

(5) The positive remarks in favour of emergence and the openness of World 1 and the incompleteness of all scientific theories. (Sections 7–9 and my [1974(z_2)].)

(6) The existence of "downward causation" has been asserted by D. T. Campbell [1974] and especially by R. W. Sperry [1969], [1973]. Sperry even suggests that any action of the mind upon the brain is merely an instance of downward causation. Examples of downward causation are given in sections 7–9. (See also pp. 540 f., below.)

(7) Any planned action such as the navigating of a ship (Plato's example) is an example not only of downward causation but also of the (indirect) causal influence of World 3 conjectures, and of moral decisions, upon World 1.

(8) Building and tuning a musical instrument is such an action. It invests a World 1 object with World 3 dispositional properties. It is this fact which makes Simmias's theory of the soul (see section 46) so interesting.

A final point which is mainly implicit in my chapters deserves to be made explicit:

(9) Natural selection, and selection pressure, are usually thought of as the results of a more or less violent struggle for life.

But with the emergence of mind, of World 3, and of theories, this changes. We may let our theories fight it out – we may let our theories die in our stead. From the point of view of natural selection, the main function of mind and of World 3 is that they make possible the application of the method of trial and the elimination of error without the violent elimination of ourselves: in this lies the great survival value of mind and of World 3. Thus in bringing about the emergence of mind, and World 3, natural selection transcends itself and its originally violent character. With the emergence of World 3, selection need no longer be violent: we can eliminate false theories by non-violent criticism. Non-violent cultural evolution is not just a utopian dream; it is, rather, a possible result of the emergence of mind through natural selection.

Bibliography to Part I

ALEXANDER OF APHRODISIAS — *Commentary on Aristotle's Metaphysics*

ALLEN R. E. C. & FURLEY D. J. (eds) [1975] *Studies in Presocratic Philosophy*, volume II, Routledge & Kegan Paul, London.

ARISTOTLE — *De anima.*
De caelo.
De generatione animalium.
Metaphysics.
Minor Works.
Nicomachean Ethics.
On Dreams.
On Memory.
Physics.
Physiognomics.
Posterior Analytics.

[1952] *Select Fragments; The Works of Aristotle*, ed. Sir David Ross, volume XII, Clarendon Press, Oxford.

ARMSTRONG D. M. [1968] *A Materialist Theory of the Mind*, Routledge & Kegan Paul, London.

[1973] *Belief, Truth and Knowledge*, Cambridge University Press, London.

ARNAULD D. & NICOLE P. [1662] *La Logique, ou l'art de penser (= Port-Royal Logic).*

AUGUSTINE ST. — *Confessions.*
De libero arbitrio.
De quantitate animae.
Soliloquia.

AUSTIN J. L. [1962] *How to Do Things With Words*, Clarendon Press, Oxford.

AYALA F. J. & DOBZHANSKY T. (eds) [1974] *Studies in the Philosophy of Biology*, Macmillan, London.

BAHLE J. [1936] *Der musikalische Schaffensprozeß*, S. Hirzel, Leipzig.

[1939] *Eingebung und Tat im musikalischen Schaffen*, S. Hirzel, Leipzig.

BAILEY C. [1926] *Epicurus: The Extant Remains*, Clarendon Press, Oxford.

[1928] *The Greek Atomists and Epicurus*, Clarendon Press, Oxford.

BELOFF J. [1962] *The Existence of Mind*, MacGibbon & Kee, London.

[1965] "The Identity Hypothesis: A Critique", in SMYTHIES (ed.) [1965], pp. 35–54.

[1973] *Psychological Sciences: A Review of Modern Psychology*, Crosby Lockwood Staples, London.

BERGSON H. [1896] *Matière et mémoire*, Alcan, Paris.

[1911] *Matter and Memory*, Macmillan, London.

BLACKMORE J. T. [1972] *Ernst Mach, His Life, Work and Influence*, University of California Press, Berkeley, Los Angeles and London.

BOHM D. [1957] *Causality and Chance in Modern Physics,* Routledge & Kegan Paul, London.

BOHR N., KRAMERS H. A. & SLATER J. C. [1924] "The quantum theory of radiation", *Philosophical Magazine, 47,* pp. 785–802.

BOSCOVICH R. [1745] *De Viribus Vivis.*

[1755] *De Lege Virium in Natura existentium.*

[1758] *Theoria philosophiae naturalis,* first edition, Vienna.

[1763] *Theoria philosophiae naturalis,* revised edition, Venice.

BRADLEY F. H. [1883] *The Principles of Logic,* Kegan Paul, London.

BÜHLER C. [1927] "Die ersten sozialen Verhaltungsweisen des Kindes", in BÜHLER, HETZER & TUDOR-HART [1927].

BÜHLER C., HETZER H. & TUDOR-HART B. H. [1927] *Soziologische und psychologische Studien über das erste Lebensjahr, Quellen und Studien zur Jugendkunde, 5,* G. Fischer, Jena.

BÜHLER K. [1918] "Kritische Musterung der neureren Theorien des Satzes", *Indogermanisches Jahrbuch, 6,* pp. 1–20.

[1934] *Sprachtheorie: die Darstellungsfunktion der Sprache,* Gustav Fischer, Jena.

BUNGE M. (ed.) [1967] *Quantum Theory and Reality,* Springer-Verlag, Berlin, Heidelberg, New York.

CAMPBELL D. T. [1974] "'Downward Causation' in Hierarchically Organized Biological Systems", in AYALA & DOBZHANSKY (eds) [1974], pp. 179–86.

CAMPBELL K. [1967] "Materialism" in EDWARDS (ed.) [1967(b)], volume 5, pp. 179–88.

CHOMSKY N. [1969] "Some Empirical Assumptions in Modern Philosophy of Language", in MORGENBESSER & others (eds) [1969], pp. 260–85.

CLIFFORD W. C. [1873] "On the hypotheses which lie at the bases of geometry", *Nature, 8,* Nos. 183–4, pp. 14–17 and 36–7. (Also in CLIFFORD [1882].)

[1879] *Lectures and Essays,* ed. L. Stephen & F. Pollock, Macmillan, London, two volumes.

[1882] *Mathematical Papers,* ed. R. Tucker, Macmillan, London.

[1886] *Lectures and Addresses,* 2nd edition, Macmillan, London.

COMPTON A. H. [1935] *The Freedom of Man,* Yale University Press, New Haven.

[1940] *The Human Meaning of Science,* The University of North Carolina Press, Chapel Hill.

COMTE A. [1830–42] *Cours de philosophie positive,* six volumes, Paris.

CRAIK K. J. W. [1943] *The Nature of Explanation,* Cambridge University Press, Cambridge.

CURTISS S. & others [1974] "The linguistic development of Genie", *Language, 50,* pp. 528–54.

DARWIN C. [1859] *The Origin of Species,* J. Murray, London.

[1959] *The Origin of Species, Variorum Text,* ed. Morse Peckham, University of Pennsylvania Press, Philadelphia.

DE GROOT A. D. [1965] *Thought and Choice in Chess,* Mouton, The Hague.

[1966] *Thought and Choice in Chess,* Basic Books, New York.

DELBRUCK M. [1974] *Anfänge der Wahrnehmung,* (Karl-August-Forster-Lectures, *10,* 1973), Akademie der Wissenschaften und der Literatur, Mainz/Franz Steiner Verlag, Wiesbaden.

DEMOCRITUS See DIELS & KRANZ [1951–2].

DENBIGH K. G. [1975] *The Inventive Universe,* Hutchinson, London.

DEREGOWSKI J. B. [1973] "Illusion and Culture", in GREGORY & GOMBRICH (ed.) [1973], pp. 161–91.

DESCARTES R. [1637] *Discourse on Method.*

[1641] *Meditations on First Philosophy.*

[1644] *Principles of Philosophy.*

[1649] *Les Passions de l'Ame.*

[1931] *The Philosophical Works of Descartes,* tr. E. S. Haldane & G. R. T. Ross, 2 volumes, Cambridge University Press.

DIELS H. (ed.) [1929] *Doxographi Graeci,* De Gruyter, Berlin & Leipzig.

& KRANZ W. (eds) [1951–2] *Die Fragmente der Vorsokratiker,* 6th edn., ed. W. Kranz, 3 vols, Weidmannsche Verlagsbuchhandlung, Berlin.

DIOGENES OF APPOLONIA See DIELS & KRANZ [1951–2].

DIOGENES LAERTIUS *Vitae philosophorum.*

DOBZHANSKY T. [1962] *Mankind Evolving,* Yale University Press, New Haven.

[1975] "Evolutionary Roots of Family Ethics and Group Ethics", in *The Centrality of Science and Absolute Values,* volume I, Proceedings of the Fourth International Conference on the Unity of the Sciences, New York, 1975, pp. 411–27.

DODDS E. R. [1951] *The Greeks and the Irrational,* University of California Press, Berkeley and Los Angeles.

ECCLES J. C. [1965] *The Brain and the Unity of Conscious Experience,* Cambridge University Press, London.

[1966(a)] "Cerebral Synaptic Mechanisms", in ECCLES (ed.) [1966(b)], pp. 24–58.

(ed.) [1966(b)] *Brain and Conscious Experience,* Springer-Verlag, Berlin, Heidelberg, New York.

[1970] *Facing Reality,* Springer-Verlag, Berlin, Heidelberg, New York.

[1973] *The Understanding of the Brain,* McGraw-Hill, New York.

EDWARDS P. [1967(a)] "Panpsychism", in EDWARDS (ed.) [1967(b)], volume 6, pp. 22–31.

(ed.) [1967(b)] *The Encyclopaedia of Philosophy,* The Macmillan Company & The Free Press, New York; and Collier-Macmillan, London.

EFRON R. [1966] "The conditioned reflex: a meaningless concept", *Perspectives in Biology and Medicine, 9,* part 4, pp. 488–514.

EINSTEIN A. [1905] "Über die von der molekularkinetischen Theorie der Wärme geforderte Bewegung von in ruhenden Flüssigkeiten suspendierten", *Annalen der Physik*, 4th series, XVII, pp. 549–60.

[1922] *The Meaning of Relativity*, Methuen, London.

[1956] *The Meaning of Relativity*, 6th edn., Methuen, London.

EPICURUS See BAILEY [1926].

ERASMUS D. [1624] *De libro arbitrio.*

ERIKSEN C. W. [1960] "Discrimination and learning without awareness", *Psychological Review, 67*, pp. 279–300.

EVANS-PRITCHARD E. E. [1937] *Witchcraft, Oracles and Magic Among the Azande*, Clarendon Press, Oxford.

FANZ R. L. [1961] "The origin of form perception", *Scientific American, 204*, May, pp. 66–72.

FEIGL H. [1967] *The 'Mental' and the 'Physical'*, University of Minnesota Press, Minneapolis.

[1975] "Russell and Schlick", *Erkenntnis, 9*, pp. 11–34.

FEIGL H. & BLUMBERG A. E. [1974] "Introduction", to SCHLICK [1974] pp. XVII–XXVI.

FEIGL H. & others (eds) [1958] *Concepts, Theories and the Mind-Body Problem, Minnesota Studies in the Philosophy of Science*, volume 2, University of Minnesota Press, Minneapolis.

FERCHMIN P. A. & others [1975] "Direct contact with enriched environment is required to alter cerebral weights in rats", *Journal of Comparative and Physiological Psychology, 88*, (1), pp. 360–7.

FISHER R. A. [1954] "Retrospect of the Criticisms of the Theory of Natural Selection", in HUXLEY & others (eds) [1954], pp. 84–98.

FLEW A. [1955] "The Third Maxim", *The Rationalist Annual*, pp. 63–6.

[1965] "A Rational Animal", in SMYTHIES (ed.) [1965], pp. 111–28.

FREEDMAN S. J. & HOLT R. A. [1975] "Tests of local hidden-variable theories in atomic physics", *Comments on Atomic and Molecular Physics, 5*, No. 2, pp. 55–62.

GIBSON J. J. [1966] *The Senses Considered as Perceptual Systems*, Houghton Mifflin, Boston.

[1968] *The Senses Considered as Perceptual Systems*, Allen & Unwin, London.

GLOBUS G. G. & others (eds) [1976] *Consciousness and the Brain*, Plenum Press, New York and London.

GOETHE J. W. *Die Wahlverwandtschaften.*

GOMBRICH E. H. [1960] *Art and Illusion*, Pantheon Books, New York.

[1962] *Art and Illusion*, 2nd edition, Phaidon Press, London.

[1973] "Illusion and Art", in GREGORY & GOMBRICH (eds) [1973].

GREGORY R. L. [1966] *Eye and Brain*, Weidenfeld & Nicolson, London.

& GOMBRICH E. (eds) [1973] *Illusion in Nature and Art*, Duckworth, London.

GUTHRIE W. K. C. [1962] *A History of Greek Philosophy: volume I, The Earlier Presocratics and the Pythagoreans*, Cambridge University Press, Cambridge.

[1969] *A History of Greek Philosophy: volume III, The Fifth-Century Enlightenment*, Cambridge University Press, Cambridge.

GUTTENPLAN S. (ed.) [1975] *Mind and Language*, Wolfson College Lectures 1974, Clarendon Press, Oxford.

HADAMARD J. [1945] *The Psychology of Invention in the Mathematical Field*, Princeton University Press, Princeton.

[1954] *The Psychology of Invention in the Mathematical Field*, Dover Books, New York.

HAECKEL E. [1878] "Zellseelen und Seelenzellen", *Deutsche Rundschau*, XVI, July – Sept. 1878, pp. 40 – 59.

HALDANE E. S. & ROSS G. R. T. [1931] See DESCARTES.

HALDANE J. B. S. [1930] *Possible Worlds*, Chatto & Windus, London.

[1932] *The Inequality of Man*, Chatto & Windus, London.

[1937] *The Inequality of Man*, Penguin Books, Harmondsworth.

[1954] "I repent an error", *The Literary Guide*, April 1954, pp. 7 and 29.

HARDIE W. F. R. [1936] *A Study in Plato*, Clarendon Press, Oxford.

[1968] *Aristotle's Ethical Theory*, Clarendon Press, Oxford.

[1976] "Concepts of consciousness in Aristotle", *Mind*, LXXXV, July 1976, pp. 388 – 411.

HARDY A. [1965] *The Living Stream*, Collins, London.

HARRÉ R. (ed.) [1975] *Problems of Scientific Revolution*, Clarendon Press, Oxford.

HARTLEY D. [1749] *Observations on Man, His Frame, His Duty and His Expectations*.

HAYEK F. A. von [1952] *The Sensory Order*, Routledge & Kegan Paul, London; University of Chicago Press, Chicago.

[1955] "Degrees of explanation", *British Journal for the Philosophy of Science*, *6*, pp. 209 – 25. (Also in Hayek [1967].)

[1967] *Studies in Philosophy, Politics and Economics*, Routledge & Kegan Paul, London.

HEFFERLINE R. F. & PERERA T. B. [1963] "Proprioceptive discrimination of a covert operant without its observation by the subject", *Science*, *139*, pp. 834 – 5.

HEISENBERG W. [1958] "The representation of nature in contemporary physics", *Daedalus*, *87*, pp. 95 – 108.

HELD R. & HEIN A. [1963] "Movement produced stimulation in the development of visually guided behaviour", *Journal of Comparative and Physiological Psychology*, *56*, pp. 872 – 6.

HILBERT D. [1901] "Mathematische Probleme", *Archiv der Mathematik und Physik*, third series, *1*, pp. 44–63 and 213–37.

[1902] "Mathematical problems", *Bulletin of the American Mathematical Society, 8*, pp. 437–79.

HIPPOCRATES *On the Sacred Disease.*

HOMER *Iliad.*

[1950] *Iliad*, tr. E. V. Rieu, Penguin Books, Harmondsworth.

Odyssey.

HOOK S. (ed.) [1960] *Dimensions of Mind*, New York University Press, New York.

[1961] *Dimensions of Mind*, Collier-Macmillan, New York.

HUME D. [1739] *A Treatise of Human Nature*, Books I and II.

[1740] *A Treatise of Human Nature*, Book III.

[1888] *A Treatise of Human Nature*, ed. L. A. Selby-Bigge, Clarendon Press, Oxford.

HUXLEY J. [1942] *Evolution. The Modern Synthesis*, Allen & Unwin, London.

HUXLEY J. & others (eds) [1954] *Evolution as a Process*, Allen & Unwin, London.

HUXLEY T. H. [1898] *Method and Results: Collected Essays Volume I*, Macmillan, London.

HYDÉN H. [1959] "Quantitative assay of compounds in isolated, fresh nerve cells and glial cells from control and stimulated animals", *Nature, 184*, pp. 433–5.

[1964] "Changes in RNA content and base composition in cortical neurons of rats in a learning experiment involving transfer of handedness", *Proceedings of The National Academy of Science, 52*, pp. 1030–5.

JACKSON J. H. [1887] "Remarks on evolution and dissolution of the nervous system", *Journal of Medical Science*, April, 1887.

[1931] *Selected Writings of John Hughlings Jackson*, 2 volumes, ed. J. Taylor, Hodder & Stoughton.

JAMES R. [1977] "Conditioning is a Myth", *World Medicine*, May 18th 1977, pp. 25–8.

JAMES W. [1890] *The Principles of Psychology*, two volumes, H. Holt, New York.

JENNINGS H. S. [1906] *The Behaviour of the Lower Organisms*, Columbia University Press, New York.

KAHN C. H. [1966] "Sensation and consciousness in Aristotle's psychology", *Archiv für Geschichte der Philosophie*, xlviii, pp. 43–81.

[1974] "Pythagorean Philosophy Before Plato", in MOURELATOS (ed.) [1974], pp. 161–85.

KANT I. [1756] *Monadologica Physica.*

[1781] *Kritik der reinen Vernunft*, first edition.

[1787] *Kritik der reinen Vernunft*, 2nd edition.

[1788] *Kritik der praktischen Vernunft.*

[1797] *Die Metaphysik der Sitten.*
Kants Werke, Akademieausgabe, 1910 etc., Georg Reimer, Berlin.
Werke, ed. E. Cassirer, 11 volumes, 1912–23, Berlin.

KAPP R. O. [1951] *Mind Life and Body*, Constable, London.

KATZ D. [1953] *Animals and Men*, Pengiun Books, Harmondsworth.

KNEALE W. [1962] *On Having a Mind*, Cambridge University Press.

KÖHLER W. [1920] *Die physischen Gestalten in Ruhe und im stationären Zustand*, Vieweg, Braunschweig.

[1960] "The Mind-Body Problem" in HOOK (ed.) [1960], pp. 3–23.

[1961] "The Mind-Body Problem", in HOOK (ed.) [1961], pp. 15–32.

KÖRNER S. & PRYCE M. H. L. (eds) [1957] *Observation and Interpretation*, Butterworths Scientific Publications, London.

KRIPKE S. [1971] "Identity and Necessity", in MUNITZ (ed.) [1971], pp. 135–64.

KUHN T. S. [1962] *The Structure of Scientific Revolutions*, University of Chicago Press, Chicago & London.

LA METTRIE J. O. DE [1747] *L'homme machine.*

[1750] *Les animaux plus que machines.*

[1960] *L'homme machine; Critical edition with an introductory monograph and notes by A. Vartanian*, Princeton University Press, Princeton N. J.

LAPLACE P. S. [1819] *Essai philosophique sur les probabilités.*

[1951] *A Philosophical Essay on Probabilities*, Dover, New York.

LASLETT P. (ed.) [1950] *The Physical Basis of Mind*, Blackwell, Oxford.

LAZARUS R. S. & MCCLEARY R. A. (See also McCleary) [1951] "Autonomic discrimination without awareness: A study of subception", *Psychological Review, 58*, pp. 113–22.

LEIBNIZ G. W. VON [1695] "Système nouveau de la nature et de la communication des substances", *Journal des Savants.*

[1717] *A Collection of Papers which passed between the late learned Mr. Leibniz and Dr. Clarke in the Years 1715 and 1716 relating to the Principles of Natural Philosophy and Religion*, London.

[1875–90] *Die philosophischen Schriften von G. W. Leibniz*, ed. C. J. Gerhardt, 7 vols. Berlin.

[1956] *Philosophical Papers and Letters*, ed. L. E. Loemker, 2 volumes, University of Chicago Press, Chicago.

LEMBECK F. & GIERE W. [1968] *Otto Loewi. Ein Lebensbild in Dokumenten*, Springer-Verlag, Berlin, Heidelberg, New York.

LETTVIN J. Y. & others [1959] "What the frog's eye tells the frog's brain", *Proceedings of the Institute of Radio Engineers 47*, pp. 1940 ff.

LEUCIPPUS — See DIELS & KRANZ [1951−2].

LEWES G. H. [1874–79] *Problems of Life and Mind*, 5 vols, esp. vol. 2.

LEWIN K. [1922] *Der Begriff der Genese in Physik Biologie und Entwicklungsgeschichte*, J. Springer, Berlin.

LLOYD G. E. R. [1966] *Polarity and Analogy*, Cambridge University Press, Cambridge.

LOCKE J. [1690] *An Essay Concerning Human Understanding*, London.

[1694] *An Essay Concerning Human Understanding*, second edition, London.

LOEWI O. [1940] "An Autobiographical Sketch", in *Perspectives in Biology and Medicine*, IV, University of Chicago Press, Chicago.

LORENZ K. [1976] "Die Vorstellung einer zweckgerichteten Weltordnung", *Österreichische Akademie der Wissenschaften, phil.-historische Klasse, 113*, pp. 37−51.

LUCRETIUS — *De rerum natura*.

LUTHER M. [1525] *De servo arbitrio*.

MCCLEARY R. A. & LAZARUS R. S. (See also LAZARUS.) [1949] "Autonomic discrimination without awareness: An interim report", *Journal of Personality, 18*, pp. 171−9.

MACE C. A. (ed.) [1957] *British Philosophy in the Mid-Century: A Cambridge Symposium*, Allen & Unwin, London.

MEDAWAR P. B. [1959] "[Review of E. SCHRÖDINGER, *Mind and Matter*]", *Science Progress, 47*, pp. 398−9.

[1960] *The Future of Man*, Methuen, London.

[1969] *Induction and Intuition in Scientific Thought*, Methuen, London.

[1974] "A Geometric Model of Reduction and Emergence", in AYALA & DOBZHANSKY (eds) [1974], pp. 57−63.

[1974(b)] "Some follies of quantification" *Hospital Practice*, July 1974, pp. 179−80.

[1977] "Unnatural science", *New York Review of Books*, February 3rd 1977, pp. 13−18.

MEDAWAR P. B. & J. S. [1977] *The Life Science*, Wildwood House, London.

MEHRA J. (ed.) [1973] *The Physicist's Conception of Nature*, D. Reidel, Dordrecht, Holland.

MEULI K. [1935] "Scythia", *Hermes. 70*, pp. 121−76.

MILL J. S. [1865(a)] *Auguste Comte and Positivism*, Trübner, London.

[1865(b)] *An Examination of Sir W. Hamilton's Philosophy*, 2 volumes, London.

MILLIKAN R. A. [1935] *Electrons, + and −, Protons, Photons, Neutrons and Cosmic Rays*, Cambridge University Press, Cambridge.

MILLNER B. [1966] "Amnesia Following Operation on the Temporal Lobe", in WHITTY & ZANGWILL (eds) [1966], pp. 109−33.

MONOD J. [1970] *L'hasard et la nécessité*, Éditions du Seuil, Paris.

[1971] *Chance and Necessity*, Alfred A. Knopf, New York.

[1972] *Chance and Necessity,* Collins, London.

[1975] "On the Molecular Theory of Evolution", in Harré (ed.) [1975], pp. 11–24.

Morgan T. H. & Bridges C. B. [1916] "Sex-linked inheritance in drosophila", *Carnegie Institute of Washington Publications No. 237.*

Morgenbesser S. & others (eds) [1969] *Philosophy, Science and Method: Essays in Honor of Ernest Nagel,* St. Martin's Press, New York.

Mourelatos A. P. (ed.) [1974] *The Presocratics,* Doubleday Anchor, New York.

Munitz M. K. (ed.) [1971] *Identity and Individuation,* New York University Press, New York.

Nadel S. F. [1952] "Witchcraft in four African societies: An essay in comparison", *American Anthropologist,* N. S. *54,* pp. 18–29.

Newton I. [1687] *Philosophiae naturalis principia mathematica,* London.

[1704] *Opticks,* London.

[1726] *Philosophiae naturalis principia mathematica,* third edition, London.

[1730] *Opticks,* 4th edition, London.

[1779–85] *Isaaci Newtoni Operae quae exstant omnia,* ed. S. Horsley, 5 vols. London.

Onians R. B. [1954] *The Origins of European Thought,* Cambridge University Press, London.

Oppenheim P. & Putnam H. [1958] "Unity of Science as a Working Hypothesis", in Feigl & others (ed.) [1958], pp. 3–36.

Oxford English Dictionary [1933] Clarendon Press, Oxford.

Parfit D. [1971] "Personal Identity", *Philosophical Review, 80,* pp. 3–27.

Passmore J. A. [1961] *Philosophical Reasoning,* Duckworth, London.

Pavlov I. P. [1927] *Conditioned Reflexes,* Oxford University Press.

Penfield W. [1955] "The Permanent Record of the Stream of Consciousness", *Proc. XIV Int. Congr. Psychol.,* Montreal, 1954, = *Acta Psychologica, 11,* pp. 47–69.

[1975] *The Mystery of the Mind,* Princeton University Press, Princeton.

Penfield W. & Perot P. [1963] "A brain's record of auditory and visual experience. A final summary and discussion", *Brain, 86,* pp. 595–696.

Pindar [1915] *The Odes of Pindar,* tr. Sir John Sandys, Loeb Classical Library, Heinemann, London.

[1947] *Carmina cum Fragmentis,* 2nd edition, ed. C. M. Bowra, Clarendon Press, Oxford.

Place U. T. [1956] "Is consciousness a brain process?", *British Journal of Psychology, 47,* pp. 44–51.

Plato *Apology.*
The Laws.
Meno.
Phaedo.

The Republic.
Timaeus.

POLANYI M. [1966] *The Tacit Dimension,* Doubleday, New York.

[1967] *The Tacit Dimension,* Routledge & Kegan Paul, London.

POLTEN E. P. [1973] *Critique of the Psycho-Physical Identity Theory* (Preface by Sir John Eccles), Mouton, The Hague & Paris.

POPPER K. R. [1934(b)]* *Logik der Forschung,* Julius Springer, Vienna.

[1940(a)] "What is dialectic", *Mind, 49,* pp. 403–26. (Also in [1963(a)].)

[1944(b)] "The Poverty of Historicism, II", *Economica, 11,* pp. 119–37. (Also in [1957(g)], [1979(z_6)].)

[1945(b) & (c)] *The Open Society and Its Enemies,* Routledge & Kegan Paul, London. (Also in [1979(z_6)].)

[1950(b) & (c)] "Indeterminism in quantum physics and in classical physics", Parts I and II, *British Journal for the Philosophy of Science, 1,* pp. 117–33 and 173–95.

[1953(a)] "Language and the Body-Mind Problem", *Proceedings of the XIth International Congress of Philosophy, 7,* North-Holland, Amsterdam, pp. 101–107. (Also in [1963(a)].)

[1957(a)] "Philosophy of Science: A Personal Report", in MACE (ed.) [1957], pp. 155–91. (Also in [1963(a)], [1981(z_{24})].)

[1957(e)] "The Propensity Interpretation of the Calculus of Probability and of the Quantum Theory", in KÖRNER & PRYCE (eds) [1957], pp. 65–70 and 88–9.

[1957(g)] *The Poverty of Historicism,* Routledge & Kegan Paul, London. (Also in [1979(z_6)].)

[1957(i)] "The aim of science", *Ratio* (Oxford). *1*, pp. 24–35. (Also in [1972(a)] and [1981(z_{13})].)

[1959(a)] *The Logic of Scientific Discovery,* Hutchinson, London. (Also in [1980(a)].)

[1963(a)] *Conjectures and Refutations,* Routledge & Kegan Paul, London.

[1966(a)] *The Open Society and Its Enemies,* fifth edition, Routledge & Kegan Paul, London. (Also in [1980(y)].)

[1967(k)] "Quantum Mechanics Without 'The Observer'", in BUNGE (ed.) [1967], pp. 7–44. (Also in [1982(b) and (d)].)

[1972(a)] *Objective Knowledge: An Evolutionary Approach,* Clarendon Press, Oxford. (Also in [1981(z^{13})].)

[1973(a)] "Indeterminism is Not Enough", *Encounter, 40,* No. 4, pp. 20–6.

[1974(b)] "Autobiography of Karl Popper", in SCHILPP (ed.) [1974], pp. 3–181. (Also in [1976(g)], [1982(g), (k)].)

* References to Popper's works (such as "[1934(b)]") follow in their numbering the "Bibliography of the Writings of Karl Popper", compiled by Troels Eggers Hansen for SCHILPP (ed.) [1974]; see also the *Select Bibliography* in POPPER [1976(g)].

[1974(c)] "Replies to my Critics" in SCHILPP (ed.) [1974], pp. 961–1197.

[1974(z_2)] "Scientific Reduction and the Essential Incompleteness of All Science", in AYALA & DOBZHANSKY (eds) [1974], pp. 259–84.

[1975(p)] "The Rationality of Scientific Revolutions", in HARRÉ (ed.) [1975], pp. 72–101.

[1976(g)] *Unended Quest: An Intellectual Autobiography,* Fontana/Collins, London.

[1979(a)] *Objective Knowledge. An Evolutionary Approach,* fifth (revised) impression, Clarendon Press, Oxford.

[1979(z_6)] *The Poverty of Historicism,* tenth impression, Routledge & Kegan Paul, London.

[1980(y)] *The Open Society and Its Enemies,* thirteenth impression, Routledge & Kegan Paul, London.

[1982(k)] *Unended Quest: An Intellectual Autobiography,* sixth impression, revised, with an extended biography, Fontana/Collins, London.

[1982(b&d)] *Quantum Theory and the Schism in Physics,* vol. III of the *Postscript* to *The Logic of Scientific Discovery,* ed. by W. W. Bartley III, Hutchinson, London.

[1981(z_{24})] *Conjectures and Refutations,* eighth impression, Routledge & Kegan Paul, London.

[1982(e)] *Logik der Forschung,* seventh edition, revised and enlarged with six new Appendices, J. C. B. Mohr, (Paul Siebeck), Tübingen.

[1982(a&c)] *The Open Universe: An Argument for Indeterminism,* vol. II of the *Postscript* to *The Logic of Scientific Discovery,* ed. by W.W. Bartley III, Hutchinson, London.

[1983(a&b)] *Realism and the Aim of Science,* vol. I of the *Postscript* to *The Logic of Scientific Discovery,* ed. by W.W. Bartley III, Hutchinson, London.

PUTNAM H. [1960] "Minds and Machines", in HOOK (ed.) [1960], pp. 148–79.

QUINE W. V. O. [1960] *Word and Object,* M. I. T. Press, Cambridge, Mass.

[1975] "Mind and Verbal Dispositions", in GUTTENPLAN (ed.) [1975], pp. 83–95.

QUINTON A. [1973] *The Nature of Things,* Routledge & Kegan Paul, London.

RAWLS J. [1971] *A Theory of Justice,* Harvard University Press, Cambridge, Mass.

RENSCH B. [1968] *Biophilosophie auf erkenntnistheoretischen Grundlage,* Gustav Fischer, Stuttgart.

[1971] *Biophilosophy,* tr. C. A. M. Sym, Columbia University Press, New York.

ROSENFIELD L. C. [1941] *From Beast-Machine to Man-Machine,* Oxford University Press, New York.

ROSENZWEIG M. R. & others [1972(a)] "Brain changes in response to experience", *Scientific American, 226,* February 1972, pp. 22–9.

[1972(b)] "Negative as well as positive synaptic changes may store memory", *Psychological Review, 79*(1), pp. 93–6.

RUBIN E. [1949] *Experimenta Psychologica,* Ejnar Munksgaard, Copenhagen.

[1950] "Visual figures apparently incompatible with geometry", *Acta Psychologica, VII,* Nr. 2–4, pp. 365–87.

RUSSELL B. [1945] *A History of Western Philosophy,* Simon and Schuster, New York; Allen & Unwin, London.

[1956] "Mind and Matter", in *Portraits From Memory,* Simon and Schuster, New York, pp. 145–65.

RUTHERFORD E. [1923] "The electrical structure of matter", *Nature, 112,* pp. 409–19

RUTHERFORD E. & SODDY F. [1902] "The radioactivity of thorium compounds II. The cause and nature of radioactivity", *Journal of the Chemical Society, Transactions,* LXXXI, Part II, pp. 837–60.

RYLE G. [1949] *The Concept of Mind,* Hutchinson, London.

[1950] "The Physical Basis of Mind", in LASLETT (ed.) [1950], pp. 75–9.

SCHILPP P. A. (ed.) [1974] *The Philosophy of Karl Popper,* vols. 14/I, 14/II, *The Library of Living Philosophers,* Open Court, La Salle, Illinois.

SCHLICK M. [1925] *Allgemeine Erkenntnislehre,* 2nd ed., J. Springer, Berlin.

[1974] *General Theory of Knowledge,* Springer-Verlag, Vienna, New York.

SCHMITT F. O. & WORDEN F. G. (eds) [1973] *The Neurosciences: Third Study Program,* M. I. T. Press, Cambridge, Mass.

SCHOPENHAUER A. [1818] *Die Welt als Wille und Vorstellung.*

[1883] *The World as Will and Idea,* Routledge & Kegan Paul, London.

[1958] *The World as Will and Representation,* Falcon's Wing Press, Indian Hills, Colo.

SCHRÖDINGER E. [1929] "Aus der Antrittsrede des neu in die Akademie eingetretenen Herrn Schrödinger", *Die Naturwissenschaften, 17,* p. 732.

[1935] *Science and the Human Temperament,* Allen & Unwin, London.

[1952] "Are there quantum jumps?", *British Journal for the Philosophy of Science, 3,* 1953, pp. 109–23; 233–42.

[1957] *Science, Theory and Man,* Dover, New York.

[1958] *Mind and Matter,* Cambridge University Press, Cambridge.

[1967] *What is Life? & Mind and Matter,* Cambridge University Press, Cambridge.

SELZ O. [1913] *Über die Gesetze des geordneten Denkverlaufs,* I, W. Spemann, Stuttgart.

[1922] *Zur Psychologie des produktiven Denkens und des Irrtums,* F. Cohen, Bonn.

[1924] *Die Gesetze der produktiven und reproduktiven Geistestätigkeit,* F. Cohen, Bonn.

SHERRINGTON C. [1906] *The Integrative Action of the Nervous System,* Yale University Press, New Haven, and Oxford University Press, London.

[1947] *The Integrative Action of the Nervous System;* reprint of 1906 edition with new preface, Cambridge University Press, Cambridge.

SMART J. J. C. [1963] *Philosophy and Scientific Realism,* Routledge & Kegan Paul, London.

SMITH A. [1759] *The Theory of Moral Sentiments,* London & Edinburgh.

SMYTHIES J. R. (ed.) [1965] *Brain and Mind,* Routledge & Kegan Paul, London.

SOLECKI R. S. [1971] *Shanidar,* Knopf, New York.

SOPHOCLES *King Oedipus.*
Oedipus at Colonus.

SPERRY R. W. [1966] "Brain bisection and mechanisms of consciousness", in ECCLES (ed.) [1966 (b)], pp. 298–313.

[1969] "A Modified Concept of Consciousness", *Psychological Review, 76,* pp. 532–6.

[1973] "Lateral specialization in the surgically separated hemispheres", in SCHMITT & WORDEN (eds) [1973].

[1976] "Mental Phenomena as Causal Determinants in Brain Function", in GLOBUS & others (eds) [1976], pp. 163–77.

SPINOZA B. DE *Ethics.*

STRAWSON P. [1959] *Individuals,* Methuen, London.

TARSKI A. [1956] *Logic, Semantics, Metamathematics,* Clarendon Press, Oxford.

THEOPHRASTUS *De sensu.*

THOMSON J. J. [1969] "The Identity Thesis", in MORGENBESSER & others (eds) [1969], pp. 219 – 34.

THOULESS R. H. & WIESNER B. [1947] "The Psi Process in Normal and Paranormal Psychology", *Proceedings of the Society for Psychical Research, 48,* pp. 177 – 96.

TURING A. M. [1950] "Computing machinery and intelligence", *Mind, 59,* pp. 433 – 60.

UNGAR G. [1974] "Molecular Coding of Information in the Nervous System", *Stadler Symposium* (University of Missouri) *6.*

VLASTOS G. [1975] "Ethics and Physics in Democritus", in ALLEN & FURLEY (eds) [1975]. pp. 381 – 408.

WADDINGTON C. H. [1961] *The Nature of Life,* Allen & Unwin, London.

WATKINS J. W. N. [1965] *Hobbes's System of Ideas,* Hutchinson, London.

[1973] *Hobbes's System of Ideas,* 2nd edition, Hutchinson, London.

[1974] "The Unity of Popper's Thought", in SCHILPP (ed.) [1974], pp. 371 – 412.

WHEELER J. A. [1973] "From Relativity to Mutability", in MEHRA (ed.) [1973], pp. 202−47.

WHITTY C. W. M. & ZANGWILL O. L. (eds) [1966] *Amnesia*, Appleton, Century, Crofts, New York.

WHORF B. L. [1956] *Language, Thought, and Reality*, ed. J. B. Carroll, M. I. T. Press, Cambridge, Mass.

WISDOM J. O. [1952] "A new model for the mind-body relationship", *British Journal for the Philosophy of Science, 2*, pp. 295−301.

WITTGENSTEIN L. [1921] "Logisch-philosophische Abhandlung", *Annalen der Naturphilosophie.*

[1922] *Tractatus Logico-philosophicus.*

[1953] *Philosophical Investigations*, Blackwell, Oxford.

WUNDT W. [1880] *Grundzüge der physiologischen Psychologie*, volumes I and II, 2nd edition, Wilhelm Engelmann, Leipzig.

ZIEHEN T. [1913] *Erkenntnistheorie auf psychophysiologischer und physikalischer Grundlage*, G. Fischer, Jena.

Part II

Preface

Far too little consideration to the neuronal machinery involved in the various manifestations of the self-conscious mind has been given in the past. Philosophers presenting physicalist theories of the brain – mind problem, such as the identity theory (Feigl [1967]) or the central-state theory (Armstrong [1968]) should build their philosophies upon the best available scientific understanding of the brain. Unfortunately, they are content with crude and antiquated information that often misleads them into espousing erroneous ideas. There is a general tendency to overplay the scientific knowledge of the brain, which, regretfully, also is done by many brain scientists and scientific writers. For example, we are told that the brain "sees" lines, angles, edges, and simple geometrical forms and that therefore we will soon be able to explain how a whole picture is "seen" as a composite of this elemental "seeing". But this statement is misleading. All that is known to happen in the brain is that neurones of the visual cortex are caused to fire trains of impulses in response to some specific visual input (see Fig. E2–6). Neurones responding to various complications of this specific visual input are identified, but there is no scientific evidence concerning how these feature-detection neurones can be subjected to the immense synthetic mechanism that leads to a brain process that is "identical" with the perceived picture.

It is not claimed here that our present scientific understanding of the brain will solve any of the philosophical problems that are the theme of this book. But it is claimed that our present knowledge should discredit the formulations of untenable theories and that it will give new insights into such fundamental problems as conscious perception, voluntary action, and conscious memory.

A full presentation of our scientific understanding of the brain up to now would be an immense task. Technically, it would be overwhelming, with a massive number of volumes. And, even it it were attempted, it would fail in our present purpose which is to give an intelligible account of the principles of operation of the brain in the various manifestations relating to self-consciousness and the self. As far as possible, Chapters E1 to E8 are based on the scientific study of the human brain, but this is necessarily incomplete; and it is supplemented in some sections where it is necessary to refer to refined electrical recording and anatomical study on mammalian brains, which generally will be primate brains.

It is recognized that even the simple level of exposition attempted in these E (Eccles) chapters may initially make too heavy a demand on the reader. For this reason each chapter is prefaced by a short résumé that gives the essential themes of the chapters and makes references to the illustrations. The text of the chapters can then serve for reference, but it is hoped that, eventually, the full text will be attempted by all readers. Chapter E7 differs from the other chapters in that it does not present scientific discoveries. A synthesis of the key findings in the other chapters is used in building a philosophical theory central to the whole theme of this book. It is a dualist – interactionist theory that is stronger that any yet propounded – a strength demanded by logical necessity. Weaker theories inevitably are reducible to materialist monism.

As mentioned above, the theme of these E (Eccles) chapters relates to neuronal machinery. This term is deliberately chosen in order to indicate the scientific assumption that the brain functions as a machine. It is essential that all considerations of the brain – mind problem take cognizance of the scientific understanding of the brain in the various activities that are believed to be concerned in the production of conscious experience. According to the dualist – interactionist philosophy presented in this book, the brain is a machine of almost infinite complexity and subtlety, and in special regions, under appropriate conditions, it is open to interaction with World 2, the world of conscious experience.

Chapter E1 The Cerebral Cortex

1. Résumé

The Introduction gives a brief description of the human cerebral cortex, both in its macroscopic (Fig. E 1 − 1) and microscopic features. There is a description of the fundamental units of the nervous system, the neurones or nerve cells, and of their connectivities by means of very intimate contacts called synapses (Fig. E 1 − 2). Activation of one type of these synapses excites the neurone and causes it in turn to discharge impulses, which are brief electrical messages travelling along its axon. Activation of the other set of synapses inhibits the neurone and tends to prevent the discharge of impulses. Each neurone has hundreds, or even thousands, of synapses on its surface and discharges impulses only when synaptic excitation is much stronger than inhibition. Impulses are almost the only means of fast transmission in the central nervous system.

The detailed micro-structure of the six layers of the cerebral cortex (Fig. E 1 − 3) allows it to be divided into over 40 discrete areas, the Brodmann areas (Fig. E 1 − 4). This subdivision will be utilized throughout the book because it is now recognized that the Brodmann subdivision coresponds quite well with the different functional performances of the areas of the cerebral cortex.

An important further subdivision of the cerebral cortex derives from its organization in columns or modules which are vertical to the surface and approximately 3 mm long and 0.1 to 0.5 mm across. These columnar arrangements were originally revealed by the finding that in the primary sensory areas of the cortex, the neurones with approximately the same performance were assembled in vertical colums. Because the columns are now recognized as forming separate functional and anatomical entities, there is a comprehensive description of the recent work of neuroanatomists in defining the neuronal composition of a column along with the conjectured interrelationships of these neurones (Figs. E1−5, 6). It is particularly important to recognize that many of the neurones are inhibitory and that the inhibitory action of these neurones is exerted on adjacent columns. A further important feature of the columnar arrangement is that the two superficial laminae of the cortex appear to be organized differently from the deeper laminae, in that they have an organization with a finer grain due to the smaller inhibitory neurones, and also in that there are less powerful and more diffuse synaptic actions upon the pyramidal cells, which are the principal cells of the column, with axons projecting to other columns in the same or opposite hemisphere and also projecting to lower levels of the central nervous system.

It is proposed that each module is a power unit designed by its internal neuronal connections to build up power within its confines so that its pyramidal cells can generate discharges of impulses that act elsewhere in the central nervous system. At the same time, it exerts a depressant action on adjacent modules by virtue of its inhibitory neurones. Thus we can think of a module as being a unit that attempts to dominate other modules by virtue of its impulse discharges. Of course, these other modules act back in their own effort at dominance. It may be estimated that within a module there are up to 10,000 component neurones, and their performance as an immensely complex ensemble is the result of a conflict between the excitatory and the inhibitory inputs from other modules. Each module can act upon hundreds of other modules and itself receive from a like number. Under normal conditions there is continued activity in the neurones of each module so the complexity of operation of the whole aggregate of about two million modules is beyond all imagination.

There is a summary of the recent work indicating the sequential activation (in cascade) that occurs from primary sensory areas through the association fibres that their columns emit to the secondary areas, and the secondary in turn to tertiary, and thence to quaternary (Figs. E1−7, 8). In this way there is a wide-spreading influence of the input that arrives at the primary sensory area by pathways activated from the receptor organs such as those of the cutaneous, the visual, and the auditory systems.

Finally, a brief account is given of the projections of these areas to the limbic system which is an ancient part of the forebrain, originally associated with olfaction (Fig. E1−9). This limbic system receives input from the various relay areas for the senses as described above, and in turn it projects back to the neocortex, particularly to the frontal lobe. The significance of these connections is described in chapter E2 in relation to the emotional content of perceptual experience.

2. Anatomical Introduction

The principal anatomical features of the human brain are the two cerebral hemispheres that are approximately symmetrical and that are linked together by a great commissural structure, the corpus callosum. The hemispheres are intimately connected by enormous tracts of nerve fibres to the next lower levels of the brain, the immense neuronal complexes of the thalamus and basal ganglia (diencephalon).Great ascending and descending pathways, composed of millions of nerve fibres, link the cerebral hemispheres and the thalamus to still lower levels, the mesencephalon, pons, cerebellum, medulla and spinal cord. A detailed description of these pathways would be out of place here, but there will be reference to some of them in the appropriate chapters on perception and control of movement, chapters E 2 and E 3 respectively.

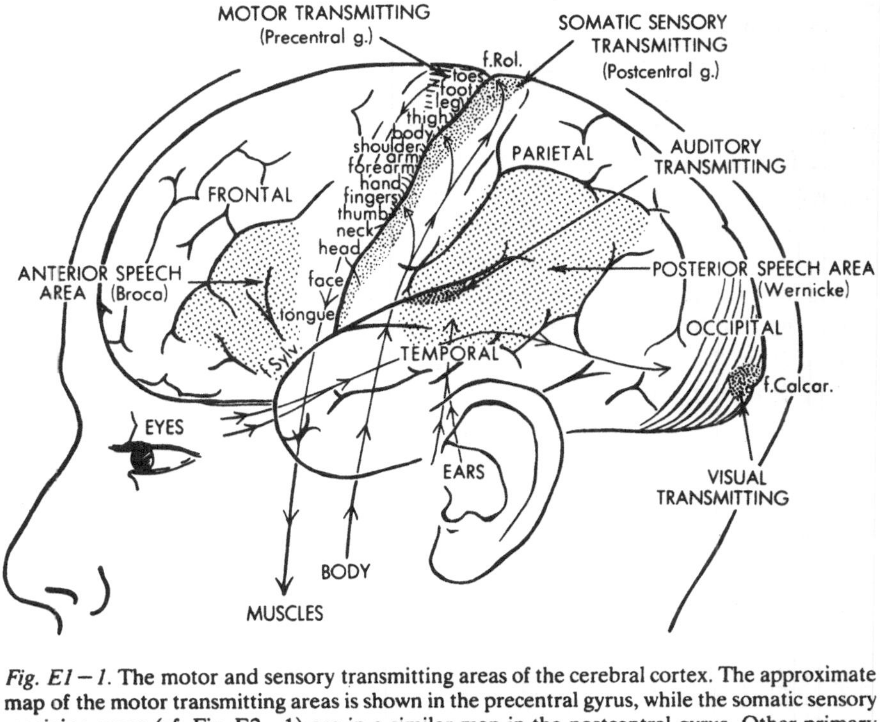

Fig. E1 – 1. The motor and sensory transmitting areas of the cerebral cortex. The approximate map of the motor transmitting areas is shown in the precentral gyrus, while the somatic sensory receiving areas (cf. Fig. E2 – 1) are in a similar map in the postcentral gyrus. Other primary sensory areas shown are the visual and auditory, but they are largely in areas screened from this lateral view. The frontal, parietal, occipital and temporal lobes are indicated. Also shown are the speech areas of Broca and Wernicke.

The cerebral hemispheres are the most recently evolved part of the forebrain, hence the designation of the great covering cortex as the neocortex. As indicated in Fig. E 1 – 1 the neocortex of each hemisphere is rather arbitrarily subdivided into four lobes, frontal, parietal, temporal, occipital. Originally the older parts of the forebrain, the archicortex and paleocortex, were specifically related to the sense of smell. These older cortices have unique structural features and connections as described below, and there will be later reference to their special functions, for example there is the mnemonic role of the hippocampus (chapter E 8) that forms the principal part of the archicortex and there is the role of other structures of the limbic system that are related to mood and emotion (chapters E 2 and E 6). For the present, attention will be concentrated on the structure of the neocortex. The cerebral hemispheres are composed of the convoluted sheet of the cerebral cortex that covers the whole folded surface, so having the large total area of about 1200 cm^2 for each hemisphere. The neocortex is about 3 mm in thickness and is a massive assemblage of neurones, about 10,000 million.

The neurones of the cerebral cortex are so densely packed that the individual neurone can be recognized in histological sections only when it is picked out by the extraordinarily fortunate staining procedure discovered by Golgi. For example in Figure E 1 – 2 A only about 1% of the neurones were stained, and several individuals can be recognized with the branching tree-like dendrites and the thin axon (nerve fibre) projecting downwards from the centre of the soma or body. In B there is shown one such neurone with short spines (s) on the dendrites, but not on the soma (p) or the axon (ax). The dendrites are truncated and are seen to be of two varieties, those arising from the apical dendrite (b) of the pyramidal cell, and those directly arising from the soma (p).

At the end of the nineteenth century it was first proposed by Ramón y Cajal, the great Spanish neuroanatomist, that the nervous system is made up of neurones which are isolated cells, not joined together in some syncytium, but each one independently living its own biological life. This concept is called the neurone theory. How then does a neurone receive information from other nerve cells? This happens by means of the fine branches of the axons of the other neurones that make contact with its surface and end in little knobs scattered all over its soma and dendrites, as indicated in Figure E 1 – 2 C. It was Sherrington's concept also at the end of the nineteenth century that these contact areas are specialized sites of communication, which he labelled synapses from the Greek word *synapto* which means to clasp tightly (Eccles [1964] chapter 1).

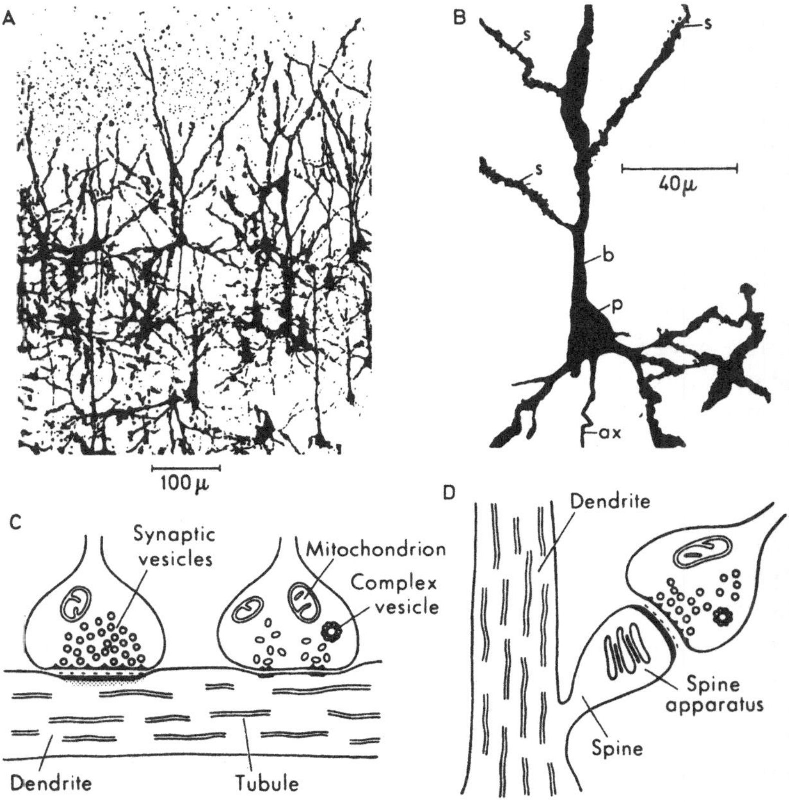

Fig. E1 −2. Neurones and synapses. A. Pyramidal and stellate cells seen in a Golgi-stained section of the cat visual cortex. B is a Golgi preparation of a neurone from cat cerebral cortex with spines *(s)* shown on apical and basal dendrites, but not on the soma *(p)*, axon *(ax)* or dendritic stumps *(b)*. C shows Type 1 (excitatory) and Type 2 (inhibitory) synapse on a dendrite with the characteristic features displayed diagrammatically. The excitatory synapse has a wider synaptic cleft with a large zone of dense staining. The synaptic vesicles are spherical for the excitatory and elongated for the inhibitory synapse. Special fixation procedures are required for this differentiation. In D there is a dendritic spine of a neocortical pyramidal cell with its spine apparatus and an associated Type 1 synapse (Whittaker and Gray, 1962).

The twentieth century dawned with these new theories being very much disputed – even for the first two or three decades. But in the last few decades the neuronal theory of Ramón y Cajal and the synaptic theory of Sherrington have been corroborated and further defined by new powerful methods of investigation. These two theories form the secure basis for all our further conceptual developments. Electronmicroscopy has revealed that the neurone is completely separated from other neurones by its enveloping membrane. At the synapse there is the close contact illustrated in Figure E 1 − 2 C, with separation by the synaptic cleft of about 200 Å. In electrically transmitting synapses the presynaptic and postsynaptic membranes are almost in direct contact; nevertheless the integrity of the neuronal membranes is maintained, there being no cytoplasmic fusion.

Transmission in the nervous system occurs by two quite distinct mechanisms. Firstly, there are the brief electrical waves called impulses that travel in an all-or-nothing manner along nerve fibres, often at high velocity. Secondly, there is transmission across synapses. In parenthesis it may be noted that also there is a decremental transmission for short distances along nerve fibres by a cable-like spread.

Impulses are generated by a neurone and discharged along its axon when it has been sufficiently excited synaptically. The impulse travels along the axon or nerve fibre and all its branches, eventually reaching synaptic knobs which are the axonal contacts with the somata and dendrites of other neurones. Figure E 1 − 2 C shows the two varieties of synapses, excitatory to the left and inhibitory to the right (Whittaker and Gray [1962]). The former act by tending to cause the recipient neurone to fire an impulse down its axon, the latter act to inhibit this discharge. There are two kinds of neurones, those whose axons form excitatory synapses and those making inhibitory synapses. There are no ambivalent neurones. For a simple account of synaptic action reference is made to chapter 3 of *The Understanding of the Brain* (Eccles [1977]). Figure E 1 − 2 D shows a synapse formed on the dendritic spine of a pyramidal cell (cp. s in Fig. E 1 − 2 B). There is now convincing evidence that all spine synapses are excitatory.

Another powerful technique for investigating synapses is the recording from the interior of nerve cells by fine microelectrodes, which has revealed not only the electrical independence of the neurones, but also the mode of operation of synapses. Each neurone has hundreds or even thousands of synapses on its surface and it discharges impulses only when the synaptic excitation is much stronger than inhibition.

Deep to the cerebral cortex is the white matter that is largely composed of the myelinated nerve fibres, which are the pathways to and from the cerebral cortices. They connect each area of the cerebral cortex to lower levels of the central nervous system, as listed above, or to other areas of the same hemisphere (the association fibres) and of the opposite hemisphere (the commissural fibres). There are about 200 million commissural fibres in the corpus callosum, which is by far the largest system connecting the two hemispheres. All parts of the neocortex have the same basic layered structure of neurones, usually six layers as indicated in Figure E 1 − 3, but there are structural

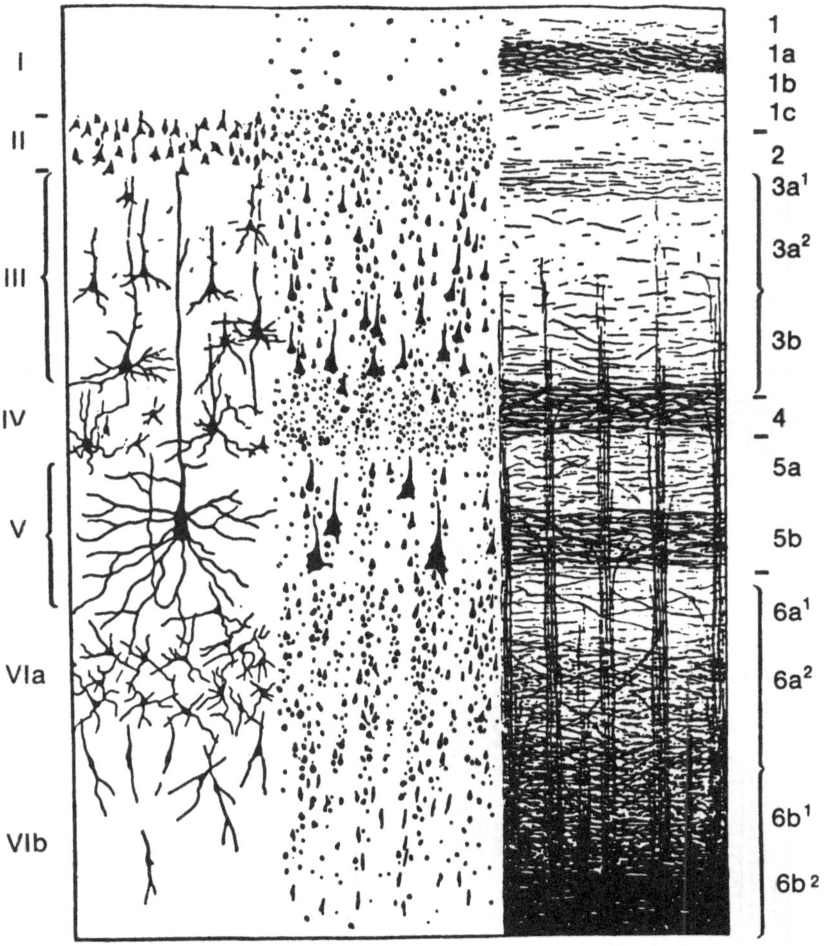

Fig. E1–3. Diagram of the structure of the cerebral cortex. *To the left,* from a Golgi preparation; *centre,* from a Nissl preparation; *to the right,* from a myelin sheath preparation. *I:* lamina zonalis; *II:* lamina granularis externa; *III:* lamina pyramidalis; *IV:* lamina granularis interna; *V:* lamina ganglionaris; *VI:* lamina multiformis. After Brodmann and O. Vogt (Brodal, 1969).

differences which allow subdivision of the human cerebral hemisphere into over 40 discrete areas, the so-called Brodmann areas which are depicted in Figure E1–4 A and B for the lateral and medial aspects respectively. Brodmann based his structural analysis on the features shown in the centre and right strips of Figure E1–3. There are many subdivisions of the six laminae and they vary greatly in the different Brodmann areas. This subdivision into Brodmann areas has a functional counterpart, many of the areas

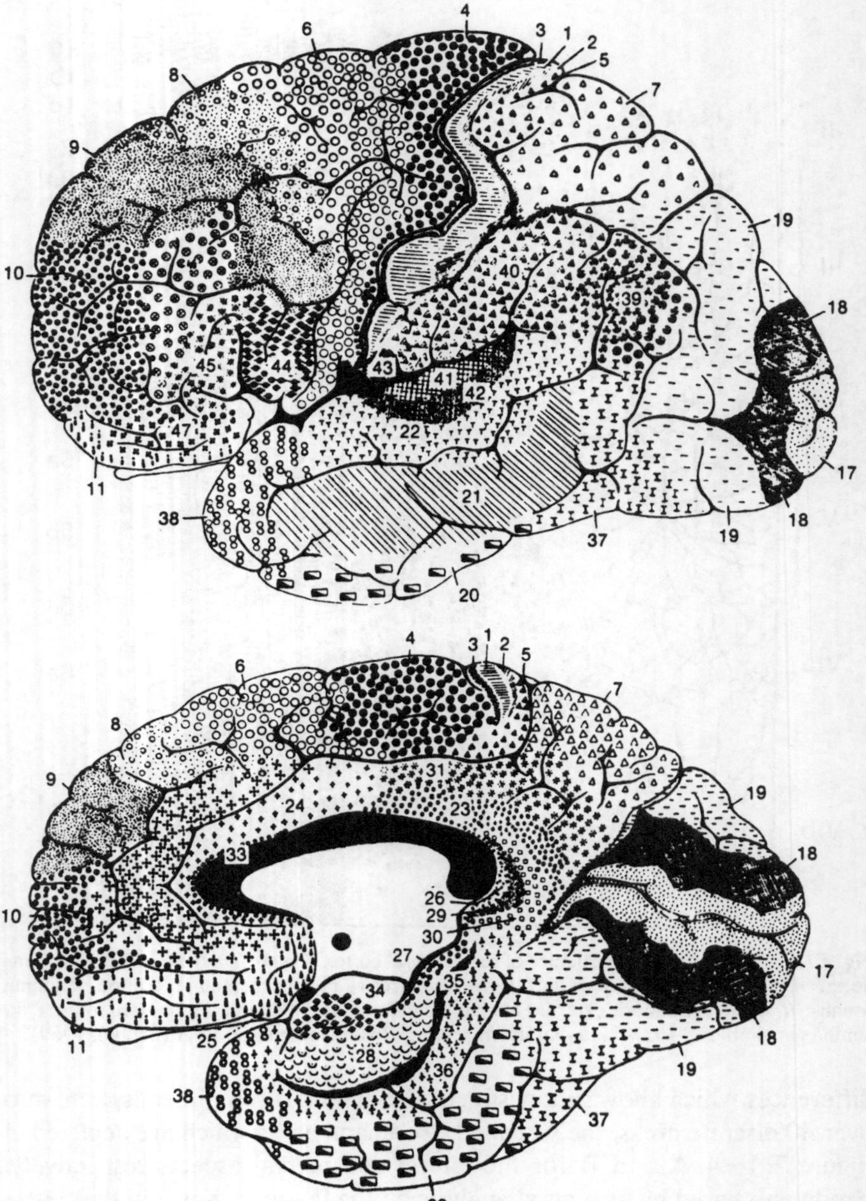

Fig. E1 – 4. Brodmann's cytoarchitectural map of the human brain. The various areas are labelled with different symbols and their numbers indicated by figures. Upper drawing is lateral view of left hemisphere, and lower is medial view of right hemisphere (Brodal, 1969).

having specific physiological properties, as will appear in subsequent chapters. The limbic system can be recognized on the medial surface. Areas 23 to 35 are classified either as in the limbic system or as paralimbic.

3. The Columnar Arrangement and the Modular Concept of the Cerebral Cortex

We owe to Ramón y Cajal [1911] the first comprehensive account of the neuronal structure of the neocortex with detailed descriptions of the pyramidal cells and of the immense population of smaller neurones. Lorente de Nó [1943] continued this detailed neurohistology, making the notable discovery that in addition to the horizontal lamination into six major layers, there was an arrangement of "vertical chains" of neurones through the whole depth of the cortex. Thus we are introduced to the modern concept of columnar arrangement that first was developed in relation to the detailed study of the responses of single neurones.

Physiological investigations by Mountcastle (Mountcastle [1957], Mountcastle and Powell [1959]) on the somaesthetic cortex and by Hubel and Wiesel [1962], [1963], [1968], [1972], on the visual cortex revealed that the cortical neurones of small sharply defined areas exhibited an approximately similar response to specific afferent inputs. The neurones were located in cortical zones forming columns orthogonal to the cortical surface (Figs. E 1−5, 6). With the somaesthetic cortex (Figs. E 1−1, somatic sensory; E 1−4, areas 3, 1, 2) the columns responded either to superficial or to deep sensation. With the primary visual cortex (Figs. E 1−1, E 1−4 A, B, area 17) the original specification of columns was by the orientation of a bright line that was optimal for exciting the neurones. The primary sensory areas are composed of a mosaic of such columns with irregular cross sections averaging about 0.1 mm^2 in area.

Recent investigations by Szentágothai [1969], [1972], [1973], [1974], [1975], Colonnier [1966], [1968], Colonnier and Rossignol [1969] and Marin-Padilla [1970] have provided important information on this columnar or modular concept by revealing its structural basis. There is now an identification of many specific types of neurones in the columns and of their probable role in the processing of information in respect both of their synaptic connectivities and of their nature as excitatory or inhibitory neurones (Creutzfeldt and Ito [1968]; Toyama & others [1974]. As a consequence we are becoming aware that the column is a complex organization of many specific cell types.

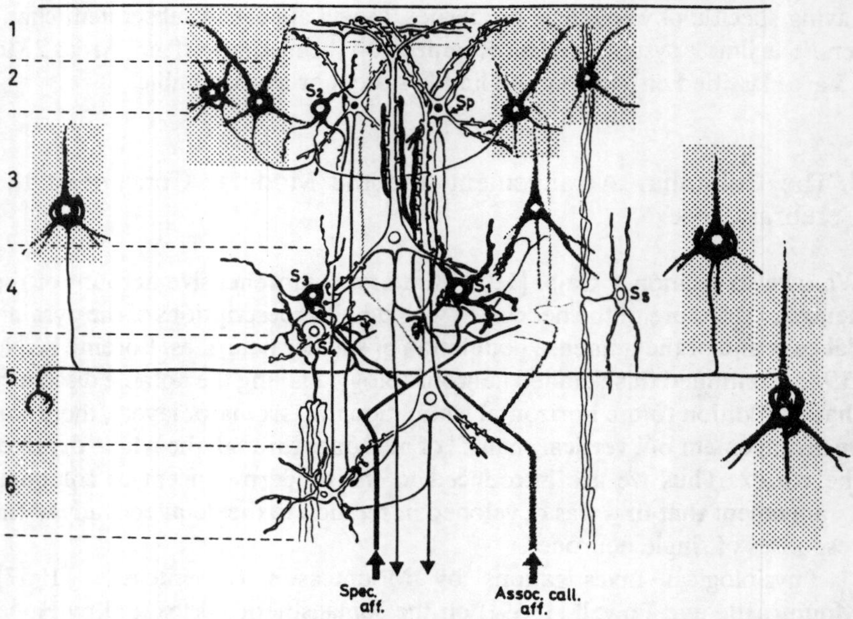

Fig. E1 – 5. Semidiagrammatic drawing of some cell types of the cerebral cortex with interconnections as discussed in the text. Two pyramidal cells are seen centrally in laminae III and V. The specific afferent fibre *(Spec. aff.)* is seen to excite a stellate interneurone S_1 (crosshatched) whose axon establishes cartridge-type synapses on the apical dendrites. The specific afferent fibre also excites a basket-type stellate interneurone, S_3, that gives inhibition to pyramidal cells in adjacent columns, as indicated by shading. Another interneurone (S_6) is shown in lamina VI with ascending axon (a Martinotti cell), and S_5 is an interneurone also probably concerned in vertical spread of excitation through the whole depth of the cortex. *Sp* are stellate pyramidal cells and S_2 are the short-axon inhibitory cells in lamina II. The afferents formed by association and callosal fibres *(Assoc. call. aff.)* are shown ascending to branch in lamina I. Further description in text (Szentágothai, 1969).

On the basis of extensive micro-structural studies Szentágothai [1972], [1973], [1974], [1975] has developed the concept that, in both the structure and function of all areas of the cerebral cortex, the column or module is the basic unit. He goes so far as to postulate that the modules are comparable to the integrated micro-circuits of electronics. The modules represent what he calls a basic neurone circuit that in its elemental form is constituted by input channels (afferent fibres), complex neuronal interactions in the module, and output channels, which are largely the axons of the pyramidal cells. Despite the diversity of the structure obtaining in different regions of the neocortex, the Brodmann areas (Fig. E1 – 4), Szentágothai [1972] finds five basic similarities:

> (1) a fairly uniform principle of lamination, (2) a relatively uniform main cell type: the pyramids, (3) certain characteristic types of interneurons or Golgi 2nd type cells, (4) an essential similarity in the organization of input channels: association afferents, commissural afferents, specific and non (or less) specific subcortical afferents, and (5) an essential similarity in the organization of the output lines, mainly the axons of pyramid neurons. This gives us the confidence that in spite of obvious differences in detailed structure and even more in connexions with other regions of the CNS, certain "units" of neocortical tissue might be built on the basis of the same fundamental principle, *i. e.*, they might be essentially similar as devices for processing neural information.

Some basic patterns of operations within and around the module are shown diagrammatically in Figures E 1–5 and 6. These figures give greatly simplified pictures of the neuronal composition of a module and its surround. According to Szentágothai there is a major functional difference between the neuronal connectivities in laminae III, IV and V on the one hand and those in laminae I and II on the other.

Figure E 1–5 shows that, in laminae III, IV and V, the afferent fibres from the thalamic complex *(spec. aff.)* form synaptic endings on the dendritic spines of excitatory interneurones (S_1, S_4) (Lund [1973] and on the dendrites of inhibitory interneurones (S_3) (Marin-Padilla [1970]). Also the association and commissural fibres *(Assoc. call. aff.)* give branches to cells in the deeper laminae on their way to their principal terminations in laminae I and II (Heimer & others, 1967). Some of the excitatory neurones (S_1) of lamina IV and the *cellule á double bouquet* (S_5) are powerfully excitatory to the apical dendrites of pyramidal cells by the so-called *cartridge type of synapse* in which the axon of this Golgi type II cell runs along the dendrites forming hundreds of synapses in a manner comparable to the climbing fibre synapses on *Purkyně* cells of the cerebellum. Some other interneurones widely distribute their excitatory synapses, both vertically and transversely. Others again (S_4 of Fig. E 1–5) are more localized. These last two types give very few synapses to any particular interneurone or pyramidal cell. The convergent action of many is required for an effective excitation. The overall result of the sequences of synaptic excitation by all of these excitatory cells is a powerful excitation of pyramidal cells within the column that is illustrated to the right in Figure E 1–6. There is a kind of amplification process. On the other hand the inhibitory neurones (S_3 in Figs. E 1–5 and E 1–6) of laminae III and IV of the module are excited by specific afferents either directly or indirectly by mediation of the excitatory interneurones, and exert their inhibitory influence on pyramidal cells in vertical slabs shown in Figure E 1–6 (Marin-Padilla [1969], [1970]) immediately adjacent to the excited columnar module, i. e. on the somata of pyramidal cells of laminae III, IV and V of adjacent modules (cp. Figs. E 1–5 and E 1–6). There is convergence of many inhibitory cells onto any one pyramidal cell soma, on which there are 50 to 100 inhibitory synapses forming a dense meshwork or basket, hence the name *basket cell* for the inhibitory neurones (Colonnier and Rossignol [1969].

In contrast to the powerful localized action of specific afferent fibres (*Spec. aff.* in Figs. E 1 − 5 and 6) in laminae III, IV and V, there is in laminae I and II the less concentrated action of the other main input lines to the module, the association fibres from other regions of the cortex and commissural fibres of the corpus callosum (cp. *Assoc. call. aff.* in Fig. E 1 − 5). These fibres, as well as the ascending axons of the *Martinotti type cells* of laminae V and VI (S_6 in Figs. E 1 − 5 and E 1 − 6), branch to form in laminae I and II tangentially running axons which have a spread of up to 5 mm in length (Fig. E 8 − 8; Szentágothai [1972]). These axons form crossing-over synapses (at about 45° angle) with ascending dendrites of pyramidal cells of the deeper laminae (cp. Figs. E 1 − 5, 6; E 8 − 8) and also of the star-pyramid cells (Sp) of laminae II. It is assumed that any one afferent fibre exerts such a limited and remote synaptic excitation by these crossing-over synapses that the summation of very many callosal or association fibre inputs is required for effective action. Thus laminae I and II are zones of diffuse mild excitatory action on pyramidal cells. Also in lamina II there are small inhibitory basket cells (S_2) with a much more limited axonal distribution to the *star-pyramidal cells* than occurs for the basket cells of the deeper laminae. This finer pattern of inhibitory action suggests that the excitatory synaptic action on star-pyramidal cells is cut to a finer grain than occurs with the large pyramidal cells in laminae III and V. However in parenthesis it should be added that there is now evidence for small inhibitory basket cells in the deeper laminae, giving there also a fine grain of inhibitory action. The more diffuse milder excitation of laminae I and II leads to the conjecture that in these superficial laminae there is a mild excitation and a fine grain inhibitory modulation of the star-pyramidal cells (Figs. E 1 − 5 and 6, Sp). However, Szentágothai [1972] states that much more systematic study is needed in order to discover if the association and callosal afferents also establish a high level of synaptic connectivity with cells in the deeper laminae (as is indicated in Fig. E 1 − 5), which presumably would be much more limited in tangential spread than in the superficial layers.

A recently discovered neurone is shown in Figure E 1 − 6 deep in lamina II (S_7). This so-called *chandelier cell* gives many inhibitory type synapses on the apical dendrites of pyramidal cells. It is conjectured by Szentágothai [1974] that this neurone inhibits specifically the excitatory synapses on the more superficial zones of these apical dendrites.

These considerations reveal that in the first place the functional integrity

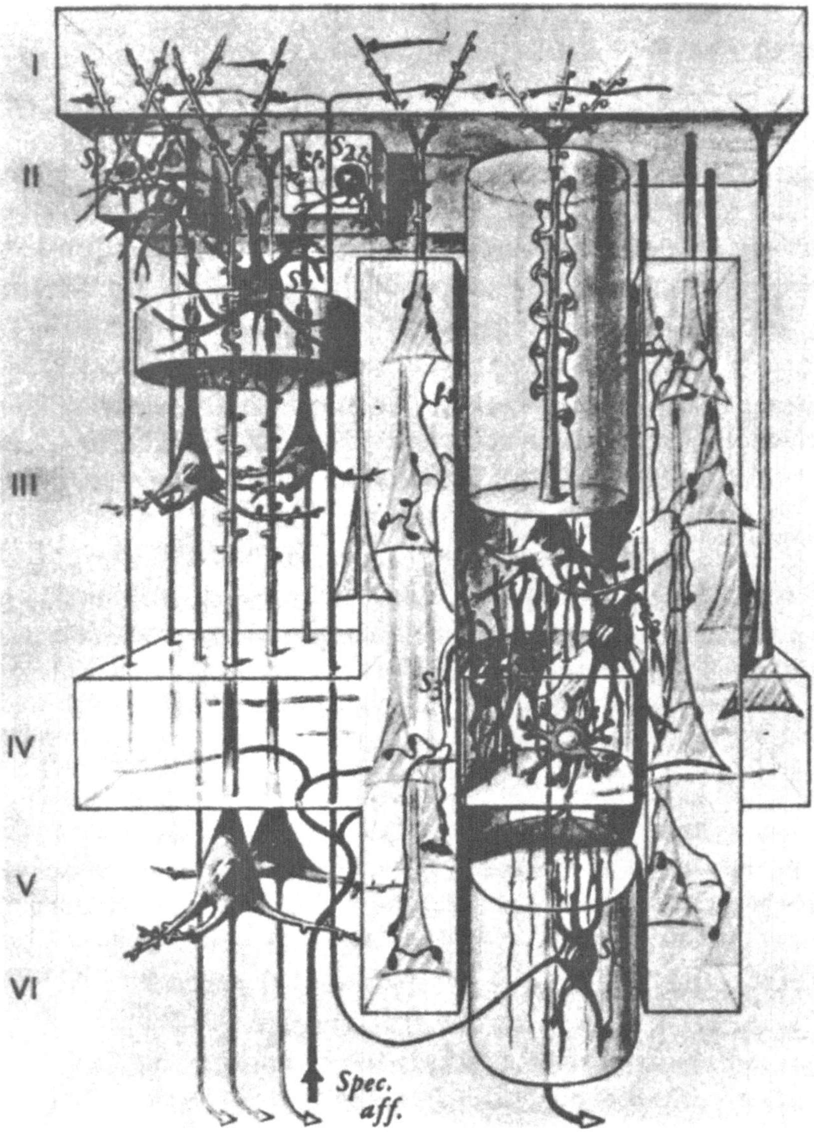

Fig. E1 – 6. Three-dimensional construct showing cortical neurones with various cell types with the same identification symbols as in Fig. E1 – 5. To the right is a column with one pyramidal cell and several varieties of stellate cell. The two inhibitory cells, S_3, are shown projecting to pyramidal cells shown in shadowy form in adjacent columns. To the left there is shown the approximate organization of neurones and synapses in laminae I and II. Further discussion in text (Szentágothai, 1975).

of a module (Figs. E 1 – 5, 6) derives from the limited range of excitatory action by the specific and other afferent fibres – in laminae III, IV and V no more than 500 μm – and from the powerful and vertically localized excitation by the interneurones (S_1, S_5 in Fig. E 1 – 5) giving the cartridge-type synapses. A further defining factor is the inhibitory surround built up by the basket cells of laminae IV. Marin-Padilla [1970] has found that the distribution of basket cells would not define a cylindrical column by the inhibitory surround, but rather a rectangular slab, resembling that proposed by Hubel and Wiesel [1972], and as will be discussed and illustrated in chapter E 2, Figure 7.

Szentágothai [1972] generalizes from the specific sensory areas, somaesthetic and visual, to the neocortex in general. One can assume that non-specific afferent fibres from the thalamus, for example, have the same distribution as the specific thalamic afferent fibre in Figure E 1 – 5. These inhibitorily defined modules in laminae III, IV and V of the neocortex are embedded, as it were, in the much more diffuse and mild excitatory and inhibitory actions of laminae I and II, which span many modules with what we may suppose to be a general modulating influence, though a finer grain would be given by the localized inhibitory action by small basket cells (S_2) on the star-pyramidal cells (Sp) of lamina II. A further complicating factor derives from the widely dispersed (up to 3 mm) axon collaterals of the pyramidal cells (Scheibel and Scheibel [1970]; Szentágothai [1972], [1974]) which appear to give a diffuse excitatory background to modules over a wide area, so constituting a wide diffuse positive feedback (Szentágothai [1974]).

Recent studies on area 17 of the monkey have disclosed fine vertical patterns of connectivity of stellate and pyramidal cells (Lund [1973]; Lund and Boothe [1975]). For example, in laminae IV the apical dendrites of deeper pyramidal cells have very few spines and the synaptic excitation is concentrated on the stellate cells. The various subdivisions of laminae III and IV appear to be zones of preferred synaptic connectivity. This most refined analysis of the laminated arrangement of dendritic input gives premonition of what is to come as we strive to understand more and more of the operative complexity of cortical modules.

4. Modular Interaction

The excitatory level built up in a module is communicated to other cortical modules from moment to moment by the impulse discharges along the association and commissural fibres formed by the axons of pyramidal cells and of the large stellate-pyramidal cells (Szentágothai [1972]). In this way powerful excitation of a module will spread widely and effectively to other modules (cp. Fig. E 7–4), but preponderantly to laminae I and II of these modules. Less powerfully excited modules will be less effective in inter-module transmission, and there will be zero action by those modules effectively inhibited by basket cell action.

There is as yet no quantitative data on module operation. However the number of neurones in a module is surprisingly large – up to 10,000, of which there would be some hundreds of pyramidal cells and many hundreds of each of the other species of neurones. The operation of a module can be imagined as a complex of circuits in parallel with summation of hundreds of convergent lines onto its constituent neurones and in addition a mesh of feedforward and feedback excitatory and inhibitory lines overpassing the simple neuronal circuitry expressed in Figure E 1–5 and 6. Thus we have to envisage levels of complexity in the operation of a module far beyond anything yet conceived, and of a totally different order from any integrated microcircuits of electronics, the analogous systems mentioned earlier. Moreover there will be an enormous range in the output from a module – from high frequency discharges in the hundreds of constituent pyramidal cells to the irregular low level discharges characteristic of cerebral cortex in the resting state (Evarts [1964]; Moruzzi [1966]; Jung [1967]). There is wide variation in the range of projection of the axons of pyramidal cells – some go only to nearby modules, other axons are association fibres to remote areas, and yet others are commissural fibres traversing the corpus callosum to areas of the other side, which tend to be in a mirror-image relationship. Finally it must be remembered that many pyramidal cells send their axons to lower levels of the central nervous system, about half a million from one motor cortex down the pyramidal tract and twenty million from one hemisphere to the brain stem. However before leaving the cerebral cortex all these axons give off extensive collaterals that would contribute positive feedback to the cerebral cortex.

It must be recognized that the evidence we have presented is based upon study of the cortices of cats and monkeys. No one has yet looked at the human cerebral cortex at the right level of electron microscopy in order to be able to recognize if there is any difference, if there is some subtle pattern of connectivity in the human cortex which distinguishes it from that in the subhuman primate brain. Another point is of course that no one has done any of the detailed microelectrode searching in the human cerebral cortex in order to discover any special features of neuronal activity in the modular arrangements. This could come quite soon. There are even some preliminary reports, and I see no insuperable difficulty. Pinneo (personal communication), for example, has investigated the electrical responses of human cerebral cortex during speech, in the speech areas, and has shown the specificity of neuronal patterns for words. They certainly are excited, as we know from the increase of circulation in the speech areas that Risberg and Ingvar [1973], Ingvar and Schwartz [1974] and Ingvar [1975] find with radio-xenon testing during talking and reading. It could be of particular interest to have a comprehensive study of the unitary responses of neurones of the speech areas during activity. Such recording, however, will need more subtle interpretation than we are yet ready for. Of more importance could be a study of the speech areas at a refined electron-microscopic level, particularly of the unique Brodmann areas 39 and 40. When this work is really at a high level, we may discover if there are subtle new properties, new connectivities, perhaps a greater number of these interconnections in laminae I and II. If something like this was discovered in the human cerebral cortex, we would be very happily placed to be able to say that here we are beginning to understand the actual structural basis of those modules with which the self-conscious mind can interact, both in receiving from and in making effective changes, as will be described in chapter E 7.

4.1. Patterns of Module Action and Interaction

In summary it can be stated that the important discovery for our purpose is that there are more or less well-defined groups of cells, perhaps up to 10,000, which are locked together by mutual connectivities, and which have as a consequence some unitary existence, building up power within themselves and inhibiting the cells of columns nearby. This is the modular concept. Now, further, the important functional property for our point of view is that there appear to be two levels of performance. There are the powerful synaptic connectivities in laminae III, IV and V, where the somata and dendrites of the large pyramidal cells are located and where the specific afferent fibres exert their main synaptic influence, partly directly, but mostly via interneurones. It may be conjectured that, for interaction with the self-conscious mind, special significance attaches to the laminae I and II, where there are synaptic connectivities with a finer grain and much less effectiveness (Szentágothai [1974]). At this level we have surmised that there are synaptic connectivities that are less demanding. We could surmise that they were just modulating the excitation of pyramidal cells in a subtle and slowly varying manner.

We propose that a module has to be regarded as a power unit. Its *raison d'etre* is to build up power at the expense of its neighbours. We think the nervous system always works by conflict – in this case by conflicts between each module and the adjacent modules. Each one is trying to overcome the other one by building up its own power by all the vertical connections which Ramón y Cajal and Lorente de Nó first described and by the projection of inhibition out to the neighbouring modules (Szentágothai [1969]; Marin-Padilla [1970]). That functional discriminatory action is really what makes a module. A module is a unit because it has a system of internal power generation and around it is the delimitation secured by its inhibitory action on the adjacent modules. Of course each of these modules in turn has its own intrinsic power and it is fighting back with a counter-inhibition to its surrounding modules. Nowhere is there uncontrolled excitation. There is an immense power interaction of excitation and inhibition. It is in this continuous interaction that we have to think of the subtlety of the whole neuronal machine of the human cerebral cortex composed perhaps of one to two million modules each with up to 10,000 component neurones. We can only dimly imagine what is happening in the human cortex or indeed in the cortices of the higher mammals, but it is at a level of complexity, of dynamic complexity, immeasurably greater than anything else that has ever been discovered in the universe or created in computer technology.

This conflict between the excitation and inhibition is actually giving all of the variation of performance from moment to moment; and superimposed on that at the level of laminae I and II there is the finer grain of inhibition. It is of finer grain because the inhibitory cells have shorter axons, only inhibiting closely adjacent cells, not the more remote inhibitory action of the inhibitory cells of the deeper laminae that project to adjacent modules. Besides this finer inhibitory grain the synaptic action is much more subtle, because in laminae I and II the synaptic excitatory power is very low, but on the other hand it is widely dispersed. There has to be a lot of convergence here because the excitatory synapses are scattered on the spines of the branching apical dendrites remote from the impulse generating sites in the somata or in the adjacent dendrites and axon (cp. Szentágothai, [1972, 1974]). There is not this powerful cartridge type of synapse along the apical dendrites of the pyramidal cell that is such a prominent feature of the deeper laminae. So we regard the synaptic influences of laminae I and II as exerting a more subtle and gentle modulating influence. It is of great interest that this proposed modulating influence is mostly exerted by the association and callosal afferent fibres. These afferents come from the pyramidal cells of other relatively remote modules and so you can think that other modules work upon this module at this gentle level and this module in turn is working back on them also at this same level (cp. chapter E 7).

5. The Connectivities of Cortical Areas

So far we have concentrated on the performance of individual modules and their interaction with adjacent modules, and have merely alluded to the pathways from the modules of one area to modules of a remote area via the association or commissural fibres. These pathways in successive stages have been most effectively studied for the primary sensory areas (cp. Fig. E 1−1): the somaesthetic (areas 3, 1, 2), visual (area 17) and auditory (Heschl's gyrus of the superior temporal gyrus). But, even within a primary sensory area there is a considerable amount of localized interaction, for example within the forelimb area, but not between forelimb and hindlimb (Jones and Powell [1969]). Furthermore, there is no direct interaction between the primary sensory areas for somaesthesis, vision and hearing. Yet interaction does occur, as for example when we identify an object felt with an object seen. Evidently it must occur in cortical areas to which these primary sensory areas project. These projections have been extensively studied for many years. The most comprehensive investigation by Jones and Powell [1970] continues this work on the primate brain and shows that there is a cascade arrangement from primary to secondary to tertiary areas and so on. This very important study will be discussed and illustrated in some detail.

As indicated in Figures E 1−7 A−D the somaesthetic pathway was investigated by a sequential degenerative technique. When the neurones in an area of the cortex are killed by the anoxia brought on by pial excision, their axons degenerate and can be traced by special staining in the serially sectioned brain several days later. For example, in the black area (S) shows that the neurones of the primary somaesthetic area, 3, 1, 2, were killed and the degenerated axonic terminals were found in the dotted areas, 5, 4 and SM (supplementary motor). Evidently areas 3, 1, 2 project to areas 5, 4 and SM and terminate there as association fibres (cp. Fig. E 1−5). In B the next stage of projection is investigated by killing neurones of area 5 in another monkey, and degeneration of axonal terminals is seen to occur in areas 6, 7 and SM. In C there is a further stage with area 7 killed and the projections are to the prefrontal cortex, areas 46 and 45, and to STS (in the depth of the superior temporal sulcus). These areas are on the outer surface of the hemisphere and on the medial surface in D there is seen to be projection to

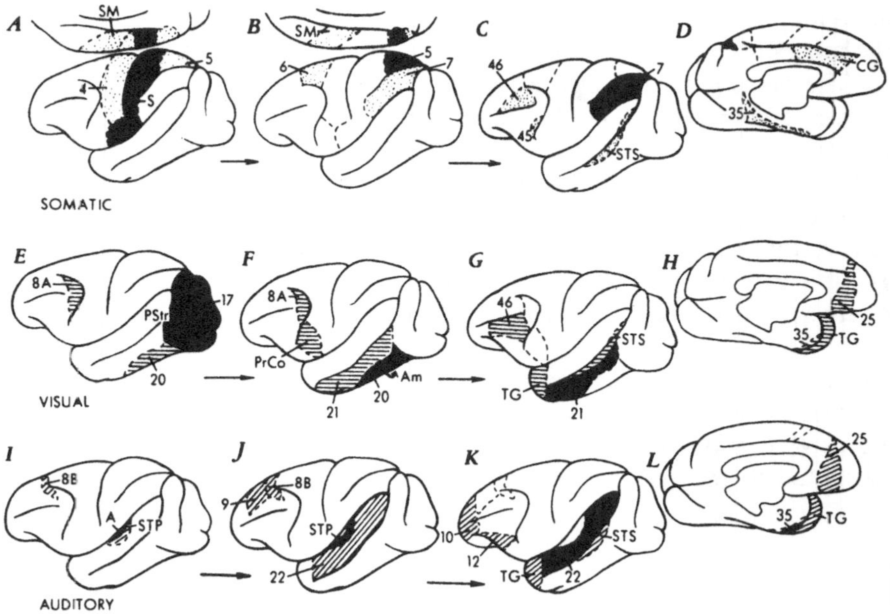

Fig. E1 – 7. A schematic diagram summarizing the outward progression of connexions from the primary somatic (A – D), visual (E – H) and auditory (I – L) areas of the cortex. Each new local step is shown in black and the further connexions of the new areas by light stippling or hatching. Notice that all sensory pathways converge in the depths of the superior temporal sulcus *(STS)*. D, H and L are the medial aspects of the hemispheres shown in C, G and K respectively (Jones and Powell, 1970).

areas 35 and CG (cingulate gyrus, areas 23 and 24 of Figure E 1 – 4 B). Areas 35 and CG are in the paralimbic zone on the way to the limbic system. Thus Figure E 1 – 7 A – D gives an illustration of the cascade of connectivities for primary to secondary to tertiary to quaternary somaesthetic areas. It will be appreciated that in Figure E 1 – 7 A – D only the main sequence (3, 1, 2) → 5 → 7 has been illustrated, and that the various secondary branches have been neglected.

The cascade of connectivities for the visual pathways is similarly illustrated in Figure E 1 – 7 E – H. In the monkey the circumstriate areas, 18 and 19, form a very slender band (the peristriate band) around the extensive primary visual area, 17, so in E the killed area included all three areas. The sequential killing was for area 20 (the inferotemporal lobe) in F, and for area 21 in G. It is of great interest that at the tertiary stage, C and G in Figure E 1 – 7, the somaesthetic and visual pathways converge onto the same cortical areas, 46 and STS, and also possibly 35 in D and H. However the two 46 areas may be contiguous at the principal sulcus and not overlapping, so STS is the principal convergent area.

The cascade of connectivities is also seen in Figure E 1 − 7 I − L from the primary auditory area (Heschl's gyrus, A in I) to STP (the superior temporal plane) to area 22, and again to STS. The further tertiary projections are again to the paralimbic areas 25 and 35.

The killing of other cortical areas in the projections adds to the complexities of the connectivities, but the diagrams of Figure E 1 − 8 A and B organize these cascades of connectivities in a way that allows certain principles to emerge. The main cascade is shown at four levels, being partly derived from Figure E 1 − 7 A − D. The primary somaesthetic area has outputs to only three areas, there being return circuits only from the motor area, 4. Next in order is the powerful projection from 5 to 7, and also from 5 to 6 and SM. Areas 4, 6 and 5 have powerful reciprocal connectivities, which can be attributed to the very effective use of the somaesthetic input for guiding

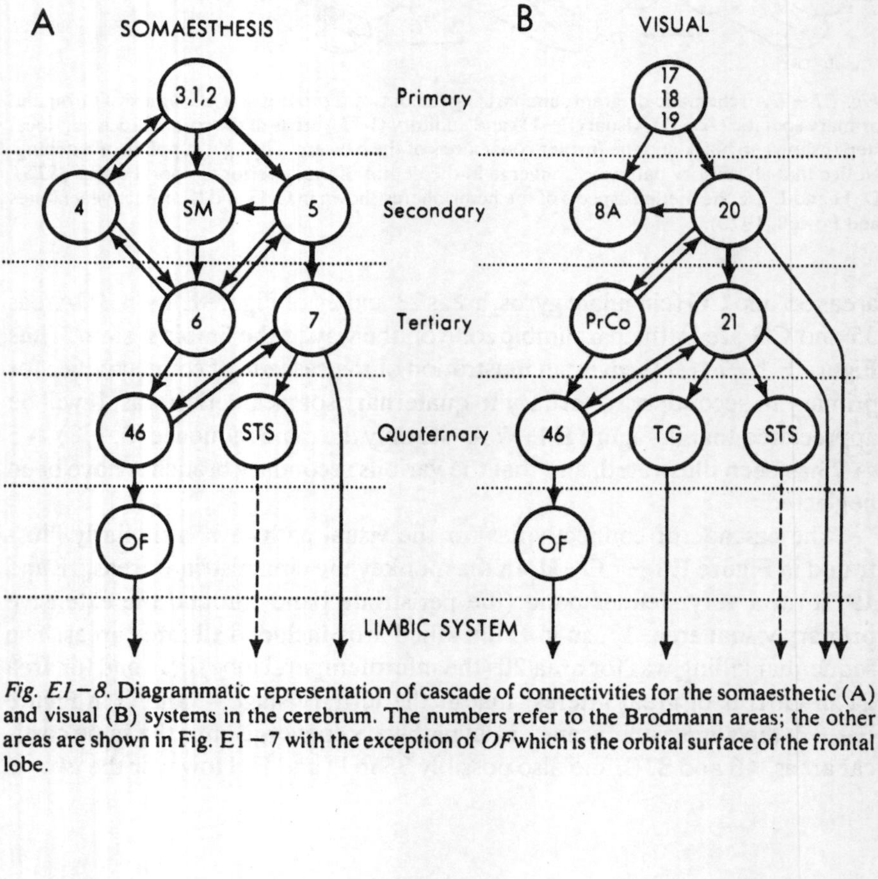

Fig. E1 − 8. Diagrammatic representation of cascade of connectivities for the somaesthetic (A) and visual (B) systems in the cerebrum. The numbers refer to the Brodmann areas; the other areas are shown in Fig. E1 − 7 with the exception of *OF* which is the orbital surface of the frontal lobe.

pyramidal cell discharges from the motor area, 4, and down the pyramidal tract to give motor action, as will be described in chapter E 3. The connection of area 5 to 7 is not reciprocal, but at the quaternary level there is reciprocity for areas 46 and 7. At the further stages there is projection to the important polymodal area STS. Also there are several projections to the limbic system either directly from 7 or via 46 or possibly STS.

In Figure E 1 − 8 B for visual pathways, areas 17, 18, 19 project at the secondary level to areas 20 and 8 A (the prefrontal eye field) with no return circuits. In the tertiary level there are reciprocal connectivities to area PrCo (the precentral agranular field), but only forward projections to 8 A and 21. Finally the principal tertiary area, 21, is reciprocal to 46, but unidirectional to STS and to the limbic system. A special feature of the visual system is a direct path from the secondary area 20 to the limbic system. There are several features common to A and B: the unidirectional paths out from the primary area; the unidirectional path from secondary to tertiary in the main sequence, 5 to 7 in A and 20 to 21 in B; the reciprocal connectivities from the two tertiary areas 7 and 21 to 46; the output from these same tertiary areas to STS; the outputs from the main tertiary areas 7 and 21 to the limbic system. In each system there are several other less direct paths to the limbic system. In both A and B the onward progressions of the secondary and tertiary projections are to both the frontal and the parieto-temporal lobes with cross linkages. The auditory projection system displays similar features but has been less studied (cp. Fig. E 1 − 7 I − L).

The connectivities displayed in Figures E 1 − 7 and 8 will be of particular interest when we come to study the cortical mechanisms involved in conscious perception in chapter E 2 and the effects of circumscribed cerebral lesions in chapter E 6. It is important to realize that each of the lines of communication in Figure E 1 − 8 represents an association pathway with enormous numbers of nerve fibres, hundreds of thousands at least, and that at each relay station there are the immense integrational systems of the modules. As shown in Figure E 1 − 5, and as repeatedly emphasized above, the input from the association fibres is largely to laminae I and II, i. e. to the operational area of the modules that is weaker and more diffuse and of finer grain.

6. Connectivities of the Limbic System (Hassler [1967]; Nauta [1971]).

There is a part of the brain developed from the old olfactory (smell) brain that has unique functions, being specially concerned in emotional experience

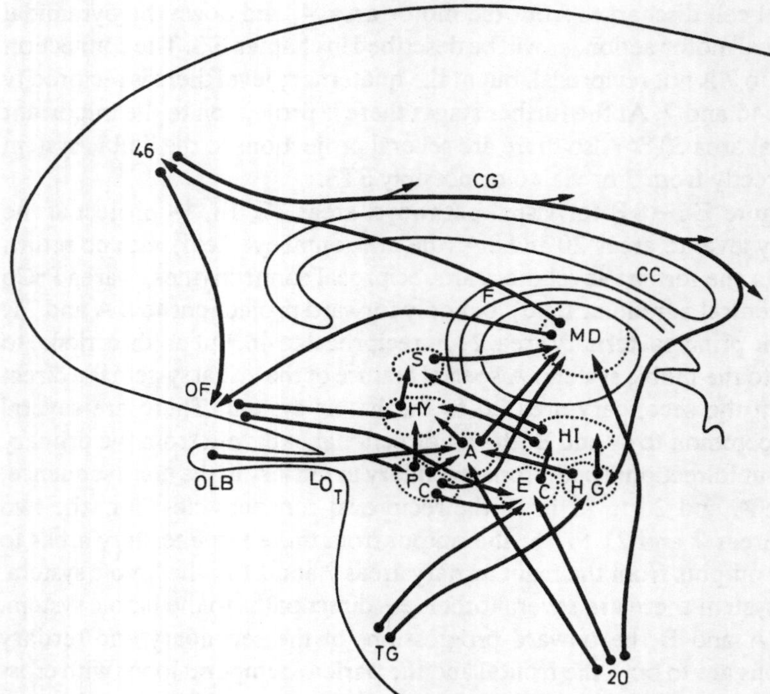

Fig. E1 − 9. Schematic drawing to show connectivities from the neocortex to and from the medio-dorsal thalamus *(MD)*. *OF* is orbital surface of prefrontal cortex; *TG*, the temporal pole; *HG*, the gyrus hippocampi; *HI*, the hippocampus; *S*, septum; *F*, fornix; *CC*, corpus callosum; *OLB*, olfactory bulb; *LOT*, lateral olfactory tract; *PC*, piriform cortex; *EC*, entorhinal cortex; *A*, amygdala; *HY*, hypothalamus; *CG*, cingulate gyrus.

(considered in chapter E 2) and also in the laying down of memories (considered in chapter E 8). It is usually known as the limbic system or the limbic lobe, terms which cover an extremely complex assemblage of structures that are still poorly understood − both structurally and functionally. It includes primitive areas of cerebral cortex that are distinct from the great newly developed neocortical areas, and that are often called archicortex. As diagrammatically shown in Figure E 1 − 9, it includes the hippocampus (HI) and the associated hippocampal gyrus (HG) including the entorhinal cortex (EC) that are also depicted in a transverse section of the brain in Figure E 8 − 6. The piriform cortex (PC in Fig. E 1 − 9) is also a primitive cortex and is on the olfactory pathway as described in chapter E 2. Besides these areas of primitive cortex there are the associated nuclei such as the amygdala (A), the septal (S) and raphae nuclei (not shown), the hypothalamus (HY) and the connectivities, particularly by the whole fornix (F) system (not shown).

Figure E 1−9 shows pathways from areas of the temporal lobe, TG and 20 (Fig. E 1−7) to the entorhinal cortex (EC) and the hippocampal gyrus (HG) and thence to the hippocampus (HI), which is the principal component of the human limbic system. It also shows two pathways from the prefrontal lobe to the limbic system, one from the convexity (area 46 in Fig. E 1−7) via a circuitous route with many branches in the cingulate gyrus (CG) to the hippocampal gyrus (HG), the other more direct from the orbital surface of the prefrontal lobe (OF, cp. Fig. E 1−8) to the hypothalamus (HY) and the entorhinal cortex (EC). Further connectivities are indicated in Figure E 1−9. Of particular interest are the pathways from PC to A and to EC, whereby olfactory information gets to the hypothalamus, the hippocampus, the septal nuclei and thence to the medio-dorsal (MD) thalamus on the way to the prefrontal cortex. The various hypothalamic nuclei (HY) concerned in sensing hunger, thirst, sex, pleasure, appear to project to the MD thalamus largely by the septal nuclei, but direct connections from the amygdala to the prefrontal cortex have now been demonstrated. The role of this flow of information in modifying and developing conscious perceptions will be considered in chapter E 2.

In Figure E 1−9 the central role of the MD thalamus is evident (cp. Nauta [1971]). The principal path from the limbic system to the neocortex is from the MD thalamus to the orbital surface of the prefrontal cortex (OF). The significance of this unique pathway cannot be overestimated. It is important to recognize that the olfactory system projects directly to the limbic system via the piriform cortex (PC) and the amygdala (A) without having to negotiate complex neocortical pathways, as do the somaesthetic, visual and auditory systems (cp. Figs. E 1−7 and E 1−8).

A final statement about the limbic system is that it is a system of sequential neuronal networks with a complexity far beyond the greatly simplified diagram of Figure E 1−9, where, for example, the whole fornix system is neglected. Nevertheless, Figure 1−9 will serve in chapter E 2 as a basis for discussion of the manner in which conscious experiences are elaborated with their emotional overtones.

Chapter E 2 Conscious Perception

7. Résumé

The fundamental design of the sensory system is described with various receptor organs for touch, vision, and hearing, for example, that signal to the central nervous system by the firing of impulses or messages that in the manner of a code transmit to the brain the place and intensity of the stimulus. The transmission is never direct but by synaptic relays (cp. Fig. E 2 – 1) which act to modify the message so that in fact the central nervous system is given a very distorted "coded image" of the peripheral stimulus. It can be thought that these transmission lines are concerned in the conversion of the original stimulus into neuronal events which can be handled and interpreted in the cerebral cortex. Each sense has the primary receiving area laid out as a map in the cortex in the appropriate Brodmann areas. For example, cutaneous sense is laid out with the surface of the body arranged as a strip map from toes to tongue along Brodmann areas 3, 1, 2 (Figs. E 1 – 1, 4).

There has been a precise anatomical study by Libet of the timing of conscious perception in relationship to events in the primary sensory area of the cerebral cortex (Figs. E 2 – 2, 3). It has been shown that conscious sensation does not occur immediately the neuronal messages reach the cerebral cortex. There is a relatively long incubation period during which there is progressive spread and complication of the neuronal patterns until they reach the appropriate level for action across the interface between the brain and the self-conscious mind. This period may be as long as 0.5 s, but the self-conscious mind is shown to be able to antedate the perception so that it is perceived to happen up to 0.5 s before the triggering neuronal events – the process of antedating. From the primary sensory area for touch, the information spreads to area 5 and then to 7, which are recognized to relate the sensory input into patterns giving the shape and the surface feel of objects palpated and also the relation to the visual experience of these objects.

There is a brief discussion of the visual pathway from the retina to the primary visual area of the cerebral cortex. It is shown in Figure E 2−4 how the left and right visual fields of both eyes are channelled by the visual pathways so that there is crossing of the left field to the right visual cortex and vice versa for the right visual field. In the primary visual area the visual field is organized as a map (Fig. E 2−5). In this map the very fine details are arranged in the cortical columns by two criteria: eye dominance and the spatial orientation of the triggering lines or edges or contours in the visual field (Figs. E 2−6, 7). Further processing in the visual cortex results in some partial reconstitution of the elements of the visual image. In the retina this visual image is of course converted simply into a mosaic of a million or so elements that project to the visual cortex in the coded manner of impulse discharges in the optic nerve fibres. There are various stages by which this punctate mosaic in the retina is eventually reconstituted in coded form by individual neurones in the tertiary and quaternary sensory areas (Figs. E 1−7 E−H, 8 B) that have feature recognition for simple geometrical forms. There is, however, no clue from this work as to how the whole visual picture is reconstituted in the conscious experience. Such recognition features as squares, triangles, rectangles, stars, for example, are very remote indeed from the reconstitution of the full picture.

Wonderful as it is, this animal experimentation still gives no clue as to how a whole visual picture can be reconstituted by the neuronal machinery of the brain. In discussing this enigma of visual perception, there is reference to chapter E 7 where a radical new hypothesis will be presented.

There is a brief account of auditory perception showing that essentially the same neuronal machinery is concerned with successive relays into other cortical areas from the primary receiving area.

Finally, there is an account of the way in which the limbic system and associated areas of the brain stem can provide the emotional colouring of conscious perception. Circuits are described from the neocortex, particularly the frontal lobe, to the limbic system and back again. It must also be recognized that there are several areas devoted to crossmodal transfer between touch, vision, and hearing, and the limbic inputs with the associated experiences of smell, taste, hunger, thirst, fear, rage, sex, pleasure, etc.

In the Epilogue, there is a quotation from Mountcastle to illustrate the extraordinary dichotomy between on the one hand what is happening in the brain as a consequence of all the inputs from receptor organs and on the other hand the conscious perceptions that each of us has as a result of these inputs.

8. Introduction

There are certain principles relating to the neural events that lead to perceptions of the various sensory experiences. Touch and vision have been most thoroughly investigated, but there is good reason to believe that all other sensory experiences are dependent upon similar neuronal mechanisms. Necessarily the crucial experimental investigation of sensory experiences must be carried out on conscious human subjects, but both the design and interpretation of these experiments are dependent on the wonderful successes that have attended investigations on animal, and particularly monkey, sensory systems in the last few decades. The powerful techniques designed for precision and selectivity of stimulation have been matched by microelectrode recording from single neurones. But just as importantly there has been the success in defining the neural pathways from receptor organs to cerebral cortex and within the cerebral cortex by precise anatomical investigations.

There is a large variety of these receptor organs with built-in properties that enable them to encode in a highly selective manner some environmental change into a discharge of nerve impulses. In general it can be stated that intensity of stimulus is encoded as frequency of discharge of impulses. In this way there are transmitted to the higher levels of the central nervous system signals from receptor organs that result in the conscious experiences of vision, hearing and touch for example. An introduction to the problem of conscious perception is best given in relation to cutaneous sensing. In the skin are receptor organs specialized for converting some mechanical stimulus such as a touch or tap into impulse discharges in nerve fibres.

The pathways from receptor organs to the brain are never direct. There are always synaptic linkages from neurone to neurone at each of several relay stations. Each of these stages gives the opportunity for modifying the coding of the "messages" from the sensory receptors. Even the simplest stimuli such as a flash of light or a tap on the skin are signalled to the appropriate primary receiving area of the cerebral cortex in the form of a code of nerve impulses in various temporal sequences and in many fibres in parallel.

Our special interest is focussed on the neural events that are necessary for giving a conscious experience. It is now generally agreed that a conscious experience does not light up as soon as impulses in some sensory pathway reach the primary sensory areas in the cerebral hemisphere. In response to some brief peripheral stimulus the initial response is a sharp potential change, the evoked response, in the appropriate primary cortical area (ER of Fig. E2 − 3 A). Immediately afterwards there is a change in the background frequency of firing of numerous neurones in this area – an increase or a decrease, or some complex temporal sequence thereof. Our present problem is to gain some insight into the neural events that have a necessary relationship to the conscious experience. In important respects the study of cutaneous sensation leads in this most challenging field of the neural sciences.

One cannot do better than to terminate this introduction by the vivid and imaginative statements by Mountcastle [1975].

> Each of us believes himself to live directly within the world that surrounds him, to sense its objects and events precisely, to live in real and current time. I assert that these are perceptual illusions, for each of us confronts the world from a brain linked to what is 'out there' by a few million fragile sensory nerve fibres. These are our only information channels, our lifelines to reality. These sensory nerve fibres are not high-fidelity recorders, for they accentuate certain stimulus features, neglect others. The central neuron is a story-teller with regard to the afferent nerve fibres; and he is never completely trustworthy, allowing distortions of quality and measure, within a strained but isomorphic spatial relation between "outside" and "inside." Sensation is an abstraction, not a replication, of the real world.

9. Cutaneous Perception (Somaesthesis)
9.1. Pathways to Primary Sensory Area in Cortex

Figure E 2 − 1 is a diagram of the simplest pathway from receptor organs in the skin up to the cerebral cortex. For example, a touch on the skin causes a receptor to fire impulses. These travel up the dorsal columns of the spinal cord (the cuneate tract for the hand and arm) and then, after a synaptic relay in the cuneate nucleus and another one in the thalamus, the pathway reaches the cerebral cortex. There are only two synapses on the way and you might say, why have any at all? Why not have a direct line? The point is that each one of these relays gives an opportunity for an inhibitory action that sharpens the neuronal signals by eliminating all the weaker excitatory actions, such as would occur when the skin touches an ill-defined edge. In this way a much more sharply defined signal eventually comes up to the cortex and there again there would be the same inhibitory sculpturing of the signal by modular interaction (cp. chapter E 1). As a consequence touch stimuli can be more precisely located and evaluated. In fact, because of this inhibition a strong cutaneous stimulus is often surrounded by a cutaneous area that has reduced sensitivity.

Also shown in Figure E 2 − 1 are the pathways down from the cerebral cortex to both of these relays on the cutaneous pathway. In this way, by exerting presynaptic and postsynaptic inhibition, the cerebral cortex is able to block these synapses and so protect itself from being bothered by

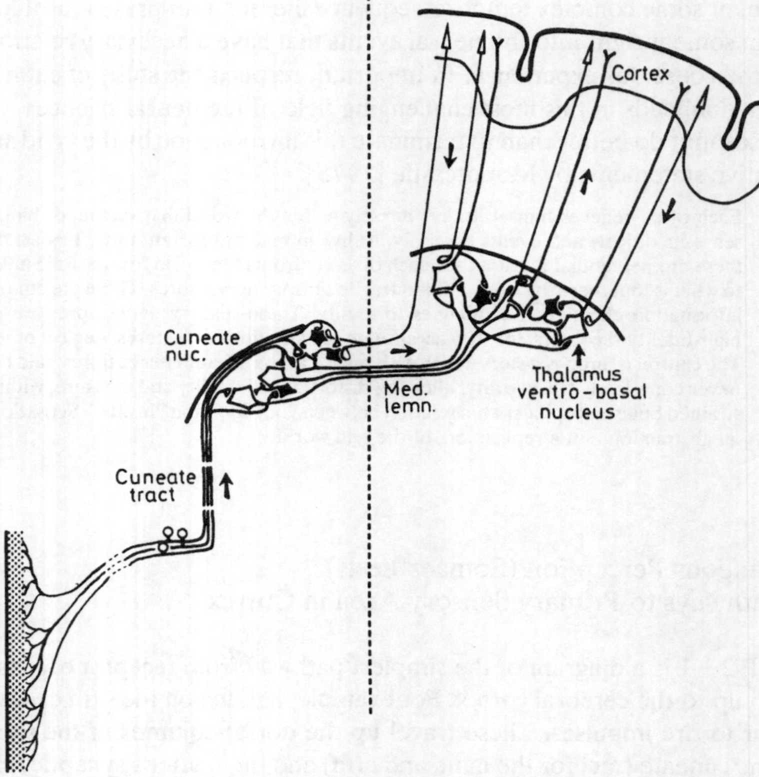

Fig. E2—1. Pathway to the sensori-motor cortex for cutaneous fibres from the forelimb. Note the inhibitory cells shown in black in both the cuneate nucleus and the ventro-basal nucleus of the thalamus. The inhibitory pathway in the cuneate nucleus is of the feed-forward type and in the thalamus it is the feed-back type. Also shown is one presynaptic inhibitory pathway to an excitatory synapse of a cuneate tract fibre. Efferent pathways from the sensori-motor cortex are shown exciting the thalamo-cortical relay cells and exciting both postsynaptic and presynaptic inhibitory neurones in the cuneate nucleus.

cutaneous stimuli that can be neglected. This is of course what happens when you are very intensely occupied, for example in carrying out some action or in experiencing or in thinking. Under such situations you can be oblivious even of severe stimulation. For example, in the heat of combat severe injuries may be ignored. At a less severe level it has long been a practice to give counter-irritation to relieve pain. Presumably in this way there is produced inhibitory suppression of the pain pathway to the brain. Thus we can account for the afferent anaesthesias of hypnosis or of yoga or of acupuncture by the cerebral and other pathways inhibiting the cutaneous pathways to the brain. In all these cases discharges from the cerebral cortex down the pyramidal tract and other pathways will exert an inhibitory blockage at the relays in the spinocortical pathways such as those diagrammed in Figure E 2 − 1. This ability of the cerebral cortex is important because it is undesirable to have all receptor organ discharges from your body pouring into your brain all the time. The design pattern of successive synaptic relays each with various central and peripheral inhibitory inputs gives opportunity for turning off inputs according to the exigencies of situations.

Conventional studies on animals and man have defined the area of cortex that is primarily involved in responding to cutaneous sense, the somaesthetic area. As shown in Figure E 1 − 1, the principal area is laid out as a long strip map in the postcentral gyrus, which is made up of three areas (Brodmann areas 3, 1, 2 in Figure E 1 − 4) distinguished by their different structures. All areas of the body surface from the extreme caudal to the extreme rostral lie in linear sequence along the postcentral gyrus from its dorso-medial end over the convex surface of the cerebral hemispheres. Area 3 b is specialized for light touch and 1, 2 for deep stimuli, skin pressure and joint movement, while 3 a, is concerned with muscle sense (see Jones and Powell [1973] for references). There is also a subsidiary somaesthetic area which is not important for the theme of this chapter. As already stated in chapter E 1, the first evidence for the columnar arrangement of the cerebral cortex was obtained by Mountcastle [1957] in his detailed topographic study of the somaesthetic area. It will be seen in Figure E 1 − 1 that cortical areas are apportioned in relationship to the fineness of discrimination of the cutaneous areas and not to their relative areas. This map has been explored in detail by two main procedures: recording in non-human primates of the cortical responses evoked by exploratory stimulation applied systematically to the whole surface of the body, limbs, neck and head; electrical stimulation of the sensory cortex in conscious human subjects who report the skin areas to which the evoked sensations are referred (Penfield and Jasper [1954]).

Usually the subjects report abnormal sensory experiences, paraesthesiae such as tingling, numbness, "pins-and-needles," though there are also reports of normal sensations − touch, tap and pressure. The paraesthesiae are plausibly explained by the outrage that the applied stimulation perpetrates on the highly organized neuronal machinery of the cerebral cortex. Even the weakest electrical stimulus will excite in a manner dependent on the relationship of the immense neuronal assemblage to the applied electrical current. As a consequence there will be "a neuronal shock wave" having little resemblance to the pattern of neuronal activation generated by a natural input from the receptor organs; hence the paraesthesia, just as when the ulnar nerve at the elbow joint is bumped — the so-called funny-bone.

9.2. Temporal Analysis of Cutaneous Perception

In our inquiry into the happenings in the cerebral hemisphere that bear a necessary relation to conscious perception, the most fundamental question may be formulated as follow: how elaborated must the spatiotemporal pattern of neuronal activity be in order that it achieves a necessary relation to a conscious experience? For example it is generally agreed that there is not even the simplest perception (the philosopher's raw feel!) when incoming impulses impinge on the neurones of the primary sensory cortex, or even when the incoming impulses trigger discharges of these neurones.

Libet's ([1973] and personal communication) investigations on cutaneous sensing of conscious human subjects have provided most surprising answers. This work has been carried out during the last 10 years, always with the informed consent of the patient and during the exposure of a cerebral hemisphere for some neurosurgical procedure. Extreme care was taken to

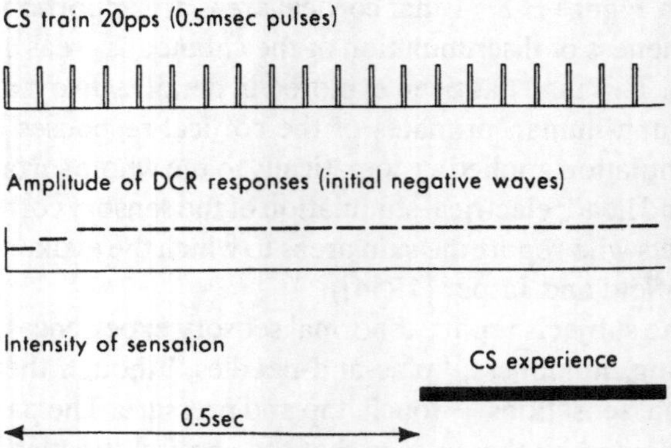

Fig. E2–2. Diagram of relationships between the train of 0.5 msec pulses at liminal intensity applied to the human postcentral gyrus, and the amplitudes of the direct cortical responses *(DCR)* recorded nearby. The third line indicates that no conscious sensory experience is elicited until approximately the initial 0.5 sec of events has elapsed and that the just-detectable sensation appearing after that period remains at the same subjective intensity while the stimulus train continues (Libet, 1966).

employ gentle electrical stimulation so that there was no injury of the exposed cerebral cortex to which the stimulation was applied.

The initial discovery was that a brief repetitive stimulation of the sensory cortex was far more effective in evoking a perceptual experience than was a single stimulus. For optimal effectiveness of a just-threshold stimulation (Figure E 2−2) the train of repetitive stimuli, each a current pulse of 0.5 ms duration, was in the range of 20/s to 120/s. Libet found that the critical pulse strength for giving a perceptual experience – often a paraesthesia – was lowest with a long train duration. As indicated by the black band in Figure E 2−2, further continuation of the train beyond 0.5 s merely gave a continuation of the perceptual experience at the just detectable level, there being no enhancement. Yet at the same time the evoked potentials recorded from the cerebral cortex showed a steady size of response to each successive stimulus of the train. Evidently with such a weak train of stimuli there can be a conscious experience only where there has been time (up to 0.5 s) for an elaboration of spatiotemporal (ST) patterns in the neuronal machinery of the sensory cortex.

In contrast to that finding with cortical stimulation, a single weak cutaneous stimulus could be perceived just as well as a train. Libet [1973] proposed that this perception occurred only after there had been time for elaboration of neuronal ST patterns, as is illustrated in Figure E 2−3 A. However, when a brief electrical pulse was applied to the skin of the hand, for example, the subject was not aware that there was this relatively long delay of up to 0.5 s before he could feel the stimulation. It is known that only a very small fraction of this time, 0.015 s, is occupied in transmission from the skin to the cerebral cortex as shown by the evoked response (ER) in Figure E 2−3 A. Libet applied very ingenious experimental procedures in testing his hypothesis. These are diagrammatically illustrated in Figure E 2−3 B−D.

The first experimental design tested the supposition that a just-threshold single skin stimulus (SS) was effective in producing a conscious sensation after the same incubation period (Fig. E 2−3 A) as a just-threshold train of cortical stimulation (CS), which is as long as 0.5 s. If that were so, when the SS was applied *during* the minimal CS train, the SS should be experienced *after* the CS; but it was usually experienced *before*! (Figure E 2−2 B). The exception was that if the SS was during the last 100 ms of the CS train, the order of awareness shifted to SS after CS. In a second experimental procedure it was found that a threshold SS often failed to be experienced when a train of CS was applied 0.2 to 0.5 s *after* the single SS (Figure E 2−3 C). This *retroactive masking* certainly suggested that a just-threshold SS was experienced only after a build-up of cortical activity for a period as long as 0.2 to

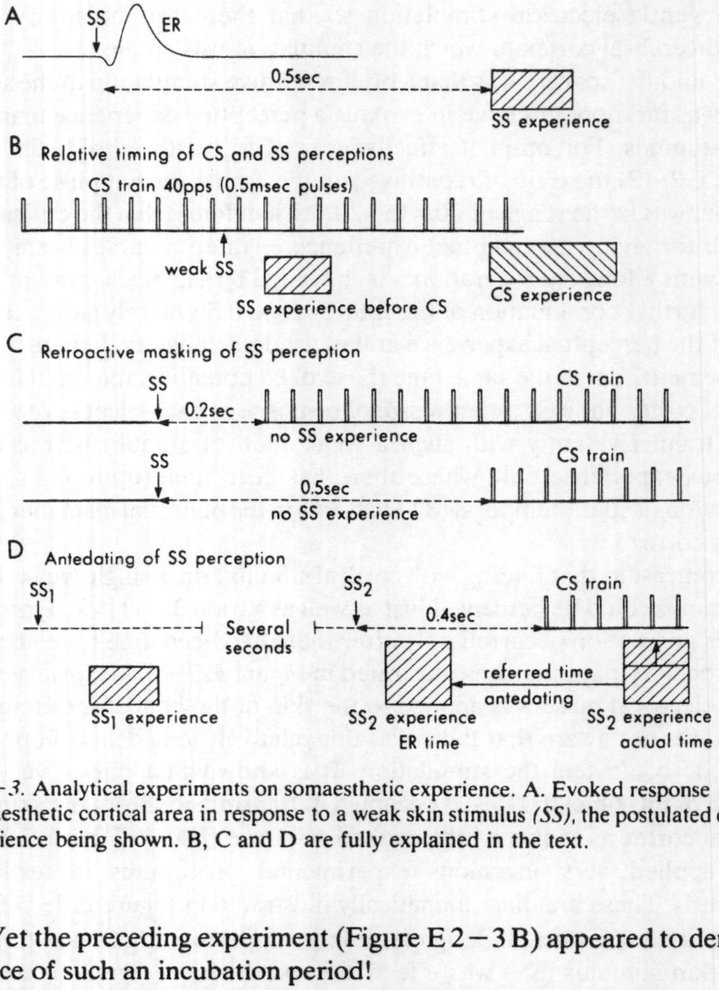

Fig. E2–3. Analytical experiments on somaesthetic experience. A. Evoked response *(ER)* of the somaesthetic cortical area in response to a weak skin stimulus *(SS)*, the postulated delayed *SS* experience being shown. B, C and D are fully explained in the text.

0.5 s. Yet the preceding experiment (Figure E 2 – 3 B) appeared to deny th existence of such an incubation period!

The final experimental procedure resolved this paradox, but raised fur ther profound problems. It is based on the finding that, when two skin stimuli SS_1 and SS_2 are applied some seconds apart, their relative intensity is recognized by the subject with surprising accuracy. After this preliminary survey, the test situation was set up with two identical stimuli SS_1 and SS_2 and with a CS train delivered 0.2 to 0.6 s *after* SS_2. Under these conditions the subject reported three experiences, SS_1, SS_2 and CS, the latter being too far to the right to be shown in Figure E 2 – 3 D. SS_2 now appeared in some cases to be stronger than SS_1 (Figure E 2 – 3 D) and in other cases it was weaker. The *retroactive enhancement* of subjective awareness of SS_2 may occur when CS starts as long as 0.6 s after SS_2. Since the conscious experience of the SS_2 stimulus can be modified by a CS starting 0.2 to 0.6 s after SS_2, it can be concluded that the neural events giving the experience to the SS_2 stimulus must continue for this time in order for there to be the requisite elaboration of neuronal spatiotemporal patterns in the cerebral cortex. Thus the activation time is comparable with that established for trains of weak CS stimuli (Fig. E 2−2). Yet at the same time, in the first experimental test described above (Figure E 2−3 B), this SS was experienced as if there was no such delay!

In order to resolve this paradox Libet developed a most interesting hypothesis, namely that, though a weak single SS requires up to 0.5 s of cortical activity before it can be experienced, *in the experiencing process* it is antedated by being referred in time to the initial evoked response of the cortex (ER in Figure E 2−3 A). Evidently, in the attempted solution of one problem, Libet has raised an even more perplexing one: what is the perceptual mechanism for this antedating? A possible solution of this problem will be suggested in chapter E 7. The initial hypothesis of Libet is corroborated by these experiments, namely, that weak skin stimuli are experienced consciously only when a period of up to 0.5 s has been spent in the cerebral cortex in the elaboration of neuronal ST patterns to the level of complexity requisite for the most primitive conscious experience, a raw feel.

In a further test of this hypothesis Libet & others (1977) have employed stimulation of the cutaneous pathway to the cerebral cortex (*med. lemn.* and *ventrobasal thalamus* in Figure E 2−1), which elicits an evoked response comparable with that produced by peripheral stimulation (ER in Figure E 2−3 A), but which, when weak, requires repetitive stimulation in order to be detected, i. e. it resembles a cortical stimulus (Figure E 2−2) in this respect. Though a train of stimuli was required, the subjective timing of the actual experience was antedated to the onset of the train, presumably because of the evoked response. It should be noted that cortical stimulation produces a diffuse weak cortical response (the DCR responses plotted in Fig. E 2−2), which is quite different from the sharp large ER response of Figure E 2−3 A.

9.3. Secondary and Tertiary Sensory Areas

Sensory experiences of touch at a more complex level are signalled by neurones of the primary sensory area that specifically respond to the direction of movement of a stimulus over the skin surface (Werner [1974]). We shall see that comparable movement sensitivities are much more highly developed in neurones of the primary visual cortex. More synthetic responses are exhibited by neurones in the secondary cortical area, 5, which is adjacent to the primary sensory areas, 3, 1, 2 in Figure E 1 – 4 A. As indicated in Figure E 1 – 7 A and 8 A, area 5 receives the principal projection from areas 3, 1, 2. Mountcastle [1975] and associates [1975] have made a most exhaustive study of the responses of individual neurones of area 5. They find that the responses of most neurones are related to the bringing about of movements in a holistic manner, the details of the movements being left to the motor areas, as will be described in chapter E 3. The neuronal machinery of area 5 contains a continually updated neuronal replicate of the position and movements of the limb in space. Complex stimulus patterns involving multiple joint and skin areas trigger responses of neurones that presumably are concerned in the synthetic sensing that occurs when an object is palpated. In palpation there is first the shaping of the hand for grasping an object, and secondly the moving of the hand over the surface of the object in an active exploration. In this way cutaneous sensing leads to feature detection that matches the visual feature detection in the inferotemporal lobe, as described below.

Area 7 is next in the main somaesthetic sequence (Figs. E 1 – 7 B, 8 A). By unitary neuronal analysis Mountcastle & others [1975] have shown that there is a considerable class of projection and of hand manipulation neurones resembling those of area 5. It was, however, unexpected to find that most neurones were related to visual exploration, discharging at high frequencies when the monkey visually fixates an object that is of great interest and within reach. Thus area 7 resembles area 5 in that the neurones are actively related to command signals for exploration of surrounding space, area 5 for manual and area 7 for both manual and visual. The relationship of area 7 to visual inputs is surprising because there are no known anatomical pathways from any of the visual areas to area 7 (cp. Jones and Powell [1970] and Figs. E 1 – 7 E, F, G and 8 A, B). Presumably more devious routes are concerned.

Figure E 1 – 7 A, B and 8 A show projections of the somaesthetic pathway in addition to the main sequence. Several of these projections are to the prefrontal lobe and to the motor areas. The latter doubtless are concerned with motor command functions and will be considered further in chapter E 3. The former may be related to the pathways in the human brain that are instrumental in giving somaesthetic conscious experiences. It is important to recognize that, although the experimental procedures of Libet are concentrated on the primary somaesthetic area (3, 1, 2), the experiences reported by the subject presumably arise in relation to neuronal activities in tertiary, quaternary or even more remote areas (cp. Fig. E 1 – 8 A).

Another important projection is to the area STS because it also receives inputs from the visual and auditory pathways (Figs. E 1 – 7 C, G, K, 8 A, B). We are led in this way to the problems of the cross-modal transfer, i. e., between visual and tactual recognition, that is possible only for man and some sub-human primates (Werner [1974]) but not for cats (Ettlinger and Blakemore [1969]). This will form the theme of a later section. The problem of antedating (Fig. E 2 – 3 D) also will be considered later in relationship to the role of the self-conscious mind in perception. The projections from somaesthetic pathways to the limbic system will be considered later in this chapter. Finally the effects of clinical lesions of areas 5 and 7 will be discussed in the section of chapter E 6 on the parietal lobes.

10. Visual Perception

10.1. Retina to Primary Visual Area in Cortex

Highly complicated and exquisitely designed structures are involved in all steps of the visual pathways. The optical system of the human eye gives an image on the retina which is a sheet of closely packed receptors, some 10^7 cones and 10^8 rods, that feed into the complexly organized neuronal systems of the retina. Thus the first stage in visual perception is a radical fragmentation of the retinal picture into the independent responses of a myriad of punctate elements, the rods and cones. In some quite mysterious way the retinal picture appears in conscious perception, but nowhere in the brain can there be found neurones that respond specifically to even a small zone of the retinal image or the observed picture. The neuronal machinery of the visual system of the brain has been shown to accomplish a very inadequate reconstitution that can be traced in many sequences (cp. Kuffler [1973]).

The initial stage of reconstitution of the picture occurs in the complex nervous system of the retina. As a consequence of this retinal synthetic mechanism the output in the million or so nerve fibres in each optic nerve is not a simple translation of the retinal image into a corresponding pattern of impulse discharges that travel to the primary visual centre of the brain, Brodmann area 17 (Figs. E 1 – 4, E 2 – 5 A). Already in the nervous system of the retina there has begun the abstraction from the richly patterned mosaic of responses by the retinal receptor units into elements of pattern, which we may call features, and this abstraction continues in the many successive stages that have now been recognized in the visual centres of the brain (Figs. E1–7E–H and 8B).

The complex interactions in the retinal nervous system eventually are expressed by the retinal ganglion cells that discharge impulses along the optic nerve fibres and so to the brain. These cells respond particularly to spatial and temporal changes of luminosity of the retinal image by two neuronal subsystems signalling brightness and darkness respectively. The brightness contrasts of the retinal image are converted into contoured outlines by several neuronal stages of information processing. One type of ganglion cell is excited by a spot of light applied to the retina over it and is inhibited by light

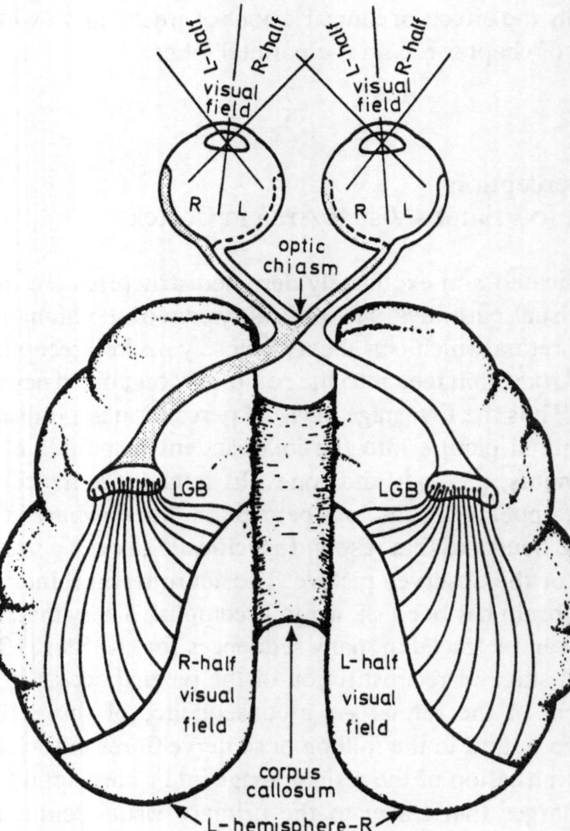

Fig. E2–4. Diagram of visual pathways showing the L-half and R-half visual fields with the retinal images and the partial crossing in the optic chiasma so that the R-half of the visual field of each eye goes to left visual cortex, after relay in the lateral geniculate body *(LGB)*, and correspondingly for left visual field to right visual cortex.

on the surrounding retina. The other type gives the reverse response, inhibition by light shone into the centre and excitation by the surround. The combined responses of these two neuronal subsystems result in a contoured abstraction of the retinal image in the visual cortex. Hence what the eye tells the brain by the million fibres of the optic nerve is an abstraction of brightness and colour contrasts.

As illustrated in Figure E 2 – 4 the optic nerves from each eye meet in the optic chiasma where there is a partial crossing. The hemi-retinas of both eyes (nasal of right and temporal of left) that receive the image from the right visual field have their optic nerve projections rearranged in the chiasma so that they coalesce to form the pathway to the left visual cortex, and vice versa for the left visual field projecting to the right visual cortex. Thus, with the exception of a narrow vertical (meridional) strip of the visual field that is directly in the line of vision, the visual imagery of the right and left fields

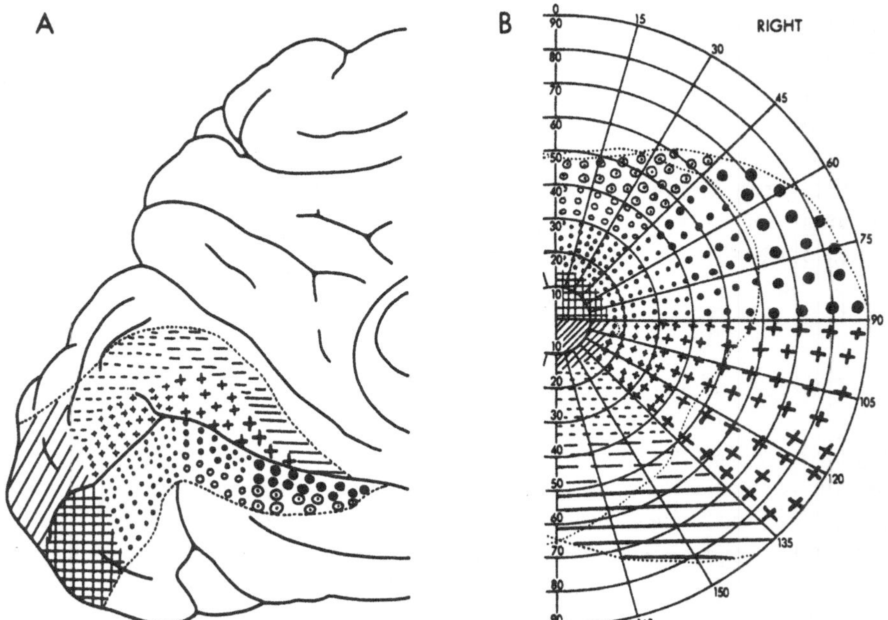

Fig. E2 – 5. Topographic relations of right visual field and left visual cortex of human cerebrum. In B there is shown the right visual field scaled in degrees from the fovea and in degrees from the upper vertical meridian. In A there is shown the projection to area 17 of the occipital lobe, that is very largely on the medial surface. There is shown by symbols the topography of the projections from the visual field to area 17. The centre of vision has a much larger representation than the periphery (Holmes, 1951).

comes to the left and to the right visual cortices respectively to form and ordered map (Fig. E 2 – 5 A) much as with the cortical map for cutaneous sensation (Fig. E 1 – 1). There is of course topographic distortion. The fine visual sensing in the centre of the visual field (oblique lines and rectangular grid) results from a much more amplified cortical projection area than for the retina concerned with peripheral vision (coarse dots and crosses etc. in Fig. E 2 – 5 A and B) (Holmes [1945]).

So far this somatotopy is based on human anatomical studies, and on the visual deprivations (scotomata) resulting from clinical lesions (cp. Teuber & others [1960]). Electrical stimulation of the human visual cortex in unanesthetized subjects gives the patient the experience of flashes of light (cortical electrical phosphenes) that are located in the visual field in correspondence to the stimulated cortical point (Penfield and Jasper [1954]; Brindley [1973]). The phosphene continues for the duration of the train of repetitive stimuli. There has been no analytic investigation of time sequences equivalent to that of Libet described above for cutaneous perceptions. There has in fact been very little detailed study of the responses of the human visual cortex and these were done only in blind people. The averaged evoked potentials from the human scalp are not very helpful (MacKay and Jeffreys [1973]). In contrast, the visual systems of mammals such as cat and monkey have been subjected to a multitude of refined electrophysiological and behavioural studies during the last two decades. A brief description of these findings is essential before we undertake the task of trying to understand the way in which our brains give us visual experiences.

10.2. Stages in Reconstitution of the Visual Image

Figure E 2 – 4 shows that, after the partial decussation of the optic chiasma, the nerve fibres from the retina reach a relay station called the lateral geniculate body. Here there is but little further sorting or synthesis. For example, a bright line in the visual field is coded as a linear arrangement of excited neurones that project on to the stellate cells in lamina IV of the primary receiving area of the visual cortex (area 17). These neurones (simple cells) are the first cortical stage in reassembly of the retinal image. They respond to a bright line in the retinal image and are selective to the orientation of this line. Moving bright lines are particularly effective.

In Figure E 2 – 6 A there is a simple cell firing impulses, having been "found" by a microelectrode which has been inserted into the primary visual

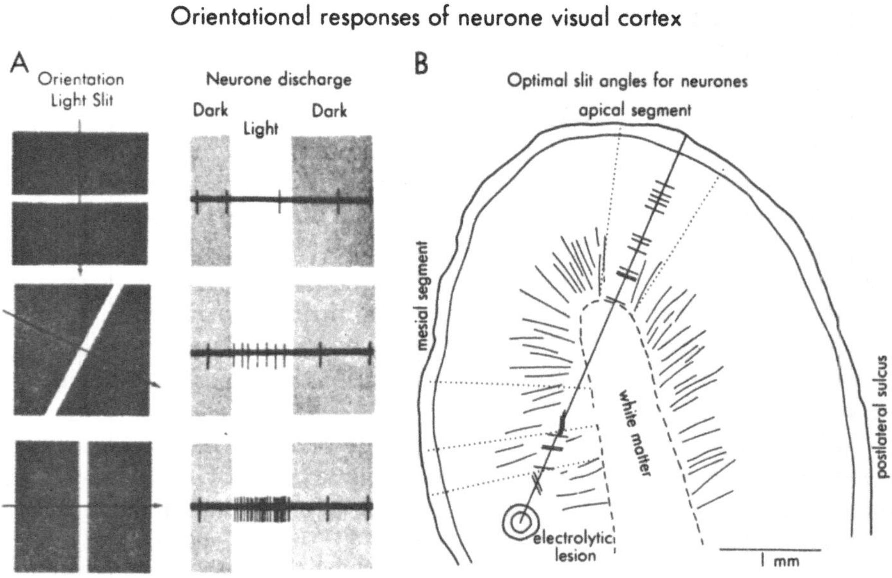

Fig. E2−6. Orientational responses of neurones in primary visual cortex of cat. Full description in text (Hubel and Wiesel, 1962).

cortex of the cat. The track of insertion is shown for example in Figure E 2−6 B as the sloping line with short transverse lines indicating the locations of many neurones along that track. With the microelectrode you can record extracellularly the impulse discharges of a single cell if you position it carefully. The cell has a slow background discharge (upper trace of Fig. E 2−6 A), but, if the retina is swept with a band of light, as illustrated in the diagram to the left, there is an intense discharge of that cell when light sweeps across a certain zone of the retina and there is immediate cessation of the discharge as the light band leaves the zone (lowest trace of Fig. E 2−6 A). If you rotate the orientation of sweep, the cell discharges just a little, as in the middle trace. Finally, if the sweep is at right angles to the most favorable orientation, it has no effect whatever (uppermost trace). It is a sign that this particular cell is most sensitive for movements of the light strip in one orientation and is quite insensitive for movements at right angles thereto. As illustrated by the direction of the lines across the microelectrode track in Figure E 2−6 B, all cells along that track have the same orientational sensitivity. This is found when the track runs down a column of cells that is orthogonal to the surface, as in the upper group of 12 cells. However, in Figure E 2−6 B the track continued on across the central white matter and then proceeded to pass through three groups of cells with quite different orientation sensitivities.

In the visual cortex, neurones with similar orientation sensitivity tend to be arranged in columns that run orthogonally from the cortical surface. Thus it can be envisaged that, in the large area of the human primary visual cortex, the population of about 400 million neurones is arranged as a mosaic of columns, each with some thousands of neurones that have the same orientation sensitivity (Hubel and Wiesel [1963]; Hubel [1963]). This arrangement can be regarded as the first stage of reconstitution of the retinal image. It will of course be recognized that this orientation map is superimposed on the retinal field map (Fig. E2−5 A), each zone of this field being composed of columns that collectively represent all orientations of bright lines or of edges between light and dark.

It has already been shown in Figure E2−4 that both the ipsilateral and contralateral eyes project to the lateral geniculate body (LGB) on the way to the visual cortex. However in the primate these projections are relayed in separate laminae, three for the ipsilateral (2i, 3i, 5i) and three for the contralateral eye (1c, 4c, 6c) (Fig. E2−7). The projection to the columns of area 17 is illustrated in highly diagrammatic form in Figure E2−7 (Hubel and Wiesel, 1972, 1974). The ipsilateral and contralateral laminae of the LGB are shown projecting to alternating columns, the ocular dominance columns. Orthogonally the columns are defined by the orientation specificities as indicated in Figure E2−6 and these can be seen to have a rotational sequence in Figure E2−7. The actual columnar elements are of course much less strictly arranged than is shown in this diagram for the monkey cortex.

At the next stage of image reconstitution are neurones at other levels in area 17 and in the surrounding secondary and tertiary visual areas (Brodmann areas 18 and 19, Fig. E 1−4 A, B). Here there are neurones that are specially sensitive to the length and thickness of bright or dark lines as well as to their orientation and even to two lines meeting at an angle. These so-called complex and hypercomplex neurones (Hubel and Wiesel [1963], [1965]) constitute a further stage of feature recognition. It is believed that these "complex" and "hypercomplex" neurones acquire their specific properties by means of a synthesis of the neuronal circuits that are activated by "simple" cells, these circuits containing inhibitory as well as excitatory components (Hubel and Wiesel [1965]; Hubel [1971]). In Figure E 2−7 there are examples of two complex cells in the upper lamina that each receive from two simple cells of different ocular dominance columns.

So far we have a relatively clear story and there is identification in the

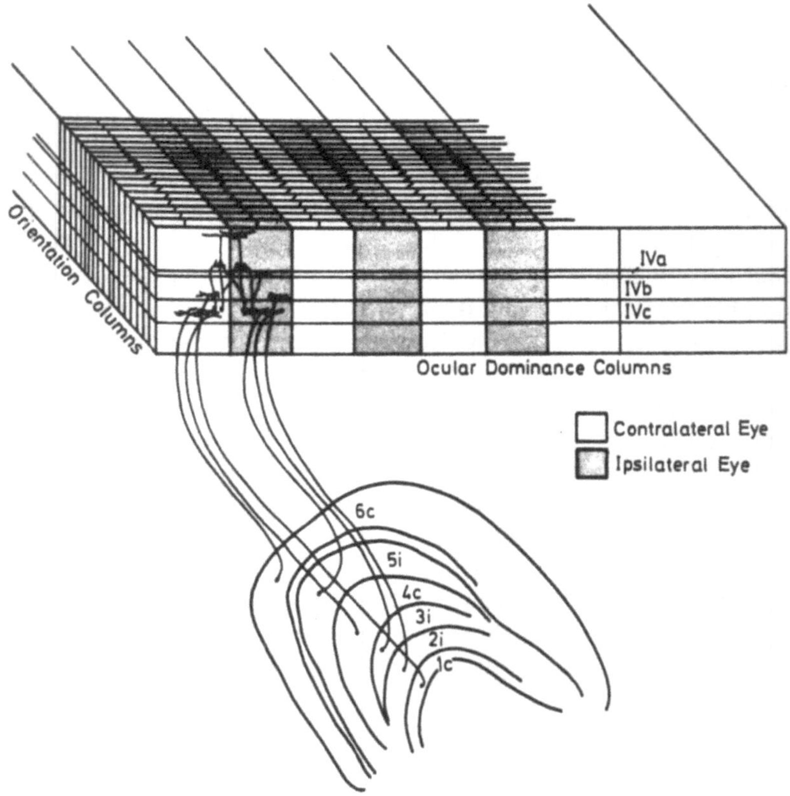

Fig. E2 – 7. Idealized diagram showing for the monkey the projection from the lateral geniculate body (LGB) to the visual cortex (area 17). The six layers of the lateral geniculate body are labelled according as they are associated with the ipsilateral (i) or contralateral (c) eye. These i and c layers project to specific areas so forming the ocular dominance columns for the ipsilateral and contralateral eyes. The stacked slab-like columns of the visual cortex are defined by the criteria of ocular dominance in one direction and orientation (shown on upper surface, cf. Fig. E2 – 6) in the other direction (Hubel and Wiesel, 1974).

visual cortex of neurones requisite for the various integrational tasks. This account is of course greatly oversimplified. For example, there has been neglect of the neural events responsible for the various contrast phenomena and for dark recognition that form the basis of many visual illusions. Colour recognition is dependent on coding by a three-colour process in the retina, beginning with red, green and blue cones that feed into relatively independent lines to the primary visual cortex (de Valois [1973]). At this stage there are various synthetic mechanisms, but we are far from understanding the neuronal mechanisms involved in colour recognition.

Since the complex and hypercomplex cells receive their inputs from various assemblages of simple cells, it would be expected that they would have inputs from a more extensive visual field. This is indeed the case, but the loss of field specificity is more than would be expected. It prompts the as yet unanswered question: how can the field specificity be recovered in the further stages of reconstitution of the visual field?

One further stage of synthesis of visual information has recently been studied physiologically (reviewed by Gross [1973]; Gross & others [1974]). As reported in chapter E 1, in monkeys the inferotemporal cortex (areas 20, 21) receives a strong input from the visual areas in the occipital lobe (Figs. E 1 – 7 E, F, 8 B). Many neurones in areas 20, 21 have more exacting stimulus requirements than the lines and angles that were adequate for the complex and hypercomplex neurones of areas 17, 18, 19. For example neurones may be fired by rectangles in the visual field and not by discs, or by stars and not by circles. Evidently some of the neurones have a remarkable feature recognition propensity. It is suggested that the feature responsivity of some neurones may be so specific that it is not discoverable in the limited testing time available in an experiment. For example one neurone appeared to be fired specifically by the silhouette of a monkey hand! In these neurones of areas 20 and 21, visual mapping is sacrificed to feature recognition even more than with neurones of areas 18 and 19. Large areas of the visual field can effectively influence one neurone, and the topography for each "feature detection neurone" always includes the centre of vision. Again it can be envisaged that this specific response to geometrical forms, such as squares, rectangles, triangles, stars, is dependent on the ordered projection onto these feature-detection neurones from complex and hypercomplex neurones sensitive to bright or dark lines or edges of a particular orientation and length and meeting at particular angles. For example, the feature detection of a triangle would be the property of a neurone receiving inputs from neurones in the extra-striate visual cortex that have angles and orientations for composing the triangle. There are two main pathways for the transmission of visual information to areas 20 and 21. The principal route is from the striate cortex via the circumstriate belt (areas 17, 18, 19). Another route is via a second visual system carrying less specific information from the superior colliculus via the pulvinar (Fig. E 5 – 6; Jones [1974]).

Weiskrantz [1974] has demonstrated the manner in which monkeys can build up a remembered three-dimensional model of an object that is repeatedly examined from only one angle. This ability is deteriorated by lesions of the infero-temporal lobe (areas 20, 21). Hence Weiskrantz postulates that this lobe is concerned in building models and categories, and so is importantly involved in visual thinking and imagination. Mishkin [1971] reports most interesting experiments which demonstrate the importance of areas 20 and 21 on the relearning of pattern discrimination.

It has long been known that in primates complete destruction of the visual areas in an occipital lobe or of the pathways thereto gives blindness in the visual half-field – hemianopia. A right occipital lobe lesion results in left-field hemianopia and vice-versa for a left lobe lesion. Partial lesions result in corresponding topographic field defects, called scotomata (Teuber & others [1960]). More subtle visual losses occur with lesions of areas 18 and 19, but there is considerable disagreement in detail (Mishkin [1972]; Pribram [1971]). Nevertheless this zone of visual cortex can be regarded as being but a station for some rather simple reconstructions of the visual image, as is evidenced even by the highest order of synthesis that is displayed in the constituent neurones. As stated in chapter E 6 the lower part of the human right temporal lobe appears to correspond in its feature detection properties to the primate inferotemporal lobes, both right and left, namely feature detection of geometrical and other more irregular shapes (Milner [1968], [1974]).

Each stage of the processing of visual information from the retina to cortical areas 20, 21 can be regarded as having a hierarchical order with features in sequential array:

(1) The visual field becomes progressively less specific. This increasing generalization results in a foveal representation for all neurones of areas 20, 21. Furthermore at this stage all neurones receive from both visual half-fields including the fovea through inputs to both occipital lobes via the splenium of the corpus callosum (cp. Fig. E 5–6).

(2) There is an increasing specificity of the adequate stimulus from a spot to a bright line or edge of particular orientation, then to lines of specified width and length and often with specificity for direction of movement, and finally to the more complex feature detection of some neurones of areas 20 and 21.

(3) There is also evidence that neurones of areas 20 and 21 have an additional response feature, namely the significance of the response to the animal, exactly as has been discovered for neurones of areas 5 and 7 of the somaesthetic system (Mountcastle [1975] and associates [1975]).

10.3. The Perceived Visual Image

Wonderful as it is, this animal experimentation still gives no clue as to how a whole visual picture can be reconstituted by the neuronal machinery of the brain. When considering the problems of visual experience in relation to the known functions of the brain, Weiskrantz [1974] states:

> "Only in the field of feature extraction is there, I believe, any reason to feel that the end of the tunnel may be sight . . . For the all-important functions of synthesizing, i. e., concocting perceptual entities such as objects and people out of detection of features, and for the imparting of perceptual constancies, I believe there has been no greying of the black box – that is, finding an assignment in the gray box of the real nervous system as opposed to speculating entirely in the realm of abstract black boxes."

Again, after a most penetrating analysis of the manner of operation of the simple and complex cells of the visual cortex, Pollen and Taylor [1974] raised the question about how objects can be recognized independently of their apparent size. Since in temporal lobe epilepsy objects in the aura may undergo size transformation (Penfield and Jasper [1954], they suggested that:

> "the normal temporal lobe may contain a mechanism that scans or zooms over the representation of visual space at a finite number of sizes, so that a number of different object sizes may be cross-correlated with the memory. Whether such zooming occurs within the temporal lobe or via temporal efferent influences on other levels of the visual system is unknown."

There is some resemblance between this proposal and the radical hypothesis that will be developed in chapter E 7. It is there conjectured that the reconstitution of the perceived image is due to the self-conscious mind that "scans and reads out" from the appropriate feature recognition elements of the visual areas. The fully reconstituted image is thus consciously perceived. It is reconstituted only in a fragmentary manner by the visual areas of the brain, though these areas of course are instrumental to the reconstitution. In this connection it should be pointed out that as yet there is no detailed investigation of the visual projections to the prefrontal lobe. These important projections are illustrated in Figure E 1 – 7 E, F, G and 8 B. It can be predicted that in these prefrontal areas the visual information will be coloured gnostically and emotionally, as will be suggested later in this chapter.

We can be overwhelmed by the immensity of high level investigation on the visual system of primates in the last two decades. However, there is no work on the visual cortex of man matching that of Libet on the human somaesthetic cortex. We have only one piece of evidence indicating that for the actual visual experience it is necessary to have a building up of neuronal

ST patterns for some tenths of a second. Crawford [1947] and others have demonstrated a backward masking effect of 0.2 s or more. An initial weak light flash is not seen if there is a stronger flash 0.2 s later. This corresponds to one of the backward masking tests of Libet.

Brindley [1973] has developed with great ingenuity a visual prosthetic device that is applied to the visual cortex of blind human subjects in the hope that the pattern of cortical electrical phosphenes generated by hundreds of stimulating sites on the area of the primary visual cortex can give the subject some crude visual experience of his surround. It will be recognized how far this stimulating technique falls short of the stimulation provided by input from the retina via the visual pathways.

In conclusion it must be emphasized that the great achievements in vision research can be regarded as only the first steps in providing an explanation of how the image on the retina that is encoded in neuronal discharges is eventually reconstituted as an observed picture. As Jung [1973] states, p. 124:

> "The sensory raw material delivered by the receptors cannot become a percept without information processing over several levels in the brain. This includes feature extraction, spatial and temporal order and memory comparison which involves some reverberation and redundant resonance of the sensory messages. The riddle of the sequential order and unity of vision may be less perplexing for the neurophysiologist when he knows that the philosophy of perception encounters similar unsolved problems."

In chapter E 7 a radical hypothesis will be presented that is essentially a new philosophy of perception that grapples with just these problems of sequential order and unity. It will build upon the feature extraction performance of the visual cortices — the striate, circumstriate and infero-temporal areas. Furthermore it builds upon the modular structure of the cortex and the conjectured performance of the exquisite neuronal machinery of modules.

11. Auditory Perception

There is a highly specialized transduction mechanism in the cochlea, where, by a beautifully designed resonance mechanism, there is a frequency analysis of the complex patterns of sound waves and conversion into the discharges of neurones that project into the brain. After several synaptic relays the coded information reaches the primary auditory area (Heschl's gyrus) in the superior temporal gyrus (cp. Figs. E 1 – 1, E 1 – 7, I, and E 4 – 4). The right cochlea projects mostly to the left primary auditory area, and vice versa for the left cochlea. There is a linear somatotopic distribution, the highest auditory frequencies being most medial in Heschl's gyrus (Fig. E 4 – 4) and the lowest most lateral. Figure E 1 – 7 I – L shows the secondary, tertiary and quaternary projections of the auditory information as determined by the sequential degeneration technique of Jones and Powell [1970]. These projections in cascade show much the same sequences as with somaesthetic and visual inputs. Similarly there are the projections to the principal secondary (STP) and teriary (22) areas of the temporal lobe and also to specific areas of the prefrontal lobe and to the limbic system (via areas 25, 35 and TG). It is not known if there is even a fragmentary reconstitution of the initiating stimulus such as occurs in the visual centres. It remains quite mysterious how a sequence of tones gives rise to a new synthesis, a melody. Nevertheless there are parallels between the connections in cascade, in Figure E 1 – 7 I – L with those for somaesthesis and vision. The projections of all three systems both to the prefrontal lobe and the limbic system will be discussed in a later section.

12. Olfactory Perception

In most lower mammals olfaction (smell) is the dominant sensory input into the forebrain, but in the evolution of primates to man olfaction became subordinated to vision and hearing, and even to somaesthesis, particularly when this became vital in manual skills. Chemical sensing in the olfactory mucosa is by receptor cells that are specialized neurones with axons that pass to the olfactory bulb where there is a processing of information by a complex nervous system much as in the retina. From the olfactory bulb (OFB) the lateral olfactory tract (LOT) passes to the brain (cp. Fig. E 1 – 9) where it has a complex distribution, only part of which is shown in Figure E 1 – 9. The principal termination is in the piriform cortex, a primitive cerebral cortex. Thence there are connections to many structures of the limbic lobe, some of which are indicated in Figure E 1 – 9. Connection to the primary receiving area of the neocortex (the orbito-frontal area) is effected only after several relays in the limbic system and is only in part via the MD thalamus (Tanabe & others [1975]). Thus the olfactory connections are quite different from the somaesthetic, visual and auditory systems, where the connections are firstly to the neocortex and after several relays reach the limbic system (Fig. E 1 – 8).

13. Emotional Colouring of Conscious Perceptions

It is a common experience that the conscious perception derived from some common sensory input is greatly modified by emotions, feeling, and appetitive drives. For example, when hungry the sight of food gives an experience deeply coloured by an appetitive drive! Nauta [1971] conjectures that the state of the organism's internal milieu (hunger, thirst, sex, fear, rage, pleasure) is signalled to the prefrontal lobes from the hypothalamus, the septal nuclei and various components of the limbic system such as the hippocampus and the amygdala. The pathways would be mainly through the MD thalamus to the prefrontal lobes (Fig. E 1−9). Thus, by their projections to the prefrontal lobes, the hypothalamus and the limbic system modify and colour with emotion the conscious perceptions derived from sensory inputs and superimpose on them motivational drives. No other part of the neocortex has this intimate relationship with the hypothalamus.

Figures E 1−7, 8 show for the somaesthetic, visual and auditory systems the many projections to the prefrontal lobes from the primary sensory and the principal secondary and tertiary areas. Simultaneously these areas project to the limbic system, and in Figure E 1−9 there are also projections from the prefrontal lobe (areas 46 and OF) to the limbic system. Thus there are pathways for complicated circuitry from the various sensory inputs to the limbic system and back to the prefrontal lobe, with further circuits from that lobe to the limbic system and back again (Nauta [1971]). From the connectivities of Figure E 1−9 it can be seen that the prefrontal and limbic systems are in reciprocal relationship and have the potentiality for continuously looping interaction. Thus by means of the prefrontal cortex the subject may be able to exercise a controlling influence on the emotions generated by the limbic system. An additional sensory input (olfaction) comes directly into the limbic system for cross-modal transfer to the other senses and thus contributes to the richness and variety of the perceptual experience. For example, the neocortical sensory systems via areas 46, OF, 20 and TG project to the hypothalamus, the entorhinal cortex and the hippocampal gyrus and so to the hippocampus, to septal nuclei and to the MD thalamus, while, after relay in the piriform cortex and amygdala, the olfactory input also goes to the hypothalamus, septal nuclei and the MD thalamus. Thus the MD nucleus is the receiving station for all inputs and it projects to the orbital and convex surfaces of the prefrontal lobe. So one can think of the prefrontal cortex as being the area where all emotive information is synthesized with somaesthetic, visual and auditory to give conscious experiences to the subject and guidance to appropriate behaviour, as will be described in chapters E 3 and

E 7. We conjecture that conscious experiences are derived from spatiotemporal patterns of neuronal activity in special modules of the neocortex (cp. chapter E 7). This conjecture is based in part on the finding that, after section of the corpus callosum, the self-conscious mind is in liaison only with the dominant hemisphere (chapter E 5).

14. Epilogue

Mountcastle [1975] gives a terse and vivid expression of the relationship of conscious perception to sensory systems and the brain:

> "Each of us lives within the universe – the prison – of his own brain. Projecting from it are millions of fragile sensory nerve fibres, in groups uniquely adapted to sample the energetic states of the world about us: heat, light, force, and chemical compositions. That is all we ever know of it directly: all else is logical inference.
> Sensory stimuli reaching us are transduced at peripheral nerve endings, and neural replicas of them dispatched brainward, to the great gray mantle of the cerebral cortex. We use them to form dynamic and continually up-dated neural maps of the external world, and of our place and orientation, and of events, within it. At the level of sensation, your images and my images are virtually the same, and readily identified one to another by verbal description, or common reaction.
> Beyond that, each image is conjoined with genetic and stored experiential information that makes each of us uniquely private. From that complex integral each of us constructs at a higher level of perceptual experience his own, very personal, view from within."

Chapter E 3 Voluntary Movement

15. Résumé

There are many hierarchical levels in the mechanisms of control of voluntary movement. At the lowest level there is the motor unit which consists of the motoneurone in the central nervous system and the nerve fibre from it to the hundred or so muscle fibres that it innervates (Fig. E 3 − 1). All movements are made up of ensembles of contractions of individual motor units. Each muscle is composed of many hundreds of these contractual units. There is brief reference to the simplest pathways involved in the reflex control of motor units (Fig. E 3 − 2). At the other extreme of the hierarchy, there is the motor cortex, area 4 of Brodmann's map, in which again there is a strip display from toes to tongue matching the sensory strip that is just posterior in areas 3, 1, 2 (Fig. E 1 − 1). Pyramidal cells of the motor cortex send their axons to innervate directly or indirectly motoneurones of muscles (Fig. E 3 − 3).

In voluntary movement specific groups of pyramidal cells are excited in order to carry out the desired action. A very perplexing problem arises in this connection: how can willing of a muscular movement set in train neural events that lead to the discharge of pyramidal cells of the motor cortex and so to activation of the neural pathway that leads to the muscle contraction giving that movement? An account is given of the experiments of Kornhuber on human subjects in which it is discovered that willing an action leads to a wide-ranging negative potential over the top of the brain, and this builds up for almost 1 s, eventually concentrating on the pyramidal cells that are appropriate for the action (Fig. E 3 − 4). It is conjectured that the self-conscious mind is in two-way communication with large numbers of modules over the surface of the hemispheres, and the consequent activity gives rise to the negative "readiness potential," as it is called. A further problem is to discover how this activity is eventually guided to the correct pyramidal cells.

A brief account is given of another major part of the brain, the cerebellum (Fig. E 3 − 5), which is concerned in the smooth and automatic control of movement. Two varieties of cerebellar action are described. One relates to movements already in train and is concerned by feedback action in moulding these ongoing movements so that they achieve their end with finesse, much as does the controlling system of a target-finding missile (Fig. E 3 − 6 A). The second cerebellar operation is concerned with the preprogramming of movements before they have actually been initiated. Areas of the cerebral cortex related to movement, particularly area 6, act on the cerebellar hemisphere by an open loop system that feeds back to the pyramidal motor cells of area 4 (Fig. E 3 − 6 B). As a consequence their impulse discharges are already a good approximation to the optimum for carrying out the desired movement. It is this preprogramming that is going on for the relatively long time of the readiness potential. In addition, there is at the same time running in parallel a loop system through the basal ganglia.

We conjecture, therefore, that the premotor association areas (area 6) and the cerebellar hemispheres and basal ganglia are responsible for preprogramming movements (Fig. E 3 − 6 B). The motor command eventually stemming from this preprogramming is discharged down the pyramidal tract to initiate the movement, and at the same time it is fed into the cerebellum (Fig. E 3 − 6 A) to update the motor command. Thus this circuit continuously exercises a feedback control that keeps the movement on target (cp. Fig. E 3 − 7).

The outstanding problem in the voluntary control of movement is of course the action across the interface between the self-conscious mind on the one hand and the modules of the cerebral cortex on the other. The existence of this influence is established by the empirical experiments of Kornhuber and associates, but there is of course no explanation of how it can come about. However, in chapter E 7 there will be formulation of a hypothesis on this problem of interaction of mind on brain.

16. Introduction

In attempting an analysis of voluntary movement and its control, it is immediately evident that there are many hierarchical levels. This was appreciated by Sherrington [1906] in his great book, *The Integrative Action of the Nervous System,* where in chapter 9, "The Physiological Position and Dominance of the Brain," he recognized the simplest reflexes with a superposition thereon of more and more complex controls at spinal, supraspinal, cerebellar, and cerebral levels.

Most important problems arise in an attempt to give an account of how we can move. How can we control our musculature to give us actions in accordance with the situations that we find ourselves in? How can I, for example, move my arm so that with my eyes shut I can smoothly put my finger on the tip of my nose? But you can think of much more complicated movements in the immense repertoire of skill that you have in games, in technology, in playing musical instruments, and most importantly and very complexly in speech and song and gesture, so that your whole personality can stand revealed. And it stands revealed simply because of your movements resulting from your muscular contractions, as for example in all facial gesture and eye movement. If you are fixed like a corpse with a mask-like face, you reveal no personality.

17. The Motor Unit

All movements are brought about by contractions induced in muscles by impulses that are discharged by specialized nerve cells called motoneurones. The impulses travel from the motoneurone along its axon that branches in the muscle to end as motor endplates (cp. Fig. E 3 − 1) so that some 100 muscle fibres are made to contract every time that the motoneurone discharges an impulse. The motoneurone and the muscle fibres it exclusively innervates form the unitary basis of all movement. Sherrington has appropriately given the name motor unit to the ensemble which is illustrated in Figure E 3 − 1 (Eccles [1973(b)]), and he arrived at the correct idea that all movements are ensembles or composites of contractions of individual motor units. Various fractions of the total number are excited, depending on the strength of contraction that is needed for any particular action. The total motoneurone pool of the muscle is fractionated from moment to moment according to needs. And the total number of motoneurones with their dependent motor units is about 200,000 for the human spinal cord. That number is responsible for the contractions of all the muscles of the limbs, body, and neck, i. e., for our total muscular performance except for that of the head. It is remarkable that we can learn to activate individual motoneurones in arm or leg muscles, and to switch now to one, now to another at will!

In Figure E 3 − 2 the afferent fibre (I a) from the annulospiral ending (AS) of the knee extensor muscle (E) enters a dorsal root of the spinal cord and acts directly (monosynaptically) on a motoneurone (E) of that muscle. It should be recognized that there are many hundreds of lines in parallel to the one drawn, giving immense scope for divergence and convergence.

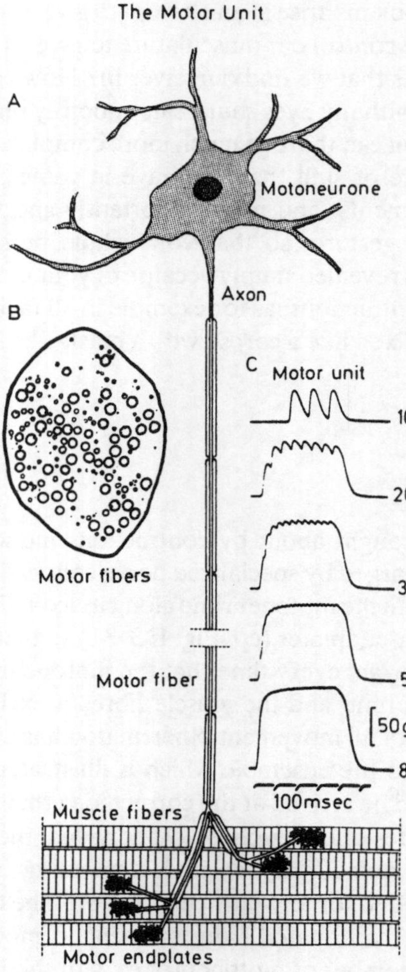

Fig. E3—1. The motor unit. A. Motoneurone with its axon passing as a myelinated nerve fibre to innervate muscle fibres. B. Transverse section of motor fibres supplying a cat muscle, all afferent fibres having been degenerated. C. Isometric mechanical responses of a single motor unit of the cat gastrocnemius muscle. The responses were evoked by repetitive stimulation of the motoneurone (cf. A) by pulses of current applied through an intracellular electrode at the indicated frequencies in cycles per second (Eccles, 1973b).

The antagonist muscle is the flexor (F) that bends the leg back at the knee. In this muscle there are the same annulospiral receptor organs (AS) and the motor endplates made by the motor nerve fibres. Impulses from the stretch

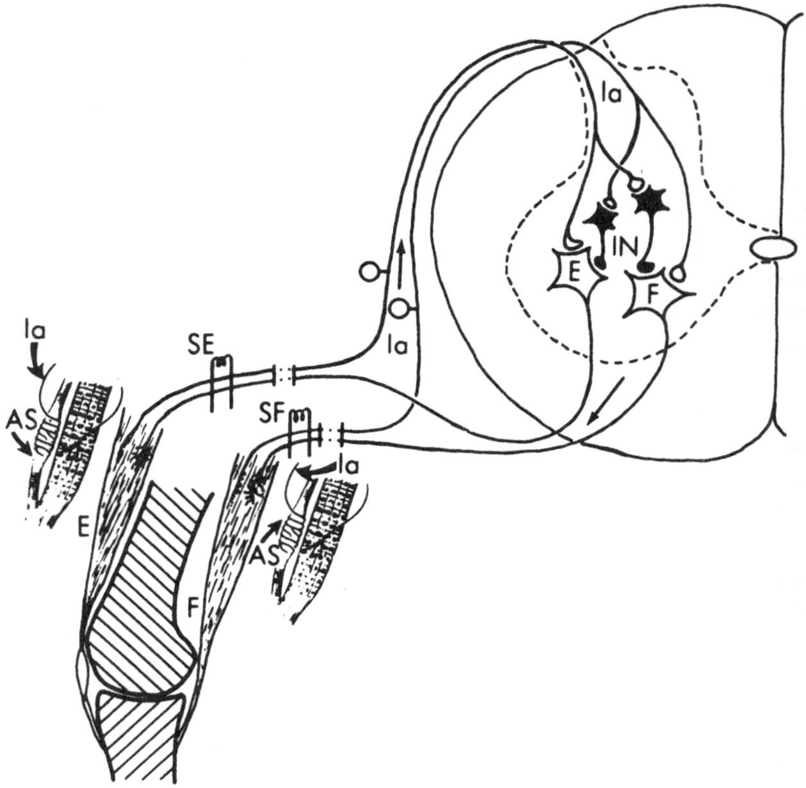

Fig. E3−2. Simple reflex pathways. A diagrammatic representation of the pathways from and to the extensor *(E)* and flexor *(F)* muscles of the knee joint. The small insets show the details of the origin of the *Ia* afferent fibres from the annulospiral endings *(AS)* of muscle spindles. In the spinal cord the *Ia* fibres branch so that the motoneurone, *E* or *F*, innervating the muscle of origin, *E* or *F*, is monosynaptically excited while the antagonist motoneurone, *F* or *E*, is inhibited via an inhibitory interneurone *(IN)*.

receptor (AS) of the flexor muscle also enter the spinal cord through the dorsal root and monosynaptically excite the motoneurone innervating the flexor muscle. So the extensor and flexor muscles have central pathways complementary to each other.

In addition there is a reciprocal arrangement in Figure E3−2. The afferent fibre from the extensor muscle (E) branches in the spinal cord so that not only does it excite its own motoneurone but it also sends a branch which excites an interneurone (IN). This neurone is shown in black and it sends its axon to the antagonist motoneurone (F) and forms inhibitory synapses on it. (Throughout this book in diagrams the black symbols are for inhibition and white for excitation, cp. Fig. E 2−1.) In the same way there is the reciprocal arrangement for the afferent fibres from the flexor muscles acting on inhibitory neurones to extensor motoneurones.

This very simple reciprocal arrangement can be given functional meaning. When you are standing with slightly bent knees your weight is stretching the knee extensor muscle (E) and the AS stretch receptors are firing into the spinal cord, exciting the knee extensor motoneurones to fire impulses so that the extensor muscle contracts and holds your weight. If this muscle contraction is inadequate, the knee gives a little, so stretching the extensor muscle more, with more firing from its AS receptors giving an increased reflex discharge to the muscle, which in this way is nicely adjusted to give a steady posture. At the same time the reciprocal inhibitory pathway prevents the antagonist motoneurones (F) from firing to give contraction of the antagonist flexor muscles (F). Such a contraction would oppose the extensors that are engaged in the essential task of weight supporting. This description of the mode of action of the pathways in Figure E 3−2 illustrates a simple reflex performance.

18. The Motor Cortex

After this introduction I will now develop the theme of this chapter. There is general agreement that voluntary control is exerted through the motor cortex of the cerebral hemisphere and the pathway (the pyramidal tract) from there to the motoneurones (Wiesendanger [1969]). Figure E 1−1 shows the position of the left motor cortex as a band across the surface of the cerebral hemisphere, being area 4 of Brodmann's map in Figure E 1−4. It lies just anterior to the central fissure (the fissure of Rolando, *f. Rol.*), and many of its constituent nerve cells are pyramidal cells whose axons are the nerve fibres running down the pyramidal tract. The motor cortex is essentially concerned in voluntary movement, but it is not the prime initiator of a movement, such as a voluntary bending of the finger. It is only the final relay station of immensely complicated activities in widely dispersed areas in the cerebral cortex, the cerebellum and the basal ganglia (Figs. E 3−6, 7). The pyramidal cells of the motor cortex with their axons passing down the pyramidal tract are important because they provide a direct channel out from the brain to the

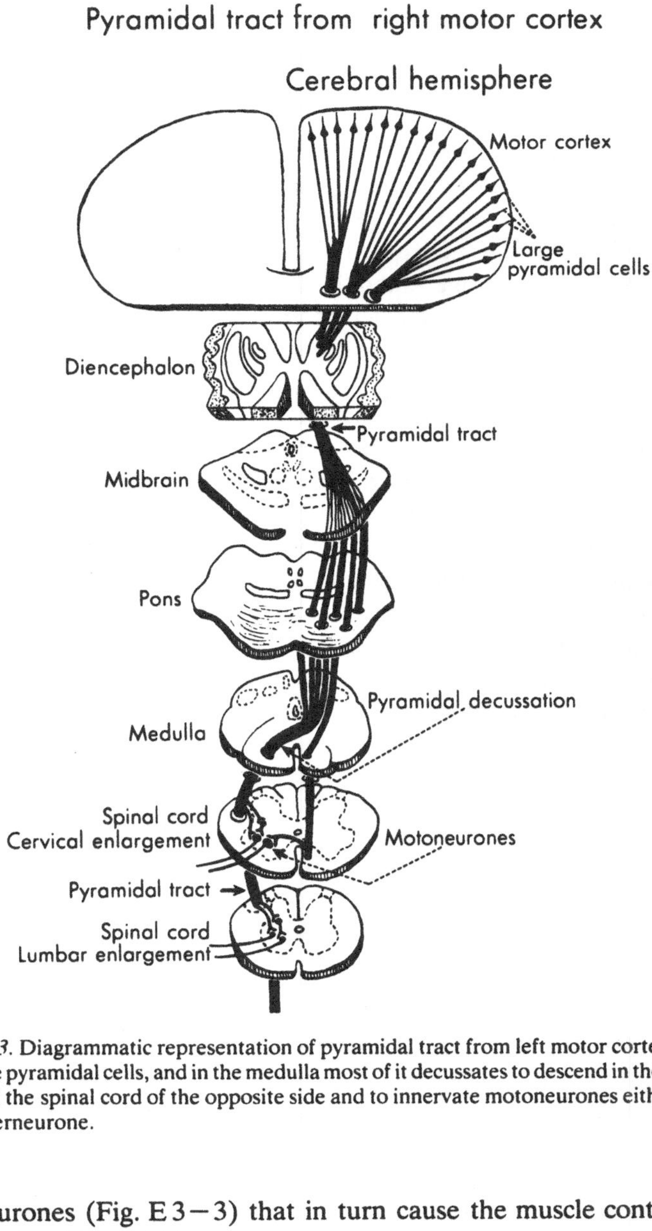

Fig. E3–3. Diagrammatic representation of pyramidal tract from left motor cortex. The origin is from the pyramidal cells, and in the medulla most of it decussates to descend in the dorsolateral column of the spinal cord of the opposite side and to innervate motoneurones either directly or via an interneurone.

motoneurones (Fig. E 3–3) that in turn cause the muscle contractions as illustrated in Figure E 3–1.

When brief stimulating currents are passed through electrodes placed on the surface of the motor cortex, there are contractions of localized groups of muscles. The first experiments were carried out on monkeys and anthropoid apes, but later the human motor cortex was explored when it was exposed in the course of a brain operation. In this way it was shown that all the various parts of the body are represented in the strip-like map of the contralateral motor cortex in Figure E 1 – 1 (Penfield and Jasper [1954]). Thereon are marked the specific areas for toes, foot, leg, thigh, body, shoulder, arm, hand, fingers and thumb, neck, head, face, etc., starting from the medial surface and progressing laterally and downwards over the surface. There is a large representation for hand, fingers, and thumb, and an even larger area for face and tongue. The motor cortex is not uniformly parcelled out in proportion to muscle size – far from it. It is skill and finesse of movements that are reflected in the areal representations!

After descending through the brain stem and giving off many branches, the pyramidal tracts cross or decussate in the medulla and so course down the spinal cord to terminate at various levels, making, with primates (Phillips [1973]; Porter [1973]), including man, strong monosynaptic connections on motoneurones (Fig. E 3 – 3). This very direct connection of the motor cortex with motoneurones is of the greatest importance in ensuring that the cerebral cortex in general, via the motor cortex, can very effectively and quickly bring about the desired movement. Nevertheless there are two fundamental problems that will be discussed in the major part of this chapter. How can your willing of a muscle movement set in train neural events that lead to the discharge of motor pyramidal cells? How do the cerebellum and other subcortical structures contribute to the finesse and skill of movement? Firstly there will be an introductory treatment of the problem of voluntary movement.

19. Voluntary Movement

I have the indubitable experience that by thinking and willing I can control my actions if I so wish, although in normal waking life this prerogative is exercised but seldom. I am not able to give a scientific explanation of how thought can lead to action, but this failure serves to emphasize the fact that, as referred to in several discussion sections, our present physics and neurobiology are too primitive for this most challenging task of resolving the antinomy between our experiences and our understanding of brain function. When thought leads to action, I am constrained, as a neuroscientist, to conjecture that in some way my thinking changes the operative patterns of neuronal activities in my brain. Thinking thus eventually comes to control the discharges of impulses from the pyramidal cells of my motor cortex (Fig. E 3 − 3) and so eventually the contractions of my muscles (Fig. E 3 − 1) and the behavioural patterns stemming therefrom. We can restate the first fundamental neurological problem outlined above: how can willing of a muscular movement set in train neural events that lead to the discharge of pyramidal cells of the motor cortex and so to activation of the neural pathway that leads to the muscle contraction giving that movement?

We are now in a position to consider the experiments of Kornhuber and associates (Deecke & others [1969]; Kornhuber [1974]) on the electrical potentials generated in the cerebral cortex prior to the actual performance of a willed action. The problem is to have an elementally simple movement executed by the subject entirely on his own volition, and yet to have accurate timing in order to average the very small potentials recorded from the surface of the scalp. This has been solved by Kornhuber and his associates who use the onset of action potentials of the muscle involved in the movement to trigger a reverse computation of the recorded potentials up to 2 s before the onset of the movement. The movement illustrated in Figure E 3 − 4 was a rapid flexion of the right index finger but many other movements of limbs have been investigated with similar results, and even vocalization. The subject initiates these movements "at will" at irregular intervals of many seconds, extreme care being taken to exclude all triggering stimuli. In this way it was possible to average 250 records of the potentials evoked at each of several sites over the surface of the skull, as shown in Figure E 3 − 4 for the three upper traces. The slowly rising negative potential, called the readiness potential, was observed as a negative wave with unipolar recording over a wide area of the cerebral surface (recorded by scalp leads against an indifferent lead), but there were small positive potentials of similar time course over the most anterior and basal regions of the cerebrum. Usually the readiness potential began *(arrows)* about 0.8 s before the onset of the muscle action potentials, and led on to sharper potentials, positive then negative, beginning at about 0.09 s before the movement. In the lowest trace there was bipolar leading from symmetrical zones over the motor cortex, that on the left being over the area concerned in the movement of the right index finger (cp. Fig. E 1 − 1). There was no detectable asymmetry until a sharp negativity developed at 0.05 s before the onset of the muscle action potentials at time zero. We can assume that the readiness potential was generated by complex patterns of neuronal discharges that originally were symmetrically distributed in the frontal and parietal lobes. Eventually, at only 0.05 s before the muscle response, the negative potential reveals that there was concentration

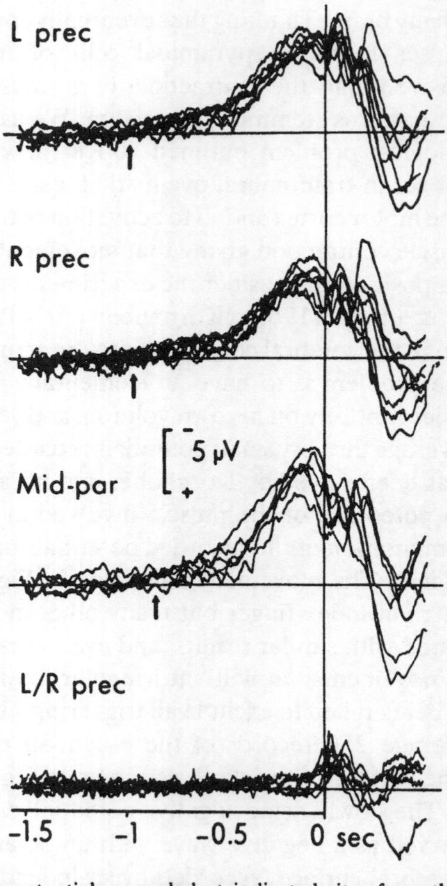

Fig. E3−4. Readiness potentials recorded at indicated sites from the scalp in response to voluntarily evoked movements of finger. Zero time is at the onset of the movement, the preceding potentials being derived by backwards computation, with averaging of 250 responses. *L prec*, left precentral; *R prec*, right precentral; *Mid-par*, mid-parietal; *L/R prec*, recording left precentral against right precentral. Further description in the text (Kornhuber, 1974).

of the neuronal activity onto pyramidal cells of the motor cortex. The time of 0.05 s is just adequate for transmission from the pyramidal cell discharge to motoneurones to muscle action potentials (cp Fig. E3−3).

These experiments at least provide a partial answer to the question: What is happening in my brain at a time when a willed action is in process of being carried out? It can be presumed that during the readiness potential there is a developing specificity of the patterned impulse discharges in neurones so that eventually there are activated the pyramidal cells in the correct motor cortical area (Fig. E 1 − 1) for bringing about the required movement. The readiness potential can be regarded as the neuronal consequence of the voluntary command. The surprising features of the readiness potential are its wide extent and its gradual build-up. Apparently, at the stage of willing a movement, the influence of the voluntary command is widely distributed onto the patterns of neuronal operation.

In attempting to arrive at a further stage of explanation of the cortical events underlying the readiness potential we have to develop hypotheses relating to the special properties of cortical modules. In chapter E 7 it will be conjectured that certain modules of the cerebral cortex (open modules) are in liaison with the self-conscious mind, which works in a weak and subtle manner giving slight deviations of the responses of these modules. This is an action across the interface between the mental world and the physical world. After commissurotomy the self-conscious mind is in liaison only with modules of the dominant hemisphere (chapter E 5), hence it has been conjectured (cp. Eccles [1973(b)]) that normally also there is a similar exclusive liaison. It will be suggested in chapter E 7 and in the discussions that this need not be so. A present problem concerns the finding that the readiness potential is bilateral, whereas the above conjecture apparently would lead to the expectation that the readiness potential would be restricted to the dominant hemisphere. However, it must be recognized that on the above hypothesis this restriction would obtain only for the primary action of the self-conscious mind. The changes produced in the open modules would be quickly transmitted by the pyramidal cell discharges from these modules to closed modules of the same and the opposite hemisphere, i. e., by the immense system of association and callosal fibres (cp. Fig. E 1 − 5). Hence a symmetrical and extensive spread of the readiness potential is to be expected. Furthermore its gradual build-up over 0.8 s can be attributed both to the cumulative effects of the slight deviations that the self-conscious mind produces in open modules and to the resultant changes in closed modules, which at a further stage also interact with one another. Additional factors aiding in the build-up of the readiness potential will be considered in the next section in relation to the preprogramming of movements.

An even more severe problem is entailed in trying to account for the moulding and guidance of the collective modular activities so that eventually there is a convergence of these activities onto those motor pyramidal cells that bring about the desired movement. All that we can conjecture at this stage derives from the hypothesis (cp. chapter E 7) that the self-conscious mind is in two-way communication with the open modules, both in acting and in receiving. Hence it could exercise a continued informed guidance during the whole of the readiness potential. Furthermore, in chapter E 7 it is conjectured that the long duration of the readiness potential is due to the extreme weakness of the action of the self-conscious mind on the open modules. At the most it would slightly deviate the course of the background activity of the neuronal discharges.

When considering the activity of the self-conscious mind in the control of movement, it is important to refer to our ability to manipulate images in the mind without there being any associated overt movement. A fascinating example has been reported by Bronowksi in an interview by Derfer [1974].

> "The idea that we actually manipulate images in mind has been unfashionable in psychology for the past generation, when operationism and functionalism and behaviorism have taken over. The current mode of behaviorism wants to disregard everything between stimulus and response.
> However, we have experimental evidence that whatever symbols or images the mind operates with are powerful. And they are operated with in ways which are indistinguishable from those that we would require if the images really were concrete objects. For instance, Roger Shepard at Berkeley has measured the time that it takes a person to rotate an unsymmetrical object in his mind so as to confirm whether or not it is a mirror image of another object that is shown to him. The time is directly proportional to the angle of rotation that is required, and is therefore directly proportional to the time taken if he actually held the object in his hand and moved it around."

20. The Cerebellar Controls of Voluntary Movement

The cerebral cortex contains all the neuronal circuits for initiating and continuing voluntary movements, but these movements are crude and irregular if there is damage of some other regions of the brain. It has long been known that severe disturbances of movement result from lesions of a large component of the brain, the cerebellum, that is shown in Figure E 3 – 5 A lying below the cerebral hemispheres and attached to the brain stem. The best studies ever made on human cerebellar lesions were carried out by Gordon Holmes [1939] on patients from the First World War who had had the cerebellum on one side destroyed by gunshot wounds with the other side normal and so available as a control. For example on the normal side the subject was able quickly and accurately to move his outstretched arm so that a pointing finger outlined a square on the wall, the finger movements being recorded photographically. In contrast on the side of the cerebellar lesion the movement was wavy and indecisive with hesitations and over-shooting in turning corners. The subject complained that "The movements of my left hand are done subconsciously, but I have to think out each movement of my

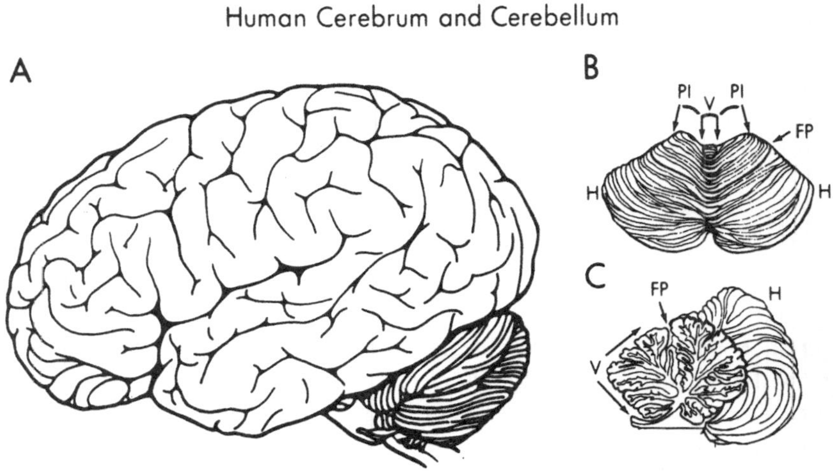

Fig. E3 – 5. A. Human cerebrum and cerebellum. In B and C the cerebellum is seen on the same scale from the dorsal aspect and after a sagittal section in the midline. *V* is the central vermis area, *PI* is the pars intermedia and *H* is the cerebellar hemisphere. *FP* in B and C is the fissura prima between the anterior and posterior parts of the cerebellum.

right arm. I come to a dead stop in turning and have to think before I start again." This shows you how much we are spared this mental concentration by the cerebellum. What you do with ordinary movements is to give a general command – such as "place finger on nose," or "write signature," or "pick up glass" – and the whole performance goes automatically.

In summary we can say that normally our most complex muscle movements are carried out subconsciously and with consummate skill. The more subconscious you are of the actual muscle contractions concerned in a golf stroke, the better it is, and the same with tennis, skiing, skating, or any other skill. In all these performances we do not have any appreciation of the complexity of muscle contractions and joint movements. All that we are conscious of is a general directive given by what we may call our voluntary command system. All the finesse and skill seems naturally and automatically to flow from that. It is my thesis that the cerebellum is concerned in all this enormously complex organization and control of movement, and that throughout life, particularly in the earlier years, we are engaged in an incessant teaching program for the cerebellum. As a consequence, it can carry out all of these remarkable tasks that we set it to do in the whole repertoire of our skilled movements, in games, in techniques, in musical performance, in speech, dance, song, and so on. It can be regarded as a remarkably successful neuronal computer, but as yet we have only general hypotheses about the way in which this immense structure with about 30.000 million constituent neurones carries out its tasks (Eccles & others [1967]; Eccles [1973(a)]).

20.1 The Closed Loop via the Pars Intermedia of the Cerebellum

Figure E 3 – 6 A illustrates one level of operation of the cerebellum (the pars intermedia, PI, in Fig. E 3 – 5 B) in its role of contributing to the smoothness and accuracy of voluntary movement (Allen and Tsukahara [1974]). There is shown by the convention of arrows merely the essential neuronal circuits, not all the detailed synaptic connectivities that occur at each stage and also at relay sites along the diagrammed circuits, where each arrow corresponds to very many thousands of nerve fibres in parallel. With respect to the motor cortex this circuit operates in a closed loop manner. When pyramidal cells of the motor cortex (area 4) are firing impulses down the pyramidal tract (PT) in order to bring about a voluntary movement (a motor command), the patterns of this discharge (the evolving movement) in all details are transmitted to the cerebellum (pars intermedia) by virtue of the collateral branches of the pyramidal tract fibres. Computation occurs in the cerebellar cortex (PI) and the resulting output is returned to the motor cortex so that there is an ongoing "comment" from the cerebellum within 10 to 20 ms of every motor command. We may regard this "comment" as being in the nature of an ongoing correction continuously provided by the cerebellum and being immediately incorporated in the modified motor commands issued by the motor cortex. Figure E 3 – 6 A also illustrates a longer feedback loop that operates through the same region of the cerebellum. When the motor command brings about a movement, this evolving movement excites a wide variety of peripheral receptors, in muscles, skin, joints, etc., and these signal back to the same regions of the cerebellar cortex *(upgoing arrow)* that were concerned in the more direct loop. A computation on the two sets of input forms the basis of the cerebellar response. Thus there is provided to the motor command centres an ongoing cerebellar comment synthesized from these two loops (Eccles [1969], [1973(a)], [1973(b)]; Allen and Tsukahara [1974]). In addition the pars intermedia has a more direct way of influencing the spinal centres via the red nucleus and the rubrospinal tract, that are shown by the descending arrow to SPC in Figure E 3 – 6 A.

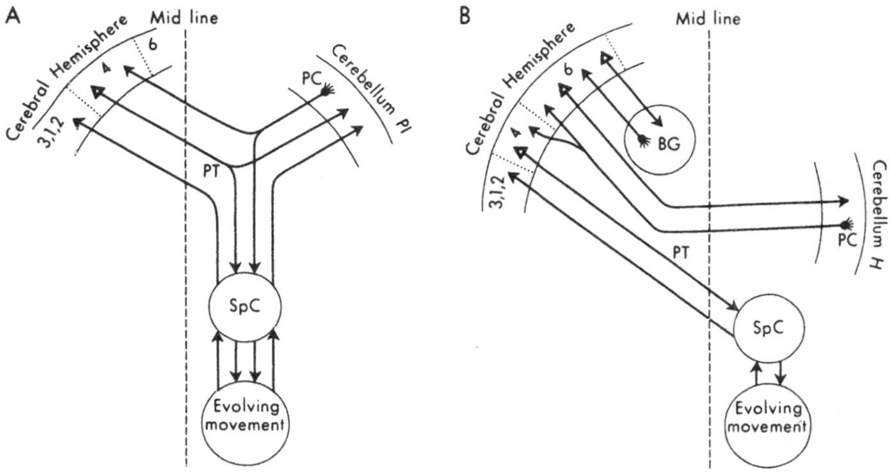

Fig. E3−6. Cerebro-cerebellar circuits in motor control are shown simplified by omission of the synaptic connectivities. A shows the circuits from pyramidal cell in motor cortex *(4)* via pyramidal tract *(PT)* to spinal cord, and so the evolving movement, and with collateral to the pars intermedia *(PI)* of the cerebellum. The Purkyně cell *(PC)* in *PI* communicates (via synaptic relays) back to the motor cortex and also down the spinal cord to the spinal centres *(SpC)*. Also shown is the projection from spinal centres to *PI* and to the somaesthetic area *(3, 1, 2)*. In B the circuits are shown from the cerebrum (principally area *6*) to the hemisphere *(H)* of the cerebellum. The return circuit from the Purkyně cell, *PC*, is back to areas *4* and *6*. From area *4* there is the projection down the spinal cord by the pyramidal tract, *PT*, as in A, and the return circuit from the evolving movement via the spinal centres to areas *3, 1, 2*. Additionally there is shown the circuit from area *6* to the basal ganglia *(BG)* and the return to the cerebrum.

In summary, we can regard the pars intermedia of the cerebellum as acting like the controlling system on a target-finding missile. It acts similarly in that it does not give a single message for correction of a movement that is off-target. Instead it provides sequences of correcting messages, so providing a continuously updating control by closed dynamic loops. The next section gives reasons for believing that it is quite otherwise with the cerebellar hemispheres.

20.2 The Open-Loop System via the Cerebellar Hemispheres

The cerebellar hemispheres comprise almost 90% of the human cerebellum (H in Fig. E3−5B, C) the principal circuits being as shown in Figure E3−6B (Allen and Tsukahara [1974]). Pyramidal cells of cortical areas other than the motor cortex, particularly the premotor area (area 6 in Fig. E 1 − 4 A), project via pontine relays to the contralateral cerebellar cortex (H), and the return circuit is partly to the motor cortex (4) but also to cortical areas (6) other than the motor cortex. Since the cerebellar hemisphere receives only a modest input from the motor cortex, it acts on the cerebral cortex principally in an open-loop manner antedating the motor command that is fired by the pyramidal cells of area 4. Because of these special features of connectivity Allen and Tsukahara [1974] have proposed that the cerebellar hemisphere is concerned in the planning of a movement rather than in its actual execution and correction by follow-up control. Its function is largely anticipatory based upon learning and previous experience. In primates there is no pathway from peripheral sense organs to the cerebellar hemispheres. Such sensory information is received into areas 3, 1, 2 (Fig. E 3 − 6 B) and is then transformed in some of the association areas, such as 6, 5 and 7 in Figure E 1 − 4 A and 8 A before being transmitted to the cerebellar hemispheres as indicated in Figure E 3 − 6 B.

21. The Open-Loop Circuits via the Basal Ganglia

In Figure E 3 − 6 B there is another dynamic loop system from cortical areas other than the motor cortex that passes through the basal ganglia, BG, which are enormous assemblages of nerve cells deep to the cerebral cortex (Brodal [1969]; de Long [1973]). This system appears to work in parallel with the cerebellar hemispheres. Its importance is indicated by the severe motor disturbances that result from lesions of the basal ganglia, the tremors and rigidity of Parkinson's disease and the wild irregular movements of Huntington's chorea. However the mode of operation of the neuronal machinery of the basal ganglia is still poorly understood, so its role in movement control is only vaguely indicated in Figure E 3 − 6 B and 7.

22. Synthesis of the Various Neuronal Mechanisms Concerned in the Control of Voluntary Movement

Figure E 3 − 7 gives an imaginative illustration of the interacting loop controls (Allen and Tsukahara [1974]). As discussed in relation to Kornhuber's experiments, the idea of a movement achieves expression in patterns of

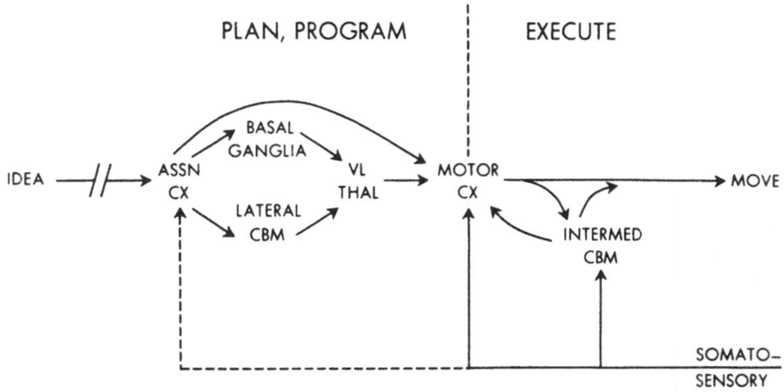

Fig. E3 – 7. Diagram showing the pathways concerned in the execution and control of voluntary movement; *ASSN CX*, association cortex; *lateral CBM*, cerebellar hemisphere; *intermed. CBM*, pars intermedia of cerebellum (modified from Allen and Tsukahara, 1974).

excitation in the association cortex, which are recognized as the readiness potential in the diffuse scalp recordings (Fig. E3–4). Thence there are the two systems of dynamic loops illustrated in Figure E3–6B with projection back to the motor cortex via the VL thalamus. In addition these loop systems project back to association cortex (area 6 in Fig. E3–6B) with the opportunity of further dynamic loop circuitry. The synthesis of all these loop inputs with the ongoing activities of the association cortex provides what we may call preprogrammed information for the motor cortex that as a consequence generates the appropriate discharges down the pyramidal tract (the motor command) for bringing about the desired movement.

Mountcastle's [1975] detailed studies on the neurones of areas 5 and 7 (cp. chapter E2) lead to concepts closely related to those expressed above. It is suggested that

> "neurones of area 5 compose a conditional command apparatus for movements of a certain kind, emitted under certain motivational sets; the command apparatus operates in a holistic manner, and does not specify the details of the movements it commands, matters left, on this hypothesis, to the apparatus of the precentral motor cortical areas (area 6). Area 5 contains a continually updated neuronal replicate of the position and movements of the limbs in space, one in which the topographical area through which an intended movement is to take place is facilitated, "lighted up" as it were, by a descending discharge corollary to the truly motor commands leading to the movement."

These corollary discharges presumably would be operating via the pathways indicated in Figure E1–8A – areas 4 $\rightleftarrows$ 6 $\rightleftarrows$ 5 $\rightarrow$ 7. Mountcastle goes on to state that:

> "we see in the holistic or gestalt command function of these parietal neurons something of that flexibility and sensitivity to motivational set and behavioral goal that all our own observations of human behavior dictate must be present: the neural drivers of adaptive behavior. Our general command hypothesis does not hold that these particular parietal command centers have exclusive control over these sets of movements. Just the opposite, I propose that there are many such command centers within the brain, and not all at cortical levels, that have access to the motor system at many of its levels"

Figures E 3 − 6 B and 7 provide illustrations of these many levels.

At the stage of motor discharge, by the two closed loops illustrated in Figure E 3 − 6 A, the pars intermedia makes an important contribution by updating the movement that is based upon the sensory description of the limb position and velocity upon which the intended movement is to be superimposed. This closed loop operation is a kind of short-range planning as opposed to the long-range planning of the association cortex and lateral cerebellum. Certainly both of these cerebellar zones must cooperate in the performance of every skilled movement (Allen and Tsukahara [1974]).

In learning a movement we first execute the movement very slowly because it cannot yet be adequately preprogrammed. Instead it is performed largely by intense cerebral concentration as well as with the constant updating via the pars intermedia of the cerebellum. With practice and the consequent motor learning, a greater amount of the movement can be preprogrammed and the movement can be executed more rapidly. With very rapid movements we rely entirely on preprogramming by the circuits to the left of Figure E 3 − 7 because there is no time for on-target correction by the pars intermedia once a fast movement has begun (Allen and Tsukahara [1974]).

Thus we may conjecture that trained movements are largely preprogrammed, whereas exploratory movements, which constitute an important fraction of our movement repertoire, are imperfectly preprogrammed, being provisional and subject to continuous revision. The role of the cerebellum, presumably the pars intermedia, in untrained or exploratory movements is attested to by the clumsiness and slowness with which they are performed when, after cerebellectomy, the cerebrum has to function in the absence of cerebellar cooperation both in preprogramming and in updating. If only the cerebellar hemisphere with the circuits of Figure E 3 − 6 B is put out of action, a tremor often results because the movement is so poorly preprogrammed that the pars intermedia ineffectually performs its normal function which is the updating of a movement that is already a good guess.

In summary, we conjecture that the pre-motor association areas and the cerebellar hemispheres and basal ganglia are responsible for preprogramming movements. The motor command so formulated is discharged down the pyramidal tract, so initiating the movement, but the pars intermedia updates the motor command and continuously exercises a feedback control, so keeping the movement on target (Allen and Tsukahara [1974]).

23. General Discussion

It is important to recognize that the long duration of the readiness potential (0.8 s) is for a very special type of voluntary movement, namely one that is initiated without any external signal. The experimental design ensures that the self-conscious mind is acting on the cerebral cortex without the help of any predisposing or determining condition of the neural machinery. The readiness potential is the small diffuse field potential built up by the complex preprogramming operation in the cerebral cortex with the cooperation of circuits through the cerebellar hemispheres and the basal ganglia, as illustrated in Figures 3 E–6 B and 7. As far as has been determined (Kornhuber [1974]), for almost its whole duration the readiness potential is non-specific, having much the same time course and spatial distribution for any voluntary movement. For example in Figure E 3–4, the local sign with the two precentral recordings does not appear until about the time of the discharge from the motor cortex down the pyramidal tract (lower trace).

It would be of particular interest to record the readiness potential in commissurotomy patients, where it would be expected to be generated only in the dominant hemisphere. Voluntary action by such patients can be initiated only by means of the dominant hemisphere (chapter E 5). All actions initiated by the minor hemisphere are not under the conscious control of the patient though often they are appropriate and intelligent responses to signals acting on receptors that transmit to the minor hemisphere.

It will be recognized that the stringent conditions for the experimental demonstration of the readiness potential are far removed from the ordinary manner of initiating and carrying out voluntary movements. The background is rarely neutral as in Kornhuber's experiments. Most voluntary movements are components of complex sequences, so that it is impossible to disentangle the components attributable to the action of the self-conscious mind and those due to learned behaviour patterns. As noted above, fully learned movements are carried out by a complex of preprogramming and updating and the details of their performance barely obtrude on the consciousness of the subject. Nevertheless it must be recognized that these movements are predominantly dependent on the memory stores of learned skills in the cortex. However, the memory stores in the cerebellum are also important, as can be recognized in the disabilities entailed by cerebellar lesions.

The restricted treatment here given to the problem of voluntary action is necessitated by the requirement that it be investigated scientifically. It is impossible to carry out any scientific study on the decision-making propensity of a human being subjected to all the complexities of a "real-life" situation even when that situation is ethically neutral – for example the decision to go home by train or bus, or which gramophone record to put on for the next playing. No doubt psychologists or philosophers could claim that in principle such decisions can be accounted for in a rigidly determined fashion by the present brain events and the stored memories. However the stringent conditions of Kornhuber's [1974] experiment preclude or negate such explanatory claims. The trained subjects literally do make the movements in the absence of determining influences from the environment, and any random potentials generated in the relaxed brain would be virtually eliminated by the averaging of 250 traces. Thus we can regard these experiments as providing a convincing demonstration that voluntary movements can be freely initiated independently of any determining influences that are entirely within the neuronal machinery of the brain. If we can regard this as established for elementally simple movements, there is no problem in extending indefinitely the range of consciously willed or strictly voluntary actions. Nevertheless there must be critical evaluation so as to exclude a large variety of automatic actions. Only rarely do we bother to exercise voluntary control of our actions. Mercifully almost all run automatically, for example breathing, walking, knitting, and one is sometimes tempted to say talking! But all of these can be voluntarily controlled if we so wish. Even breathing can be controlled within limits. We may hyperventilate, or breathe to a chosen rhythm, or cease breathing for as long as one minute.

The outstanding problem in the voluntary control of movement is of course the action across the interface between the self-conscious mind on the one hand and the modules of the cerebral cortex on the other. The existence of this influence is established by the empirical experiments of Kornhuber and associates, but there is of course no explanation of how it can come about. However, in chapter E 7 there will be formulation of a hypothesis on this problem of interaction of mind on brain.

Chapter E 4 The Language Centres of the Human Brain

24. Résumé

There is firstly an account of the areas of the cerebral cortex that are concerned in speech, the anterior speech area of Broca, and the large posterior speech area of Wernicke (Fig. E 4 − 1). These areas were originally defined by astute inferences from cortical lesions in patients that suffered various kinds of aphasia. The remarkable discovery was that about 95% of aphasics have lesions in their left cerebral hemisphere. Experiments on exposed human brains have confirmed these earlier clinical studies and sharpened the localizations of the speech area, showing in particular that the Wernicke area extended up into areas 39 and 40 of the parietal lobe (Fig. E 4 − 3).

Another important investigation has been by the dichotic listening test in which two different auditory stimuli are presented by headphones, one to the right ear and the other to the left ear. Since each ear predominantly feeds into the auditory cortex on the contralateral side (Fig. E 4 − 4), it could be established in this way that the inputs of words were much better recognized by the right ear than with the left because there was projection more directly to the linguistic areas of the left hemisphere.

The commissurotomy investigations described in the next chapter are important because they have shown that the hemisphere containing the speech centres has the amazing property of being in liaison with the self-conscious mind of the subject in respect both of giving and receiving. Recenr investigations have shown that the linguistic areas of the hemisphere are associated with enlargements of cortical areas with respect to the symmetrical zones on the other hemisphere (Fig. E 4 − 5). Particular importance is attached to Brodmann's areas 39 and 40, which came very late in evolution, being barely recognizable in nonhuman primates. These are the areas specifically concerned in cross-modal associations, that is associations from one sensory input, say touch, to another, say vision (cp. area STS in Figs. E 1−7 and 8). It is postulated that language comes when you have the association between objects that you feel and objects that you see, and which you then name. There is a brief reference to the evolution of language and its great importance in human activity. Language provides the means of representing objects abstractly and for manipulating them hypothetically in one's mind.

Despite the recent advances in recognition of asymmetries of the dominant hemisphere arising from the hypertrophy of areas associated with speech (Fig. E 4−4), there is still no detailed microscopic analysis of the cortical structure of speech areas. Nor is there any advanced physiological study of the neuronal activity in speech areas during their activity.

Finally, there is an account of the extraordinary disability suffered by a girl who was kept isolated from any linguistic experience until she was 13½ years old. Because of this long period of inactivity of the speech areas, grave disabilities have been revealed in response to the efforts to train her to speak. Even after 3 years her linguistic performance is quite limited, but meaningful sentences can be generated. Though right-handed, she utilizes the right hemisphere for speech. This is an indication that the areas of the cerebral cortex built in readiness for speech require utilization in the earlier years in order to allow effective development of the wonderful potentialities for speech.

25. Introduction

The representation of language in the cerebral cortex has been investigated by four methods: firstly, the study of linguistic disorders arising from cerebral lesions (reviewed by Geschwind [1965(a)], [1970], [1972], [1973]); secondly, the effects of stimulation of the exposed brain of conscious subjects and of the transient aphasias resulting from this exposure (Penfield and Roberts [1959]; thirdly, the effects of intracarotid injections of sodium amytal (a neural depressant) (Serafetinides & others [1965]); fourthly, the dichotic listening tests of Broadbent [1954] and Kimura [1967].

26. Aphasia

As described by Penfield and Roberts [1959] and Geschwind [1970], for over a century disorders of speech (aphasia) have been associated with lesions of the left cerebral hemisphere (Fig. E 4−1). There was firstly the motor

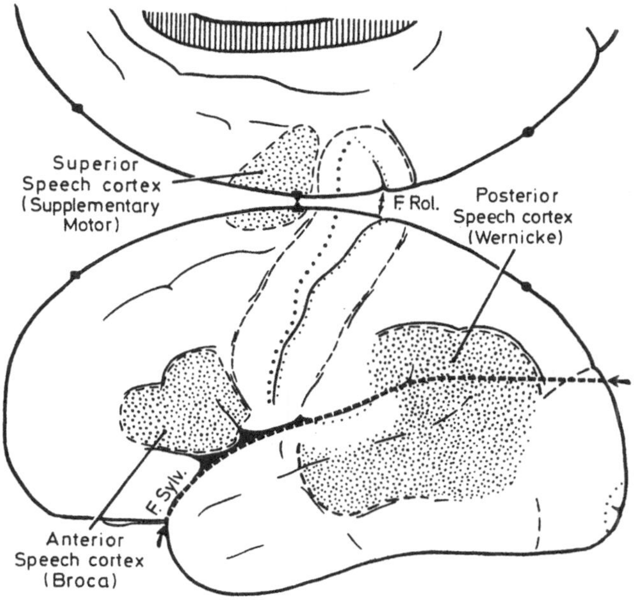

Fig. E4–1. Cortical speech areas of dominant left hemisphere. Note that the view is of left hemisphere from both lateral and medial aspects. *F. Rol.* is fissure of Rolando and *F. Sylv.* is fissure of Sylvius (Penfield and Roberts, 1959).

aphasia described by Broca [1861], as arising from lesions of the posterior part of the third frontal convolution, an area that we now call the anterior speech centre of Broca. The patient had lost the ability to speak although he could understand spoken language. Broca's area lies just in front of the cortical areas controlling the speech muscles; nevertheless motor aphasia is due not to paralysis of the vocal musculature, but to disorders in their usage.

Much more important, however, is the large speech area, lying more posteriorly in the left hemisphere. On the basis of evidence from lesions, it was originally thought by Wernicke [1874] to be only in the superior temporal convolution, but now it is recognized (Penfield and Roberts [1959]) as having a much more extensive representation on the parieto-temporal lobes (Fig. E 4–1). We now call this area the posterior speech centre of Wernicke and it is specially associated with the ideational aspect of speech. The aphasia is characterized by failure to understand speech – either written or spoken. Although the patient could speak with normal speed and rhythm, his speech was remarkably devoid of content, being a kind of nonsense jargon. In the great majority of patients lesions anywhere in the right hemisphere

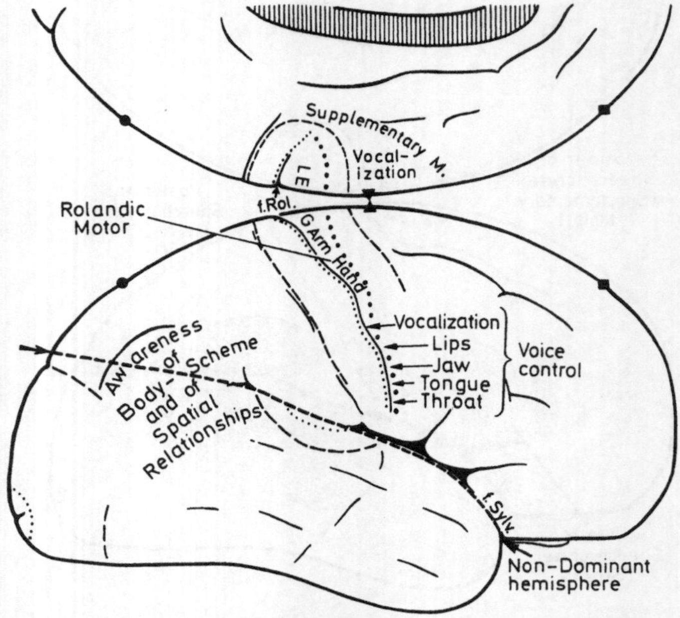

Fig. E4—2. Vocalization areas of minor right hemisphere. As with Fig. E4—1, the view is both of lateral and medial aspects. The various effects were evoked by electrical stimulation (Penfield and Roberts, 1959).

(Fig. E4—2) do not result in serious disorders of speech. Minor defects in linguistic expression will be described in chapter E6. Even lesions of the motor areas for vocalization cause little disability because the speech muscles are bilaterally represented.

Aphasia itself has been subjected to most detailed and diverse descriptions and classifications. Areas specialized for reading and writing have been, for example, recognized by the alexia or agraphia resulting from their destruction (Geschwind [1965(a)], [1965(b)], [1970]; Hécaen [1967]; Milner [1967], [1968], [1974]). It is essential to recognize the incredible complexity of the encoding and decoding in speech (cp. Teuber [1967]). As an illustration we can consider the neural events concerned in some simple linguistic performance.

For example, in reading aloud, black marks on white paper are projected from the retina to the brain, in the encoded form of impulse frequencies in the optic nerve fibres, and so eventually to the primary visual cortex (area 17 in Fig. E4—3, cp. chapter E2, Figs. E2—4 and 5). The next stage is the transmission of the encoded visual information to the visual association areas

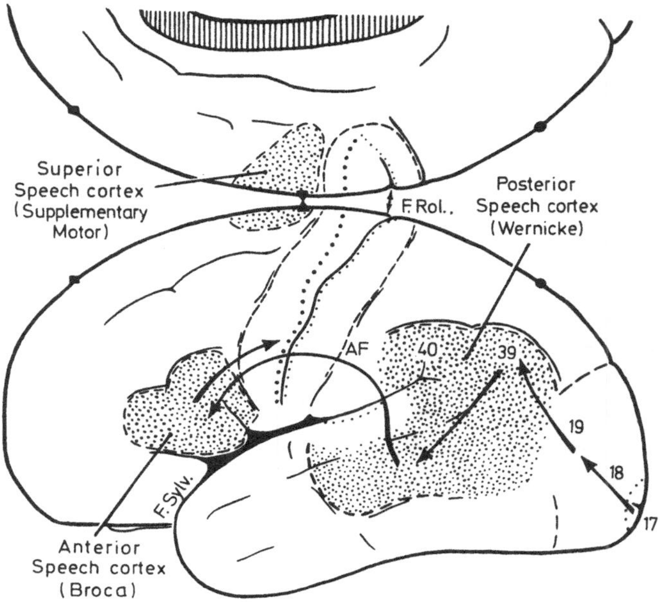

Fig. E4–3. Redrawing of left hemisphere as in Fig. E4–1 but with angular and supramarginal gyri labelled as Brodmann areas 39 and 40 (cf. Fig. E1–4). Also shown by arrows is the pathway from area 17 to 18, 19 to 39 (angular gyrus) to the Wernicke speech area, thence by the arcuate fasciculus *(AF)* to Broca's area, and so to the motor cortex for speech.

(Brodmann areas 18, 19), where there is a further stage of reconstitution of the visual image. As described in chapter E 2, this reconstitution is still most inadequate. Neurones specifically respond to simple geometrical forms, the so-called feature recognition neurones. However, at the next stage, lesions of the posterior part of Wernicke's area (the angular gyrus, area 39 in Fig. E 4–3) result in dyslexia, suggesting that the relay from the visual association neurones provides information that is converted into word patterns and that these in turn are interpreted as meaningful sentences in the process of conscious recognition. It is our thesis that this occurs because the self-conscious mind is able to interact with the open modules in this cortical area (chapter E 7). Lesions result in Wernicke's aphasia. The further stage in the process of reading aloud is via the arcuate fasciculus (AF in Fig. E 4–3) to the motor speech area (Broca's area). Lesions of the arcuate fasciculus result in conduction aphasia (Geschwind [1970]). There is comprehension of spoken language but a gross defect in its repetition and in normal speaking. At the terminal stage appropriate patterns of neural activity in Broca's area lead to the motor areas for vocalization and so to the coordinated contractions of the speech muscles. A comparably complex chain of encoding and decoding is involved in writing out language that is heard.

As a general summary, it can be stated that great difficulties arise in a sharp classification of aphasias because of the irregular destructive action of clinical lesions. For our present purpose it is not necessary to go into all of the detailed disputation between the various experts on the many types of aphasia or on the causative cerebral lesions (cp. Geschwind [1965(a)], [1970], [1973]). The remarkable discovery is that the enormous proportion of aphasics have lesions in their left cerebral hemisphere. Only rarely is a right cerebral lesion associated with aphasia. There was originally a general belief that right-handed patients had their speech centres on the left side and vice versa for the left-handed patients. This has proved to be untrue. The majority of left-handed subjects also have their speech centres in the left cerebral hemisphere (Penfield and Roberts [1959]; Zangwill [1960]; Serafetinides & others [1965]; Piercy [1967]).

27. Experiments on Exposed Brains

In the hands of Penfield and his associates stimulation of the cerebral cortex has been responsible for quite remarkable discoveries relating to the localization of speech centres. Stimulation of the motor areas in either hemisphere (Fig. E4−2) innervating structures concerned in sound production such as tongue and larynx cause the patients to produce a variety of calls and cries (vocalization) but not recognizable words. These are the motor areas of voice control and are bilateral. Only rarely does a similar stimulation in animals give vocal responses. On the other hand, stimulation of the speech areas (Fig. E4−1) results in an interference with speech or an arrest of speech. For example, if the subject is engaged in some speech production, such as the counting of numbers, his voice may be slurred or distorted, or the same number may be repeated. Often the application of the gentle stimulating current to the speech areas causes a cessation of speech, which is resumed as soon as the stimulation stops; or there is a temporary inability to name objects during the stimulation. One can imagine that the stimulus has caused a widerspread interference with the specific spatiotemporal patterns of neuronal activity that are responsible for speech. In this way Penfield and his associates have been able to delimit the two speech areas that have been recognized from clinical studies of aphasia, namely the anterior and posterior speech areas, and also a subsidiary third area (Fig. E4−1).

Inadvertent sequelae to operative procedures have been important in demonstrating the cerebral hemisphere that is responsible for speech – whether it is the right or the left hemisphere of the subject. It has been observed, that, after a cerebral operation involving exposure of one cerebral hemisphere, a transient aphasia often develops some days after the operation and continues for 2 or 3 weeks. This is attributed to the neuroparalytic oedema resulting from brain exposure. A systematic study of the neuroparalytic aphasia of patients by Penfield and Roberts [1959] showed that it developed in over 70% of patients with left hemisphere operation regardless of whether they were right- (157) or left-handed (18). By contrast with operations on the right hemisphere, aphasia was very rare, occurring in only one of 196 right-handed and in one of the 15 left-handed subjects. These observations indicate the very strong dominance of speech representation (over 98%) in the left hemisphere regardless of handedness. Other investigators using various techniques are in general agreement with these results, but give a less strong bias for the left-handed patients, which in their figures have right hemisphere representation of speech more frequently, though still not as frequently as left hemisphere representation (reviewed by Zangwill [1960]; Piercy [1967]).

28. Intracarotid Injections of Sodium Amytal

A new method of determining speech representation and relating it to handedness was developed by Wada with the injection of sodium amytal into the common or internal carotid arteries of subjects in whom it was important preoperatively to identify the speech hemisphere (Serafetinides [1965]). This work has been analyzed by Milner & others [1964]. There was likewise the overwhelming dominance of the left hemisphere representation of speech for right-handed subjects and a considerable dominance also for the left-handed subjects, but the left dominance was less marked than that reported by Penfield and Roberts [1959]. Similar results have been reported by other investigators. One difficulty about the Wada test is that it is dependent upon a very strict lateralization of vascular distribution. In some cases it has been recognized that this is not so, and other observations at variance with the strict unilateral representation of speech may be attributed to such vascular abnormalities. There are a few reports of speech being located in both hemispheres (Zangwill [1960]; Milner [1974]; Sperry [1974]). What seems more certain is that in infancy damage to the left hemisphere may result in the development of speech areas in the right hemisphere, as will be described in chapter E 6 (Milner [1974]). There appears to be considerable neural plasticity at this early age. Basser [1962] presented evidence that speech in very young children was bilateral, the left hemisphere gradually assuming dominance over the first few years of life. Using the dichotic listening test Kimura [1967] showed that by 4 to 5 years speech had become fully lateralized.

29. The Dichotic Listening Test

A powerful technique has recently been employed for the study of cerebral asymmetry: the dichotic listening test (Broadbent [1954]; Kimura [1967], [1973]). The great advantage of this test is that it permits investigations in healthy subjects. It thus expands enormously the source of potential test subjects and eliminates the uncertainties entailed in aiming at physiological goals through the study of diseased brains. The subject receives simultaneously through headphones two different auditory stimuli, one to the right ear, the other one to the left ear. The test was first tried on word recognition. Three pairs of digits (say 2, 5 then 3, 4 then 9, 7) were presented dichotically to normal subjects in rapid succession, after which the subject was asked to report in any order as many of the digits as he could. It was surprising to find that those digits presented to the right ear were more accurately reported than those to the left ear, although it was shown that there were no differences in the respective sensory auditory channels.

The asymmetry in normal auditory recognition is explained by the peculiarities of the neural pathways along which the signals presented to the ears are transmitted to the brain. As in the visual system, there is a crossed connexion from the ear to the primary auditory sensory area, that is to Heschl's gyrus in the temporal lobe (Fig. E 4−4). However, the situation differs from that in vision, where the connections of one visual field to the respective primary visual cortex are entirely crossed (Fig. E 2−4). There exist also ipsilateral connexions from one ear to Heschl's gyrus of the same side. However, this ipsilateral connexion is much weaker than the contralateral (Bocca et al. [1955]); furthemore, the ipsilateral pathways are suppressed by the contralateral during dichotic presentation (Milner & others [1968]; Sparks and Geschwind [1968]), presumably by inhibition in the cerebral cortex. Thus we would attribute the right ear advantage in the dichotic digits test to the fact that the right ear has a more direct access to that

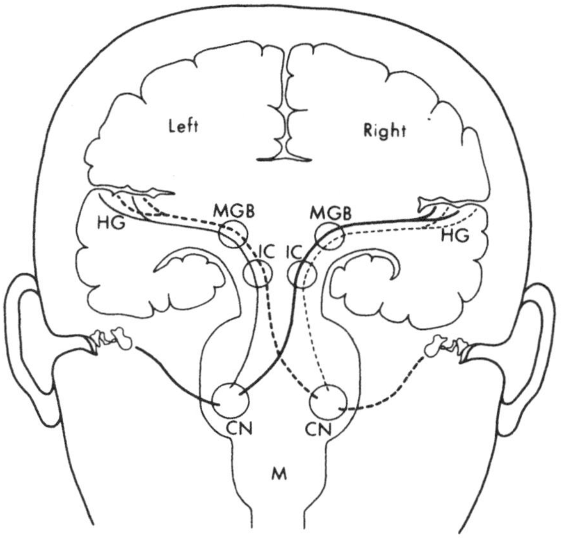

Fig. E4−4. Schematic drawing of the auditory pathways to the Heschl's gyri *(HG)* on each side, showing by the thicker lines the dominance of the crossed connections. *CN*, cochlear nucleus, *IC*, inferior colliculus, *MGB*, medial geniculate body, *M*, medulla oblongata.

hemisphere in which the encoded auditory input is decoded into recognizable words, viz to the left hemisphere, the speech hemisphere.

As yet we have not defined the range of sensory input that could be classified as verbal. Some significant data have been obtained from dichotic presentation of nonsense speech played backwards. In this case also the right ear was superior and hence presumably also the left hemisphere. Thus the left hemisphere is specially concerned with a stage in the processing of acoustic information that is even prior to the recognition of its conceptual content. The situation in the auditory cortex is therefore analogous to that in the visual cortex, as would be expected from the cascade organizations illustrated in Fig. E 1−7 (Jones and Powell [1970]).

Studdert-Kennedy and Shankweiler [1970] found a right ear superiority for syllables consisting of consonant-vowel-consonant, but for vowels alone no significant ear advantage has been established (Darwin [1969]). Obviously vowels are more readily processed on the basis of their musical content. It is postulated by Studdert-Kennedy and Shankweiler [1970] that, at the level of word recognition, the left hemisphere displays its linguistic superiority, but the auditory areas of both hemispheres perform equally well at the earlier stage of auditory pattern analysis.

30. The Self-Conscious Mind and Speech

We will see in chapter E 5 that with human subjects callosal transection (commissurotomy) reveals that the left hemisphere is the speech hemisphere for all subjects so far investigated (Fig. E 5–4). In fact there is an identification of the speech hemisphere with the dominant hemisphere and an association of this hemisphere with the conscious experiences of all the subjects, both as regards receiving from the world and acting upon it. There is thus strong evidence that we have to associate the dominant hemisphere, i. e. the speech hemisphere, with the amazing property of being able to give rise to conscious experiences in perception (chapter E 2), and also to receive from them in the carrying out of willed movements (chapter E 3). *Moreover, the most searching investigation of commissurotomy patients discloses that the minor hemisphere does not have in the smallest degree this amazing property of being in liaison with the self-conscious mind of the subject in respect either of giving or receiving* (chapter E 5). One would predict with assurance that in subjects with the rarely occuring right hemispheric representation of speech, the right hemisphere would be dominant, as revealed after the callosal transection, and be predominantly associated with the conscious experiences of the subject. That leaves us of course with the acute problem of what would happen if there were callosal transection of brains in which there is bilateral representation of speech, as has been claimed to occur as a rare abnormality (Zangwill [1960]; Milner [1974]).

In 1965 Serafetinides & others reported that relatively slow intracarotid injections of sodium amylobarbitone resulted not only in aphasia but also in a loss of consciousness for some minutes when given on the side of the dominant speech hemisphere. By contrast, with intracarotid injection to the minor hemisphere, there was at the most a brief unconsciousness. These results would be in good accord with the present hypothesis of a unique association of the dominant hemisphere with the self-conscious mind. However, the experimental results have been criticized by Rosaldini and Rossi [1967], who found that unconsciousness occurred only when the greater part of both hemispheres was functionally inactivated. They concluded that there is no evidence to associate consciousness with the neuronal mechanisms responsible for speech. In interpreting these results it must be recognized that normally each hemisphere is subjected to an intensive barrage of impulses traversing the corpus callosum. Inactivation of the minor hemisphere would thus be expected to disturb the dominant hemisphere because of the silencing of this trans-callosal barrage. Evidently more definitive technical procedures are required before the intracarotid injections can be employed to test the hypothesis that, with intact corpus callosum, the dominant hemisphere is uniquely concerned in the phenomena of self-consciousness.

31. Anatomical Substrates of Speech Mechanisms

The exclusive association of speech and consciousness with the dominant hemisphere after commissurotomy gives rise to the question: Is there some special anatomical structure in the dominant hemisphere that is not matched in the minor hemisphere? In general, the two hemispheres have been regarded as being mirror images at a crude anatomical level, but recently it has been discovered that in about 80% of human brains there are asymmetries with special developments of the cerebral cortex in the regions both of the anterior

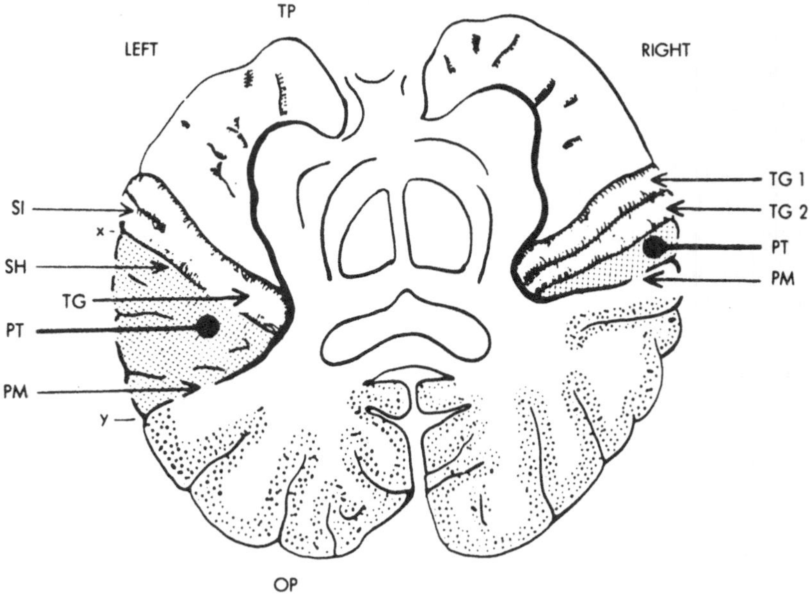

Fig. E4—5. Asymmetry of human superior temporal lobes. Upper surfaces of human temporal lobes exposed by a cut on each side as illustrated by the broken lines in Figs. E4—1 and E4—2. Typical left-right differences are shown. The posterior margin *(PM)* of the planum temporale *(PT)* slopes backward more sharply on the left than on the right, so that end *y* of the left Sylvian fissure lies posterior to the corresponding point on the right. The anterior margin of the sulcus of Heschl *(SH)* slopes forward more sharply on the left. In this brain there is a single traverse gyrus of Heschl *(TG)* on the left and two on the right *(TG_1, TG_2)*. *TP*, temporal pole; *OP*, occipital pole; *SI*, sulcus intermedius of Beck (Geschwind and Levitsky, 1968).

and posterior speech areas (Geschwind and Levitsky [1969]; Geschwind [1972], [1973]; Wada & others [1973]). In Figure E 4 – 5 there is displayed the superior surface of the temporal lobe after removal of the frontal and parietal lobes of both hemispheres by cutting along the dotted lines in Figure E 4 – 1 and E 4 – 2. There is seen to be hypertrophy of a part of the left superior temporal gyrus in the region of the posterior speech area of Wernicke (the planum temporale shown as the cross-hatched area). It is just posterior to the primary auditory area, Heschl's gyrus (TG). This asymmetry was observed with the left side larger in 65% of brains, but in 11% the right planum temporale was larger and on the remainder (24%) there was approximate equality.

Evidence supporting the independence in location of speech and handedness comes also from a recent observation of Wada & others [1973] who found the left-right asymmetries of the planum temporale not only in infants who died at birth, but also in a 29-week-old foetus. Thus the speech localization appears to be genetically determined, the speech centres being built in preparation for their eventual usage after birth. On the other hand, handedness would appear to be much more flexible and to be at least in part determined by environmental habits.

An important enquiry concerns the location of the Wernicke speech area. Why was this region of the inferior parietal lobule (Brodmann areas 39, 40) utilized for language in addition to the cortical areas specially related to hearing, namely area 22 in the superior temporal gyrus (cp. Figs. E 1 – 7 K, L)? Geschwind [1965(a)] makes the most interesting suggestion that areas 39 and 40 were developed to enhance the ability for cross-modal associations. In the monkey the STS area has been shown to be the site where somaesthetic, visual and auditory information converge (Figs. E 1 – 7 and 8). According to Jones and Powell [1970] this area is homologous with areas 39 and 40 in the human brain. Lesions of these areas are the most critical in the production of agnosias, which are characterized by apraxia for the minor hemisphere and dyslexia, agraphia and other aphasias for the dominant hemisphere. Geschwind [1965(a)] goes so far as to state that

> "the ability to acquire speech has as a prerequisite the ability to form cross-modal associations [cp. chapter E 2]. In sub-human forms the only readily established sensory-sensory associations are those between a non-limbic (i. e. visual, tactile or auditory) stimulus and a limbic stimulus. It is only in man that associations between two non-limbic stimuli are readily formed and it is this ability which underlies the learning of names of objects."

Teuber's [1967] very challenging remarks on this same theme are worth quoting in full.

> Undoubtedly one of the crucial aspects of Language, beyond its formal characteristics described by the linguist, is the labeling of objects. Language imposes order on events by permitting their classification, and it provides a tool for representing absent objects and for manipulating them hypothetically 'in one's mind.' For all this, it would seem essential that there be some central mechanism for transcending the division between the different senses, for identifying an object felt with an object seen, and both with the object we can name; there should be some form of cross-modal processing resulting in supramodal, more that sensory, categories, extracted from or imposed upon experience. Language frees us to a large extent from the tyranny of the senses. . . It gives us access to concepts that combine information from different sensory modalities and are thus intersensory or suprasensory, but the riddle remains as to how this is achieved. To say that language is needed to 'mediate' suprasensory objects requires that we understand how we know in the first place that a thing seen is identical with that same thing felt. The paradox here was posed by the many studies reviewed for us which seemed to indicate nearly complete absence of any transfer from one sense modality to the other, in monkeys, and even under some conditions in man.

In the light of these insights into the nature of the neuronal machinery that forms a necessary substratum for linguistic development, it can be conjectured that, in the evolution of skilled movements involving cross-modal associations, there arose special skills in expression in sound and gesture. These skills were associated with the developing areas of cross-modal association, area STS, and eventually there developed out of STS areas 39 and 40 which come to occupy such a large part of the parietal lobe (Figs. E 1 – 4 and E 4 – 3). The lateralization of speech in the dominant hemisphere is a further problem, but I think less acute now that it is recognized that speech is initially bilaterally represented, dominance being established in the first few years of life. And even later there is some speech ability latent in the minor hemisphere that can be developed after destruction of the speech areas of the dominant hemisphere (chapters E 5 and E 6).

Zaidel [1976] has formulated a most interesting hypothesis. Up till 4 or 5 years both hemispheres develop together in linguistic competence, but the great increase in linguistic ability and skill coming on at that age demands fine motor control in order to give well-formed speech. It is at this stage that one hemisphere, usually the left, becomes dominant in linguistic ability because of its superior neurological endowment. Meanwhile the other hemisphere, usually the right, regresses in respect to speech, but retains its competence in understanding. This understanding is particularly valuable when there are gestalt concepts to be interpreted. We suggest also that the right hemisphere is important for expressiveness and rhythm in speech, particularly in song, which is well preserved after dominant hemispherectomy and lost after minor hemispherectomy. This hypothesis accounts well for the transfer of speech to the minor hemisphere when there is severe damage to the linguistic areas of the dominant hemisphere before the age of 5, and the progressive limitation of transfer at later ages.

In addition to these discoveries at a macro-level, one must assume that there are specially fine structural and functional properties as the basis for the linguistic performance of these speech areas. Undoubtedly most exciting work awaits the investigation by electron-microscopic techniques, and eventually by electrophysiological analysis, of the ongoing events in the speech areas of conscious subjects whose brains are exposed for some therapeutic purpose. In the evolution of man there must have been most remarkable developments in the neuronal structure of the cerebral cortex that has made possible the evolution of speech. One can imagine that progressively more subtle linguistic performance gave primitive men the opportunities for very effective survival, which may be regarded as a strong evolutionary pressure. As a consequence there were the marvellously rapid evolutionary changes transforming in several million years a primitive ape to the present human race. The evolution of language will be extensively treated in the discussions (II, IV, V, VI).

In respect of the anatomically represented speech area, and the associated linguistic ability and self-consciousness, the human brain is unique. Undoubtedly the experimental investigations on chimpanzees both with respect to their developing a sign language (Gardner and Gardner [1969], [1971]; Fouts [1973]) and a symbol language (Premack [1970]) show that the chimpanzee brain exhibits considerable levels of intelligent and learned performance, but this chimpanzee communication is at a different level from human speech (Bronowski and Bellugi [1970]; Chomsky [1968]). The tests reported by Lenneberg [1975] are of particular relevance. He trained normal high school students with the procedures described by Premack, replicating Premack's study as literally as possible. Two human subjects were quickly able to obtain considerably lower error scores than those reported for the chimpanzee. However, they were unable to translate correctly a single sentence, completed by them, into English. In fact, they did not understand that there was any correspondence between the plastic symbols and language; instead, they were under the impression that their task was to solve puzzles. Further, they tended to forget the solution to a task almost as soon as they were confronted with new tasks. Lenneberg has suggested that the comprehension of Premack's chimpanzee should be tested by more general and objective methods than heretofore.

Moreover, the linguistic performance of chimpanzees is at a lower level than that exhibited by the minor hemisphere in experiements by Sperry and associates on the commissurotomy patients (chapter E5). There will be a discussion of the subject of animal consciousness in chapter E 7, and in several sessions of the conjoint discussion (sections II, VII, VIII).

Relevant to the attempts to train chimpanzees in the use of human language is the evidence that Brodmann areas 39 and 40 cannot be recognized in the brains of monkeys (Jones and Powell [1970]) and appear to be poorly developed in anthropoid apes (Mauss [1911]; Vogt and Vogt [1919]; Bailey & others [1943]; Critchley [1953]; Geschwind [1965(a)]). It is most important to reinvestigate the chimpanzee brain in order to discover how far this brain shares in the tremendous hypertrophy of the areas of cross-modal association (39 and 40) that appears to play a key role in the evolution of human language.

32. The Acquisition of Language

The relationship of speech to human cognitive ability has been intensely studied using the normal acquisition of language in childhood. Recently a remarkable study has been carried out on the victim of a tragic family situation (Curtiss & others [1974]). The girl, Genie, had been kept in isolation and without any linguistic experience until she was discovered and rescued at the age of 13½ years. She had then no language and scored at only 15 months on a non-verbal cognitive test. Over a period of 2 years she has developed a considerable linguistic and cognitive ability, but her language is still very defective. Starting with monosyllables she developed a two-word grammar and she can now construct strings of 3 or 4 words that have meaning. Her word sequences show that her performance is not imitative, but that she is actually generating sentences. She, however, has difficulties in sentence construction. For example she cannot insert the negatives "not" or "no" into her sentences. They have an invariable position at the beginning.

The dichotic listening test was applied by Kimura and revealed that the delayed linguistic development of Genie was located in the right hemisphere despite her right handedness. All auditory processing appears to be accomplished by the right hemisphere, which suggests that there was a functional atrophy of the left hemisphere because of the enormously prolonged absence of linguistic usage. Consequently the extremely delayed linguistic development was handled by the right hemisphere. This functional atrophy could parallel that observed at a much simpler level in the transfer of ocular dominance that results from deprivation of visual input by one eye of kittens (Wiesel and Hubel [1963]).

In summary, the tragic and prolonged deprivation of all linguistic inputs has revealed the fundamental role of language in creating a human person with cognitive and creative abilities. The deprived brain was still able to recover some of its latent abilities, albeit in the other hemisphere from that which almost certainly would have been used in normal development. However Genie's greatly delayed linguistic development was beset by many difficulties and it is still very inadequate. The final comment in the progress report of Curtiss et al. [1974] is worth quoting.

> "Her language acquisition so far shows that, despite the tragic isolation which she suffered, despite the lack of linguistic input, despite the fact that she had no language for almost the first fourteen years of her life, Genie is equipped to learn language and she is learning it. No one can predict how far she will develop linguistically or cognitively. The progress so far, however, has been remarkable, and is a tribute to the human capacity for intellectual achievement."

Chapter E5 Global Lesions of the Human Cerebrum

33. Résumé

In this chapter there is an account of the performance of the human brain after massive lesions either in some operative procedure or as a result of injury. The study of the disabilities resulting from these lesions helps us to understand the normal functioning of the brain.

The most remarkable study has been that of Sperry and his associates on patients that have had the corpus callosum sectioned in the treatment of intractable epilepsy. The corpus callosum is an immense assemblage of nerve fibres, about 200 million, linking almost all parts of one hemisphere with mirror image areas of the other hemisphere (Fig. E5 – 1). These commissurotomy patients have been systematically investigated in a most skilled and careful manner by Sperry and his associates (Fig. E5 – 2), who have amassed a wealth of observations that have been confirmed again and again in the sequence of patients. By taking advantage of the fact that the left visual half-field projects to the visual area of the right hemisphere (Figs. E2 – 4, 5) and vice versa for the right visual field and the left hemisphere, Sperry has been able to investigate the responses of the right hemisphere to inputs that specifically go to it and not to the other hemisphere (Fig. E5 – 3). All patients have their linguistic areas in the left hemisphere (cp. chapter E4) which, for this reason, is termed the dominant hemisphere (Fig. E5 – 4). *The outstanding discovery in the investigations of these subjects is the uniqueness and exclusiveness of the dominant hemisphere in respect of conscious experience.* The friends and relatives recognize that the expression by the subject in language and in memory is not greatly disturbed by the operation. The unity of self-consciousness or the mental singleness that the patient experienced before the operation is retained, but at the expense of unconsciousness of all the happenings in the minor, right, hemisphere. Despite this failure of the right hemisphere to give any conscious experiences to the self-conscious subject, it can carry out remarkably skilled and purposive movements, particularly in the spatial and pictorial tests (Fig. E5 – 5). However, it is almost devoid of linguistic ability, so it is impossible to communicate with it at the symbolic level that is requisite for discovering if it has conscious experiences of its own.

There is an account of the most interesting investigative procedures that have been carried out by Sperry and his colleagues with great ingenuity and insight. In the light of these remarkable discoveries made with commissurotomized subjects we may now ask: how does the minor hemisphere function in the normal brain? It is postulated that in normal subjects activities in the minor hemisphere reach consciousness very largely after transmission to the dominant hemisphere, which very effectively occurs via the immense impulse traffic in the corpus callosum, as is illustrated in Figure E5 – 7 by the numerous arrows. Complementarily, it is postulated that the neural activities responsible for voluntary actions are generated in the dominant hemisphere by some willed action of the conscious self (see downward arrows in Fig. E5 – 7). Normally these neural activities spread widely over both the dominant and minor hemispheres giving the "readiness potential," described in chapter E3. At a further stage there is concentration of neural activity onto the area of the motor cortex that projects by the pyramidal tracts to bring about the willed movement.

There is a discussion of the status of the minor hemisphere. Undoubtedly it displays performance and skill superior to the brain of an anthropoid ape because before the commissurotomy it was part of an intact human brain with the memories and performances that that hemisphere specializes in, as will be described in chapter E6. Further reference to the remarkable findings of Sperry and his colleagues will be made in chapter E7, where the brain-mind problem will be considered in relationship to all the findings on the effects of lesions on the human brain.

The other massive lesions that are considered in this chapter result from the complete removal of one or other hemisphere. The removal of the minor hemisphere results in the disabilities of a severe hemiplegia, but the subject retains reasonable linguistic ability. The removal of the dominant hemisphere has much more serious sequelae. Besides the hemiplegia, there is a grave loss of linguistic ability, and communication with older patients becomes very difficult. The younger the patient, the more remarkable the recovery, and cases have been described of the ages of 10 and 14 where there was some linguistic recovery. Infants present a much more encouraging situation because there is a remarkable plasticity, the linguistic function of the dominant hemisphere being fairly effectively transferred to the other hemisphere up to 5 years of age. In fact there is some bilateral representation of speech up to that age. There is, as a consequence, considerable linguistic ability in these hemispherectomized patients, but there is a penalty in that the other functions of the minor hemisphere, such as the pictorial and spatial, suffer because of the crowding by the invasion of the newly developing linguistic areas.

34. Introduction

It is a general principle of biology that an understanding of some biological mechanism is greatly aided by a systematic study of this mechanism under various imposed disorders. In this chapter there will be an account of the performance of the human brain after global lesions which often are made in some therapeutic procedure, but which also happen inadvertently from some accidental injury. Lesions result in some deficiency in performance when it is measured relative to a normal intact brain. A systematic study of these deficiencies leads to the building up of ideas on the performance of the multitude of specialized areas of the brain that have been described in chapter E1. The more circumscribed lesions will be treated in the next chapter. It is proposed here to give firstly a critical account of the work of Sperry and associates on the "split-brain" patients, because this work provides the most illuminating insights on the functioning of the human brain, particularly in its relationship to conscious experience.

35. Investigations on the Human Brain After Commissural Section — Commissurotomy

This work has been published and discussed on many occasions by Sperry and his colleagues (Sperry [1964], [1968], [1970], [1974]; Bogen [1969 (a)], [1969 (b)]; Gazzaniga [1970]), but it is our thesis that the extraordinary implications of this work for the self-brain problem have not yet been fully realized by philosophers and scientists. This has occurred because the climate of opinion is not yet ready for a searching evaluation of these most surprising and revolutionary results.

The operative transection of the corpus callosum has so far been carried out in about 20 cases for therapeutic reasons and has often resulted in a remarkable amelioration of the intractable epilepsies suffered by these subjects. In parenthesis it may be noted that complete section of the corpus callosum had been carried out by other investigators in a series of human subjects many years earlier, but, because of the less rigorous post-operative testing procedures, the remarkable disabilities were overlooked.

This transection of the corpus callosum and of the anterior and hippocampal commissures is a severe cerebral lesion, and it was not performed on patients until experiments with equivalent lesions in non-human primates had been fully investigated by Sperry [1964] and Myers [1961] for many years, and shown not to result in severe disabilities. It is important to realize that this transection differs from any other lesion that has been produced in the brain by surgical intervention because ideally it inflicts a quite clear and sharp lesion restricted to commissural nerve fibres. There is no surround of injury invading adjacent neural territories, such as occurs for example with a cortical resection. It is important, furthermore, to realize that the corpus callosum is a tremendous tract, there being an estimated 200 million fibres crossing through it from one hemisphere to the other and linking almost all of the cortical areas of one hemisphere to the mirror-image areas of the other (Fig. E5 – 1). The exceptions are the primary visual area and most of the somaesthetic area, areas 17 and 3, 1, 2 respectively of Figure E1 – 4. It is of importance also that there is crossed representation for most inputs to the cerebrum from sense organs and also for its motor action via the pyramidal tracts. In particular, because of the partial decussation in the optic chiasma, the left cerebral hemisphere receives from the right visual fields of both eyes, as illustrated in Figure E2 – 4, and vice versa for the right hemisphere and the left visual fields. Because of decussation of the motor and sensory pathways, crossed representation also obtains for the limbs. The left hemisphere is in sensory and motor communication with the right arm and leg, the right hemisphere with the left arm and leg. The midline brain section does not of course extend to lower levels. The fibre crossings between the cerebral hemispheres by indirect pathways at the level of the diencephalon and mesencephalon remain intact. Only the direct commissural connections via the corpus callosum and the anterior commissure are severed.

These commissurotomy patients have been systematically investigated in a most skilled and careful manner by Sperry and his associates, who have amassed a wealth of observations that have been confirmed again and again in the sequence of patients. Great care has been exercised throughout in the experimental design in order to eliminate all inadvertent crosscueing. For example, in the main series of investigation all presentation of visual data has been to one or other visual half-field by flashes no more than 0.1 s in duration

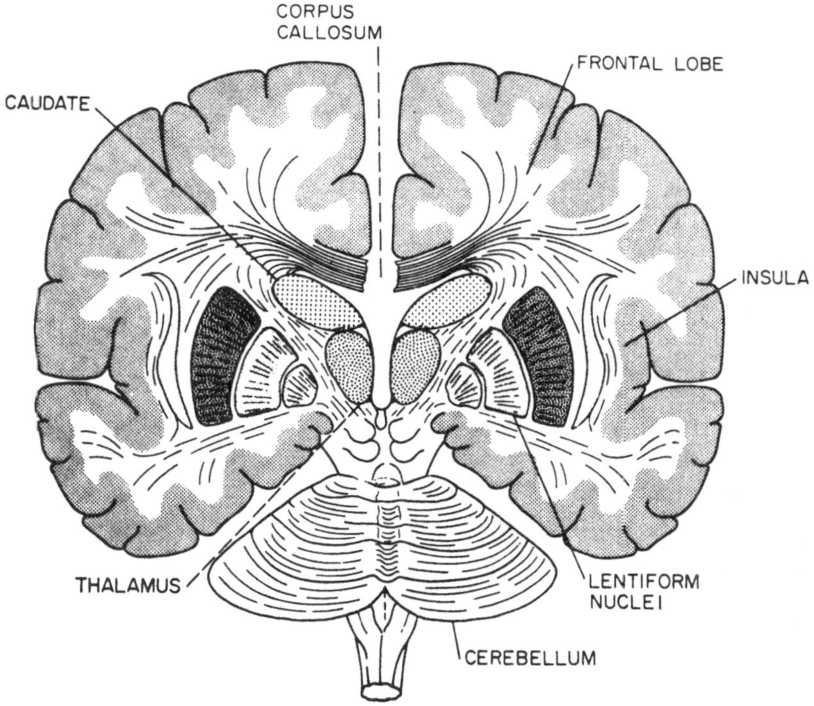

Fig. E5—1. Separation of the two cerebral hemispheres produced by section of the corpus callosum in the primate brain (Sperry, 1974).

in order to prevent eye movements from deviating the visual data to the other visual half-field. Moreover, in the usual experimental procedure the hands are screened from view as they search for objects and recognize them by touch. One other point to note at the outset is that, in the eight patients experimentally investigated, the speech centres were demonstrated post-operatively to be in the left hemisphere. Because of this location of the linguistic areas, the left hemisphere has been termed the dominant hemisphere.

The outstanding discovery in the investigations of these subjects is the uniqueness and exclusiveness of the dominant hemisphere in respect of conscious experience. The friends and relatives recognize that the expression by the subjects in language is not greatly disturbed by the operation and the conscious self reports a good memory of its preoperative life. The unity of self-consciousness or the mental singleness (Bremer [1966]; Eccles [1965])

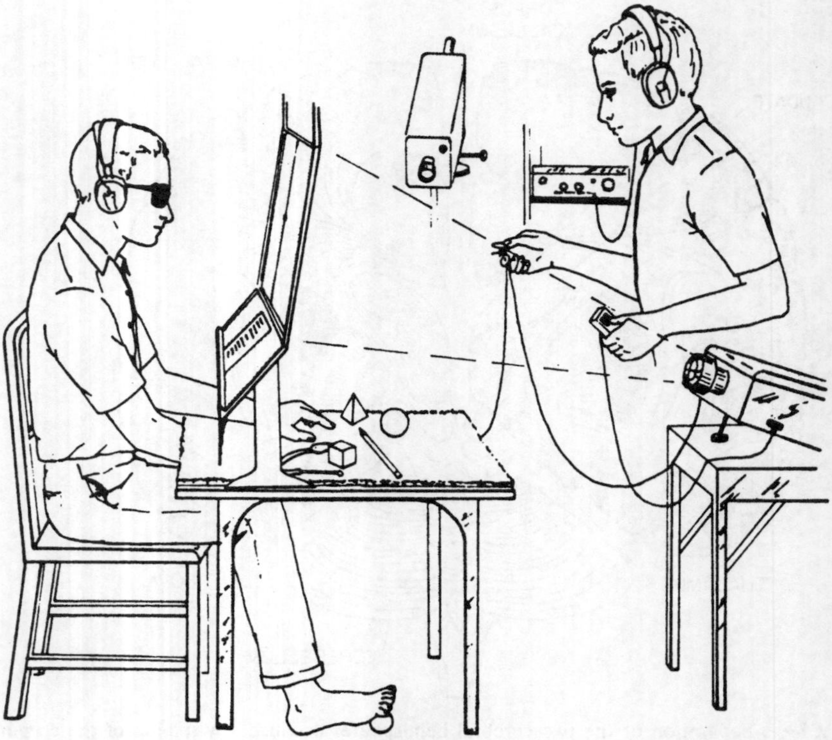

Fig. E5−2. Arrangement of general testing unit in demonstrating symptoms produced by commissural section (From Sperry, 1970).

that the patient experienced before the operation has been retained, but at the expense of unconsciousness of all the happenings in the minor, right, hemisphere. This minor hemisphere continues to perform as a very superior brain with a refined ability in stereognosis, and in pattern recognition and copying, yet none of the goings-on in that hemisphere gives conscious experiences to the patient, except by delayed and very diffuse pathways in the brain, or by sensory recognition of movements brought about by the minor hemisphere. It is remarkable to see the superior stereognostic performance programmed by the minor hemisphere to the left har d, all unbeknown to the subject who sees it with amazement and chagrin. These tests can be carried out in full visual view, not screened in the usual manner. In this respect the conscious performance of the patient using the dominant hemisphere and the right hand is greatly inferior to that carried out by the minor hemisphere. For

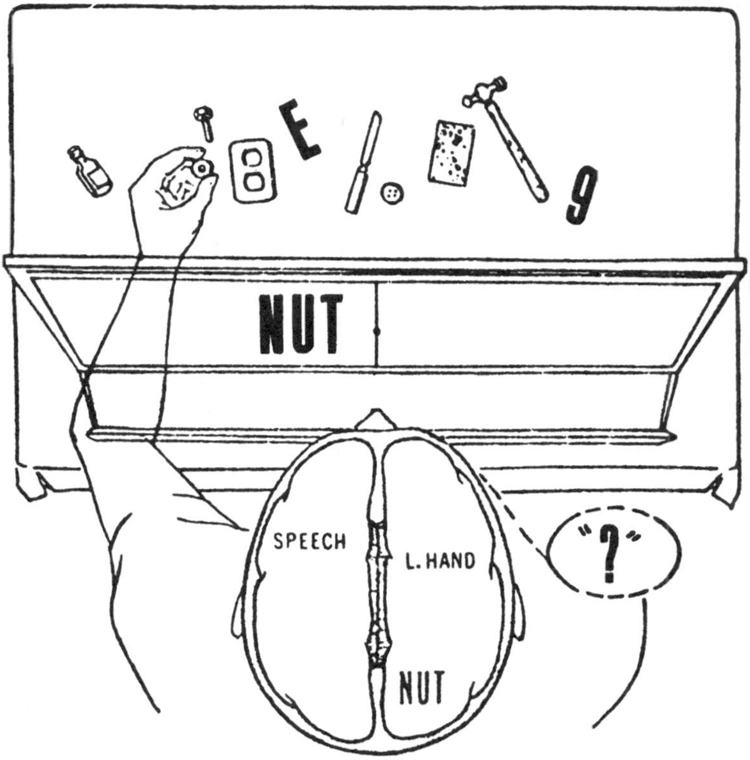

Fig. E5–3. Names of objects flashed to left half-field can be read and understood but not spoken. Subject can retrieve the named object by touch with the left hand, but cannot afterwards name the item or retrieve it with the right hand (Sperry, 1970).

example, there is failure in the attempt to match a simple geometrical design by a composite made up by assembling coloured blocks, a task quickly and accurately performed by the minor hemisphere programming the left hand (Gazzaniga [1970]).

Bogen [1969 (a)] has illustrated the superior performance of the left hand in copying drawings such as a Necker cube or a Maltese cross or in copying a written script. A related ability is demonstrated by the superior tactile pattern recognition by the left hand of the commissurotomized subject. This has been tested by the time during which a figure of bent wire can be remembered after an initial tactile recognition, the remembrance being tested by its retrieval from a set of four such figures each of a different shape. Even after rigorous training, the right hand usually fails completely at a test interval of a few seconds, whereas the left usually succeeds even after an interval of 2 min (Milner, 1974).

In other respects the minor hemisphere is deficient not only in that it has an extremely limited linguistic performance, which of course would be expected because it lacks the language centres of the brain, but also in its extremely poor ability in calculation and in ideation. Nevertheless it has a limited "reading" ability, when printed names of common objects are flashed onto the left visual field in the manner illustrated Figure E5 – 2, and so are transmitted to the minor hemisphere. For example in Figure E5 – 3 the word NUT in the left visual fields is "recognized" by the right hemisphere. This hemisphere displays an intelligent understanding of common names so that it can programme the left hand to search for and discover manually the object named amongst an assortment presented to it under the screen and even to demonstrate its correct usage. Also names spoken to the subject can initiate successful search and recognition by the left hand. However, the extremely limited linguistic ability is displayed by the failure to react when verbs such as "point," "wave," "nod," "wink" are flashed on the left visual field. Word recognition is limited to names of common objects and on occasion to a few verbs.

This recognition transcends a simple name-object identification in that it discloses a language comprehension, e.g., "measuring instrument" for ruler, "for lighting fires" for match. In this manner the minor hemisphere can exhibit not only appreciation of words but can also display a simple learning in new situations. Despite all this apparently intelligent behaviour, the subject never derives any conscious experience from the goings-on in the minor hemisphere in all of its operative procedures. In fact, as stated above, the subject disclaims responsibility for these appropriate and intelligent actions programmed from his minor hemisphere.

Sperry [1970] has shown in diagrammatic form (Fig. E5 – 4) the essential performances of the right and left cerebral hemispheres, as revealed by these investigations on patients with complete sectioning of the corpus callosum. The projections of the right (R) and left (L) visual fields to the left and right occipital cortices are shown, and some of the functions of the hemispheres are inscribed on them. It will be noted that hearing is bilateral, but mostly crossed, whereas olfaction is strictly ipsilateral.

Remarkable examples of the complementary functions of the dominant and minor hemispheres have been revealed by the chimeric studies of Levy & others [1972]. Chimeric figures were formed by splitting pictures, for example of a face as in Figure E5 – 5. The faces are numbered 1 to 8 and chimeric stimuli are shown by four combinations in A, B, C, D. One of these combinations is flashed on the screen while the subject fixes the mid-point of the screen, for example the chimeric stimulus A formed from faces 7 and 2. The

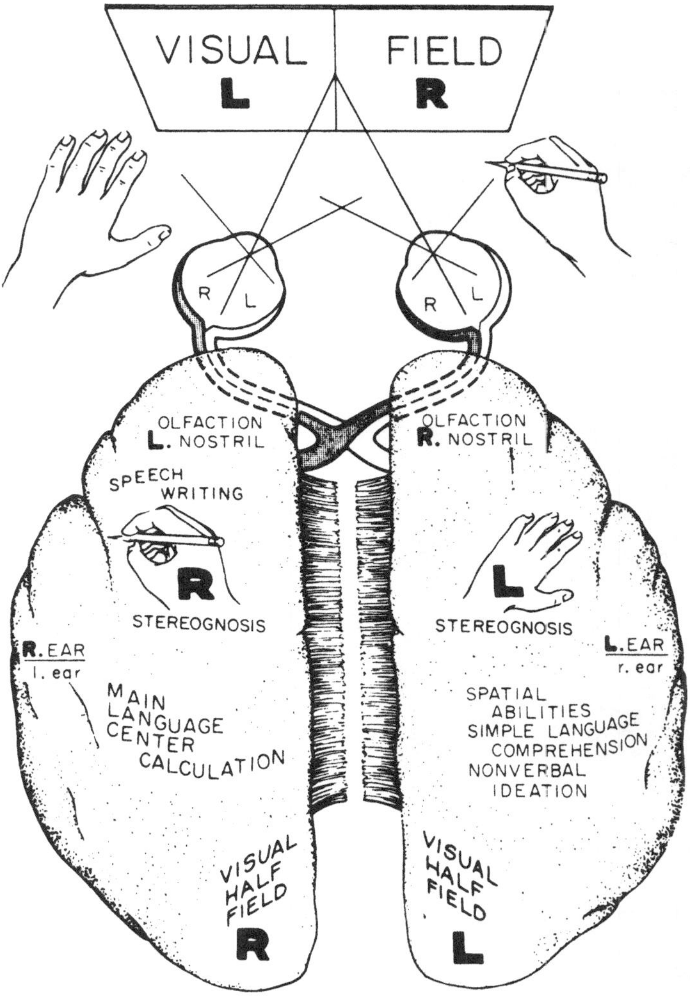

Fig. E5–4. Schema showing the way in which the left and right visual fields are projected onto the right and left visual cortices, respectively, due to the partial decussation in the optic chiasma (cf. Fig. E2–4). The schema also shows other sensory inputs from right limbs to the left hemisphere and that from left limbs to the right hemisphere. Similarly, hearing is largely crossed in its input, but olfaction is ipsilateral. The programming of the right hand in writing is shown pictorially to come from the left hemisphere (Sperry, 1974).

image in the left visual field (half of 7) is projected to the right hemisphere. Similarly the right visual field projects with half of image 2 to the left hemisphere. Because of the absence of commissural communication there is processing of information in each hemisphere that leads to a completion of

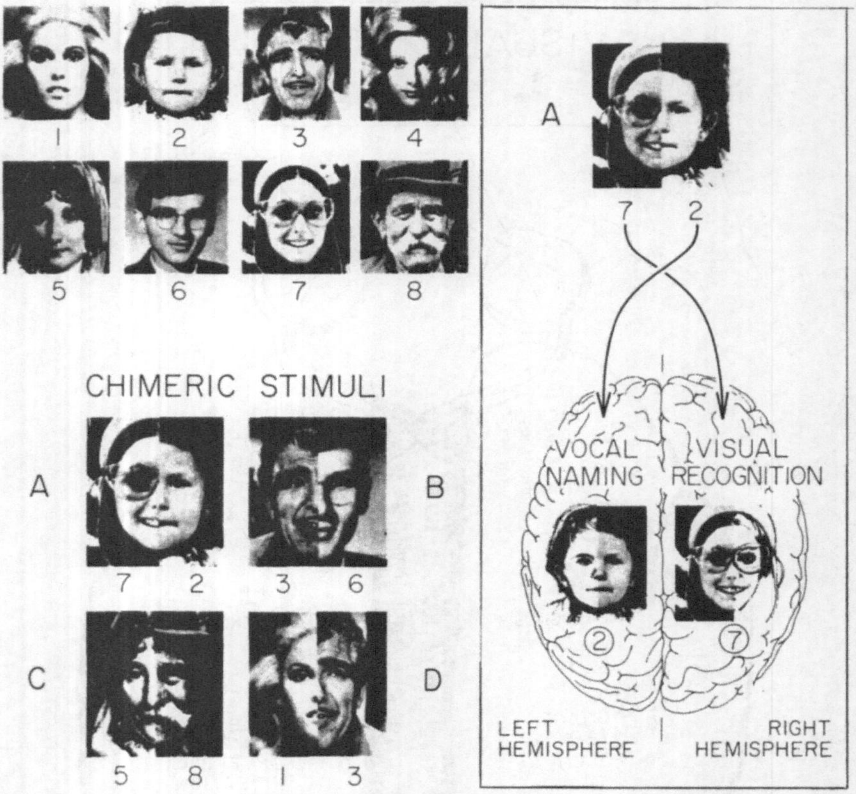

Fig. E5–5. Composite face stimuli (chimeras) for testing hemispheric specialization for facial recognition. Full explanation in text (Sperry, 1974).

the image as shown by the images inscribed on each hemisphere. The chimeric nature of the total visual input is not recognized, but each hemisphere displays responses in accord with its specific functions. Thus if a verbal response is required, the vocal naming is in accord with the image completed in the left hemisphere. On the other hand if there is a visual recognition response by pointing by the left hand to the array of eight faces, face 7 is indicated. There have been many variants of this chimeric testing with various objects besides faces. Always the results illustrate the complete separation of the two hemispheres in their perceptual responses. If a verbal response is required, the left hemisphere dominates with its perception of the right visual field. The right hemisphere dominates if the required perception is for complex and nondescript patterns (cp. Fig. E6–2) and if there is a manual readout, for example by pointing. Thus the chimeric testing confirms the distinctive functions of the two hemispheres as indicated in Figures E5–4, E6–6.

The finer detailed investigations of Sperry and his colleagues have shown that some sensory information from the left side is projected to the dominant hemisphere, presumably by the uncrossed pathways that have been recognized anatomically and physiologically. The simplest example is in the auditory system where the input from one ear goes to both hemispheres, though preponderantly to the contralateral hemisphere (Fig. E4–4). Similarly there is bilateral representation in the hemispheres for much of the midline regions of the body, head and neck. Marginal ipsilateral representation goes even further and the dominant hemisphere is able to receive from the proximal parts of the limbs and to cause motor actions certainly in the shoulder and hip muscles of the ipsilateral side. The exclusive crossed representation for perception and for action by the cerebral hemispheres holds particularly for the visual system and for the forearm and hand and the leg and foot.

Another kind of ipsilateral transfer consists in vague and diffuse conscious experience. If, for example, the left visual field is illuminated suddenly, the subject has a vague experience of this increase of illumination although it has not occurred in the right visual field. When injurious skin stimulation is applied to the left hand, for example, it is experienced as a discomfort without localisation, with the statement "I am being hurt somewhere."

Of more general interest are the emotional reactions that can be transferred to a limited degree. A picture of a female nude presented to the minor hemisphere through the left visual field caused the subject to experience a vague emotional state of embarrassment with blushing that she could not explain. Similarly the reactions of fear may be subconsciously conveyed to the conscious subject by a terrifying picture presented to the left visual field. Presumably this cross-communication is effected through subcortical structures such as the superior colliculus, thalamus, hypothalamus and basal ganglia whose commissural connections remain intact (Sperry [1974]). In all cases it can be assumed that the conscious experience results from a neural communication to the dominant hemisphere through pathways that give only vague information. There is no evidence that it arises in the minor hemisphere. Transmission of information by these subcortical commissural pathways will now be discussed.

So far the experimental tests have shown that there are quite distinct inputs from the right and left visual fields, the former to the left occipital lobe, the latter to the right. The experimental procedures were standardized with testing signals only a few degrees from the centre of vision. Quite other results were obtained by Trevarthen and Sperry [1973] when the testing signals were applied in the field of peripheral vision, about 40 ° laterally. Then the commissurotomized subjects were able usually to recognize objects in the left visual field as well as the right, and to combine them into unified percepts which they could cross-integrate across the vertical meridian. In addition they reported correctly about attributes of stimuli such as colour and size that were far out in the left visual field. These results were obtained while subjects maintained steady central fixation, and in the absence of any acts capable of giving cross-cueing between the hemispheres. Thus ambient vision remains undivided after callosal section. Fortunately anatomical pathways decussating at subcortical levels provide a plausible explanation of the way in which left visual field inputs eventually reach the left hemisphere, there to be consciously recognized by the subject. As shown in Figure E5 − 6 the pathway of this second visual system (open and cross-hatched arrows) is from the left visual field of the right eye to the superior colliculus of the mid-brain and thence via the pulvinar to the visual association cortex of the left hemisphere (cross-hatched arrows). Decussation occurs both at the collicular and pulvinar levels, hence the left visual field projects to the left visual cortex. Thus this investigation conforms to the general conclusion that

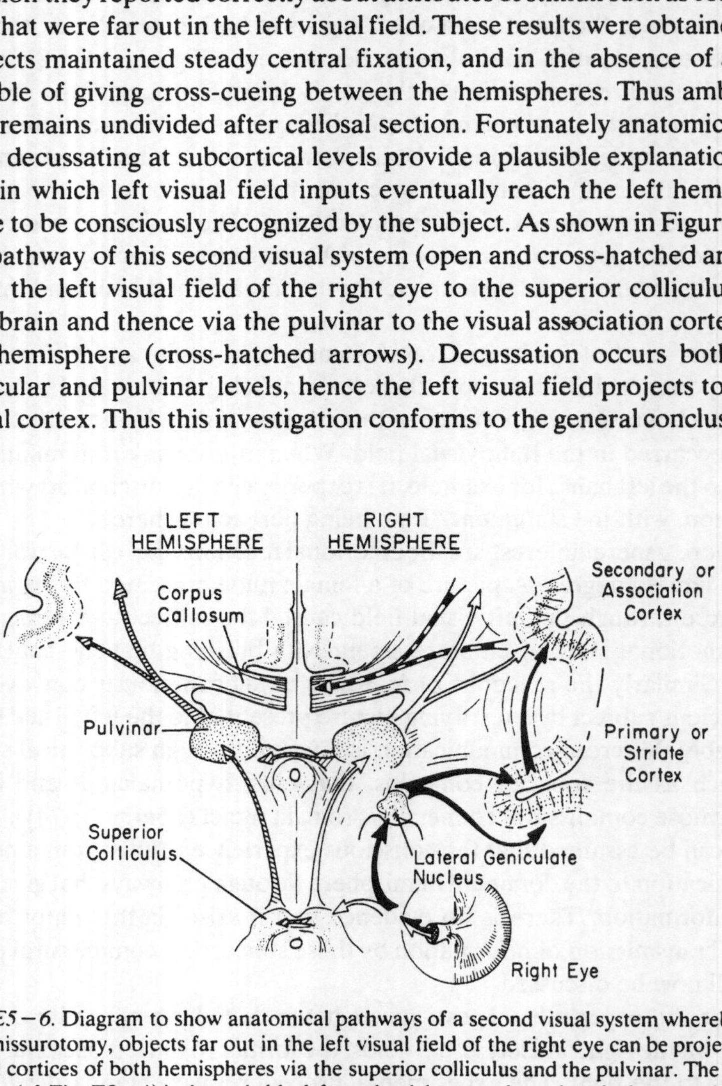

Fig. E5 − 6. Diagram to show anatomical pathways of a second visual system whereby, despite commissurotomy, objects far out in the left visual field of the right eye can be projected to the visual cortices of both hemispheres via the superior colliculus and the pulvinar. The first visual system (cf. Fig. E2 − 4) is shown in black from the right eye to lateral geniculate to striate (visual) cortex (Trevarthen and Sperry, 1973).

only the events of the dominant hemisphere give conscious experience to the split-brain subject.

All of the very fine work with flash testing has been superseded by a new technique (Zaidel and Sperry [1972 (a)], [1972 (b)]; Zaidel [1973]) in which a contact lens is placed in the right eye with an optical device that limits the input into that eye to the left visual field no matter how the eye is moved. At the same time, an eye shield prevents the left eye from being used. In this way there can be up to 2 h of continuous investigation of the subject, which gives opportunity for much more sophisticated testing procedures than with the flash testing. The tests have been concerned with the ability of the right (minor) hemisphere to understand complex visual imagery, as shown by appropriate reactions with the left hand.

For example, in experimental sessions witnessed through the kindness of Drs Sperry and Zaidel, strip cartoons made up of four to six pictures randomly arranged were sorted by the left hand and arranged in correct sequence despite the fact that the subject verbally reported that he had no idea either of what was being presented in the left visual field or of the reactions of the left hand thereto. There was elimination of all input to the brain from the right visual field, consequently the conscious subject was quite blind. He reported no conscious visual experiences except a general sense of luminosity or at times of colour.

Other examples of the pictorial understanding of the right hemisphere are given by testing procedures in which there is a picture, say, of a cat and, below, the words "cat" and "dog." The subject with the left hand can correctly point to the appropriate word. Symmetrically, if there are two pictures, a cup and a knife, and below one word "cup," the subject will point to the correct object (cup) with the left hand. An even more sophisticated test of picture identification is provided by a drawing of landscapes with below a correct and an incorrect name. For example below the picture were the names "summer," and "winter" and the subject was able to point to the name "winter" rather than "summer" in correct identification of the picture. Yet all of these visual inputs to the brain give no conscious experiences to the subject.

Despite this intelligent performance with pictorial and verbal presentation to the minor hemisphere, this hemisphere is completely unable to complete sentences, even the simplest, when tested in the manner illustrated by the verbal arrangement given below.

Mother loves

nail baby broom stone

The subject points with the left hand as the sentence is read: "Mother loves" and then sequentially to the four words below for identification. The subject then tries to complete the sentence using the left hand to point to one or other of the four words below, and only at random chance chooses "baby." The evidence from language testing of chimpanzees indicates likewise that they are unable to complete sentences, though some dubious claims have been made. This of course arises from the fact that neither the minor hemisphere nor the chimpanzee brain has a Wernicke area that provides the necessary semantic ability.

These more rigorous testing procedures (Zaidel [1976]) have shown that after commissurotomy the right hemisphere has access to a considerable auditory vocabulary, being able to recognize commands and to relate words presented by hearing or vision to pictorial representations. It is particularly effective in recognition of pictorial representations that occur in common experiential situations. It was also surprising that the right hemisphere responded to verbs as effectively as to action names. Response to verbal commands was not recognized by the flash technique. Despite all this display of language comprehension, the right hemisphere is extremely deficient in expression in speech or in writing, which is effectively zero. It is also incapable of understanding instructions that include many items which have to be remembered in correct order. The highly significant finding is the large difference between comprehension and expression in the performance of the right hemisphere.

The operative lesion of commissurotomy merely interrupts the direct commissural connections between the two hemispheres, leaving intact all their communication to and from the lower centres. Hence, for example, the two hemispheres exhibit the same sleep-wake cycles, for this is dependent on the arousal influences probably from mesencephalic and diencephalic structures that are interconnected across the midline and that act bilaterally. Even more important is the very effective integration of the postural and automatic movements of the body and limbs of both sides. For example, the patients can walk, stand and swim normally, because the neural machinery governing such actions has commissural connections at subcortical levels and so is not split by the callosal section.

In the rare human cases of congenital absence of the corpus callosum (Saul and Sperry [1968]), there must have been developed in the embryo compensatory connections between the two hemispheres at subcortical levels. As a consequence such a subject responded to the battery of cross-integration tests essentially as a normal control subject. Also of interest was the experimental evidence that speech had been developed in both hemispheres with the unfortunate sequel of defectiveness of other functions. It is another example of the dominance of linguistic function in diminishing the cerebral representation of other functions.

36. Discussion on Commissurotomy

These remarkable investigations on commissurotomized subjects are of the greatest interest for our enquiry into *The Self and Its Brain,* as illustrated in Figure E5–4. It can be conjectured that the distinctive performances of the "separated" hemispheres provide reliable evidence for their specific functions when linked normally by the corpus callosum. Thus the dominant hemisphere performs with almost complete control of expression in speech, writing and calculation. It is also more aggressive and executive in the control of the motor system. It is the hemisphere with which one ordinarily communicates.

In the commissurotomized subject

> the mute, minor hemisphere, – seems to be carried along much as a passive, silent passenger who leaves the driving of behavior mainly to the left hemisphere. Accordingly, the nature and quality of the inner mental world of the silent right hemisphere remains relatively inaccessible to investigation, requiring special testing measures with non-verbal forms of expression. (Sperry [1974])

Yet Sperry [1974] regards it as

> a conscious system in its own right, perceiving, thinking, remembering, reasoning, willing, and emoting, all at a characteristically human level, and that both the left and the right hemisphere may be conscious simultaneously in different, even in mutually conflicting, mental experiences that run along in parallel.
>
> Though predominantly mute and generally inferior in all performances involving language or linguistic or mathematical reasoning, the minor hemisphere is nevertheless clearly the superior cerebral member for certain types of tasks. If we remember that in the great majority of tests it is the disconnected left hemisphere that is superior and dominant, we can review quickly now some of the kinds of exceptional activities in which it is the minor hemisphere that excels. First, of course, as one would predict, these are all nonlinguistic nonmathematical functions. Largely they involve the apprehension and processing of spatial patterns, relations and transformations. They seem to be holistic and unitary rather than analytic and fragmentary, and orientational more than focal, and to involve concrete perceptual insight rather than abstract, symbolic, sequential reasoning.

In the light of these remarkable discoveries made with commissurotomized subjects we may now ask: how does the minor hemisphere function in the normal brain? Some years ago I formulated (Eccles [1973]) the radical hypothesis that, even before section of the corpus callosum, the goings-on in the minor hemisphere did not directly give the subject any conscious experiences, a hypothesis that had been suggested several years earlier (Eccles [1965]). In order to make this hypothesis of brain-mind interaction explicit we present a diagram (Fig. E5 – 7) that portrays the flow of communication between major subdivisions of the brain and also to and from the outside world. Some special features of this diagram will be explained elsewhere in this book when formulating hypotheses relating to the origin and development of language and culture. For present purposes we will concentrate on the neural pathways from receptors to the cerebrum and reciprocally from the cerebrum to muscles. Due to the decussations of the neural pathways, the left cerebral hemisphere in general receives from and acts upon the right side, e.g. right visual field and right arm, and vice versa for the right cerebral hemisphere and the left visual field and left arm. However, as shown in Figure E5 – 7, not all of the pathways are crossed. For example, there is a significant ipsilateral input for somaesthesis. In Figure E5 – 7 there are also shown small ipsilateral motor projections from each cerebral hemisphere.

The rigorous testing of the subjects who have been subjected to section of the corpus callosum has revealed that conscious experiences of the subject arise only in relationship to neural activities in the dominant hemisphere. This is shown in Figure E5 – 7 by the arrows leading from the linguistic and ideational areas of the dominant hemisphere to the conscious self that is represented by the circular area above. It must be recognized that Figure E5 – 7 is an information flow diagram and that the location of the conscious self is for diagrammatic convenience. It is of course not meant to imply that the conscious self is spatially located above the dominant hemisphere!

It was postulated that in normal subjects activities in the minor hemisphere reach consciousness only after transmission to the dominant hemisphere, which very effectively occurs via the immense impulse traffic in the corpus callosum, as is illustrated in Figure E5 – 7 by the numerous transverse arrows. Complementarily, it was postulated that the neural activities responsible for voluntary actions are generated in the dominant hemisphere by some willed action of the conscious self (see downward arrows in Fig. E5 – 7). Normally these neural activities spread widely over both the dominant and minor hemispheres giving the "readiness potential" described in chapter E3. At a further stage there is concentration of neural activity onto the area of the motor cortex that projects by the pyramidal tracts to bring about the willed movement.

It must be recognized that this transmission in the corpus callosum is not a simple one-way transmission. The 200 million fibres must carry a fantastic wealth of impulse traffic in both directions. For example, a conservative

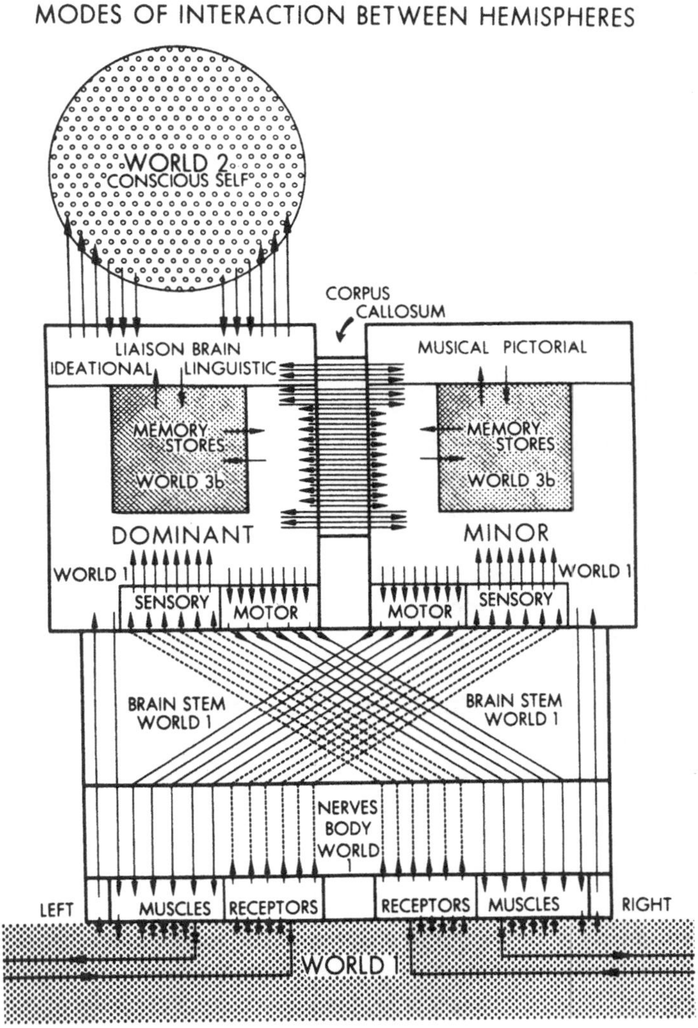

Fig. E5 – 7. Communications to and from the brain and within the brain. Diagram to show the principal lines of communication from peripheral receptors to the sensory cortices and so to the cerebral hemispheres. Similarly, the diagram shows the output from the cerebral hemispheres via the motor cortex and so to muscles. Both these systems of pathways are largely crossed as illustrated, but minor uncrossed pathways are also shown by the vertical lines in the brain stem. The dominant left hemisphere and minor right hemisphere are labelled, together with some of the properties of these hemispheres that are found displayed in Fig. E6 – 6. The corpus callosum is shown as a powerful cross–linking of the two hemispheres and, in addition, the diagram displays the modes of interaction between Worlds 1, 2, and 3, as described in the text, and also illustrated in Fig. E7 – 1.

estimate of the average impulse frequency in a fibre would be 20 Hz, which gives a total traffic of 4×10^9 impulses in a second. In the normal operation of the cerebral hemispheres, activity of any part of a hemisphere is as effectively and rapidly transmitted to the other hemisphere as to another lobe of the same hemisphere. The whole cerebrum thus achieves a most effective unity. It will be appreciated from Figure E5—7 that section of the corpus callosum gives a unique and complete cleavage of this unity. The neural activities of the minor hemisphere are isolated from those cerebral areas that give and receive from the conscious self. As we have mentioned already, all other surgical or pathological lesions of the cerebrum are crude and imperfect by comparison.

On this hypothesis we can regard the minor hemisphere as having a status superior to that of the non-human primate brain. It displays intelligent reactions, even after delays of many minutes, and learning responses; and it has many skills, particularly in the spatial and auditory domain that are far superior to those of the anthropoid brain, but it gives no conscious experience to the subject, being in this respect in complete contrast to the dominant hemisphere. Moreover there is no evidence that this brain has some residual consciousness of its own. Sperry [1974] and Bogen [1969 (a)], [1969 (b)] postulate that there is another mind in this brain, but it is prevented from communicating to us because it has no speech. We would agree with this statement if it were linked with the further statement that in this respect the minor hemisphere resembles the brain of a non-human primate, though its performance is superior to that of the brains of the highest anthropoids. In both of these cases we lack communication in a rich linguistic level, so it is not possible to test for the possibility of some consciously experiencing being. We therefore must be agnostic about the question of mental activities and consciousness.

The superiority of the minor hemisphere over non-human primate brains is demonstrated, for example, by the time of many minutes during which an initial signal can be held in its memory before a successful retrieval (Sperry & others [1969]). It is also superior to a non-human brain in respect of cross-modality transfer of information. A visual or auditory signal can be very effectively used to signal an object to be retrieved using kinaesthetic sensing, and this retrieval can be effected with intelligence and understanding. For example, the flash of a dollar sign results in retrieval of some coin — 25 c or 10 c — when no dollar notes are available, or the flash of a picture of a wall clock results in retrieval of the only related object available — a child's toy watch. By contrast, rhesus monkeys cannot be trained to perceive objects as the same when they are seen in the light and also palpated by touch in the dark (Ettlinger and Blakemore [1968]); however chimpanzees can succeed (Davenport [1975]).

It is opportune here to expose erroneous interpretations of the commissurotomy experiments. The assertion is made that the intelligent performance of the minor hemisphere establishes that the activities of the minor hemisphere are associated with a consciousness that is equivalent to that of the dominant hemisphere, merely differing because of linguistic disability. This view was extravagantly developed by Puccetti [1973] in that he raised the question: "if we cerebrally intact twin-brained [sic] human beings are really compounds of two persons, which is me?" The erroneous interpretations of Puccetti [1973], Zangwill [1973], Doty [1975] and Savage [1975] occur because they fail to distinguish between the self-consciousness associated with the dominant hemisphere, as reported by the conscious subject, and the consciousness that is assumed to be associated with the minor hemisphere because of its skilled responses that display insight and intelligence.

A gedanken experiment reveals the fundamental difference between the responses of the dominant and minor hemispheres. After commissurotomy with left hemisphere dominance the conscious subject has voluntary control of the right forearm and hand, but not of the left, yet the left forearm and hand can carry out skilled and apparently purposive movements. In our gedanken experiment the left hand inadvertently grabs a gun, fires it and kills a man. Is this murder or manslaughter and by whom? If not, why not? But no such questions can be asked if the right hand does the shooting and killing. The fundamental difference between the dominant and minor hemispheres stands revealed on legal grounds. Commissurotomy has split the bihemispheric brain into a dominant hemisphere that is exclusively in liaison with the self-conscious mind and controlled by it and a minor hemisphere that carries out many of the performances previously carried out by the intact brain, but it is not under control by the self-conscious mind. It may be in liaison with a mind, but this is quite different from the self-conscious mind of the dominant hemisphere — so different that a grave risk of confusion results from the common use of the words "mind" and "consciousness" for both entities.

37. Investigations on the Human Cerebrum After Gross Lesions

The investigations on patients subjected to commissurotomy have provided far more definitive and challenging information than have other cerebral lesions. Nevertheless the conclusions derived from the commissurotomy investigations can be subjected to testing procedures applied to patients with global or circumscribed cerebral lesions. The most radical are the hemispherectomized patients, where either the minor or the dominant hemisphere has been radically removed in the treatment of a gross cerebral tumour. In the subsequent chapter we will give an account of the investigation on patients with circumscribed lesions that result from excisions of large areas of one or the other lobes of a cerebral hemisphere. All of these investigations are of direct relevance to our present enquiry into *The Self and Its Brain*. They supplement the more definitive observations on the commissurotomy patients, and are in general agreement therewith.

Lesions of the brain stem and medial thalamus may result in coma of man and animals (Cairns [1952]; Sprague [1967]). This complete and permanent loss of consciousness is probably due to damage to the reticular activating system. However, these lesions of the brain cannot be regarded as providing evidence with respect to the location in the brain of the "seat of consciousness." Unconsciousness results because of the removal of background excitation of the cerebral cortex that is requisite for wakefulness, i.e., it would seem that these lesions involve structures whose activity is necessary but not sufficient for consciousness. Comparable observations on lesions resulting in unconsciousness led Penfield [1966] to postulate that there is in the base of the brain an area of the diencephalon (the centrencephalic area) specially concerned in giving conscious experiences to the subject. As pointed out by Sperry [1974] this theory is falsified by the finding that, after section of the corpus callosum, the self-consciousness is derived only from the neuronal activities of the dominant hemisphere. The postulated centrencephalic area and its connections to the cerebral hemispheres are not affected by the commissurotomy operation. It may be a necessary, but it is not a sufficient condition for consciousness.

38. Hemispherectomy

We now turn to the human cerebral cortex in order to study the possible regions concerned in consciousness. It is remarkable that excision of the minor hemisphere under local anaesthesia gives rise to no loss of the patient's consciousness or self-awareness. This even occurs during the actual operation when it is performed under local anaesthesia, as reported by Obrador [1964] and Austin & others [1972]. These investigators as well as Gardner &

others [1955] report (seven cases) that excisions of the minor hemisphere result in symptoms that, except for the hemiplegia and the absence of far-out left visual field recognition, are not appreciably different from those described in detail by Sperry in his study of patients with brain bisection, and that are reported above. Interestingly, in one left-handed subject of Gardner & others [1955] it seemed that the right hemisphere was dominant, and, as would be expected, the same results were observed after left hemispherectomy. Thus minor hemispherectomy gives a result in complete agreement with the postulate that self-consciousness is derived only from neural activities in the dominant hemisphere. One of the two cases of minor hemispherectomy reported by Gott [1973 (a)] is remarkable because it occurred in a young woman who was a music major and an accomplished pianist. After the operation there was a tragic loss of her musical ability. She could not carry a tune, but could still repeat correctly the words of familiar songs.

The left (dominant hemisphere) excisions in the adult have much more serious sequelae. In the four cases that have been reported there seem to be some traces of residual consciousness and some slight recovery in very primitive linguistic ability. Patients were very difficult to study as they were almost completely aphasic. Smith [1966] reported that his patient could use expletives and simple words in a song that he used to know. He had extreme restriction in language usage. Nevertheless, the isolated minor hemisphere had more linguistic ability than occurs in the minor hemisphere of Sperry's patients, where it is overshadowed by the dominant hemisphere. One wonders how much transfer of dominance had occurred in this patient before the operation because there had been a severe lesion of the dominant hemisphere for at least 2 years, from age 45 to age 47 at the time of the operation.

Hillier [1954] gave a much more encouraging account of dominant hemispherectomy in a boy of 14 who survived about 2 years. This boy achieved a good recovery in general performance, but linguistically was very handicapped. Hillier reports:

> Comprehension of the spoken word is quite accurate. The motor aphasia shows a constant improvement. He is capable of reading individual letters, but cannot formulate words. He is at times unable to name an article in an advertisement, but yet can tell the radio program and describe the artists who advertise the particular product.

Again one suspects that there was some transfer of dominant hemisphere functions before operation, and the youthfulness of the patient could help in his recovery. Despite the rather optimistic tone of this report it can be recognized that there was a tragic linguistic disability, a sequel that is to be expected after excision of the Wernicke speech area.

A better recovery was reported by Gott [1973 (b)] in a girl who had complete hemispherectomy (dominant) at age 10. At age 8 there had been an excision of a tumour from that hemisphere, the final operation 2 years later being for a recurrence in the parietal area. At age 12 the patient had a linguistic ability gravely reduced, but surpassing those of the cases of dominant hemispherectomy considered above. It is suggested by Gott that there was a better recovery because at the age of 7 to 8 language may already be in the process of transfer from the damaged dominant hemisphere. It was remarkable that despite the very limited speaking ability, the patient could sing well and liked to do so, usually with the correct words. Despite the grave linguistic handicap it cannot be doubted that this girl had retained a self-conscious mind after the dominant hemispherectomy.

Infants present a much more encouraging situation. There is good evidence of a remarkable plasticity, the functions of the dominant hemisphere being effectively transferred up to 5 years of age. There is evidence that, at this early age, linguistic ability normally is well developed in the right as well as the left hemisphere (Basser [1962]). Then, over the first few years of life cerebral dominance is established with regression of the linguistic ability of the minor hemisphere.

Krynauw [1950] reported 12 cases of hemispherectomy for infantile hemiplegia, and White [1961] added 2 more and reviewed an extensive literature. Krynauw suggests that the language was already transferred from the dominant hemisphere because of its damage at birth, so that in all cases he was removing the minor hemisphere! The age at which effective transfer can occur is usually given as up to 5 years, but Obrador [1964] suggests a time as long as 15 years. McFie [1961] reviews the extensive literature on hemispherectomy and speaks of this transfer of functions, but warns of the danger of crowding (cp. Milner [1974]; Sperry [1974]). When speech is transferred to the minor hemisphere, it is always defective, and there is in addition a deterioration of the normal functions of the minor hemisphere. Thus McFie concludes that there is a limit to the capabilities of the remaining hemisphere so that it is deficient in mediating its normal functions and in accepting the functions from the other hemisphere. Later there will be further discussion of this important hypothesis of "crowding."

Complete removal of the dominant hemisphere gives somewhat enigmatic results. The very exhaustive investigations on the split-brain patients by Sperry and his associates have led to the formulation of the hypothesis in chapter E7 that normally self-consciousness is derived exclusively from spatiotemporal patterns of neuronal activity in certain areas of the dominant hemisphere. This hypothesis would predict that dominant hemispherectomy would result in a patient lacking self-consciousness, just as strikingly as does the minor hemisphere in the split-brain cases. Yet, so far as tests are possible in these almost completely aphasic cases, there seems to be some residual self-consciousness. Certainly, years after "dominant" hemispherectomy in the first 5 years of life, tests reveal that the "minor" hemisphere has taken over linguistic functions and hence assumed a "dominant" status, at least to a partial extent. Possibly a small transfer of this kind occurs even in adults because of the destruction of large areas of the dominant hemisphere in the years preceding the operation.

39. Summary of Linguistic Abilities Disclosed by Global Lesions

After commissurotomy the right hemisphere seems mute and after left hemispherectomy the isolated right hemisphere is severely aphasic. However, in both cases the right hemisphere has a substantial comprehension of language. This is particularly so in linguistic usage associated with pictures. The right hemisphere can also comprehend short verbal instructions but not beyond three words, and it lacks semantic ability to complete sentences. In these respects the linguistic competence of the right hemisphere differs from that of a child, where comprehension and expression develop together.

Zaidel [1976] suggests that at each stage in the acquisition of language there is a complex interhemispheric interaction. Also there is evidence that the right hemisphere lends support in auditory comprehension to an aphasic left hemisphere. It is extraordinary that, despite its considerable verbal comprehension, the right hemisphere is so deficient in verbal expression, except when it has been isolated at such a young age that there can be a considerable transfer of linguistic ability. This will be considered further in chapter E6.

Chapter E6 Circumscribed Cerebral Lesions

40. Résumé

Lesions confined to large parts of one or another lobe of a cerebral hemisphere give opportunity for discovering the functions of the missing zones. Many of these lesions have resulted from operative excision of damaged cerebral cortex, so there is a fairly accurate location of the excised area.

With the temporal lobe, aphasias of various kinds result from lesions of the speech areas, so operative removal of such areas is contraindicated. With the minor hemisphere it has been shown that there are disorders of musical appreciation and this correlates with the tests by dichotic listening. With these testing procedures it is shown that the dominant hemisphere (usually the left) is better for recognition of words or word sounds, whereas the minor hemisphere specializes in musical recognition (Fig. E6 − 1). It has also been found that nonverbal visual memory is represented in the temporal lobe of the minor hemisphere. The results of the various testing procedures are described in the text and they relate to the discovery that the inferotemporal lobe is specially concerned in visual discrimination tasks (Figs. E6 − 2, 3 and 4). In summary, these tests show that the right temporal lobe is importantly concerned in both musical and spatial recognition.

With parietal lobe lesions distinction must be made between the primary somaesthetic area in Brodmann areas 3, 1, 2 and the areas more posterior which are concerned with the processing of the cutaneous information and its integration with visual inputs. There is a description of the extraordinary performance of patients with right parietal lobe lesions, the pantomime of neglect! The right parietal lobe is also concerned with fine control of movement, apraxias resulting from excision of areas 39 and 40. On the left side these areas are of course concerned with reading and the understanding of language (semantics). Besides these specific deficits, right parietal lobe lesions result in a variety of cognitive disorders.

Occipital lobe lesions result in visual deficits with areas of blindness (scotomata) and defects in visual cognitive performances.

Frontal lobe lesions have a much deeper influence on the personality of the subject. The posterior part of the frontal lobe is of course concerned with motor functions that have been considered in chapter E3. This present chapter is concerned with lesions of the prefrontal cortex. There is shown to be a complementary relationship between the frontal and the temporal lobes on the same side. On the left side the temporal lobe is important for verbal recognition, and the frontal lobe for verbal recency, namely the recognition of temporal sequences of verbal presentations. On the right side there is failure, as already mentioned, of pictorial recognition in the temporal lobe and picture recency in the frontal lobe. Besides these specific disabilities, the subjects suffer from more general disabilities as is illustrated, for example, by the perseveration in the card sorting test (Fig. E6–5). As indicated by this test, the prefrontal lobe patients have difficulty in stabilizing their behaviour and in general lack purpose in their actions. An additional disability comes from the intimate relationship of the prefrontal lobe with the limbic system. As already conjectured in chapter E2, the reciprocal communication to the limbic system and the hypothalamus gives the prefrontal lobe the unique function of associating the somaesthetic, visual and auditory experiences with the emotional input from the limbic system and hypothalamus. Also linked in this association is the olfactory system that projects directly into the limbic system from the sensory pathway. As already indicated in chapter E2, the limbic system with the associated hypothalamus gives colour, drive, vividness and emotion to the sensory experiences.

Finally, in this chapter there is a section on the dominant and minor hemispheres (Fig. E6–6). The subdivision has already been indicated in chapter E5 in relationship to the commissurotomy patients. It has been further studied with the dichotic testing procedures. In general, the evidence indicates that the dominant hemisphere is specialized in respect of fine imaginative details in that it is analytic and sequential; but, very importantly, it is verbal, and even more importantly, it is in direct liaison with the self-conscious mind. The minor hemisphere on the other hand is superior in pictorial and pattern sense and in musical sense, its synthetic abilities matching the analytical abilities of the dominant hemisphere. However, it must be realized that there has been a tendency to overdo the antithesis between the two hemispheres. When separated by commissurotomy, each hemisphere is much poorer in the performance of its own specific functions. There is a brief account of the evolutionary significance of hemispheric specialization and also an account of the development of specialization during the first few years of life.

41. Introduction

There is an immense literature on patients with cerebral lesions that inadvertently result from a vascular accident. Subsequent autopsy revealed the site and extent of the cerebral destruction. Amongst the most remarkable discoveries were the recognition of the motor (Broca [1861]) and sensory (Wernicke [1874]) speech areas. Since this pioneer work of more than a century ago, the study of lesional aphasia has become a great field of clinical neurology as reviewed for example by Geschwind [1965 (a)], [1965 (b)] and Hécaen [1967]. An adequate treatment of this extremely complex subject is beyond the scope of this book, but has been dealt with in its special relation to consciousness in the section on speech (chapter E4). We will here concentrate on the study of patients subjected to excisions of quite large areas of one cerebral hemisphere. This study is simpler in interpretation in that the lesion is circumscribed and accurately located, which contrasts with the indeterminate nature of most clinical lesions. It is convenient to organize this account in relation to lesions of the major lobes of the cerebral hemisphere, that are illustrated in Figure E1 – 1 and 4. The present account will concentrate on the human brain. But reference has to be made to the important supporting experimental evidence on other mammalian brains, particularly primate brains.

42. Temporal Lobe Lesions

Most interesting work has been done by Milner [1974] and her associates [1964] on the contrasting functions of the left and right temporal lobes. In about 95% of subjects the left has a special linguistic function by virtue of being centred in the Wernicke area (Fig. E4 – 1), as has been described in chapter E4. Complementarily the right temporal lobe has been shown to be specially concerned in the appreciation of music and in spatial pattern recognition (Scheid and Eccles [1975]). Advantage has been taken of subjects who are to have the temporal lobe removed on one or the other side for treatment of epilepsies that arise from areas of extensive brain damage. Altogether in this very important test series there was excision of the left or right temporal lobe with or without the hippocampus in 21 and 26 patients respectively. Controls were provided by normal subjects and by patients with extensive excisions of the left or right frontal lobes.

When studying the effects of temporal lobe lesions on musical appreciation, it was found that subjects with right temporal lobe lesions did not differ from normal in respect of simple pitch or rhythm discrimination. However, differences were revealed when these patients were tested for two subtests of the Seashore tests, viz. the timbre and tonal memory tests (Milner [1967]). For example in the tonal memory test a short sequence, four or five notes, was played twice in rapid succession, after which the subject had to decide which note was changed in pitch at the second playing. After right temporal lobectomy many more errors were made in this test for melody recognition than before, whereas left temporal lobectomy hardly changed the score (Fig. E6−1).

Further evidence of the association of the right temporal lobe with musical appreciation was provided by Shankweiler [1966] using memory of traditional tunes. After listening to a few bars, the subject was required either to continue the tune by humming or to name it. Subjects with right temporal lobectomies gave abnormally poor performance on both these tests. As would be expected, subjects with left temporal lobectomies performed well with the humming, but, because of the linguistic defect, were abnormally poor in the verbal task of naming the tune. Perhaps the most striking evidence relating musical appreciation to the right temporal lobe is the recent

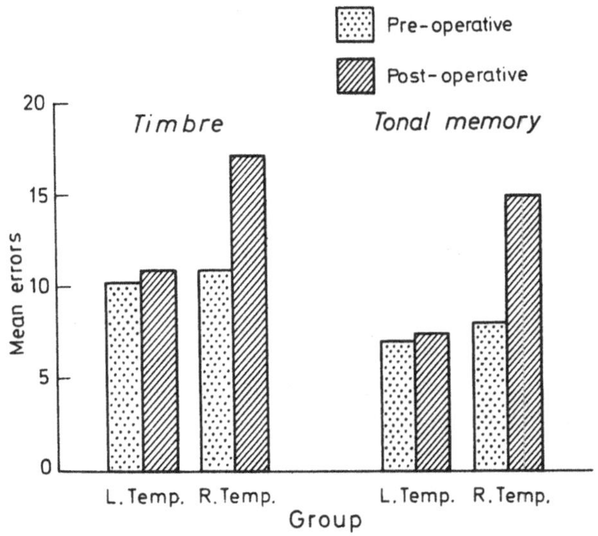

Fig. E6−1. Seashore Timbre and Tonal Memory tests: mean error scores before and after operation for left *(L. temp)* and right *(R. temp.)* temporal-lobe groups, showing postoperative impairment after right temporal lobectomy but not after left (Milner, 1967).

report (as yet unpublished) of a gifted musician that he suddenly lost all the aesthetic feelings associated with his performances. Clinical investigations revealed a vascular lesion of the right temporal lobe. The importance of the right hemisphere for the musical performance of the brain is also convincingly shown by the tragic results of a right hemispherectomy in a musically gifted young woman (Gott [1973]), as reported in chapter E5. A more complex case of musical disability was exhibited by Ravel, who had a widespread bilateral involvement of parietal and temporal lobes resulting in both aphasia and apraxia (Alajouanine, 1948).

All of this lesional evidence for the representation of musical appreciation in the minor hemisphere has been corroborated by the evidence derived from dichotic listening tests on normal subjects (Kimura [1967], [1973]). In these tests a headset with earphones is used to play simultaneously two short melodies, one into each ear. The subject was then asked to pick out these two melodies from an assemblage of four melodies, that were heard sequentially in a normal manner. There was a significantly higher score for the melodies played into the left ear, which indicates a superiority in recognition of the right hemisphere over the left because each ear signals predominantly into the acoustic area of the contralateral temporal lobe (Fig. E2). When sequences of words or numbers were applied by this same method of dichotic listening, there is, as expected, a better recognition of the right ear input, which would preponderantly go to the left temporal lobe for processing and verbal recognition.

It has also been shown by Milner ([1967], [1971], [1974]) and her associates Kimura [1963] and Corsi that right temporal lobe lesions give a consistent impairment in perception of irregular patterned stimuli, particularly those not identifiable verbally. Of the three tests used, the facial recognition test is of particular importance to the patient. Photographs of 12 faces are initially examined at leisure by the subject and then have to be identified in a larger assemblage of 25 faces in which the original 12 are randomly arranged (Milner [1968]). After right temporal lobectomy there was poor performance in this test, but in part it was dependent on the extent of the hippocampal excision associated with the temporal lobectomy, as will be further discussed in chapter E8.

A second important test for non-verbal visual memory is the so-called recurring nonsense figures test designed by Kimura [1963], in which the subject is tested for memory of unfamiliar designs, geometrical or irregular curvilinear (Fig. E6 – 2A). In a pile of successively presented cards a number of these designs recur randomly, and the subject has to say "yes" or "no" according to whether he thinks that he has seen it before or not. When

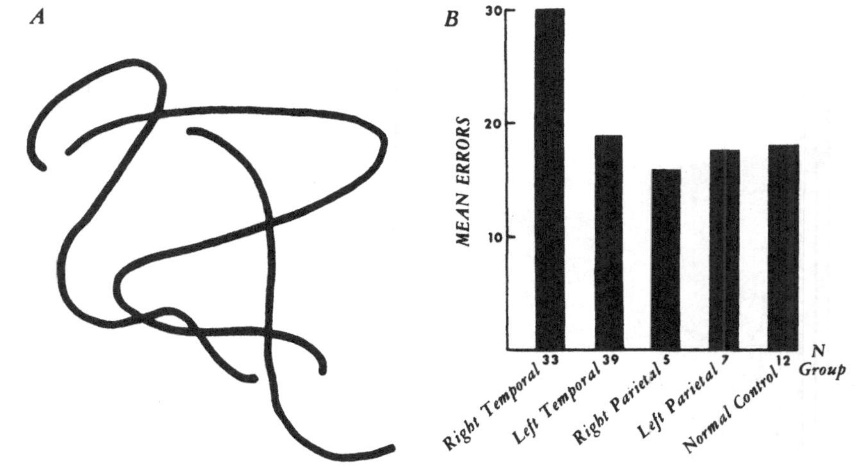

Fig. E6−2. A. Example from Recurring Nonsense Figures test. B. Mean error scores (sum of false positive or negative responses) for different lesion groups, showing significant impairment after right temporal lobectomy (Milner, 1967).

Kimura subjected to this test patients with lesions in right or left parietal or temporal lobes, she could clearly show that the mean error score was significantly higher in the right temporal lobe group than in all other patients (Fig. E6−2B), there being no difference between the latter patients and the normal control group. The results of this and of similar tests suggest that lesions in the right temporal lobe interfere with the ability to process information that may be defined as visual pattern recognition. In similar tests Milner [1967] found impairments in many other visual tasks. Thus the patients with right temporal lobe lesions cannot easily organize patches of black and white into distinct patterns, such as a human face shown in a cartoon representation. Indeed, as revealed by the test described above, they have difficulties in recognizing photographic portraits that they had carefully inspected less than 2 minutes earlier.

In another interesting test by Milner and Corsi (Milner [1974]), the subject has to point to a small circle at a specific place on a line (Fig. E6−3A) and has later to replicate the location of that circle on another line of the same length and orientation, the first line being meanwhile screened from view (Fig. E6−3B). The performance is quantitatively evaluated by addition of errors in location in four tests. Again, subjects with the right temporal lobectomy failed badly on this test relative to normal controls and left temporal lobectomy patients (Fig. E6−4A). There was a similar relative failure when a mental distraction was interpolated between the inspection

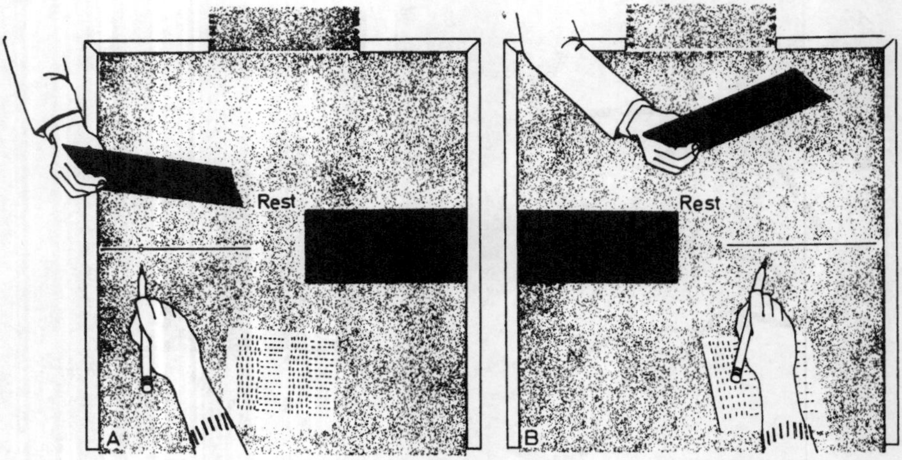

Fig. E6−3. A and B, sketches illustrating the procedure used by Corsi to test memory for visual location. (A) The patient marks the circle indicated on the exposed 8-inch line. (B) After a short delay, he tries to reproduce this position from memory as accurately as possible, on a similar 8-inch line. The sign *REST* means that the patient does nothing during the interval, in contrast to *WORK* trials in which a distracting activity is interpolated (Milner, 1974).

and the test (Fig. E6−4B). Corsi found that the deficiencies resulting from right temporal lobectomies were related to the extent of the associated hippocampal excisions.

This human lesion work implicates the right temporal lobe as being specially concerned in visual feature detection. Thus this lobe parallels the monkey inferotemporal lobe, as described in chapter E2, the only difference being the bilateral representation in the monkey brain. With monkeys bilateral inferotemporal lesions produce a severe deficit in the performance of visual discrimination tasks (Gross [1973]), much as described above for human lesions. This defect is restricted to visual tests involving pattern, brightness or colour, and correlates with the feature detection described in chapter E2 for neurones of the primate inferotemporal lobe. These visual performances of the inferotemporal lobe can be correlated with the anatomical pathways depicted in Figure E1−7E−G for the secondary and tertiary relays from the primary visual area to areas 20 and 21 of the inferotemporal lobe.

Thus we may conclude that in man and monkey the temporal lobe (right side only for man) is involved in higher order perceptual detection for visual inputs. Lower level visual functions such as visual acuity and the topography of visual fields are not affected by temporal lobe lesions. The hippocampus

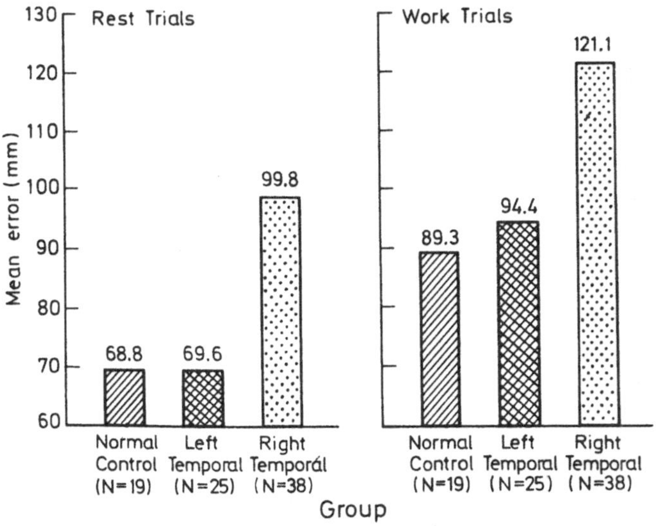

Fig. E6 – 4. Corsi's results for the spatial memory task, showing impairment after right temporal lobectomy but not after left. The score is the total error (in mm) for four trials, without regard to sign, averaged across three retention intervals (Milner, 1974).

usually was removed to a greater or lesser extent with the human temporal lobe excision. The resultant severe memory defects will be described in the chapter on memory (chapter E8).

In summary, these tests show that the right temporal lobe is importantly concerned in both the musical and the spatial recognition and recall performances of the human brain. It is not claimed that the right temporal lobe is alone concerned in such performances, only that it is the area principally concerned. It will be our thesis throughout these enquiries into cerebral localization that functions are widely distributed over the cerebral hemispheres. These functions of the human right temporal lobe counterbalance to some extent the massive involvement of the left temporal and parietal lobes in linguistic performance (cp. chapter E4). The musical representation in the right temporal lobe can be correlated with the secondary and tertiary relays depicted in Figure E1 – 7I,J for the auditory pathway, namely areas STP and 22.

43. Parietal Lobe Lesions

Hécaen [1967] reviewed the effects of lesions of the parietal lobes of the human cerebrum. The anterior parts of both parietal lobes are constituted by the somaesthetic areas, both the primary area (Brodmann areas 3, 1, 2 in Fig. E1–4) in the postcentral gyrus and the association area (Brodmann 5) lying immediately posterior. Lesions of the primary area give sensory losses in the cutaneous regions corresponding to the somatotopic map (Fig. E1–1), there being a preponderant crossed effect. With more posterior lesions of the parietal lobe there are distinct differences between the dominant (left) and the minor hemispheres. However with both lobes there are zones of integration of sensory inputs of different modalities, somaesthetic, visual and auditory, in areas adjacent to the temporal and occipital lobes. Mountcastle [1975] gives a good summary:

> Humans with parietal lesions display profound disturbances of behavior. The common feature is an alteration of the perception of the body form, and its relation to surrounding space; especially, in stereotactic and visual exploration of the immediate extrapersonal space.
> The syndromes can be divided into:
> (1) Those in which a unilateral lesion produces changes in function that are purely contralateral, and
> (2) Those in which even unilateral lesions produce more global disorders affecting both sides of the body.

The contralateral syndrome (1) is usually associated with a right (minor) parietal lobe lesion. It results in the most bizarre behaviour patterns that Hécaen [1967] appropriately refers to as a "pantomime of massive neglect." The subject may neglect or deny the existence of the contralateral limbs and even neglect to clothe them. There is often failure to observe objects in the contralateral half-field of visual space. The contralateral limbs are rarely moved, yet are not paralysed. There is a failure of command performance as described in chapter E3. The patient tends to withdraw from and avoid the contralateral half-field of space. Yet despite this pantomime of neglect the patient may deny that he is ill at all! A remarkable case of neglect of the left side has been described by Jung [1974] in a painter whose self-portraits after the lesion were almost restricted to the right side of the face.

The bilateral syndrome (2) may occur when there is a large lesion of the right (minor) hemisphere. The patient has difficulties in orienting to the surrounding space, as for example in map-reading and route-finding, tasks that involve the coordination of somaesthetic and visual cues that are especial minor hemisphere functions. The subject also fails in copying drawings and in constructing three-dimensional forms by block assemblage. A wide variety of global disorders also results from extensive lesions of the left (dominant) parietal lobe. There are associated disorders of language and all manner of failure of communication from the sensory inputs. The failure also extended to the initiation and control of movements, as if the patient was lacking ideas.

In the left parietal lobe there is integration of sensory data with language. This is revealed by finding that lesions result in disorders of gesture, of writing, of arithmetic and of verbal knowledge of both sides of the body. As a consequence there are disabilities of motor action (apraxia), of constructive ability and of calculation. Parietal lobe lesions abutting on the temporal lobe result in aphasia, so much so that the Wernicke area is shown extending into the left inferior parietal region (Fig. E4−1 and 3). With lesions of the angular gyrus (Brodmann, 39) there is loss of word and symbol recognition (alexia). Nevertheless, patients with left parietal lobectomy score reasonably well on tests of auditory and visual verbal recall, being much better than those with left temporal lobe lesions (Milner [1967]).

On the other hand the right parietal lobe is specially concerned in the handling of spatial data and in a non-verbalized form of relationship between the body and space. It is specially concerned in spatial skills. Lesions result in loss of skills dependent on finely organized movements, apraxia. The disability in handling spatial data appears in writing, where the lines are wavy with the words unevenly spaced and often deformed by perseveration, e.g. the proper double letter appearing tripled, as "lettter" for letter. There seem also to be more subtle disorders of linguistic expression, with deteriorations in fluency, and in vocabulary. Patients suffer from an abnormal level of linguistic fatigue. The distinguished neuroanatomist Prof. Brodal suffered from a right parietal lobe lesion in April 1972. About a year later he wrote a most interesting account of the disabilities he has experienced and of his gradual recovery (Brodal [1973]). In addition to the above account he reported losses of higher mental functions. There was reduction in power of concentration, in consecutive sentence memory, and in short-term memory for abstract symbols such as numbers. Clearly there is more linguistic performance in the right hemisphere than has been believed hitherto.

Hécaen (1967) summarizes the difference between the two parietal lobes:

> Right brain injury disorganizes the spatial reference of various activities, while left injury causes disturbances of the systems of signs, codes and categorizing activity. Thus we believe that an organizing role of verbal mediation in activities of the major (dominant) hemisphere must be postulated.

There will be further reference to the differences between the functions of the two lobes when dealing more generally with the dominant and minor hemispheres.

As already mentioned in chapters E1 and E2 the principal transmission from the primary sensory areas 3, 1, 2 is to the secondary area, 5, and thence to the tertiary area 7. There is no cross-modal communication in area 5, and, although most neurones of area 7 respond to both somaesthetic and visual inputs (Mountcastle & others [1975]), there is apparently no direct pathway from the visual areas in the occipital lobe, as is illustrated in Figure E1−7E−H (Jones and Powell [1970]). The concept of immediate extrapersonal space derives from both somaesthetic and visual inputs, and for this there must be cross-modal communication. The findings of Jones and Powell [1970] indicate that this integration occurs first in the STS area (cp. Fig. E1−7). In the human brain this region of the left temporal lobe has been appropriated as a central part of the great posterior speech area. Mountcastle [1975 (personal communication)] suggests that the STS area must serve as the simian prologue for the huge development of the angular and supramarginal gyri in man, regions intimately concerned with communication, language, imagery, and hemispheric specialization. These great areas (Brodmann 39 and 40 in Figs. E1−4, E4−3) are stated to be poorly developed in anthropoid apes (cp. chapter E4) (Mauss [1911]; Goldstein [1927]; Critchley [1953]; Geschwind [1965 (a)]; Jones and Powell [1970]).

44. Occipital Lobe Lesions

Reference has already been made to the visual defects arising from occipital lobe lesions (chapter E2). For example, excision of the left occipital lobe results in blindness for the right visual field of each eye, which is called a right hemianopia, and similarly for the right occipital lobe and left hemianopia. Less severe destructions cause blind patches of the visual field that are called scotomata. The classical investigations have been carried out by Teuber & others [1960] on visual field defects after penetrating missile wounds. The detailed study of scotomata gives reliable mapping of the relation of retina to visual cortex (Fig. E2−5), and also of the various compensations in visual interpretation by the subject.

Milner [1967] reported that lesions of the right occipital lobe decreased the speed of reading as much as lesions of the speech area in the left temporal lobe. Yet tests for the ability to recall words or sentences in set tasks (verbal memory) revealed that these right occipital lobectomy patients performed as well as those with right temporal lobectomies. The left temporal lobectomies failed as badly in this test as in the speed of reading. Milner [1967] reports a very interesting case of a radical left occipital lobectomy. This girl had good verbal memory scores both for auditory and visual presentation, but she had severe defects in reading and in calculation. Evidently a severe handicap was introduced because of the necessary transfer from the right occipital lobe to the verbal and calculating centres of the left parietal-temporal lobes: A general conclusion is that speed of reading is dependent on both occipital lobes.

Subtle visual losses occur with lesions of the visual association cortex (areas 18, 19), but there is considerable disagreement in detail. This zone of visual cortex can be regarded as functioning in some rather simple reconstruction of the visual image, as is evidenced by the high level of synthesis that is displayed by the constituent neurones (complex and hypercomplex cells). As reported in chapter E2 there is a still higher level of feature detection in the next relay area in the right inferotemporal lobe.

45. Frontal Lobe Lesions

The lesional studies described in this section are for the frontal lobe anterior to the motor areas 4 and 6, i.e. for what is called the prefrontal lobe. The function of areas 4 and 6 has been discussed in chapter E3. There have now been many systematic studies of patients with large ablations of the right or left prefrontal lobes (reviewed by Teuber [1964], [1972]; Milner [1967], [1968], [1971], [1974]). These subjects score at normal level in linguistic tests, in both the auditory and the visual forms; yet subjects with left prefrontal lesions tend to speak very little spontaneously and to have significantly low scores with word fluency tests (Milner [1967]).

A related defect is disclosed by the so-called verbal recency test. On cards there are printed two spondaic words (e.g. cow-boy or rail-road). The subject reads sequentially through a stack of such cards, and at times a question mark appears between the two words. The subject has to indicate which of the words he has read most recently, or alternatively, if only one was previously seen, to recognize which word. Thus two verbal memories are tested: verbal recency and verbal recognition. Left prefrontal lobe excisions impair recency but not recognition, whereas, in accord with a wide range of studies of the speech centres, left temporal lobe excisions impair recognition, but, surprisingly, not recency.

Patients with right prefrontal lobe excisions do not have any linguistic disability, but have a defect in sequential picture recognition. The tests resemble those for words. A sequence of cards each with two abstract pictures is presented to the subject, and at times two pictures turn up with a question mark between them. The subject has to recognize whether he has seen either picture before; and, if he has seen both, which was the most recent one in the series. In conformity with the tests described above, the recognition test is related to the right temporal lobe and patients fail badly after right temporal lobectomy. On the other hand, the recency test is not affected by right temporal lobectomy, but is seriously disturbed by right prefrontal lobectomy.

In summary there is a complementary relationship between the temporal and frontal lobes of the same side. On the left side they give, respectively, verbal recognition and verbal recency, and, on the right side, picture recognition and picture recency. Each frontal lobe has the function of providing a temporal ordering of the events that have been recognized and evaluated by means of the corresponding temporal lobe. Frontal lobe excisions thus result in a memory loss for the sequential order of experiences.

Besides these relatively specific functions, patients with prefrontal lesions display disabilities in carrying out tasks involving insight and flexibility. The Wisconsin card sorting test has been employed by Milner [1963]. As indicated in Figure E6−5 the patient is presented 4 "stimulus" cards with characteristics of colour, number and shape, and is given a pack of 128 cards which vary in those three respects. For example, the specimen card on the top of the pack could be placed under A for colour, B for number or C for shape. The procedure of the test is that the subject is instructed to place sequentially each card of the pack under a stimulus card which may be chosen for one or other of these three characteristics, colour, number or shape. The strategy of the experimenter is to decide on a particular characteristic, say colour, and only inform the subject if each card placement is "right" or "wrong" on this criterion. The subject has to get as many cards "right" as he can. After ten consecutive "right" placements the strategy is shifted without warning or explanation to some other criterion, say number, colour responses being forthwith labelled "wrong," and number "right." After ten consecutive correct placements the strategy is again shifted to shape and so on. This procedure tests for a flexibility in problem solving, that is dependent on learning.

In comparison with patients having various cerebral lesions including even orbito-frontal lesions, patients with dorsolateral frontal lobe lesions on either side displayed a grave disability, which has been called perseveration. The subject performs quite well in recognizing the initial strategy, but, when the strategy is changed, he fails badly with mounting errors because he tends to persevere with the original strategy. The subjects recognize their errors, but show a "curious dissociation between the ability to verbalize the requirements of the test and the ability to use this verbalization as a guide to action" (Milner [1974]).

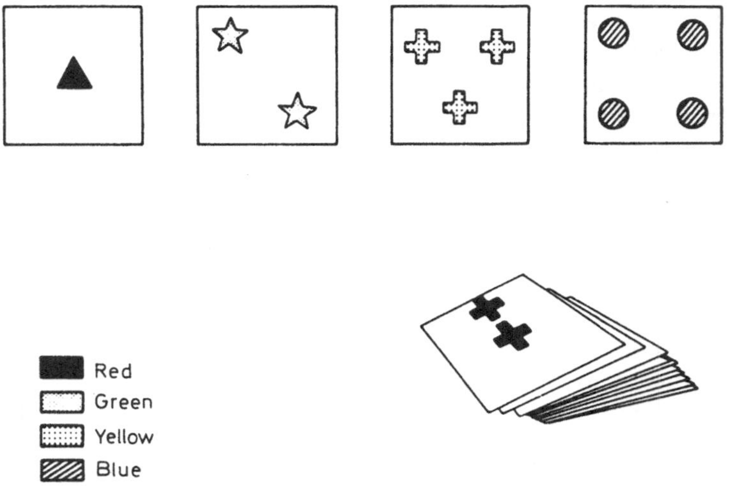

Fig. E6–5. Drawing showing the Wisconsin Card Sorting test. Full description in text (Milner, 1963).

Nauta [1971] summarizes the frontal-lobe disorder as being:

> characterized foremost by a derangement of behavioral programming. One of the essential functional deficits of the frontal-lobe patient appears to lie in an inability to maintain in his behaviour a normal stability-in-time: his action programs, once started, are likely to fade out, to stagnate in reiteration or to become deflected away from the intended goal. The fact that even his self-admitted awareness of a mismatch between the purpose and the result of his actions fails to affect his strategy suggests an inadequate "internalization" of all those error – or error-approach signals, including even self-directed verbal commands, that normally modulate the evolvement of behavioral programs.

In fact, loss of foresight is the characteristic disabling consequence of massive frontal lobe lesions on both sides and is attributable to a memory deficit. This loss correlates with the failure of the subjects in the simple recency tests described above.

These investigations on patients with frontal lobe lesions have to be considered in relation to the very extensive studies on primates. The early experiments provided surprisingly clear demonstrations of memory losses after frontal lobe lesions. The delayed reaction test of Jacobsen [1936] gave the simplest evidence for failure of memory. The chimpanzee observed through a grating some food being placed under one of two cups, then an opaque screen was lowered for a time ranging from a few seconds to several minutes. On raising the screen even after 4 s the animal with bilateral frontal lobectomy failed to remember under which cup the food was placed, whereas a normal chimpanzee or one with a unilateral lesion succeeded even when screened from viewing the cups for as long as 5 min. Monkeys with bilateral prefrontal lesions in the area approximately corresponding to area 46 in Figure E1 – 7 displayed a disability to a comparable delayed testing procedure almost as severe as with excision of both prefrontal lobes (Mishkin [1957]). A more complex task involved learning to use a short stick to secure longer sticks that could eventually pull in food far out of reach. The sticks and the food were on platforms so widely separated that they could not be observed simultaneously. This task involved memory of recent sensory experiences and could quickly be learnt by normal chimpanzees and by those with unilateral frontal lobectomy; but with bilateral lesions the failure was profound (Jacobsen & others [1935]). Since that time there have been many investigations on memory deficits arising from frontal lobe lesions in primates. Reference may be made to the Symposium *The Frontal Granular Cortex and Behaviour,* edited by J. M. Warren and K. Akert [1964] for a survey of the complexity of the experimental findings that go far beyond the scope of this book. The role of the prefrontal lobe in memory will be dealt with extensively in chapter E8.

Nauta [1971] has attempted to correlate the functions of the prefrontal lobe with the communication systems linking it with other regions of the cerebral hemispheres (cp. Pandya and Kuypers [1969]). There are firstly the lines of communication to and from the temporal and parietal lobes, as depicted in outline in Figure E1 – 7 and 8. As indicated in Figure E1 – 8, many of these pathways are reciprocal. By these pathways the prefrontal lobes can enter into the domain of temporal sequence in the handling of somaesthetic, visual and auditory information. Lesions of the prefrontal lobes thus can result in the various defects of temporal judgement as described above. In this respect the prefrontal lobes participate in the sensory effector mechanisms.

But a more significant and unique performance of the prefrontal lobes derives from their reciprocal relations with the limbic system. As already illustrated in Figure E1 – 7 and 8, the secondary area 20, and the tertiary areas 7, 21 and 22 project to the limbic system. Thus all three afferent systems, somaesthetic, visual and auditory, communicate to the limbic system from widely dispersed areas of the parietal and temporal lobes. However, the most important projection is from the prefrontal lobe (Figs. E1 – 8 and 9; Pandya and Kuypers [1969]; Nauta [1971]). By contrast the only direct projection from the limbic system to the neocortex is to the prefrontal lobes (Jones and Powell [1969], [1970]; Nauta [1971]). This unique connection comes to the prefrontal cortex via a large nucleus of the thalamus, the MD nucleus, which does not project to any other neocortical areas

(Fig. E1 – 9). This projection preponderantly goes to the orbital surface of the prefrontal lobe, but also is widely dispersed over the convexity (Nauta [1971]). As already conjectured in chapter E2, the reciprocal communication to the limbic system and the hypothalamus gives the prefrontal lobe the unique function of associating the somaesthetic, visual and auditory experiences with the emotional input from the limbic system and hypothalamus. Also linked in this association is the olfactory system that projects directly into the limbic system from the sensory pathway (Fig. E1 – 9, OLB, LOT).

Nauta [1971] suggests that

> the failure of the affective and motivational responses of the frontal-lobe patient to match environmental situations that he nonetheless can describe accurately could thus be tentatively interpreted as the consequence of a loss of a modulatory influence normally exerted by the neocortex upon the limbic mechanisms via the frontal lobe.

As a consequence these patients display unfortunate mood and character changes such as euphoria and lack of initiative.

46. Limbic System Lesions

The limbic system has an extensive and complex topography, being in its principal feature a large ring, or gyrus fornicatus, that encircles the black and white area in the centre of Figure E1 – 4. Important lines of communication are indicated in Figure E1 – 9. The memory defects arising from circumscribed lesions of the principal component, the hippocampus, will be described in chapter E8. The most revealing evidence on the function of the limbic system is provided by a description of the experiences of patients with psychomotor epilepsy in which the epileptogenic focus is in or near to the limbic system.

> During the initial epileptic discharge, patients typically experience one or more of a wide variety of vivid affects. The basic and specific affects include feelings of hunger, thirst, nausea, suffocation, choking, cold, warmth, and the need to defecate or urinate. Among the general affects are feelings of terror, fear, sadness, depression, foreboding, familiarity or strangeness, reality or unreality, wanting to be alone, paranoid feelings, and anger. Sometimes a patient will experience an alternation of opposite feelings . . . (MacLean [1970]).

In general these symptoms indicate the strong emotional and visceral experiences that are given by activity of the limbic system. The manner in which the limbic system with the associated hypothalamus gives colour, urgency, vividness and emotion to the sensory experiences has already been described in chapter E2.

47. The Dominant and Minor Hemispheres

Teuber [1974] has remarked that "the concept of the unilateral dominance of left over right hemisphere in man has been abandoned and replaced by one of complementary specialization." The evidence for this statement has been presented in its essentials in the preceding sections. However, I will continue here to use the dominant-minor terminology because I believe that hemispheric dominance is clearly established by the linked functions of speech and self-consciousness. As Teuber [1974] points out, the enhanced status of the minor hemisphere has been derived from three quite distinct modes of investigation: the analysis both of total hemispherectomy (chapter E5) and of unilateral and circumscribed cortical lesions (this chapter), notably by Milner and her associates; the intensive study of patients with complete section of the corpus callosum (commissurotomy), notably by Sperry and his associates (chapter E5); the further application of the dichotic technique of Broadbent ([1954], [1974]) by Kimura and her associates (Kimura [1967], [1973]) (this chapter).

The dichotic technique is valuable in that it is applied to normal subjects, and corroborates the findings from lesions. It also gives evidence of a more general kind showing that there is strong inter-hemispheric action in tasks that had appeared to be localized in one or the other hemisphere. There have been many experimental tests of this interference between hemispheres. For example Broadbent and Gregory [1965] employed a simple manual reaction of finger movement in response to a finger tap and showed that, during this "reflex" reaction elicited every 5 s, the subject had a diminished memory for spoken letters of the alphabet, also presented once every 5 s. Also during this stimulus combination the finger reaction time was slowed even if it was in the left hand and thus driven by the right hemisphere, which would not be immediately concerned in the simultaneous linguistic test. The interference between these two testing procedures reveals that they are *not* utilizing two quite distinct cerebral mechanisms. Similarly it can be shown that there is interference between two complex tasks, that, at the first level of interpretation, could be considered as being carried out by distinct cortical areas, for example, repeating aloud speech that is heard (left hemisphere) and playing the piano by sight-reading (right hemisphere). As Broadbent [1974] points out, under these conditions the interference is much less than would be the case if the subject was responding to two simultaneous linguistic messages.

Reaction time studies have also been employed in demonstrating the difference in hemispheric functions of normal subjects. For example Berlucchi [1974] has shown that, with flash inputs of letters to the left or right visual field, the reaction time is significantly less (mean difference 18.5 ms) for inputs to the right field and hence directly to the left hemisphere. By contrast the reaction times for recognition of faces are shorter (mean difference 15.5 ms) with flash presentation to the left visual field and so directly to the right hemisphere. These latency differences are of the order to be expected for interhemispheric transfer via the corpus callosum on the pathway from the visual cortex to the hemisphere concerned in the discriminative processing of the information. Surprisingly, it was immaterial which hand was used for signalling the response.

Despite the bilateral hemispheric involvement in tasks that are predominantly the function of one, it is possible to compose lists of functions for the dominant and minor hemispheres, that are valuable for our further discussion. Figure E6–6 is derived from recent publications of Levy-Agresti and Sperry [1968], Levy [1973] and Sperry [1974], but there are additions from the studies that have been reported in the sections above on global and localized hemispheric lesions.

In general the dominant hemisphere is specialized in respect to fine imaginative details in all descriptions and reactions, i.e., it is analytic and sequential – properties that seem essential for verbal feature extraction and for arithmetic. And so it can add and subtract and multiply and carry out other computer-like operations. But of course its dominance derives from its verbal and ideational abilities and its liaison to self-consciousness (the World 2 of Popper, cp. chapter E7). Because of its deficiencies in these respects the minor hemisphere deserves its title, but in many important properties it is preeminent, particularly in respect of its spatial abilities with a strongly developed pictorial and pattern sense. For example, after commissurotomy the minor hemisphere programming the left hand is greatly superior in all kinds of geometrical and perspective drawings (Bogen [1969 (a)]). This superiority is also evidenced by the ability to assemble coloured blocks so as to match a mosaic picture (Gazzaniga [1970]). The dominant hemisphere is unable to carry out even simple tasks of this kind and is almost illiterate in respect to pictorial and pattern sense, at least as revealed by its copying disability. It is an arithmetical hemisphere, but not a geometrical hemisphere. It is quite surprising how sharply these distinctions can be made. It could never have been predicted before the commissurotomy patients were scientifically studied by Sperry and his associates: Bogen, Gazzaniga, Levy-Agresti and Zaidel.

Figure E6–6 shows that in their properties the two hemispheres have a complementary relationship. The minor is coherent and the dominant is detailed. Furthermore, the minor hemisphere is specialized in relationship to

DOMINANT HEMISPHERE	MINOR HEMISPHERE
Liaison to consciousness	No such Liaison
Verbal	Almost non-verbal
Linguistic description	Musical
Ideational Conceptual similarities	Pictorial and Pattern sense Visual similarities
Analysis over time	Synthesis over time
Analysis of detail	Holistic — Images
Arithmetical and computer-like	Geometrical and Spatial

Fig. E6—6. **Various specific performances of the dominant and minor hemispheres as suggested by the new conceptual developments of Levy-Agresti and Sperry (1968) and Levy (1973). There are some additions to their original list.**

pictures and patterns, and it is musical. Music is essentially coherent and synthetic, being dependent on synthesis of a sequential input of sounds. A coherent, synthetic, sequential imagery is made for us in some holistic manner by our musical sense.

Bogen [1969 (b)] summarizes his extensive investigation on the same commissurotomy patients as those investigated by Sperry by the statement that the dominant hemisphere is predominantly symbolic and propositional in its function, having specialization for language with syntactical, semantic, mathematical, and logical abilities. By contrast he designates the minor hemisphere as being appositional, with the property of apposing or comparing perceptions and schemas in some Gestalt manner, which is far beyond our present understanding.

Those areas of the two cerebral hemispheres that are concerned with the simplest operations, namely the primary sensory areas and the motor areas (cp. Fig. E1—1), are composed of a mosaic of columns or modules (cp. Figs. E1—5, 6) that are in parallel on the input or output pathways. Moreover there is very little commissural cross-connection of these primary areas. At all higher cerebral levels there is commissural connection in an approximate mirror-image manner, and some complementary hemispheric performance is discovered when the testing procedures are sufficiently sensitive (Dimond and Beaumont [1973]; Levy [1973]; Trevarthen [1973]). For example, reference has already been made both to the primitive linguistic performance of the minor hemisphere after commissurotomy, and to the losses in linguistic ability that result from circumscribed lesions of the right parietal lobe. Complementarily, although the right hemisphere is greatly superior to the left in visual and tactile pattern recognition, after commissurotomy its performance is greatly inferior to normal subjects using either hand (Milner [1974]). The separation of the hemispheres reveals that the left hemisphere normally adds to the performance of the right, perhaps by providing some valuable verbal symbolism.

This hemispheric specialization is unique to man. The homologous cortical areas of non-human primates show no evidence of any asymmetry of function (Milner [1974]). During human evolution hemispheric specialization must have developed in response to the unique demands made by language and perhaps, to a lesser degree, for the development of unique abilities in spatial and pattern recognition, as for example in tool construction and usage. It is difficult to overestimate the complexity and immensity of the neuronal machinery required for language in its fullest development, not only for the overt performances of hearing, speaking, reading, writing, but more importantly on the cognitive side in thinking, imagining and in the storage and retrieval processes involved in memory. This large demand on hemispheric space, if we may so call it, could be met only by eliminating the redundancy of bilateral representation, and having some separation of functions. In the evolutionary development of the hominid brain we can conjecture that it was biologically efficient (cp. Levy [1973]) to have one hemisphere specialized, by the subtle microstructure of its neuronal machinery, for linguistic, analytic, calculating, and ideational tasks. Complementarily the other hemisphere by a slightly different microstructural design would be specialized for synthetic, holistic, pictorial and spatial tasks. It is remarkable that such hemispheral differentiation of function is maintained in the face of the wealth of commissural cross-connections. This raises the perplexing problem of the function of these commissural connections, and their mode of operation. There was reference to this problem when discussing the microstructure of the cerebral cortex in chapter E1.

There is evidence that this separation of hemispheric functions is genetically coded (Levy [1973]), though of course a large contribution is made by usage, particularly at the plastic stage of early life. As already reported, Geschwind and Levitsky [1969] found that in 65% of human brains there was an enlargement of the planum temporale of the left hemisphere (Fig. E4–3), which lies at the centre of the posterior speech area. Wada & others [1973] confirmed these observations and in addition reported that this asymmetry of the planum temporale was just as evident in children at birth, and even could be observed as early as the 29-week-old foetus.

It might therefore be concluded that the building of the brain by genetic instructions determines irrevocably that the left hemisphere will be used for speech in the large majority of babies. But this is not so. In the first place Basser [1962] has produced good evidence from the study of lesions that, in children under 6 years, both hemispheres are concerned in the learning and production of speech. Thereafter, in over 90%, there is a gradual taking over of speech by the left hemisphere, which in this way assumes dominance. Dichotic listening studies on children suggest that already by age 4 or 5 left hemispheral dominance of speech is well established (Kimura [1967]).

Convincing evidence for plasticity at an early age has been given by Milner [1974]. The investigated patients had suffered in infancy circumscribed excisions of large areas of the left hemisphere in the surgical treatment of epilepsy. Where there had been removal of all or almost all of the normal putative speech areas, the subjects in later life were found by the sodium amytal test to have their speech transferred to the right hemisphere. In the control group with just as massive left hemispheric excisions, but with sparing of the normal speech areas, the speech remained in the left hemisphere. Exceptionally there appeared to be bilateral representation of speech.

Unfortunately there is an "intellectual price" to pay for this plastic relocation of the speech area in early life. Sperry [1974] and Teuber [1974] find that, when speech is crowded into the right hemisphere, it tends to develop at the expense of the other cognitive abilities normally there, and even speech suffers from the inadequacy of the available neuronal territory. The dominating cerebral demand of speech is well illustrated by these untoward effects of plastic relocation. The other message is that the linguistic areas that are normally built by genetic coding do not have a microstructure uniquely specified for linguistic performance. At the most they have a structure which biases the normal speech areas to assume the full linguistic performance at the expense of the primordial linguistic developments in the right hemisphere. To an important extent nurture can be regarding as taking over from nature in the development of the hemispheral partition of functions that is discovered in the adult human brain.

Chapter E7 The Self-conscious Mind and the Brain

48. Résumé

This chapter is devoted to the development of a new theory relating to the manner in which the self-conscious mind and the brain interact. It is a very strong dualism and raises the most severe scientific problems in relationship to the interface between the world of matter-energy, in the special instance of the liaison area of the brain, and the world of states of consciousness that is referred to as the self-conscious mind. This dualist-interactionist explanation has been specially developed for the self-conscious mind and the human brain, in particular the dominant hemisphere, as disclosed by the experiments on commissurotomy patients. Its role for animals and for the minor hemisphere is debatable.

There is firstly an introductory section on the three-world hypothesis of Popper (chapter P2 and Fig. E7−1) because it is in terms of this hypothesis that the theory has been developed; and, furthermore, this hypothesis provides a very interesting explanation of the development of the self-conscious mind. It is argued that the world of the self-conscious mind (World 2) of each individual self is developed in relationship to the World 3 influence on that self. World 3 includes the whole of the cultural heritage, most importantly language.

Briefly, the hypothesis is that the self-conscious mind is an independent entity (Fig. E7−2) that is actively engaged in reading out from the multitude of active centres in the modules of the liaison areas of the dominant cerebral hemisphere. The self-conscious mind selects from these centres in accord with its attention and its interests and integrates its selection to give the unity of conscious experience from moment to moment. It also acts back on the neural centres (Fig. E7−2). Thus it is proposed that the self-conscious mind exercises a superior interpretive and controlling role upon the neural events by virtue of a two-way interaction across the interface between World 1 and

World 2 (Fig. E7 – 2). It is proposed that the unity of conscious experience comes not from an ultimate synthesis in the neural machinery but in the integrating action of the self-conscious mind on what it reads out from the immense diversity of neural activities in the liaison brain (Figs. E7 – 3 and 4).

There is a detailed discussion of the problems arising in relationship to this hypothesis and of the various testing procedures which provide empirical evidence relating to the many aspects of this hypothesis. Both in this chapter and in the discussion sections an attempt is made to show how the operative features of modules of the cerebral cortex can result in properties of such subtlety that they could be recipients of the weak actions that are postulated to be exerted by the self-conscious mind across the interface. These actions are evidenced by voluntary movements as described in chapter E3 and also by the recall of memories on demand by the cognitive processes, as described in chapter E8.

In further aspects of the theoretical development, it is conjectured that some modules are open to interaction with World 2, and others are closed (Fig. E7 – 3). However, there is no rigid separation between these two categories. For example, according to the inputs to the liaison brain from the various sensory processes, some modules can be raised to a level of activity that makes them open to interaction with World 2. It is thus envisaged that from time to time the modules are sometimes open and sometimes closed, and this is dependent upon the integrative operations of the neuronal machinery. It is even conjectured that, although the open modules of the liaison are predominantly in the left (dominant) hemisphere, activity across the corpus callosum may lift modules in the minor hemisphere to be in liaison with the self-conscious mind, although this is not the case after commissurotomy.

This treatment of the self-conscious mind in relationship to the brain gives opportunity for an interpretation of sleep and dreams, and also in the unconscious states resulting from anaesthesia, comas of various kinds, and, finally, in brain death. On the opposite side of this picture there is the loss of consciousness resulting from the strongly driven activities of the cortical modules that occur in epileptic seizures.

In a final section there is mention of the implications of this strong dualist-interactionist hypothesis. Its central component is that primacy is given to the self-conscious mind which during normal life is engaged in searching for brain events that are in its present interest and in integrating these into the unified conscious experience that we have from moment to moment. We can regard it as having a scanning operation over the hundreds of thousands of cortical modules that potentially are capable of being open to interaction with World 2. In the discussions there will be treatment of the fundamental problems arising from this dualist-interactionist hypothesis. In particular, of course, the most challenging problem relates to the possibility that the action of the mind on the brain comes into conflict with the first law of thermodynamics. This will be considered in dialogues VII, X, XI and XII.

49. Introduction

One of us (J. C. E.) – at 18 years old – had a sudden overwhelming experience. He wrote no account of it, but his life was changed because it aroused his intense interest in the brain-mind problem. As a consequence he has spent his life in the neural sciences with some continuing involvement in philosophy. Years later he found that Pascal in his inimitable style had described the predicament of an unbeliever in words that expressed so well the poignancy of that adolescent experience.

> When I consider the short extent of my life, swallowed up in the eternity before and after, the small space that I fill or even see, engulfed in the infinite immensity of spaces unknown to me and which know me not, I am terrified, and astonished to find myself here, not there. For there is no reason why it should be here, not there, why now rather than at another time. Who put me here? By whose order and design have this place and time been allotted to me? . . . The eternal silence of those infinite spaces strikes me with terror. (Pascal, translated by J. M. Cohen [1961])

The investigations of Sperry and his associates on commissurotomy patients (chapter E–5) have provided the most illuminating discovery on the problem under discussion in this chapter. Their very early investigations led to the conclusion that the self-consciousness of the subject arose only in relationship to the activities of the dominant hemisphere. At subsequent stages there appeared at times to be evidence that the subject experienced some vague diffuse consciousness from events in the minor hemisphere. However, more rigorous investigations have shown that the observations do not warrant this conclusion. For example, the diffuse discomfort felt when a sharp object was pressed into a left finger is now attributed to a diffuse non-specific pathway from the ipsilateral limb to the left (dominant) cerebral cortex. The emotional reaction experienced in response to the nude photo projected to the right hemisphere has already been explained in a comparable manner (chapter E5). An account has also been given of the pathways whereby objects far out in the left visual field cause an input into the left hemisphere (Trevarthen and Sperry [1973]), and so are consciously perceived (Fig. E5–6). In summary of all this more recent work it can be stated that it corroborates the exclusive claim that in the commissurotomy patients self-conscious experiences arise only in relationship to activities in the dominant hemisphere (chapter E5).

From this evidence there is derived the concept that only a specialized zone of the cerebral hemispheres is in liaison with the self-conscious mind. The term liaison brain denotes all those areas of the cerebral cortex that potentially are capable of being in direct liaison with the self-conscious mind. Later in this chapter it is conjectured that from moment to moment only minute fractions are actually in this state of direct liaison. In the commissurotomy patient this liaison brain is restricted to the dominant hemisphere, presumably encompassing the linguistic areas of that hemisphere, though doubtless extending more widely to encompass areas that are concerned with non-verbal modes of conscious experiences, for example the pictorial, the musical, and the polymodal areas described in chapter E2, and very importantly the prefrontal lobes. However, normally there may well be some liaison areas of brain in the minor hemisphere (cp. Fig. E7–5).

50. Self-conscious Mind and the Brain

In general terms there are two theories about the way in which the behaviour of an animal (and a man) can be organized into the effective unity, which it so obviously is.

Firstly, there is the explanation inherent in monist materialism plus all varieties of parallelism. In current neurological theory the diverse inputs into the brain interact on the basis of all the structural and functional connectivities to give some integrated output of motor performance. The aim of the neural sciences is to provide a more and more coherent and complete account of the manner in which the total performance of an animal and of a human being is explicable on those terms. Without making too dogmatic a claim, it can be stated that the goal of the neurosciences is to formulate a theory that can in principle provide a complete explanation of all behaviour of animals and man, including man's verbal behaviour (cp. Barlow [1972]; Doty [1975]). With some important reservations I (J. C. E.) share this goal in my own experimental work and believe that it is acceptable for all automatic and subconscious movements, even of the most complex kind. However, I believe that the reductionist strategy will fail in the attempt to account for the higher levels of conscious performance of the human brain.

Secondly, there is the dualist-interactionist explanation which has been specially developed for the self-conscious mind and human brains. Its role for animals and for the minor hemisphere is debatable. It is proposed that superimposed upon the neural machinery in all its performance, as outlined in chapters E1, E2, E3, E4, E5 and E6, there are at certain sites of the cerebral hemisphere (the liaison areas) effective interactions with the self-conscious mind, both in receiving and in giving.

It is desirable to make brief reference to the philosophical basis of my discussion. As illustrated in Figure E7–1, everything in existence and in experience is subsumed in one or other of three worlds: World 1, the world of physical objects and states; World 2, the world of states of consciousness and subjective knowledge of all kinds; World 3, the world of man-made culture, comprising the whole of objective knowledge (Popper [1972]). Furthermore it is proposed that there is interaction between these worlds. There is reciprocal interaction between Worlds 1 and 2, and between Worlds 2 and 3 generally (see dialogue XI) via the mediation of World 1. When the objective knowledge of World 3 (the man-made world of culture) is encoded on various objects of World 1 – books, pictures, structures, machines –, it can be consciously perceived only when projected to the brain by the appropriate receptor organs and afferent pathways. Reciprocally the World 2 of conscious experience can bring about changes in World 1, in the first place in the brain, then in muscular contractions, World 2 in that way being able to act extensively on World 1. This is the postulated operation in voluntary movement that has been considered in chapter E3. We may formulate the conjec-

WORLD 1	WORLD 2	WORLD 3
PHYSICAL OBJECTS AND STATES	STATES OF CONSCIOUSNESS	KNOWLEDGE IN OBJECTIVE SENSE
1. INORGANIC Matter and energy of cosmos 2. BIOLOGY Structure and actions of all living beings human brains 3. ARTEFACTS Material substrates of human creativity of tools of machines of books of works of art of music	Subjective knowledge Experience of perception thinking emotions dispositional intentions memories dreams creative imagination	Cultural heritage coded on material substrates philosophical theological scientific historical literary artistic technological Theoretical systems scientific problems critical arguments

Fig. E7–1. Tabular representation of the three worlds that comprise all existents and all experiences as defined by Popper (Eccles, 1970).

tured interactions of the trialist-interactionist hypothesis as: World 1 ⇄ World 2 and World 3 ⇄ World 1 ⇄ World 2, where World 2 → World 1 contains the problem of voluntary action (chapter E3) and World 1 → World 2, the problem of conscious perception (chapter E2). However, when the self-conscious mind is engaged in creative thinking on problems or ideas, there would seem to be a direct interaction of World 2 and World 3, as has been conjectured in dialogue XI.

Figure E7 – 2 defines the mind-brain problem more succinctly in terms of the three major components that are generally recognized for World 2 (cp. Polten [1973]). There is firstly the outer sense which relates specifically to the perceptions given immediately by the inputs of the sense organs, visual, auditory, tactile, smell, taste, pain, etc. Secondly, there is inner sense which comprises a wide variety of cognitive experiences: thoughts, memories, intentions, imaginings, emotions, feelings, dreams. Thirdly, and at the core of World 2, there is the self or the ego that is the basis of the personal identity and continuity that each of us experiences throughout our lifetime, spanning for example the diurnal gaps of consciousness in sleep. Each day consciousness returns to us with its continuity essentially unbroken by the hours of unconsciousness in sleep.

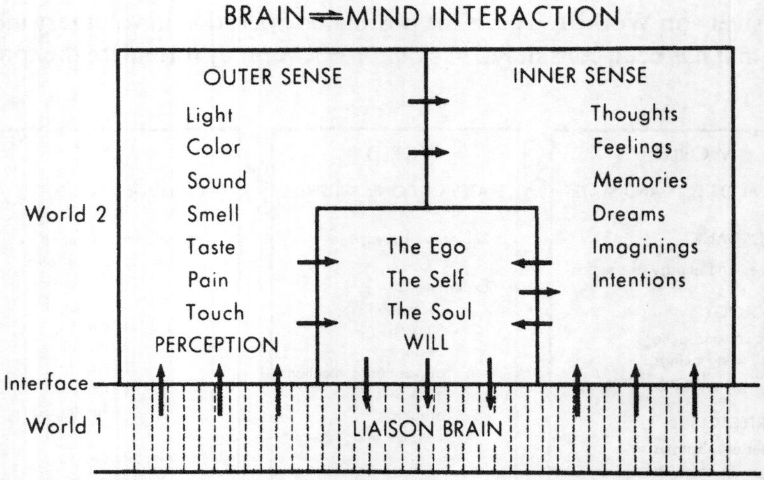

Fig. E7 – 2. Information flow diagram for brain-mind interaction. The three components of World 2: outer sense, inner sense and the ego or self are diagrammed with their connectivities. Also shown are the lines of communication across the interface between World 1 and World 2, that is from the liaison brain to and from these World 2 components. The liaison brain has the columnar arrangement indicated (cf. Figs. E1 – 5 and 6; E2 – 6 and 7). It must be imagined that the area of the liaison brain is enormous, with open modules numbering a hundred thousand or more, not just the two score here depicted.

51. Hypothesis of Interaction of Self-conscious Mind and the Liaison Brain

It is important now to develop an hypothesis on the mode of interaction between the self-conscious mind and the brain that is much stronger and more definitive than any hypothesis that has hitherto been formulated in relation to what we may term the dualistic postulates. In formulating a strong dualistic hypothesis we build upon the following evidence.

(1) There is a *unitary character* about the experiences of the self-conscious mind. There is concentration now on this, now on that, aspect of the cerebral performance at any one instant. This focussing is the phenomenon known as *attention* (cp. Paschal [1941]; Berlyne [1969]; Dichgans and Jung [1969]).

(2) We can assume that the experiences of the self-conscious mind have a relationship with neural events in the liaison brain, there being *a relationship of interaction giving a degree of correspondence, but not an identity.* In our discussions and in chapter P3 there has been strong criticism of the parallelist claim that there is identity (Feigl [1967]; Armstrong [1968]; Smart [1962]; Pepper [1962]; Laszlo [1972]; Barlow [1972]). The psychoneural identity hypothesis has been effectively criticized on philosophical grounds (Polten [1973]). The neurophysiologist Barlow [1972] states his parallelistic belief succinctly and dogmatically: "Thinking is brought about by neurons, and we should not use phrases like 'unit activity reflects, reveals, or monitors thought processes,' because the activities of neurons, quite simply, *are* thought processes." No scientific evidence is presented for this identity. It is surprising to find that he expresses a belief in the operational effectiveness of single neurones. "A high impulse frequency in a given neuron corresponds to a high degree of confidence that the cause of the percept is present in the external world." In an effort to stress neuronal parsimony there is a neglect of all the anatomical and physiological evidence that, at the higher levels of the nervous system, effective neuronal action is secured by large assemblages of neurones arranged in colonies or modules (chapters E1, E2, E3). In the higher levels of the central nervous system neuronal parsimony is a myth. The operation of the brain can be understood only in terms of *neuronal prodigality* in the constitution of myriads of spatiotemporal patterns. The neurophysiologist Doty [1975] appreciates neuronal prodigality very well, but in the end opts for a strange psychoneural identity, consciousness being linked with the immense and incessant traffic in the corpus callosum. The importance of this traffic in relationship to consciousness is attested by the investigations on commissurotomy patients (cp. chapter E5), but it seems

inconceivable that all-or-nothing impulses in myelinated fibres could be directly involved in the liaison with the self-conscious mind. It should also be noted that, in the clinical condition of agenesis of the corpus callosum (cp. chapter E5), the absence of the corpus callosum apparently does not result in any disturbances of the conscious experiences.

(3) *There can be a temporal discrepancy between neural events and the experiences of the self-conscious mind.* This is shown particularly clearly with the experiments of Libet, as described above (chapter E2), for example the phenomena of backward masking and of antedating. It also occurs in the slowing down of experienced time in acute emergencies (dialogue X).

(4) *There is the continual experience that the self-conscious mind can effectively act on the brain events.* This is most overtly seen in voluntary action (chapter E3), but throughout our waking life we are deliberately evoking brain events when we try to recall a memory or to recapture a word or phrase or to express a thought or to establish a new memory (chapter E8).

A brief initial outline of the hypothesis may be stated as follows. The self-conscious mind is actively engaged in reading out from the multitude of active centres at the highest level of brain activity, namely the liaison areas of the dominant cerebral hemisphere. The self-conscious mind selects from these centres according to attention, and from moment to moment integrates its selection to give unity even to the most transient experiences. Furthermore the self-conscious mind acts upon these neural centres modifying the dynamic spatiotemporal patterns of the neural events. Thus we propose that the self-conscious mind exercises a superior interpretative and controlling role upon the neural events.

A key component of the hypothesis is that the unity of conscious experience is provided by the self-conscious mind and not by the neural machinery of the liaison areas of the cerebral hemisphere. Hitherto it has been impossible to develop any neurophysiological theory that explains how a diversity of brain events comes to be synthesized so that there is a unified conscious experience of a global or gestalt character. The brain events remain disparate, being essentially the individual actions of countless neurones that are built into complex circuits and so participate in the spatiotemporal patterns of activity. This is the case even for the most specialized neurones so far detected, the feature detection neurones of the inferotemporal lobe of primates (chapter E2). Our present hypothesis regards the neuronal machinery as a multiplex of radiating and receiving structures: *the experienced unity comes, not from a neurophysiological synthesis, but from the proposed integrating character of the self-conscious mind.* We conjecture that in the first place the self-conscious mind is developed in order to give this unity of the self in all of its conscious experiences and actions.

In refining the conjecture we have to imagine that in the liaison areas of the cerebral hemisphere some sensory input causes here and there an immense ongoing dynamic pattern of neural activity. As described in chapter E1 the primary sensory areas project to secondary and these to tertiary and so on (cp. Figs. E1–7 and 8). In these further stages the different sensory modalities project to common areas, the polymodal areas. In these areas most varied and wide-ranging information is being processed in the unitary components, the modules of the cerebral cortex (cp. chapter E1). We may ask how is this to be selected from and put together to give the unity and the relative simplicity of our conscious experience from moment to moment? As an answer to this question it is proposed that the self-conscious mind plays through the whole liaison brain in a selective and unifying manner. An analogy is provided by a searchlight in the manner that has been suggested by Jung [1954] and by Popper [1945]. Perhaps a better analogy would be some multiple scanning and probing device that reads out from and selects from the immense and diverse patterns of activity in the cerebral cortex and integrates these selected components, so organizing them into the unity of conscious experience. Thus we conjecture that the self-conscious mind is scanning the modular activities in the liaison areas of the cerebral cortex, as may be appreciated from the very inadequate diagram in Figure E7–2. From moment to moment it is selecting modules according to its interest, the phenomenon of attention, and is itself integrating from all this diversity to give the unified conscious experience. Available for this read-out, if we may call it so, is the whole range of performance of those areas of the dominant hemisphere which have linguistic and ideational performance or which have polymodal inputs. Collectively we will call them *liaison areas*. Brodmann areas 39 and 40 and the prefrontal lobes (cp. Fig. E1–4) are probably most important in this respect.

It might be claimed that this hypothesis is just an elaborated version of parallelism – a kind of selective parallelism. However, that would be a mistake. It differs radically in that the selectional and integrational functions are conjectured to be attributes of the self-conscious mind, which is thus given an active and dominant role. There is a complete contrast with the passivity of conscious experience postulated in parallelism (cp. Feigl [1967]). Furthermore the active role of the self-conscious mind is extended in our hypothesis to effect changes in the neuronal events. Thus not only does it read out selectively from the ongoing activities of the neuronal machinery but it also modifies these activities. For example, when following up a line of thought or trying to recapture a memory, it is proposed that the self-conscious mind is actively engaged in searching and in probing through specially selected zones of the neural machinery and so is able to deflect and mould the dynamic patterned activities in accord with its desire or interest. A special aspect of this intervention of the self-conscious mind upon the operations of the neural machinery is exhibited in its ability to bring about movements in accord with some voluntary desired action, what we may call a motor command. The readiness potential is a sign that this command brings about changes in the activity of the neural machinery (chapter E3, Fig. 4).

The essential feature of the hypothesis is the active role of the self-conscious mind in its influence on the neural machinery of the liaison brain. Recent experimental investigations provide evidence on the time relations of this influence. The experiments of Libet on the human brain (chapter E2) show that direct stimulation of the somaesthetic cortex results in a conscious experience after a delay as long as 0.5 s for weak stimulation, and a similar delay is observed for a sharp, but weak, peripheral skin stimulus. As described in chapter E2, although there is this delay in experiencing the peripheral stimulus, it is actually judged to be much earlier, at about the time of cortical arrival of the afferent input (cp. Fig. E2−3D). This antedating procedure does not seem to be explicable by any neurophysiological process. Presumably it is a strategy that has been learnt by the self-conscious mind. Two comments may be made. In the first place these long recognition times of up to 0.5 s (Fig. E2−2) are attributable to the necessity for building up an immense and complex patterned neuronal activity before it is detectable by the scanning self-conscious mind. Secondly, the antedating of the sensory experience is attributable to the ability of the self-conscious mind to make slight temporal adjustments, i.e. to play tricks with time (Fig. E2−3D). The patterned neuronal activity is detectable by the scanning process of the self-conscious mind at the time that there is the requisite build-up of the neuronal activity. The antedating is effected by the self-conscious mind in a compensation for the tardy development of weak neuronal spatiotemporal patterns to the threshold level for conscious recognition. In this way all experienced events may have a time correction so that the experiences will have a time sequence corresponding to the initiating stimuli, whether they be strong or weak. We suggest that Libet has discovered a temporal adjustment attributable to the self-conscious mind.

Another temporal property of the self-conscious mind is displayed by the long duration of the readiness potential (Fig. E3−4). In the light of the hypothesis it can now be proposed that, when willing brings about a movement, there is continuous action of the self-conscious mind on a neuronal field of great extent. As a consequence of this action there is an increase in neuronal activity over this wide area of the cerebral cortex, and then a long and complex moulding process leading to the eventual homing in on the motor pyramidal cells that are appropriate for bringing about the desired movement. The self-conscious mind does not effect a direct action on these motor pyramidal cells. Instead, the self-conscious mind works remotely and slowly over a wide range of the cortex so that there is a time delay for the surprisingly long duration of 0.8 s. When evaluating such times we should refer to the scale of neuronal time, transmission from one neurone to the next occuring in about 1 ms. The readiness potential indicates that the sequential activity of many hundreds of neurones is involved in the long incubation time of the self-conscious mind in eventually evoking discharges from the motor pyramidal cells. Presumably this time is employed in building up the requisite spatiotemporal patterns in millions of neurones in the cerebral cortex. It is a sign that the action of the self-conscious mind on the brain is not of demanding strength. We may regard it as being more tentative and subtle and as requiring time to build up patterns of activity that may be modified as they develop (cp. chapter E3). Furthermore we have to remember that during the readiness potential there will be the complex neuronal circuitry involved in preprogramming activity as described in chapter E3, circuits that include the cerebellum and the basal ganglia (Figs. E3−6 and 7). In summary, our hypothesis helps to resolve and redefine the problems involved in accounting for the long duration of the readiness potential that precedes a voluntary action.

52. The Hypothesis of Cortical Modules and the Self-conscious Mind

We can now ask the question: What neural events are in liaison with the self-conscious mind both for giving and receiving? The question concerns the World 1 side of the interface between World 1 and World 2. We reject the hypothesis that the agent is the field potential generated by the neural events. The original postulate of the gestalt school was based on the finding that a massive visual input such as a large illuminated circle resulted in some topologically equivalent potential field in the visual cortex, even a closed loop! This crude hypothesis need not be further considered. However a more refined version has recently been proposed by Pribram [1971] in his postulate of micro-potential fields. It is assumed that these fields provide a more subtle cortical response than the impulse generation by neurones. However, this field potential theory involves a tremendous loss of information because hundreds of thousands of neurones would be contributing to a micro-potential field across a small zone of the cerebral cortex. All the finer grain of neuronal activity would be lost in this most inefficient task of generating a minute electrical potential by current flow in the ohmic resistance provided by the extracellular medium. In addition we have the further problem that there would have to be some homunculus to read out the potentials in all their patterned array! The assumed feedback from micro-potential fields onto the firing frequencies of neurones would be of negligible influence because the currents would be extremely small.

We must believe that there is an essential functional meaning in all the discrete neuronal interactions in spatiotemporal patterns, otherwise there would be great losses of information. In this context, we must consider the organization of the cortical neurones in the anatomical and physiological entity that is called a module (chapter E1, Figs. E1−5 and 6). In the first place it is inconceivable that the self-conscious mind is in liaison with single nerve cells or single nerve fibres as has been proposed by Barlow [1972]. These neuronal units as individuals are far too unreliable and ineffective. In our present understanding of the mode of operation of neural machinery we emphasize ensembles of neurones (many hundreds) acting in some collusive patterned array. Only in such assemblages can there be reliability and effectiveness. As described in chapter E1 the modules of the cerebral cortex (Figs. 5 and 6) are such ensembles of neurones. The module has to some degree a collective life of its own with as many as 10,000 neurones of diverse types and with a functional arrangement of feed-forward and feedback excitation and inhibition. As yet we have little knowledge of the inner dynamic life of a module, but we may conjecture that, with its complexly organized and intensely active properties, it could be a component of the physical world (World 1) that is open to the self-conscious mind (World 2) both for receiving from and for giving to. We can further propose that not all modules in the cerebral cortex have this transcendent property of being "open" to World 2, and thus being the World 1 components of the interface. By definition there would be restriction to the modules of the liaison brain, and only then when they are in the correct level of activity. Each module may be likened to a radio transmitter-receiver unit. Szentágothai has suggested that the module may be thought of as an integrated microcircuit of electronics, only vastly more complicated (cp. chapter E1).

Figure E7−3 gives a diagrammatic illustration of the conjectured relationship of open and closed modules as viewed by looking down at the surface of the cortex. A convenient diagrammatic liberty is to show the columns as separate discs, and not in the close contiguity that is the actual relationship (cp. chapters E1, Figs. 5, 6; E2, Fig. 7). Furthermore it has to be recognized

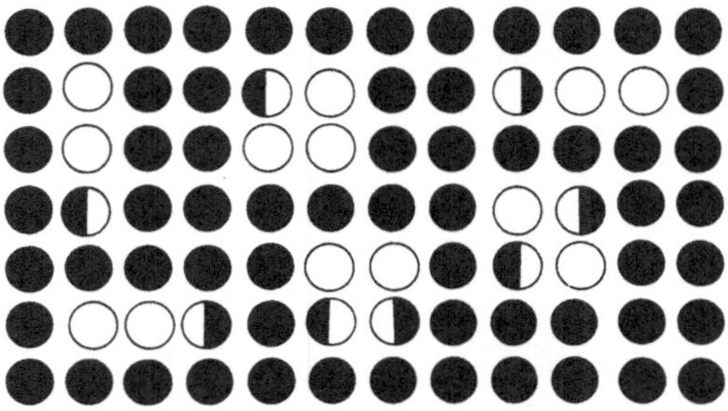

Fig. E7−3. Diagrammatic plan of cortical modules as seen from the surface. As described in the text the modules are shown as circles of three kinds, open, closed (solid black) and half open. Further description in text.

that the normal intensely dynamic situation is frozen in time. The convention is that open modules are shown as open circles, closed as solid circles and that there are also partly open modules. It can be conjectured that the self-conscious mind scans this modular array, being able to receive from and give to only those modules that have some degree of openness. However, by its action on open modules, it can influence closed modules by means of impulse discharges along the association fibres from the open modules, as already described (chapter E1), and may in this manner cause the opening of closed modules. It can be conjectured that there is an intense dynamic interaction between modules. Interaction would be by inhibitory action on the immediately adjacent modules (cp. chapter E1, Figs. 5 and 6) and by the excitatory actions of association and commissural fibres for the more remote modules. Figure E7−4 shows in an extremely simplified form how sequential excitatory action by association fibres can result in some spatiotemporal patterns of modular interaction with even a closed loop. Since each module has some hundreds of pyramidal and stellate pyramidal cells with axons passing out of the module to other modules (chapter E1), the impulses discharged by a module would project to many other modules, as indicated by the radiating arrows, and not just the one or two drawn in Figure E7−4. It may even be projecting to hundreds, altering their activity, and these in turn to hundreds of others. The complexity of the spreading pattern of activation is beyond all imagination, and would result in convulsive seizures were it not for the controlling inhibitory actions between modules as described in chapter E1.

The simplest hypothesis of mind-brain interaction is that the self-conscious mind can scan the activity of each module of the liaison brain — or at

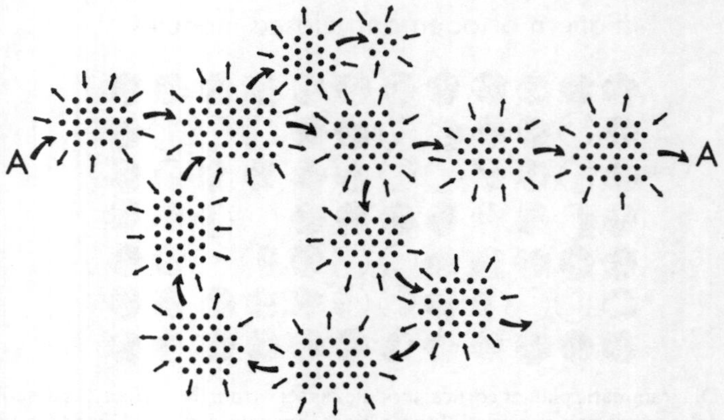

Fig. E7 – 4. In this schema of the cerebral cortex looked at from above, the large pyramidal cells are represented as dots that are arranged in clusters, each cluster corresponding to a column or module as diagrammed in Figs. E1 – 5 and 6, where only two large projecting pyramidal cells are shown of the hundreds that would be in the column. The arrows symbolize impulse discharges along hundreds of lines in parallel, which are the mode of excitatory communication from column to column. Only a minimal system of serially excited columns is shown.

least those modules tuned in to its present interests. We have already conjectured that the self-conscious mind has the function of integrating its selections from the immense patterned input it receives from the liaison brain – the modular activities in this present hypothesis – in order to build its experiences from moment to moment. The modules selected in this way constitute for the moment the World 1 side of the interface between World 1 and World 2. This interface is thus a constantly changing territory within the extensive area of the liaison brain. We have even presented evidence in chapter E2 that the self-conscious mind can make slight temporal adjustments in order to correct for perceptual delays. In this way events from the external world come to be experienced in the correct temporal relationships regardless of their strength, which is an ability of vital significance, for example, in playing a percussion instrument such as a piano.

As argued in chapter E1, only the afferents that have come in from the thalamic nuclei (*spec. aff.* in Fig. E1 – 5) preponderantly exert their influences at the power level (laminae III, IV and V). So it is conjectured that in the dynamic control and poise of the operating cerebral cortex there are all kinds of levels of subtlety and sensitivity in which activity is changed slightly, not with a "bash." Presumably the self-conscious mind does not act on the cortical modules with some bash operation, but rather with a slight deviation. A very gentle deviation up or down is all that is required. It may be conjectured that this effect builds up at the superficial laminae (I and II) and modulates and controls the discharges of pyramidal cells, which of course work on other modules. They are all playing this interacting game with one another. Furthermore we would conjecture that the self-conscious mind is weak relative to the power of the synaptic mechanisms in laminae III, IV and V that are activated by the thalamic inputs. It is simply a deviator, and modifies the modular activity by its slight deviations.

We have to consider the arrangements for modular interaction through association and commissural fibres (chapter E1, Fig. 5), which are axons of the pyramidal cells of other modules. Thus each module is projecting to many others and they in turn are firing back. So we have long and complex patterns of this mutual interaction. We conjecture that the self-conscious mind acts in modifying slightly some of these modules, presumably hundreds, and that the modules collectively react to these modifications which are transmitted by the circuits of the association fibres and the callosal fibres. In addition the self-conscious mind is all the time apprehending or perceiving the responses that it is making in this subtle manner and the neuronal build-up therefrom. It is an essential feature of the hypothesis that the relations between modules and the self-conscious mind are reciprocal, the self-conscious mind being both an activator and a receiver in the manner that has been extensively treated in this chapter and that will be further discussed in chapter E8 on memory.

As a consequence of the investigations (chapters E 5, E 6) on global and circumscribed lesions of the human brain we may conjecture that the liaison brain comprises a large part of the dominant hemisphere, particularly the linguistic areas and the polymodal areas as well as a large area of the prefrontal lobe. These extensive areas probably are composed of several large continuous sheets of cerebral cortex. However, the actual interface of open cortical modules of interest to the self-conscious mind at any moment would probably have a spotty or patchy character. The reading out by the self-conscious mind would be concerned not with anatomical contiguity, but with the modules in functional communication by association or even by commissural fibres. The integrational operation of the self-conscious mind in giving the unity of conscious experience would not be aided by the spatial proximity of modules. It is their functional interconnection that is important.

In further developing the hypothesis of some modules being open to World 2 in the guise of the self-conscious mind, we may suppose that the self-conscious mind does not make a superficial pass over the module, as may be imagined if it merely sensed the micropotential fields in the area. Rather we have to envisage that it "probes" into the module, reading out and influencing the dynamic patterns of the individual neuronal performances. We can assume that this is done from moment to moment over the whole scattered assemblage of those modules processing information of immediate interest (attention) to the self-conscious mind for its integrational performance.

Another important feature of the interaction of self-conscious mind with modules is that, by its interaction with "open" modules, the self-conscious mind can indirectly interact with "closed" modules.

Since the self-conscious mind is in liaison with open modules of the left hemisphere that project through the corpus callosum, we conjecture that there is a way into the right hemisphere for the self-conscious mind via open modules of the left hemisphere through the corpus callosum into all of the specialized but closed modules of the right hemisphere. These modules in turn will feed back into the open modules of the left hemisphere in a symmetrical two-way operation. Thus the self-conscious mind can be engaged in the active processing of information in the right hemisphere. There is a wealth of association and commissural connections whereby modules communicate very effectively both within a hemisphere and to the other hemisphere via the corpus callosum. There must be a very rich connectivity, and this is revealed by the losses of brain performance when the corpus callosum is sectioned, or when large areas of brain are ablated. For example, both speech and verbal memory suffer after commissurotomy or after minor hemisphere lesions (chapters E 5, E 6; Sperry [1970], [1974]; Brodal [1973]; Milner [1974]). Surprisingly, section of the anterior 80% of the corpus callosum had as deleterious effect on memory as complete section (Sperry [1974]). The intact posterior segment appears to be ineffective for memory transfer; nevertheless such patients displayed no evidence of commissurotomy by the tests described in chapter E 5.

53. Sleep, Dreams and Various Forms of Unconsciousness

We do know that, as sleep comes on, both the level of the cerebral activity and the patterns of neuronal discharges are changing. In the patterns normally running, the successive interspike intervals have a random arrangement about some mean value, which may fluctuate up or down. The ordinary rhythms of the electroencephalogram (EEG) show that. When you record from neurones during sleep you find out that they have lost their normal waking patterns. Some are going slow, some faster; and there is some chaos taking over, with firing in bursts. Sleep doesn't mean cessation of activity, but it is something much more like disordered activity (Evarts [1964]). When this happens, I would say that the self-conscious mind finds there is nothing to read out. All modules are closed to it. Suddenly it is deprived of data and this is unconsciousness. Reading nothing gives nothing.

But every now and then during the night, every 2 or 3 hours, we know that some organized cerebral activity is assumed with the rapid low voltage waves in the EEG. This is what is called paradoxical sleep. There are rapid eye movements with various muscle actions corresponding and then the self-conscious mind finds again an ability to read out from active modules a dream with strange and even bizarre conscious experiences, but always recognizably its own dream. During the dream cycle it may be conjectured that the self-conscious mind is reading out from the neuronal activities in the brain, even from the most disordered neuronal happenings, yet nevertheless they are assimilated to itself. They may relate to its past experiences and often are reminiscences or playback to other experiences of earlier life. Sometimes there are such bizarre experiences that the dream seems not at all assimilable to anything that happened in the remembered life, but which may have some deeper meaning that we don't know, as Freud conjectured. In any case this is the way the self-conscious mind is working in relationship to the brain. With waking up, the self-conscious mind seems gradually to pull itself together, finding some organized open modules, an illumination here or there in patterned operation, and soon the dawning consciousness of the new day comes in patches and in limited experiences and gradually there is assemblage together. You remember where you are, you remember the plans already made for the coming day, you remember what you immediately have to do; and you then resume the full waking day.

I think all of this has to be thought of as if the self-conscious mind has probably been, as it were, probing over or scanning over the cerebral cortex all through the sleep, searching for any modules that are open and which can be utilized for an experience. We also know that quite a lot of "dreams" go on in the self-conscious mind, which no doubt is scanning continuously and effectively over the liaison brain, but they are not remembered on waking, perhaps hours later. A dream can be recalled if the subject is wakened while the associated neural events can be seen going on in the recorded EEG and eye movements. If you wake him up 10 minutes or more later, he usually has no recall of any dream, yet a dream state was indicated by the records. Moreover you can statistically be sure that the records are reliable indicators of dreams because, if you awaken the subject during or just after the paradoxical sleep signalled by the electroencephalogram, a dream is reported in about 90% of the cases. These findings give important information about the way the self-conscious mind is related to the brain. I suggest it is always there scanning the brain, but the brain is not always in a communicative state for it!

A characteristic feature of most dreams is that the subject of the dream feels a most disturbing impotence. He is immersed in the dream experience, but feels a frustrating inability to take any desired action. Of course he is acting in the dream, but with the experience that in doing so he is a puppet. His self-conscious mind can experience but not act effectively, which is exactly the position of the parallelists, such as the identity theorists. The difference between dream states and waking states constitutes a refutation of parallelism. A parallelist world would be a dream world!

I will now consider other unconscious states. For example, what happens to the self-conscious mind in the much more severe states of cerebral depression that occur, first of all in deep anaesthesia, or secondly in comas of different kinds? We know that in deep coma there is cessation of all neuronal discharges. There can be for a considerable time no EEG. If this occurs for as long as 30 minutes it is likely to be irreversible, in which case the cerebral hemispheres have died, the so-called brain death. During these severe states of unconsciousness, we may ask if the self-conscious mind is still trying to scan and find some little focus which could give an experience or not? What happens is beyond our understanding and may be unknowable.

The next cerebral condition for consideration is the opposite state, convulsions. In an epileptic seizure a most intense driven activation of the constituent neurones is travelling over the brain. We know that at a certain level of involvement, a certain mass of involvement of the brain, the subject loses consciousness. He can be conscious with seizures occupying perhaps 50% of the cerebral cortex, but no more. Then he loses consciousness and there is a long period before recovery comes. After the seizure is over, the brain gradually recovers from its intense convulsive activity. For some time it is in disorder, and again the subject has no record of what is happening. We can think that the self-conscious mind is scanning to no effect.

Finally, of course we come to the ultimate picture, what happens in death? Then all cerebral activity ceases permanently. The self-conscious mind that has had an autonomous existence in a sense in World 2 now finds that the brain that it has scanned and probed and controlled so efficiently and effectively through a long life is no longer giving any messages at all. What happens then is the ultimate question.

54. Plasticity of "Open" Modules

We have proposed that there is some unique dynamic performance in the modules of the liaison brain that makes them open to transmit to and to receive from the self-conscious mind. We can now consider the situation at the plastic state which seems to occur in early life, where both the left and right hemispheres have linguistic ability, and where damage to the linguistic areas of the left hemisphere may result in transfer of dominance to the right hemisphere (Milner [1974]). At that early stage we can conjecture that some modules of both hemispheres have the property of being "open" to World 2 and that damage to such modules in the left hemisphere results in the further development of such modular properties in the right hemisphere, along with the transfer of speech. We are therefore introduced to the problems of the plasticity of modular properties in their unique relationship to World 2. During the early years of life, when the left hemisphere assumes dominance with almost the monopoly of speech, is there regression of the "open" modules of the right hemisphere? We may further ask if the scanning operation of the self-conscious mind somehow is restricted to "open" modules, and are there no "open" modules in the right (minor) hemisphere, as is indicated in Figure E 5 – 7? Alternatively there could be "open" modules, as indicated by the arrows with broken shafts in the upper part of Fig. E 7–5, but they lose this property after the trauma of commissurotomy which permanently interrupts the powerful lines of communication (the 200 million fibres), so that the minor hemisphere loses its liaison with World 2 (cp. chapter E 5). There is further discussion in dialogues V, VII and IX.

55. Summary

We can now briefly consider the implications of the strong dualist hypothesis that we have formulated. Its central component is that primacy is given to the self-conscious mind. It is proposed that the self-conscious mind is actively engaged in searching for brain events that are of its present interest, the operation of attention, but it also is the integrating agent, building the unity of conscious experience from all the diversity of the brain events. Even more importantly it is given the role of actively modifying the brain events according to its interest or desire, and the scanning operation by which it searches can be envisaged as having an active role in selection. Sperry [1970] has made a similar proposal.

> "Conscious phenomena in this scheme are conceived to interact with and to largely govern the physiochemical and physiological aspects of the brain process. It obviously works the other way round as well, and thus a mutual interaction is conceived between the physiological and the mental properties. Even so, the present interpretation would tend to restore mind to its old prestigious position over matter, in the sense that the mental phenomena are seen to transcend the phenomena of physiology and biochemistry."

It has been suggested here that this interaction of the self-conscious mind and the brain is dependent on the arrangement of the cerebral neurones in the modules that are defined by anatomical and physiological studies. It is proposed that each module has an intense and subtle inner dynamic life based upon the collective interaction of its many thousands of constituent neurones. These components of the physical world (World 1) come in this way to be momentary constituents of a fundamental interface, being "open" to two-way influences from another world, the self-conscious mind of World 2. Not all of the modules of the cerebral hemispheres are "open" in this way. After the commissurotomy operation the self-conscious mind is in liaison only with the dominant hemisphere, and it is proposed that the liaison area is further restricted to the linguistic areas in the widest sense, to the polymodal sensory areas, particularly of the prefrontal lobe and to the ideational areas whereby the self-conscious mind communicates non-verbally, as for example pictorially and musically. We propose that the self-conscious mind can read out at will from the modules of that great area of neuronal activation in the dominant hemisphere. From moment to moment only a minute fraction is so sampled, and much that is read is held only for seconds in the short-term memory (cp. chapter E 8). Thus the greater part of our conscious experiences are ephemeral. However, concentration on special deliverances of the self-conscious mind can start neuronal processes of storage that are the basis of intermediate and long-term memories (chapter E 8). We would conjecture that the self-conscious mind is actively engaged in the process of laying down this memory storage and in retrieving from it. We will develop these ideas in chapter E 8.

It can be claimed that the strong dualist-interactionist hypothesis that has been here developed has the recommendation of its great explanatory power. It gives in principle at least explanations of the whole range of problems relating to brain-mind interaction. It also aids in the understanding of some aspects of memory and illusion and creative imagination (see discussions). But most importantly it restores to the human person the senses of wonder, of mystery and of value. In the discussions there will be many exchanges with respect to the manner in which the World 3 $\rightleftarrows$ World 2 interaction is necessary for the creation of a human person — necessary but not sufficient.

MODES OF INTERACTION BETWEEN HEMISPHERES

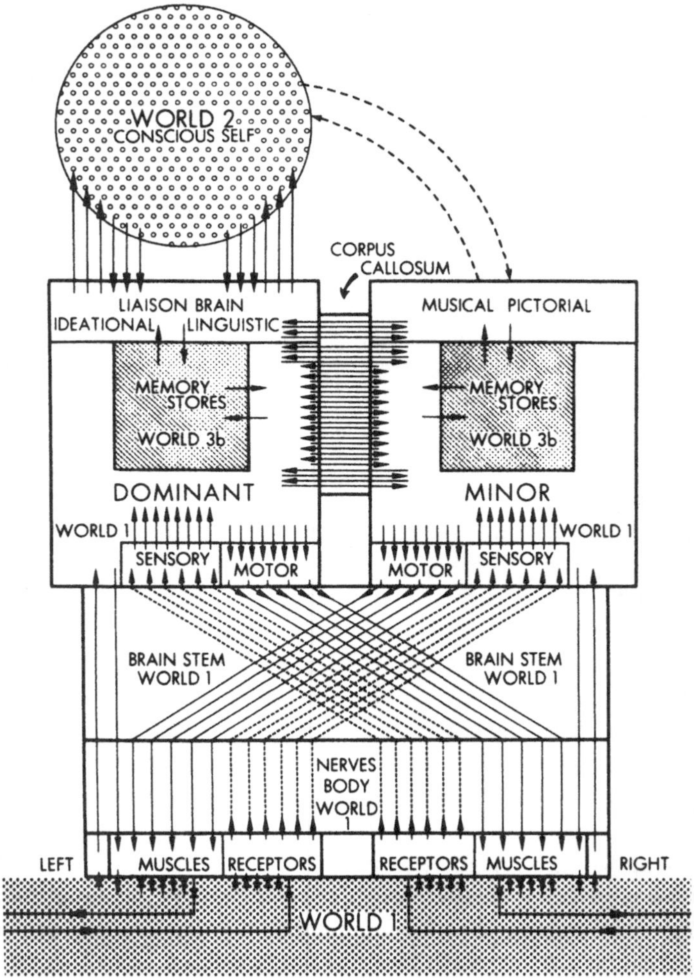

Fig. E7–5. The same diagram as in Fig. E5–7, but with addition (broken lines) of possible lines of communication from World 2 to the minor hemisphere.

Finally it can be claimed that the hypothesis belongs to science because it is based on empirical data and is objectively testable. It must be emphasized that, just as with other scientific theories of great explanatory power, the present hypothesis has to be subjected to empirical testing. However, it is claimed that it is not refuted by any existing knowledge. It can be predicted optimistically that there will be a long period of remodelling and development, but not an irretrievable falsification.

The philosophical implications of this hypothesis of brain-mind liaison will be further considered in many places of the discussion (dialogues V, VI, VII, VIII, IX, X, XII). There will also be consideration there (dialogue X) of the thermodynamic implications of these conjectured actions across the interface between brain and mind as diagrammed in Figure E 7−2.

If as conjectured the self-conscious mind is not a special part of World 1, that is of the physical and biological worlds, it is likely to have different fundamental properties. Though it is in liaison with special zones of the neocortex, it need not itself have the property of spatial extension. Apparently it integrates instantaneously what it reads out from diverse scattered elements of the active neocortex, largely of the dominant hemisphere, but probably also from the minor hemisphere of the normal brain (cp. Fig. E 7−5). But the question: where is the self-conscious mind located? is unanswerable in principle. This can be appreciated when we consider some components of the self-conscious mind. It makes no sense to ask where are located the feelings of love or hate, or of joy or fear, or of such values as truth, goodness and beauty which apply to mental appraisals. These are experienced. Abstract concepts such as in mathematics have no location per se, but can be materialized, as it were, in specific examples or demonstrations. Similarly a location of the self-conscious mind appears when its actions become materialized in its interactions with the liaison brain. It is otherwise with the question: does the self-conscious mind have some specific temporal properties? Experienced time does transcend clock time by its slowing in acute emergencies and in the experiments of Libet on antedating (Fig. E 2−3 D). It also transcends clock time in the recall and reliving of past experiences and in the imaginative prediction of happenings in the future, which can be experienced emotionally, for example with joyous anticipations or with dire forebodings. But, in our general waking experiences, experienced times and clock times are virtually synchronized, as well they must be for the effective control of actions in response to present situations. Thus for practical purposes experienced time and clock time are closely locked together. We can thus envisage that World 2 has a temporal property, but not a spatial property. However, much more investigation is needed into these deep questions.

Chapter E8 Conscious Memory: The Cerebral Processes Concerned in Storage and Retrieval

56. Résumé

In this chapter there is an attempt to answer the question: How can we recover or re-experience some events or some simple test situation as, for example, a number or a word sequence? This problem is discussed in two levels. In the first level it is a problem of neurobiology concerned with the structural and functional changes in the brain that form the basis of memory. It is attractive to conjecture that with memories enduring for years there is some structural basis in the way of changed connectivities in the neuronal machinery. This would explain that there is a tendency for the replay of the spatiotemporal patterns of neural activity that occurred in the initial experience. This replaying in the brain would be accompanied by remembering in the mind. The second level concerns the role of the self-conscious mind. This is essentially a development of the theory formulated in chapter E7.

The neurobiological level of memory is illustrated by a study of synaptic structure and synaptic action under conditions either of enhanced activity (Figs. E8−1, 2 and 3) or of disuse. In this way it is shown that there are modifiable synapses that could be responsible for memory because they are greatly enhanced by activity and depleted by disuse (Fig. E8−4). It is concluded that the excitatory spine synapses (chapter E1, Fig. 2D) are probably the modifiable synapses concerned in memory. There is further consideration of the manner in which activity could result in growth and increased effectiveness.

It is generally recognized that the memory processes are composite in time, there being very short memories of a few seconds, probably intermediate memories of seconds to hours and, finally, long-term memories of hours to a lifetime. This composite is illustrated in Figure E8−7. In short-term memory of a few seconds, it can be recognized that the remembered event has to be perceived by continual verbal rehearsal as, for example, when one is reading and then dialing a telephone number. It is conjectured that such brief memories are retained in the self-conscious mind because it is reading out from the continued activity in neuronal circuits that carry the information to be recovered.

Remarkable evidence for this brief memory is derived from patients in which there has been bilateral removal of the hippocampi (Fig. E8 – 6). This was carried out for bilateral epileptic seizures involving the hippocampi. It was not recognized that a tragic memory loss would result. Such patients have not lost the memories from before the operation, but they have an almost complete failure to establish any new memories. Brief descriptions are given of the extraordinary disabilities resulting from this loss of all memories except those of the shortest duration. It is concluded that the hippocampus is necessary for bringing about the storage processes for all memories except those of the verbal rehearsal type, but it is not itself the site of the storage.

It is conjectured that the hippocampus participates in the consolidation of memory by virtue of the operation of circuits especially from the prefrontal lobe to the hippocampus and back again to the neocortex (Figs. E1 – 9, E8 – 7). It is further suggested that the pathway from the hippocampus to the neocortex may act in an instruction-selection manner analogous to that of the climbing fibre pathway to the cerebellum (Fig. E8 – 9). These proposed operative circuits (Figs. E8 – 8, E8 – 10) are already known anatomically but have not been studied physiologically. It is suggested that the hippocampus plays a key role in this memory storage because it has been shown to be very susceptible to moderate levels of activation. Under such conditions, the transmitting synapses display a greatly increased and prolonged effectiveness (Figs. E8 – 1, 2 and 3). There are many challenging types of investigation deriving from this general theory of memory storage and the role of the hippocampus.

Particularly important in conscious memory is the role of the self-conscious mind that commands, as it were, the storage data banks in the cerebral cortex by virtue of its action across the interface between World 2 and World 1 (Fig. E7 – 2). The self-conscious mind can bring about activities in the brain which are effective in the retrieval of information from the data banks that probably are widely distributed over the cerebral cortex. The retrieved information is read out from the liaison areas of the brain and checked against the expected result by what we may call the recognition memory function of the self-conscious mind. By virtue of this memory recognition, the self-conscious mind may discover that the retrieval from the data bank is erroneous and institute a further search through the data banks of the brain in the attempt to secure a memory that is recognized as being correct. It is evident that a continual interaction between the self-conscious mind and the liaison brain is just as necessary in memory retrieval as in voluntary action.

Some evidence about location and operation of data banks in the brain is derived from the fascinating discoveries of Penfield in respect of the experiential memories that are recovered by gentle electrical stimulation on the surfaces of the brains of unanesthetized subjects (Fig. E8−5). The preferred areas for this phenomenon are largely in the temporal lobes, particularly in the minor hemisphere. Experiences of the kind described in the text are not evoked by stimulation of normal brains, but only the brains of patients subject to epileptic seizures.

There is a brief discussion of the durations of the various kinds of memories, it being suggested that at least three separate memory processes are concerned in giving us the continuity of memory that we normally experience (Fig. E8−7). There are firstly the brief rehearsal memories of seconds, secondly the longer memories for hours, probably of a physiological kind (post-tetanic potentiation) that bridge the gap between the very short memories and the slowly developing memories that are dependent upon synaptic growth and that normally require times measured in hours for effective development.

At the end of the chapter there is a treatment of neuronal performances related to memory, namely the plastic responses that occur in the brain subjected to specific inputs and the active responses to these inputs (Fig. E8−8).

57. Introduction

The theme of this chapter is conscious memory. It is an attempt to answer the question: How can we recover or re-experience some events, or some simple test situation, as for example a number or word sequence? It will be recognized that two distinct problems are involved — storage and retrieval, or in relation to our present problem of conscious memory, learning and remembering. It is proposed to deal with these problems at two levels.

Firstly, it will be considered as a problem of neurobiology, namely the structural and functional changes which form the basis of memory. It is generally supposed that the recall of a memory involves the replay in an approximate manner of the neuronal events that were responsible for the experience that is being recalled. There is no specially difficult problem with short-term memories for a few seconds. It can be conjectured that this is effected by the neural events continuing during the verbal or pictorial rehearsal. The distinctive patterns of neuronal activity that are suggested in Figure E7–4 thus continue to recirculate for the whole duration of these brief memories and are available for read-out. On the other hand, with memories enduring for minutes to years, it has to be discovered how the neuronal connectivities are changed so that there tends to be stabilized some tendency for replay of the spatiotemporal patterns of neuronal activity that occurred in the initial experience, and that have meanwhile subsided.

Secondly, the role of the self-conscious mind has to be considered. We have conjectured in chapter E7 that a conscious experience arises when the self-conscious mind enters into an effective relationship with certain activated modules, "open" modules, in the cerebral cortex. In the willed recall of a memory the self-conscious mind must again be in relationship to a pattern of modular responses resembling the original responses evoked by the event to be remembered, so that there is a reading out of approximately the same experience. We have to consider how the self-conscious mind is concerned in calling forth the neuronal events that give the remembered experience on demand, as it were. Furthermore the self-conscious mind acts as an arbiter or assessor with respect to the correctness or relevance of the memory that is delivered on demand. For example the name or number may be recognized as incorrect by the self-conscious mind, and a further recall process may be instituted, and so on. Thus the recall of a memory involves two distinct processes in the self-conscious mind: firstly that of recall from the data-banks in the brain; secondly the recognition memory that judges its correctness.

58. Structural and Functional Changes Possibly Related to Memory

There have been theories of long-term memory based upon a supposed analogy with genetic or immunological memory. For example it has been conjectured that memories are encoded in specific macromolecules, in particular RNA (Hydén [1965], [1967]), or that it is analogous to immunological memory (Szilard [1964]). These theories fail for various reasons (cp. Eccles [1970]; Szentágothai [1971]) and need not here be further discussed. A brief account will now be given of the evidence for the generally accepted growth theory of learning in the central nervous system.

In general terms following Sherrington [1940], Adrian [1947], Lashley [1950] and Szentágothai [1971] we have to suppose that long-term memories are somehow encoded in the neuronal connectivities of the brain. We are thus led to conjecture that the structural basis of memory lies in modifications of synapses (cp. Eccles [1970]; Szentágothai [1971]). In mammals there is no evidence for growth or change of major neuronal pathways in the brain after their initial formation. It is not possible to construct or reconstruct major brain pathways at such a gross level. But it should be possible to secure the necessary changes in neuronal connectivity by microstructural changes in synapses (cp. Eccles [1976]). For example, they may be hypertrophied or they may bud additional synapses, or alternatively they may regress. Since it would be expected that the increased synaptic efficacy would arise because of a strong conditioning synaptic activation, experiments such as those illustrated in Figure E8 – 1 have been carried out on many types of synapses.

Figure E8 – 1B is remarkable in showing that repetitive stimulation results in a large increase (up to six times) in the excitatory post-synaptic potentials, EPSPs, monosynaptically produced in an α motoneurone by

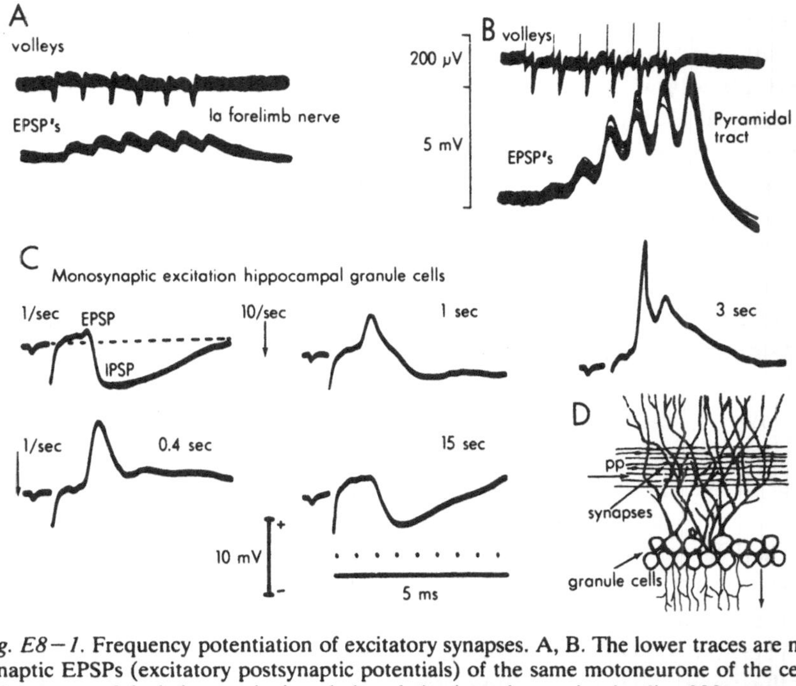

Fig. E8 – 1. Frequency potentiation of excitatory synapses. A, B. The lower traces are monosynaptic EPSPs (excitatory postsynaptic potentials) of the same motoneurone of the cervical enlargement of the baboon spinal cord, there being in each case six stimuli at 200 per second to the Ia afferent pathway in A and to the pyramidal tract in B. (Landgren, S., Phillips, C. G., and Porter, R., J. Physiol., 161:91 [1962].). C shows frequency potentiation of monosynaptic EPSPs of hippocampal granule cells (shown in D) when the frequency of stimulation of the perforating pathway (*pp* of D) was increased from 1 to 10 per second, and its decline on return to 1 per second (Bliss and Lømo, 1973).

pyramidal tract fibres (cp. Fig. E3 – 3). By contrast in Figure E8 – 1A the EPSPs generated monosynaptically in that same motoneurone by I a fibres from muscle spindles (cp. Fig. E3 – 2) were not potentiated. Evidently the pyramidal tract synapses display an extreme range of modifiability by what we may call *frequency potentiation*. The synaptic mechanism involved in this potentiation is not understood, but at least we can be sure that it is due to an equivalent increase in emission of the synaptic transmitter substance. Many types of synapses at the higher levels of the brain have this ability to build up operationally during intense activation.

The series of Figures E8 – 1C, D gives another example for synapses in a primitive part of the cerebrum, the hippocampus (cp. chapter E1). The hippocampus is of particular interest because it is believed to be important in the laying down of memory traces, as will be described below. Part D shows the excitatory synapses from the perforating pathway (pp) onto the dendrites of the granule cells. In C the intracellular record from a granule cell during the initial series at 1 per second stimulation of pp showed a very small initial EPSP followed by a large IPSP. With the stimulus frequency raised to 10 per second, already within 1 s there was a large potentiation of the EPSP that counteracted to some extent the IPSP. After 3 s of this stimulation the very large EPSP completely submerged the IPSP and is seen to generate an impulse discharge from the cell. On again slowing the stimulation to 1 per second, the frequency potentiation had already considerably declined at 0.4 s and had disappeared in 15 s. It is attractive to think that synapses responding so enthusiastically during and for some seconds after moderate activation (post-tetanic potentiation) could be the *modifiable synapses* responsible for the phenomena of learning and memory.

Figure E8 – 2 shows a much more enduring kind of post-tetanic potentiation in those same synapses of the hippocampus. A very mild stimulation of 20 per second for 15 s (300 pulses) was applied at the first arrow *(below)*. The plotted points show that there was only a small transient potentiation. But, with successive repetitions (at the later arrows) of this mild stimulation about every half-hour, there was a progressive increase in the potentiation so that after the fifth there was an enormous potentiation of the impulse discharge from the granule cells. Actual records are given in the insets, where three test responses may be compared with the three controls below that are given by the other side. The plotted measurements are of the sharp downward extracellular spikes marked by the arrows in these test responses. This large potentiation continued for 3 h. This amazing effect was observed in many such experiments, potentiations being fully maintained even for 10 h in acute experiments (Bliss and Lømo [1973]). In chronic experiments with im-

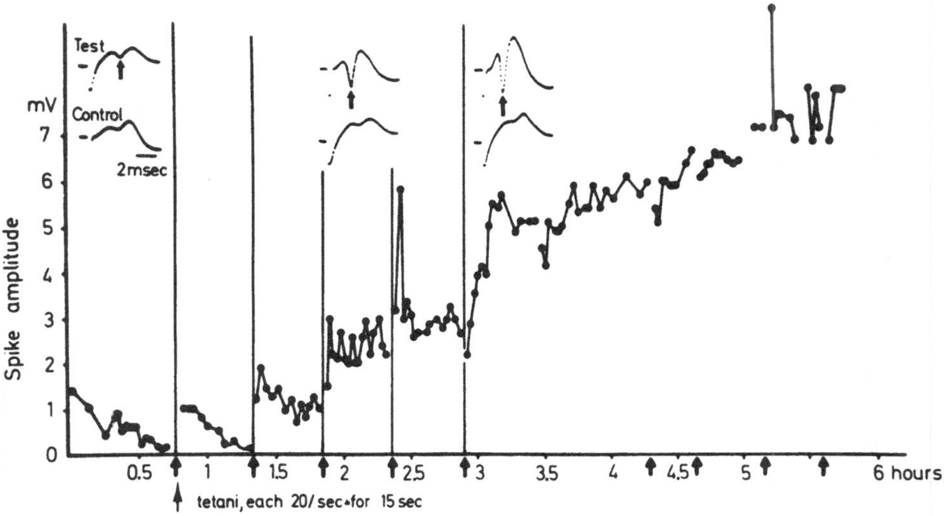

Fig. E8–2. Post-tetanic potentiation of hippocampal granule cells. The measurements were made on the extracellular recording of the positive spike shown in the specimen records above by arrows, and it may be taken to be a measure of the number of granule cells firing impulses in the zone sampled by the recording electrode. Further description in text (Bliss and Lømo, 1973).

planted electrodes a similar potentiation was observed for several weeks after conditioning by six brief trains of stimulation, 15/s for 15 s (Bliss and Gardner Medwin [1973]). In Figure E8–3A the potentiation was built up as in Figure E8–2, but only by the episodes of 60 V stimulation, and is seen in B to have declined to about half by 12 h, but it declined little further at 1 day, 6 days and 16 weeks thereafter. We can conclude that in these experiments there is good evidence that the spine synapses on the dendrites of the hippocampal granule cells are modifiable to a high degree and exhibit a prolonged potentiation that could be the physiological expression of the memory process.

Physiological experiments have thus indicated that the *modifiable synapses* which could be responsible for memory are excitatory and are specially prominent at the higher levels of the brain. In the cerebral cortex the great majority of excitatory synapses on pyramidal cells are on their dendritic spines, as illustrated in Figures E1–2 and 5. There is also much evidence by Valverde [1968] and others that these spine synapses regress during disuse (cp. Eccles [1970]). Hence it is conjectured that these spine synapses on the dendrites of such neurones as the pyramidal cells of the cerebral cortex and the hippocampus, the granule cells of the hippocampus and the Purkyně cells of the cerebellum are the modifiable synapses concerned in learning. These

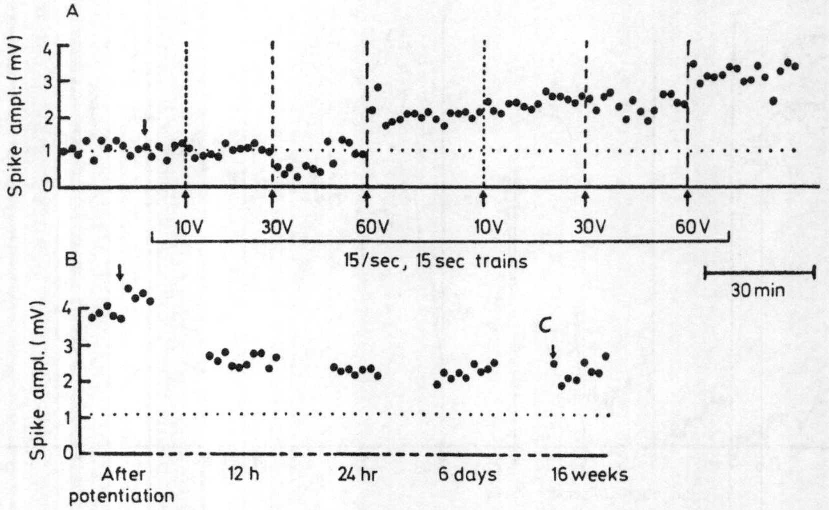

Fig. E8–3. Post-tetanic potentiation of hippocampal granule cells. Measurements of spike amplitudes as in Fig. E8–2 (from averages of 16 responses to 30 V stimuli) plotted as several trains of stimuli (15/sec for 15 sec) were given at the indicated strengths, and at various indicated times afterwards. The approximate mean spike amplitude before the conditioning trains is shown by the dotted lines. Further description in text (Bliss and Gardner-Medwin, 1973).

would be the synapses displaying the indefinitely prolonged potentiation illustrated in Figure E8–2 and 3. One can imagine that the superior performance by these synapses was indefinitely prolonged because a growth process had developed in the dendritic spines giving a structural change which could have great endurance. There is as yet no convincing demonstration of this growth in electronmicrographs, but there is much circumstantial evidence. The conjectured changes are diagrammatically shown in Figure E8–4, where A represents the normal state and B and C the hypertrophied states. An alternative to the synaptic spine hypertrophy of Figure E8–4B is shown in C where an increase in synaptic potency has been secured by branching of the spines to form secondary spine synapses as reported by Szentágothai.

We are on much surer histological grounds in showing the effects of disuse in causing a regression and depletion of spine synapses (Fig. E8–4D). This has been beautifully demonstrated by Valverde [1967] on the dendrites of the pyramidal cells in the visual cortex of mice raised in visual deprivation, and indeed similar demonstrations have been made with other spine synapses, and even with excitatory synapses in the spinal cord (Szentágothai,

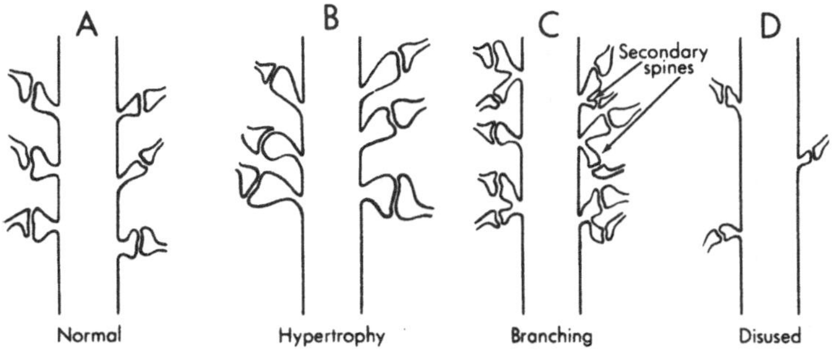

Fig. E8−4. Plasticity of dendritic spine synapses. The drawings are designed to convey the plastic changes in spine synapses that are postulated to occur with growth in B and C and with regression in D. Further description in text.

1971). So it can be assumed that normal usage results in the maintenance of the dendritic spine synapses at the normal level depicted in Figure E8−4A.

It can be concluded that the excitatory spine synapses are probably the modifiable synapses concerned in memory, but much more rigid experimental investigation with systematic electronmicroscopic examination is urgently needed to test this hypothesis. It is surprising that there has as yet been no such systematic study of synapses in the hippocampus under conditions that would be expected to show synaptic hypertrophy.

59. The So-Called Growth Theory of Learning

If synaptic growth is required for learning, there must be an increase in brain metabolism of a special kind with the manufacture of proteins and other macromolecules required for the increases in membranes and in chemical transmission mechanisms. Presumably, in the synaptic growth theory of learning, it must be assumed that RNA is responsible for the protein synthesis required for growth. However, this assumed growth would not be the highly specific chemical phenomenon conjectured in Hydén's [1967] molecular theory of learning, where the coding of memories is attributed to specific macromolecules, each memory being associated with unique macromolecules. Instead the specificities would be encoded in the structure, particularly in the synaptic connections of the nerve cells, which are arranged in the unimaginably complex pattern that has already been formed in development. From then onward, all that seems to be required for the functional reorganization that is assumed to be the neuronal substrate of memory is merely the microgrowth of synaptic connections already in existence as indicated in Figure E8 – 4B,C, which can be regarded as models of the spine synapses on pyramidal cells and Purkyně cells (Eccles [1966], [1970], [1972]). The flow of impulses from receptor organs into the nervous system (cp. chapter E2, Figs. 1, 4) will result in the activation of specific spatiotemporal patterns of neurones linked by sequential impulse discharges. The synapses so activated will grow to an increased effectiveness and even sprout branches to form secondary synapses; hence, the more a particular spatiotemporal pattern of impulses is replayed in the cortex, the more effective become its synapses relative to others. And by virtue of this synaptic efficacy, later similar sensory inputs will tend to traverse these same neuronal pathways and so evoke the same responses, both overt and psychic, as the original input.

However, frequent synaptic excitation alone could hardly provide a satisfactory explanation of synaptic changes involved in learning. Because of the incessant discharging of impulses by most neurones, such "learned" synapses would be too ubiquitous! This criticism of the simple "growth theory" of learning can perhaps be contained by the recent suggestion of Szentágothai [1968] and Marr [1969] that synaptic learning is a dual or dynamically linked happening, namely that activation of a special type of synapse provides instructions for the growth of other activated synapses on the same dendrite. This may be called the "conjunction theory of learning." It was originally suggested that the unique operation of climbing fibres on the Purkyně cell dendrites of the cerebellum (Fig. E3 – 5) was to give "growth instructions" to the spine synapses that are simultaneously activated by the parallel fibres. Though the word instruction has been used, the proposed process is analogous to the "selection" theory of immunity (Jerne [1967]) in that a selection of existing synapses is given an increased potency.

By most ingenious experiments Ito and Miyashita [1975] have provided the first evidence in favour of the conjunction theory of learning. When animals are rotated on a vertical axis, mossy fibre and climbing fibre inputs to a special lobe of the cerebellum (the flocculus) are concerned in controlling the eye movements so that the visual picture suffers a minimum of disturbance. When climbing fibre input from the visual pathways is superimposed on the mossy fibre input from the vestibular pathway, a plastic change results so that the vestibular input becomes more effective in the control of the eye movements. It appears that the climbing fibre input has resulted in a selection of the Purkyně cells learning to respond more effectively to their mossy fibre inputs (cp. Eccles [1977 (a)]). Later we shall suggest an analogous learning system for the cerebral cortex.

Libet & others [1975] have very recently proposed a model for a synaptic memory process that is also a conjunction process between two different synapses on a sympathetic ganglion cell.

> A heterosynaptic interaction takes place between two types of synaptic inputs to the same neurone; the memory trace is initiated by a brief (dopaminergic) input in one synaptic line, while 'read-out' of the memory consists simply in the enhanced ability of the postsynaptic unit to produce its specific response to another (cholinergic) synaptic input. This arrangement provides for a "learned" change in the response to one input as a result of an "experience" previously carried by way of the other input.

This model is based on carefully controlled responses of sympathetic ganglion cells, which display a doubling of response to acetyl-β-methyl choline for many hours after a brief exposure to the other transmitter, dopamine. Furthermore it is shown that cyclic AMP is concerned in the metabolic pathway that gives the heterosynaptic potentiation. It is evident that this discovery is of great significance in relation to the conjunction theory of learning.

In neurochemistry and neuropharmacology there have now been many fine studies by Barondes ([1969], [1970]), Agranoff ([1967], [1969]) and others, which reveal that long-term learning (beyond 3 h) does not occur when either cerebral protein synthesis or RNA synthesis is greatly depressed by poisoning of the specific enzymes by cycloheximide or puromycin. It is conjectured that, in the process of learning, synaptic activation of neurones leads first to specific RNA synthesis and this in turn to protein synthesis and so finally to the unique structural and functional changes involved in the synaptic growth that encodes the memory. Unfortunately the crucial step is not yet understood, namely how synaptic activation can trigger the activities of the appropriate enzymes. However, it is known (Barondes [1970]) that the critical protein synthesis in the brain is in action during the learning process and within minutes has apparently been effective in laying down the memory traces. These experiments suggest that long term memory can be established only if there is an intact protein-synthesizing capacity, an appropriate "state of arousal" and an availability of the information in a short-term memory store (Barondes [1970]).

60. The Role of the Self-conscious Mind in Short-Term Memory

Let us consider some simple and unique perceptual experience, for example the first sight of a bird or flower hitherto unknown to us or of a new model of a car. Firstly, there are the many stages of encoded transmission from retinal image to the various levels of the visual cortex with feature recognition as the highest interpretive level so far recognized, as described in chapter E2. At a further stage we propose the activation of modules of the liaison brain that are "open" to World 2 (chapter E7), the consequent read-out by the self-conscious mind giving the perceptual experience with all its sensual richness. This read-out by the self-conscious mind involves the integration into a unified experience of the specific activities of many modules, an integration that gives the pictured uniqueness to the experience (chapter E7). Furthermore, it is a two-way action, the self-conscious mind modifying the modular activity as well as receiving from it, and possibly evaluating it by testing procedures in an input-output manner. It must further be conjectured that there is an intense patterned interaction of "open" modules with each other and with closed modules, there being for this purpose the immense connectivities provided by association and commissural fibres as described in chapter E1. Moreover we have to postulate closed self-re-exciting chains in these ongoing patterns of modular interaction (cp. chapter E7, Fig. 4). In this way there is a continuation of the dynamic patterned activity in time.

As long as the modular activities continue in this specific patterned interaction, we assume that the self-conscious mind is continuously able to read it out according to its interests and attention. We may say that in this way the new experience is kept in mind – as for example when we try to remember a telephone number between the time of looking it up and dialling. We propose that the continued activity of the modules can be secured by continuous active intervention or reinforcement by the self-conscious mind, which in this way can hold memories by processes that we experience and refer to as either verbal or non-verbal (pictorial or musical, for example) rehearsal. As soon as the self-conscious mind engages in some other task, this reinforcement ceases, that specific pattern of neuronal activities subsides and the short-term memory is lost. Recall now becomes dependent on memory processes of longer duration. McGaugh [1969] measures short-term memory in seconds. It is for example the total memory performance in patients with bilateral ablation of the hippocampus, as will be described in the next section of this chapter (Milner [1966], [1968], [1970], [1972]). Under special conditions that allowed prolonged undivided attention such patients could hold a memory for as long as 15 min, but this does depend on a continual process of rehearsal, which we assume to be due to the continuous reinforcement of modular activities by the self-conscious mind.

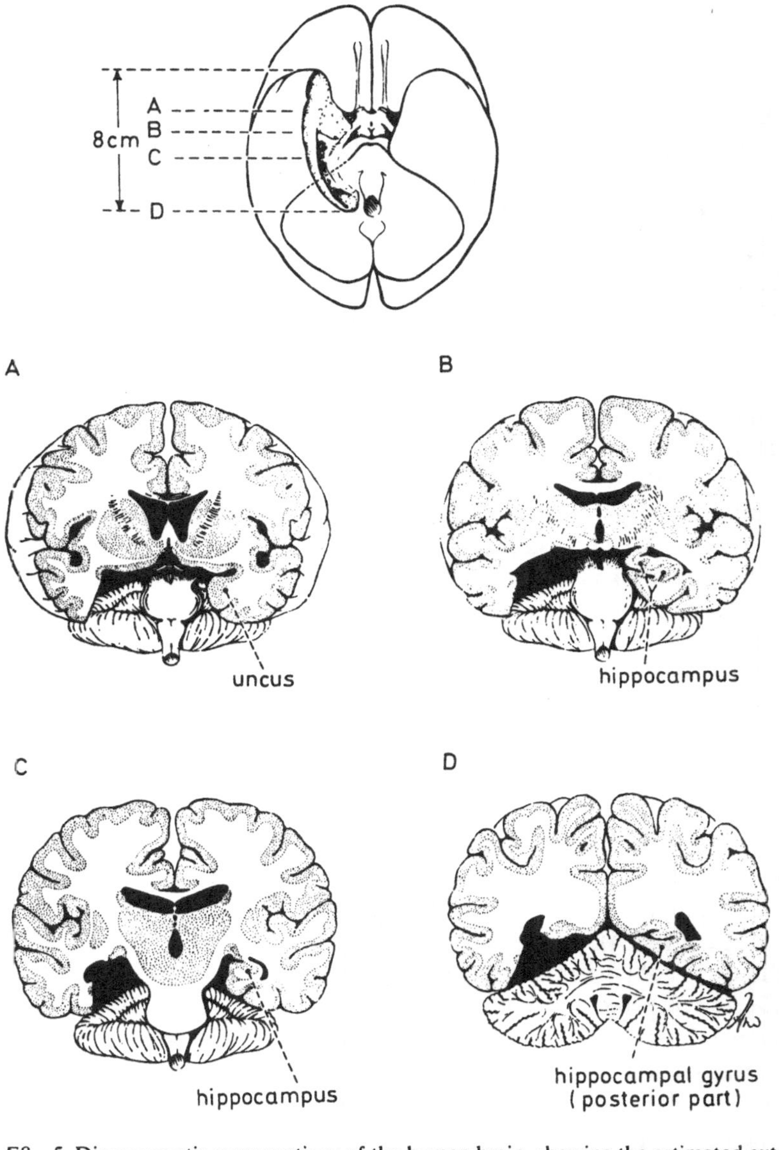

Fig. E8–5. Diagrammatic cross sections of the human brain, showing the estimated extent of removal in Scoville's medial temporal ablation in the case discussed in the text. The anterior-posterior extent of the hippocampus is shown in the upper drawing of the brain as seen from below with A, B, C and D indicating the level of the transverse sections below. For illustrative purposes the removal is shown on the left side only, but the removal was made on both sides in a single operation (Milner, 1972).

61. The Role of the Hippocampus in Learning and Memory

Good evidence is provided by study of patients having operative resections that the left hippocampus is concerned in the laying down or consolidation of verbal memories and the right for pictorial and spatial memories. The stylus maze test[1] is an interesting example of a test dependent on right hippocampal function (Milner [1967], [1972], [1974]). The more radical the hippocampal resection, the more fleeting is the memory.

Quantitative evaluation of memory has been achieved by Corsi (reported by Milner [1974]) in the location test of dot on line described in the section on lesions of the temporal lobe (Fig. E6 – 3). Another valuable test for the right temporal lobe and hippocampus utilizes the memory for irregular shapes made from bent wire. Following a complete resection of the right hippocampus very little of the test memory remains after 20 s, whether it be visual or tactual (Milner [1972], [1974]).

Similarly, lesions of the left hippocampus were tested by Corsi by a verbal memory test – for example, memorizing a group of three consonants, such as XBJ, there being some distracting activity to prevent continual verbal rehearsal. Left temporal lobe lesions resulted in a poor performance, and left hippocampal resection was implicated in this memory loss, the more complete the resection, the more fleeting the memory (Milner [1972], [1974]).

As described below, memory deficits are more severe with bilateral hippocampectomy, so it is concluded that there is some hippocampal support across the midline, which could occur via the hippocampal commissure that links equivalent areas of the hippocampi on the two sides. The unilateral ablations therefore provide evidence in accord with the still more severe memory losses (the amnestic syndrome) that result from bilateral hippocampectomy, or from lesions on the pathways to or from the hippocampus (Kornhuber [1973]).

Milner [1966] describes a remarkable case of a young man in whom Scoville had resected the medial parts of both temporal lobes for treatment of incessant bilateral epilepsy that was uncontrolled by drugs and that completely incapacitated him. The hippocampus was removed along with a small medial area of the temporal lobe on both sides (Fig. E8 – 5) (Milner [1972]). This man has had since that time an extremely severe loss of ability to lay down memory traces. There is an almost complete failure of memory for all happenings and experiences *after* the lesion, i.e. he has a complete antero-

[1] In this test the subject has to learn to retrace by a stylus the correct path that wanders across a rectangular pattern of visible "stepping stones."

grade amnesia. He lives entirely with short-term memories of a few seconds duration and with the memories retained from before the operation. Milner [1966] gives a graphic account of his memory loss.

> "His mother observes that he will do the same jigsaw puzzles day afer day without showing any practice effect, and read the same magazines over and over again without ever finding their contents familiar. The same forgetfulness applies to people he has met since the operation, even to those neighbours who have been visiting the house regularly for the past six years. He has not learned their names and he does not recognize any of them if he meets them in the street."
>
> "His initial emotional reaction may be intense, but it will be short-lived, since the incident provoking it is soon forgotten. Thus, when informed of the death of his uncle, of whom he was very fond, he became extremely upset, but then appeared to forget the whole matter and from time to time thereafter would ask when his uncle was coming to visit them; each time, on hearing anew of the uncle's death, he would show the same intense dismay, with no sign of habituation."

He can keep current events in mind so long as he is not distracted. Distraction completely eliminates all trace of what he has been doing only a few seconds before. There are cited many remarkable examples of his failure to remember as soon as he is distracted. Milner [1966] sums up this by stating that:

> "Observations such as this suggest that the only way in which this patient can hold on to new information is by constant verbal rehearsal, and that forgetting occurs as soon as this rehearsal is prevented by some new activity claiming his attention. Since in daily life attention is of necessity constantly shifting, such a patient shows a continuous anterograde amnesia. One gets some idea of what such an amnesic state must be like from the patient's own comments, repeated at intervals during a recent examination. Between tests, he would suddenly look up and say, rather anxiously:
> "Right now, I'm wondering. Have I done or said anything amiss? You see, at this moment everything looks clear to me, but what happened just before? That's what worries me. It's like waking from a dream; I just don't remember."

There are three other recorded cases where a comparable severe anterograde amnesia resulted from destruction of both hippocampi (Milner [1966]). There was almost no recovery, even after 11 years. However the variable retrograde amnesia, i.e. the memory of events preceding the hippocampal destruction, showed a continued recovery. There are two other reported cases where unilateral hippocampectomy resulted in a comparable anterograde amnesia, but there was evidence that the surviving hippocampus was severely damaged. We can conclude that the severe anterograde amnesia only occurs with grave bilateral hippocampal deficiency. Supporting evidence has been provided by Milner [1966] with cases of unilateral hippocampectomy in which the remaining hippocampus and the cerebral hemisphere on that side were temporarily knocked out by the brief anaesthesia provided by sodium amytal injection into the carotid artery in the Wada test (cp. chapter E4). A severe anterograde amnesia was produced that persisted after the transient anaesthesia. It is important to recognize that the hippocampus is not the seat of the memory traces. Memories from before the hippocampectomy are well retained and recalled. The hippocampus is merely the instrument responsible for the laying down of the memory trace or engram, which presumably is very largely located in the cerebral cortex in the appropriate areas. There is no obvious impairment of intellect or personality in these subjects despite the acute failure of memory. In fact, they live either in the immediate present or with remembered experiences from before the time of the operation. Recently Marlen-Wilson and Teuber [1975] have shown by a testing procedure of prompting that a minimal storage of information even occurs for experiences after the operation, but it is of no use to the patient.

There is one small relieving feature, namely that they still have some ability to learn motor acts. Thus the subject can build up skills in motor performances such as drawing a line in the narrow space between the double line drawings of a five pointed star using only the guidance provided by the view in a mirror of his hand and the double star; but he has no memory of how he learned the skill! Partial amnestic syndromes have been observed in patients with a variety of lesions in structures related to the hippocampus: the cingulate gyrus, the fornix, the anterior and medio-dorsal nuclei of the thalamus (Victor & others [1971]), and the prefrontal lobe (chapter E6). We are now in a position to consider the neuronal pathways concerned in the laying down of memory traces in the neocortex.

We can conclude this brief review of memory defects associated with hippocampal lesions by three statements, which are in accord with the concepts developed by Kornhuber [1973]. (1) In retrieving the memory of an event that is not being continuously rehearsed in the short-term memory process, the self-conscious mind is dependent on some consolidation or storage process that is brought about by hippocampal activity. (2) The hippocampus is itself not the site of the storage. (3) We conjecture that the hippocampal participation in the consolidation process is dependent on neuronal pathways that transmit from the modules of the association cortex to the hippocampus and thence back to the prefrontal lobe.

In chapter E1 there was a brief reference to the various pathways whereby the primary sensory areas for somaesthesis and vision projected to the limbic system, the major routes being diagrammed in Figure E1−8 on the basis of the sequential lesion studies (Fig. E1−7) by Jones and Powell [1970]. In both cases there is a more direct route to the limbic system and a route through the prefrontal lobe via the orbital cortex (OF). In the limbic system these various inputs eventually can reach the hippocampus (HI in Fig. E8−6), which is a finding of great interest in view of the evidence presented above for its key role in the consolidation of memory traces. Similar pathways have been recognized also in the case of the less studied auditory system (cp. Fig. E1 – 7 I – L). The olfactory system is specially privileged because it projects directly into the limbic system (Fig. E1 – 9).

The postulated role of the hippocampus in consolidation of memory requires that there be also return circuits from the hippocampus to the neocortex. One well-known circuit is from the hippocampus to the MD thalamus and thence to the orbital surface (OF) and the convexity of the prefrontal lobe (Akert [1964]; Nauta [1971]; Fig. E8 – 6). Another major output line from the hippocampus is to the anterior thalamic nucleus (not shown in Fig. E8 – 6), thence via the cingulate gyrus (areas 23 and 24 in Fig. E1 – 4B) to the wide areas of the neocortex via association fibres (Brodal [1969]). There is need for a more detailed study of these pathways in primates so that the clinical evidence on lesions of the hippocampus and related structures can be interpreted with confidence.

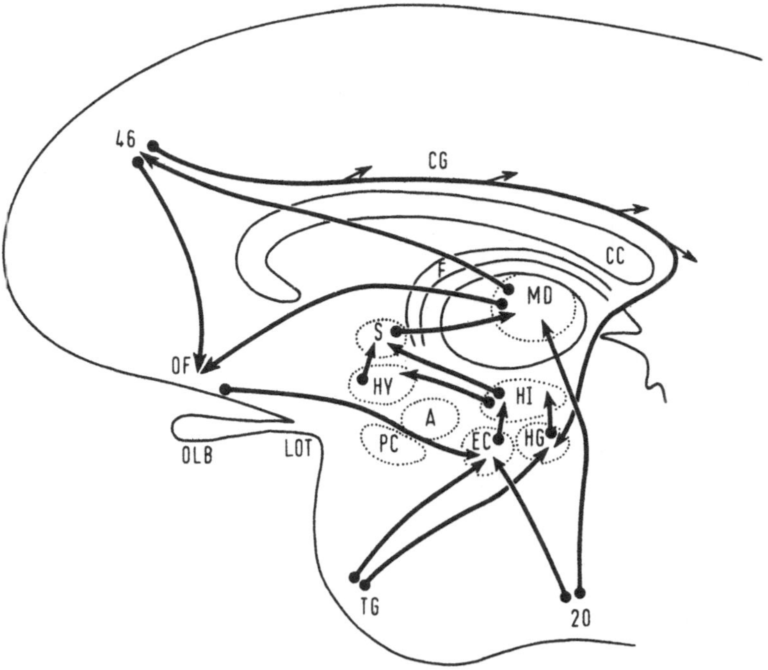

Fig. E8 – 6. Schematic drawing simplified from Fig. E1 – 9 to show connectivities from the neocortex to and from the medio-dorsal thalamus *(MD)*. OF is orbital surface of prefrontal cortex; *TG*, the temporal pole; *HG*, the gyrus hippocampi; *HI*, the hippocampus; *S*, septum; *F*, fornix; *CC*, corpus callosum; *OLB*, olfactory bulb; *LOT*, lateral olfactory tract; *PC*, piriform cortex; *EC*, entorhinal cortex; *A*, amygdala; *HY*, hypothalamus; *CG*, cingulate gyrus.

62. Hypotheses of Neuronal Happenings in Memory Storage (cp. Kornhuber [1973]; Eccles [1978])

The theory here proposed is developed from Kornhuber's theory [1973], which is illustrated in Figure E8 – 7. The sensory association areas play a key role, being firstly on the input pathway to the limbic system and frontal cortex and secondly in an intimate two-way relationship to the frontal cortex that receives a "selection input" from the limbic system. It is to be noted that the hippocampus is given a dominant role in the two limbic circuits. One circuit is the so-called Papez loop: hippocampus, mammillary body, anterior thalamic nucleus, cingulate gyrus, parahippocampus, hippocampus. The other circuit is of special interest because it leads from the association cortices to the hippocampus via the cingulate gyrus and thence via the medio-dorsal (MD) thalamus to the prefrontal lobe (cp. Fig. E8 – 6). Kornhuber [1973] conjectures that with special neurones of the sensory association areas: ". . . the synapses of afferents coming (directly or indirectly) from the limbic system are essential for forming long term memory, while other synapses on the same neurons are essential for information processing and for recall." He even conjectures that "long term memory could involve coincidence of

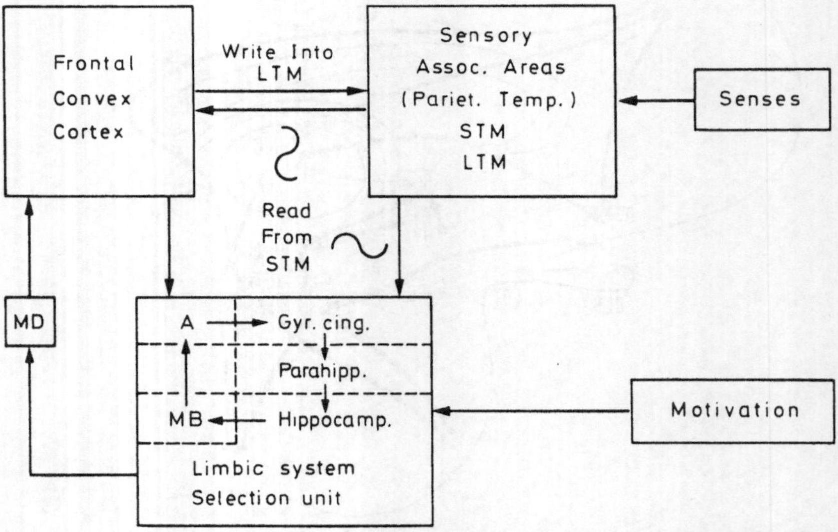

Fig. E8 – 7 Scheme of anatomical structures involved in selection of information between short term memory (STM) and long term memory (LTM)
MB = mamillary body, *A* = anterior thalamic nucleus,
MD = mediodorsal thalamic nucleus (Kornhuber, 1973).

thalamic and cortico-cortical afferents at a given cortical neuron or cell column." These theoretical developments by Kornhuber provide the basis for the further developments here described.

Figure E8 – 6 gives a more detailed picture of the pathways in both directions from neocortex to hippocampus (HI). Firstly pathways to the hippocampus are shown relaying in the hippocampal gyrus (HG) or a special zone of it called the entorhinal cortex (EC). In addition to the pathway from area 46 via the cingulate gyrus (CG) shown in Figure E8 – 6, there are also pathways from temporal areas 20 and TG and from the orbital zone of the prefrontal lobe (OF). On the output side the hippocampus projects to the MD thalamus via the septal nucleus (S) and thence to areas 46 and OF of the prefrontal lobe, but probably the projections have a much wider distribution. The role of the prefrontal lobe in memory is described in chapter E6.

In general there are remarkable similarities between the dual input systems to the Purkyně cells of the cerebellum on the one hand and to the pyramidal cells of the neocortex on the other. There is much experimental evidence supporting the instruction-selection role of the climbing fiber on the parallel fiber input to the Purkyně cell, as briefly described above (cp. Eccles [1977 (a)]), which has been developed on analogy with the selection theory of immunity by Jerne [1967]. The question arises: does the dual input system to the pyramidal cells of the neocortex function similarly in learning, and can this be linked with the role of the hippocampus?

In Figure E8 – 7 two pathways are shown converging on the frontal cortex – that from the sensory association areas directly and that indirectly via a detour through the limbic system and the MD thalamus. In the frontal cortex we would propose that the indirect input would be via non-specific thalamic afferents from the MD thalamus that would excite the spiny stellate cells forming the cartridge type of synapse (cp. Figs. E1 – 5 and 6 and Fig. E8 – 8), while the direct input would be the association fibers that terminate as horizontal fibers in laminae 1 and 2 and that are particularly well shown in Figure E8 – 8. On analogy with the cerebellum it is proposed that the cartridge-type synapse on a pyramidal cell acts similarly to the climbing fibers in selecting from the input of about 2000 horizontal fibers on the apical dendrites of that same pyramidal cell. This selection would be dependent on conjunction of the two inputs in some specific time relationship, as yet undefined, and would result in an enduring potentiation of the selected synapses on the apical dendrite. Just as with parallel fibers, it is assumed that several association, commissural and Martinotti fibers would be selected from the 2000 as forming the context of the cartridge synaptic activity on that pyramidal cell (Marr [1970]; Eccles [1977 (b)]). Thus activity of the cartridge

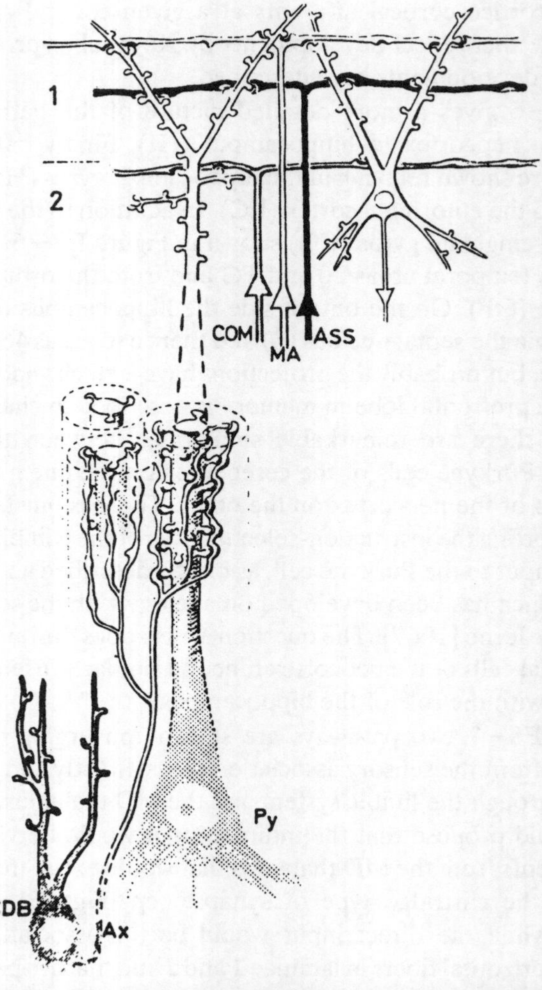

Fig. E8−8. Simplified diagram of connectivities in the neocortex (cf. Figs. E1−5 and E1−6). In laminae 1 and 2 there are shown horizontal fibers arising as bifurcating axons of commissural *(COM)* and association *(ASS)* fibers and also of Martinotti cells *(MA)*. The horizontal fibers make synapses with the apical dendrites of a pyramidal and a stellate-pyramidal cell. Deeper there is shown a spiny stellate cell *(CDB)* making cartridge synapses with the shafts of apical dendrites of pyramidal cells (Szentágothai, 1970).

system is the instruction that selects for potentiation those horizontal fiber synapses that are activated in the appropriate temporal conjunction. As indicated in Figure E8−8, Szentágothai [1972] proposes that a single cartridge system comprises the apical dendrites of about three pyramidal cells,

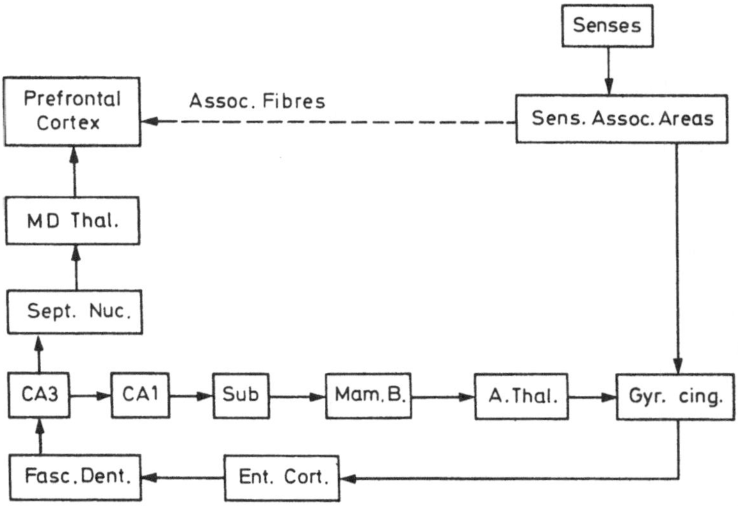

Fig. E8−9. Fig. E8−7 is redrawn to show the two circuits emanating from the *CA3* and *CA1* hippocampal pyramidal cells. The connections within the hippocampus are as follows: entorhinal cortex by perforating pathway to fascia dentata; granule cells of fascia dentata by mossy fibres to *CA3* pyramidal cells; axon collaterals of *CA3* pyramidal cells (Schaffer collaterals) to *CA1* pyramidal cells; *CA1* to subiculum *(Sub)* to mamillary bodies; *CA3* by fimbria to septal nucleus to mediodorsal thalamus.

which thus form a unitary selection system. For further quantitative consideration see Eccles [1977 (b)]. Possibly the Papez circuit (cp. Fig. E8−7) functions to provide the reverberatory activation of the hippocampus with its CA3 output through the septal nucleus to the MD thalamus, as is indicated in Figure E8−9.

Before we consider further the proposed mode of selective action of the hippocampal output on the immensely complex neuronal connectivities in the association cortex (cp. Figs. E1−7, E1−8), we should enquire into the neuronal circuitry of the hippocampus in order to see if it is built so as to work in a highly selective manner with respect to the inputs it receives from the neocortex. Recent investigations by Andersen and associates [1971], [1973] have shown to an amazing degree that the hippocampus is indeed organized in a series of narrow transverse lamellae which function independently through all the complex connectivity. This discrimination is maintained in the output line of the CA3 pyramidal cells by a strict segregation of the CA3 axons, according to location in the fimbria, the more rostral being medial and the more caudal lateral. It can be presumed that this segregation leads on to a segregation in the septal nucleus. Andersen & others [1971] sum up their findings: "A point source of entorhinal activity projects its impulses through the four-membered pathway along a slice, or lamella, of hippocampal tissue oriented normally to the alvear surface and nearly sagittally in the dorsal part of the hippocampal formation."

The diagrammatic representation in Figure E8 – 7 gives deep meaning to the fundamental design feature discovered by Andersen & others [1973], namely that the CA3 and CA1 pyramidal cells of the hippocampus are sharply discriminated by their distinctive projections as indicated in Figure E8 – 9. One of the synaptic links in the circuits of Figure E8 – 9, the entorhinal cortex to the granule cells of the fascia dentata *(Fasc. Dent.)*, exhibits remarkable responses to repetitive stimulation, which would make it function very effectively in a reverberating loop such as that proposed for the Papez circuit in Figures E8 – 7 and E8 – 9. There is very large potentiation during repetitive stimulation at 10 per second (Fig. E8 – 1C) and with repeated short episodes there is a progressive build-up of a potentiation that is maintained for hours (Fig. E8 – 2); and even for days (Fig. E8 – 3). Thus this synaptic transmission would operate with greatly increased potency during reverberating circuit action. As shown in Figure E8 – 9 this potentiation would also be on the circuit from CA3 neurones to the prefrontal lobe and so be of importance in causing a progressive build-up in the activation of the cartridge synapses.

It is interesting that motivation comes into Kornhuber's circuit diagram (Fig. E8 – 7). This implies attention or interest in the experiences that are coded in the neuronal activities of the association cortex and that are to be stored. It implies a process of mind-brain interaction. We are all cognizant that we do not store memories of no interest to us and to which we do not pay attention. It is a familiar statement that a single sharp experience is remembered for a life-time, but it overlooks the fact that the intense emotional involvement is re-experienced incessantly immediately after the original, highly charged emotional experience. Evidently there has been a long series of "replays" of the patterns of cortical activity associated with the original experience, and this activity would particularly involve the limbic system as indicated by the strong emotional overtones. Thus there must be built into the neuronal machinery of the cortex the propensity for the reverberating circuit activity which would cause the synaptic potentiation giving the memory.

In the further development of our hypothesis of long-term conscious memory we would propose that the self-conscious mind would enter into this transaction between the modules of the liaison brain and the hippocampus in two ways: firstly, by keeping up the modular activity by the general action of interest or attention (the motivation system of Kornhuber [1973]) so that the hippocampal circuit would be continuously reinforced; secondly, in a more concentrated manner by probing into the appropriate modules to read out their storage and if necessary to reinforce it or modify it by direct action on the modules concerned. Both of these proposed actions are from the self-conscious mind to those modules that have the special property of being "open" to it. However, as already proposed, by its direct action on open modules the self-conscious mind can exercise an indirect action on those "closed" modules to which the open modules project (chapter E7). Evidence for this supportive action by closed modules has been presented by Sperry [1974]. He finds that there is a pronounced impairment of verbal memory of the left cerebral hemisphere after the commissurotomy. This would be expected if the closed modules of the minor hemisphere were indirectly active in the memory storage and retrieval, as here proposed. Sperry [1974] makes a related comment: "Any storage, encoding or retrieval process dependent normally on integration between symbolic functions in the left hemisphere and spatio-perceptual mechanisms in the right would also be disrupted by commissurotomy."

It is of great interest that after commissurotomy each hemisphere can learn and remember its own particular tasks: the left hemisphere for verbal and numerical tasks; the right hemisphere for spatial, musical and pictorial tasks. As already indicated, the respective left and right hippocampi are concerned in this memory storage. Each hippocampus would work alone because the hippocampal commissure is also sectioned in the commissurotomy. A further interesting finding is that, in the modified commissurotomy with sparing of the posterior 20%, the memory defect is almost as severe as with total commissurotomy (Sperry [1974]). There is no explanation at present for the severe memory defect after partial commissurotomy.

63. Memory Retrieval

In retrieval of a memory we have further to conjecture that the self-conscious mind is continuously searching to recover memories, e.g. words, phrases, sentences, ideas, events, pictures, melodies by actively scanning through the modular array, and that, by its action on the preferred open modules, it tries to evoke the full neural patterned operation that it can read out as a recognizable memory rich in emotional and/or intellectual content. Largely this could be by a trial-and-error process. We are all familiar with the ease or difficulty of recall of one or another memory, and of the strategies we learn in order to recover memories of names that for some unknown reason are refractory to recall. We can imagine that our self-conscious mind is under a continual challenge to recall the desired memory by discovering the appropriate entry into module operation that would by development give the appropriate patterned array of modules.

It is proposed that there are two distinct kinds of conscious memory. Data-bank memory is stored in the brain and its retrieval from the brain is often by a deliberate mental act. Then another memory process comes into play – what we may call recognition memory. The retrieval from the data banks is critically scrutinized in the mind. It may be judged erroneous – perhaps a slight error in a name or in a number sequence. This leads to a renewed attempt at retrieval, which may again be judged faulty – and so on until the retrieval is judged to be correct, or until the attempt is abandoned. It is therefore conjectured that there are two distinct kinds of memory: (1) *brain storage memory* held in the data banks of the brain, especially in the cerebral cortex; (2) *recognition memory* that is applied by the self-conscious mind in its scrutiny of the retrievals from the brain storage memories. There is further discussion of memory retrieval in dialogues VI and VII.

Penfield and Perot [1963] gave a most illuminating account of the experiential responses evoked in 53 patients by stimulation of the cerebral hemispheres during operations performed under local anaesthesia. These responses differed from those produced by stimulation of the primary sensory areas, which were merely flashes of light or touches and paraesthesia (chapter E2), in that the patients had experiences that resembled dreams, the so-called dreamy states. During the continued gentle electrical stimulation of sites on the exposed surface of their brains, the patients reported experiences that they often recognized as being recalls of long forgotten memories. As Penfield states, it is as if a past stream of consciousness is recovered during this electrical stimulation. The most common experiences were visual or auditory, but there were also many cases of combined visual and auditory. The recall of music and song provided very striking experiences for both the patient and the neurosurgeon. All of these results were obtained from brains of patients with a history of epileptic seizures. Figure E8 – 10 shows the sites of stimulation that evoked experiential responses in the whole series of patients. It is noteworthy that the temporal lobes were the preferred sites, and that the minor hemisphere was more effective than the dominant. It also will be recognized that the primary sensory areas are excluded.

In summary of these most interesting investigations it is stated that the experiences are those in which the patient is an observer not a participator, just as in dreams.

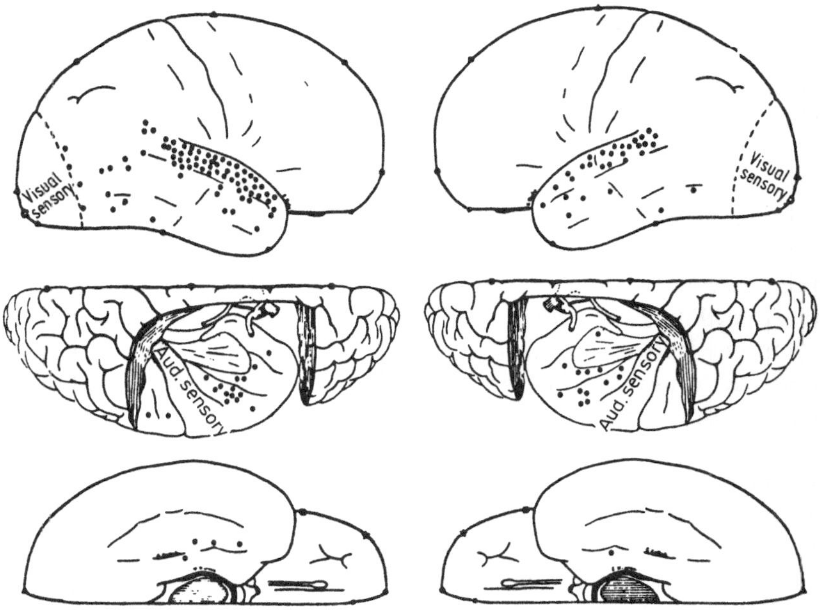

Fig. E8 – 10. Drawings of human brain to show sites (dots) from which experiental responses were produced by electrical stimulation in the total experimental series. In the upper row are the right and left hemispheres seen from the lateral aspect. In the middle row the view is from above and the parietal and frontal lobes are cut away to show the superior aspect of the temporal lobes. In the lowest rows the view is from below (Penfield and Perot, 1963).

> The times that are summoned most frequently are briefly these: the times of watching or hearing the action and speech of others, and times of hearing music. Certain sorts of experience seem to be absent. For example, the times of making up one's mind to do this or that do not appear in the record. Times of carrying out skilled acts, times of speaking or saying this and that, or of writing messages and adding figures – these things are not recorded. Times of eating and tasting food, times of sexual excitement or experience – these things have been absent as well as periods of painful suffering or weeping. Modesty does not explain these silences. (Penfield and Perot [1963]).

It can be concluded that the stimulation acts as a mode of recall of past experiences. We may regard this as an instrumental means for a recovery of memories. It can be suggested that the storage of these memories is likely to be in cerebral areas close to the effective stimulation sites. However it is important to recognize that the experiential recall is evoked from areas in the region of the disordered cerebral function that is displayed by the epileptic seizures. Conceivably the effective sites are abnormal zones that are thereby able to act by association pathways to the much wider areas of the cerebral cortex which are the actual storage sites for memories.

64. Durations of Memories

An analysis of the durations of the various processes involved in memory provides evidence for three distinct memory processes (cp. McGaugh [1969]). We have already presented evidence for the short-term memory, usually of a few seconds, that can be attributed to the continual activity in neural circuits that holds the memory in a dynamic pattern of circulating impulses. The patients with bilateral hippocampectomy have almost no other memory. Secondly there is the long-term memory that endures for days to years. According to the growth theory of learning, this memory (or memory trace) is encoded in the increased efficacy of synapses that have been hyperactive during and after the original episode that is being remembered. In the present context of conscious memory it can be conjectured that this synaptic growth would occur in multitudes of synapses in patterned array in the modules strongly reacting in response to the original episode that sets in train the operation of the reverberatory circuits through the hippocampus. As a consequence of this synaptic growth, the self-conscious mind would be able to develop strategies for causing the replay of modules in a pattern resembling that of the original episode, hence the memory experience. Moreover this replay would be accompanied by a renewed reverberatory activity through the hippocampus resembling the original, with a consequent strengthening of the memory trace.

However we are confronted with the urgent problem of filling in the temporal gap between the short-term memory of seconds and the hours required for the synaptic growth of long-term memory. Barondes [1970] reviews the experiments testing for the time course of action of substances, cycloheximide for example, that prevent protein synthesis in the brain, which at the same time is unable to learn. The approximate time of about 30 min to 3 h seems to be required for the synaptic growth giving long-term memory. McGaugh [1969] has proposed an intermediate-term memory to bridge the gap of seconds to hours between the end of short-term memory and the full development of synaptic growth giving the long-term memory as is diagrammed in Figure E8−11. We would propose that the post-tetanic potentiation described earlier (Figs. E8−1C, 2, 3) is exactly fitted for bridging this gap. It would be induced by the repetitive synaptic activations of short-term memory and would immediately follow those actions, utilizing the same hippocampal loop circuitry as for long-term memory. It would be restricted to the activated synapses and be graded in accord with their action. In Figures E8−2 and 3 post-tetanic potentiations enduring for hours followed quite mild repetitive stimulation of hippocampal synapses. As that physiological

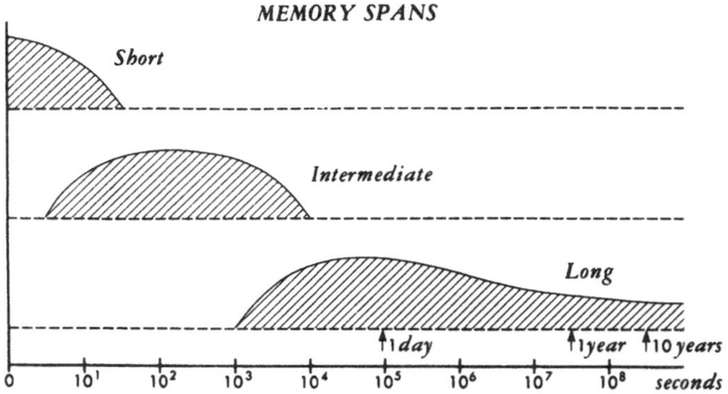

Fig. E8—11. Diagrammatic representation of the durations of the three memories described in the text. Note the logarithmic time scale and the conjectured rise and fall of the memories with time.

process of synaptic potentiation declines, the metabolically induced synaptic growth supervenes to provide an enduring basis for the strategic read-out by the self-conscious mind.

65. Plastic Responses of Cerebral Cortex

There are special examples of plastic responses of the nervous system of young animals that can be regarded as examples of learning. A remarkable discovery has been reported by Blakemore [1974] when he exposed young kittens (3 to 14 weeks) to horizontal or vertical stripes for several hours each day, the remaining time being in darkness. Even after a few hours of this exposure there was a conversion of visual cortical cells to a high preference for the line orientation to which they had been exposed, e.g. vertical or horizontal (cp. chapter E2). If the exposures were to vertical and horizontal stripes in alternating periods the visual cortical cells were of two types, those with horizontal and those with vertical orientations. Blakemore suggests that these adaptive responses are analogous to the fundamental process underlying learning and memory. It is certainly remarkable that such relatively brief exposures result in the development of specific connectivities within a visual column (cp. chapter E2) that are responsible for the observed orientation specificities.

A related plastic response of visual cells of kittens soon after birth was discovered by Wiesel and Hubel [1963] and fully discussed by Kuffler and

Nicholls [1976]. When one eye was closed for a few days after the normal time of opening, it was found that the pathways from the other eye dominated almost all visual cells in both visual cortices. Normally in the kitten there is a partition of these visual cells over the whole range of dominance by one or other eye with all degrees of convergence. At the most sensitive age of 3 to 4 weeks after birth the activated pathways from the uncovered eye established dominant connections to all visual cells to the exclusion of pathways from the closed eye. With younger or older kittens the effects were less severe. These effects are due to changes in the synaptic action on visual cortical cells, not in the retina and in the pathways to the cortex (cp. Figs. E2−4 and E2−7). Here again we have plastic changes in connectivities resulting from usage, and hence the effects can be regarded as a special type of learning.

A further illustration of the way in which learning can transform the interpretation of visual information is provided by Stratton's experiments [1897], in which a system of lenses was placed in front of one of his eyes (the other being covered), so that the image on the retina was inverted with respect to its usual orientation. For several days the visual world was hopelessly disordered. Since it was inverted, it gave an impression of unreality and was useless for the purpose of apprehending or manipulating objects. But as a result of 8 days of continual effort, the visual world could again be sensed by him correctly, and then became a reliable guide for manipulation and movement. If no active effort is made, no learning occurs. There have been several experimental confirmations of Stratton's remarkable findings, and many additional observations, particularly by Kohler [1951]. Subjects with inverted retinal images have even learned to ski, which requires a very accurate correlation of visual with kinaesthetic experiences. Recently Gonshor and Melvill Jones [1976 (a)], [1976 (b)] have reported a quantitative evaluation of the learning process in subjects that had a horizontal inversion of their visual fields by means of dove prisms worn continuously for several days.

These observations and many others of like kind establish that, as a consequence of active or trial-and-error learning, the brain events evoked by sensory information from the retina are interpreted so that they give a valid picture of the external world that is sensed by touch and movement, i.e. the world of visual perception becomes a world in which one can effectively move.

The most elegant and delightful example of the role of activity in visual learning is provided by the experiments of Held and Hein [1963]. Littermate kittens spend several hours a day in a contraption (Fig. E8−12) which allows one kitten fairly complete freedom to explore its environment actively, just as a normal kitten. The other is suspended passively in a gondola that by a simple mechanical arrangement is moved in all directions by the exploring litter mate so that the gondola passenger is subjected to the same play of visual imagery as the active kitten, but none of this activity is initiated by the passenger. Its visual world is provided for it just as it is for us on a TV screen. When not in this contraption both kittens are kept with their mother in

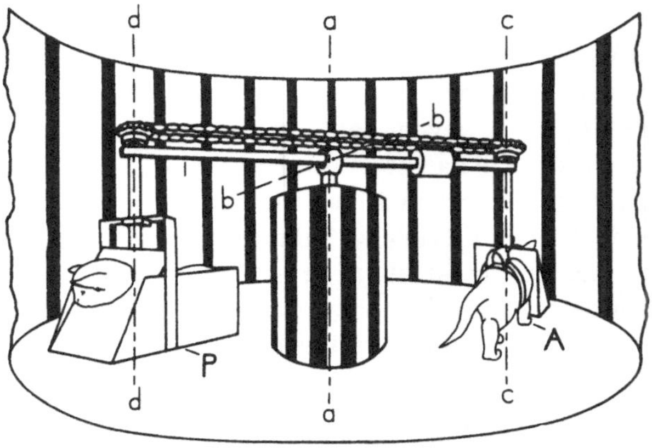

Fig. E8–12. Apparatus for equating motion and consequent visual feedback for an actively moving kitten *(A)* and a passively moved one *(P)* (Held and Hein, 1963).

darkness. After some weeks, tests show that the active kitten has learnt to utilize its visual fields for giving it a valid picture of the external world for the purpose of movement just as well as a normal kitten, whereas the gondola passenger has learnt nothing. One simple example of this difference is displayed by placing the kittens on a narrow shelf which they can leave either on one side with a small drop, or on the other side with an intimidating fall. Actually a transparent shelf prevents any untoward damage in getting off on the dangerous side. The actively trained kitten always chooses the easy side, the "gondola" kitten chooses either in random manner.

The conclusion from these and many other experiments on animals and man is that continually active exploration is essential even if adults are to retain their existing visual discriminations or to learn new ones. The most remarkable physiological and anatomical problems are raised by these intriguing experiments on perception and behaviour, but as yet we can only formulate the problems in the vaguest terms.

66. Retrograde Amnesia

It is a common observation that loss of memory results fom a severe trauma of the brain, as for example from mechanical damage giving unconsciousness (concussion), or from the convulsive seizures resulting from electroshock therapy. The retrograde amnesia is usually complete for events immediately before the trauma, and becomes progressively less severe for memories of earlier and still earlier events. Depending on the severity of the trauma, retrograde amnesia may cover periods of minutes, hours or days.

Animal investigations have used the memory built up by training procedures to test for retrograde amnesia produced by trauma applied at various times after training. The trauma could be by electroshock or by various chemical agents. These experiments indicate that the memory storage process is consolidated during 6h. after the training period. With shorter times the memories are progressively more sensitive to trauma. It can be envisaged that the growing of synapses that results in long-term memory is very sensitive to trauma for many hours, presumably until the whole growth process is completed (cp. McGaugh [1969]; Barondes [1970]).

Following hippocampectomy there was not only the severe anterograde amnesia for events following the operation, but there was also a severe retrograde amnesia, i.e. for events preceding the operation by hours or days (Milner [1972]). Apparently the trauma of the operation caused this retrograde amnesia, which in the course of time became less severe, i.e. events preceding the operation were better remembered.

Bibliography to Part II

Adam G. (eds) [1971] *Biology of Memory, Symposia Biologica Hungarica, 10,* pp. 21–25.

Adrian E. D. [1947] *The Physical Background of Perception,* Clarendon Press, Oxford, p. 95.

Agranoff B. W. [1967] "Agents That Block Memory", in Quarton, Melnechuk & Schmitt (eds) [1967], pp. 756–64.

[1969] "Protein Synthesis and Memory Formation", in Bogoch (eds) [1969], pp. 341–53.

Akert K. [1964] "Comparative Anatomy of the Frontal Cortex and Thalamocortical Connections", in Warren & Akert (eds) [1964], pp. 372–96.

Alajouanine T. [1948] "Aphasia and artistic realization", *Brain, 71,* pp. 229–41.

Allen G. I. & Tsukahara N. [1974] "Cerebrocerebellar communication systems", *Physiological Reviews, 54,* pp. 957–1006.

Andersen P., Bland B. H. & Dudar J. D. [1973] "Organization of the hippocampal output", *Experimental Brain Research, 17,* pp. 152–68.

Andersen P., Bliss T. V. P. & Skrede K. K. [1971] "Lamellar organization of hippocampal excitatory pathways", *Experimental Brain Research, 13,* pp. 222–38.

Armstrong D. M. [1968] *A Materialist Theory of the Mind,* Routledge London.

Austin G., Hayward W. & Rouhe S. [1972] "A Note on the Problem of Conscious Man and Cerebral Disconnection by Hemispherectomy", in Smith (eds) [1972].

Bailey P., Bonin G. von, Garol H. W. & McCulloch W. S. [1943] "Functional organisation of temporal lobe of monkey (Macaca Mulatta) and chimpanzee (Pan Satyrus)", *Journal of Neurophysiology, 6,* pp. 121–28.

Barlow H. B. [1972] "Single units and sensation: A neuron doctrine for perceptual psychology?", *Perception, 1,* pp. 371–94.

Barondes S. H. [1969] "The Mirror Focus and Long-Term Memory Storage", in Jasper, Ward & Pope (eds) [1969], pp. 371–74.

[1970] "Multiple Steps in the Biology of Memory", in Schmitt (eds) [1970], volume 2, pp. 272–78.

Basser L. S. [1962] "Hemiplegia of early onset and the faculty of speech with special reference to the effects of hemispherectomy", *Brain, 85,* pp. 427–60.

Berlucchi G. [1974] "Cerebral Dominance and Interhemispheric Communication in Normal Man", in Schmitt & Worden (eds) [1974], pp. 65–9.

Berlyne D. B. [1969] "The Development of the Concept of Attention", in Evans & Mulholland (eds) [1969], pp. 1–26.

Blakemore C. [1974] "Developmental Factors in the Formation of Feature Extracting Neurons", in Schmitt & Worden (eds) [1974], pp. 105–13.

BLISS T. V. P. & GARDNER-MEDWIN A. R. [1973] "Long-lasting potentiation of synaptic transmission in the dentate area of the unanaesthetized rabbit following stimulation of the perforant path", *Journal of Physiology*, London, *232*, pp. 357–74.

BLISS T. V. P. & LØMO T. [1973] "Long-lasting potentiation of synaptic transmission in the dentate area of the anaesthetized rabbit following stimulation of the perforant path", *Journal of Physiology*, London, *232*, pp. 331–56.

BOCCA E., CALEARO C., CASSINARI V. & MIGLIAVACCA F. [1955] "Testing 'cortical' hearing in temporal lobe tumors", *Acta Oto-Laryngolica*, Stockholm, *45*, pp. 289–304.

BOGEN J. E. [1969a] "The other side of the brain I. Dysgraphia and dyscopia following cerebral commissurotomy", *Bulletin of the Los Angeles Neurological Societies*, *34*, pp. 73–105.

[1969b] "The other side of the brain II. An appositional mind", *Bulletin of the Los Angeles Neurological Societies*, *34*, pp. 135–62.

BOGOCH S. (eds) [1969] *The Future of the Brain Sciences*, Plenum Press, New York.

BREMER F. [1966] "Neurophysiological Correlates of Mental Unity", in ECCLES (eds) 1966 pp. 283–297.

BRINDLEY G. S. [1973] "Sensory Effects of Electrical Stimulation of the Visual and Paravisual Cortex in Man", in JUNG (eds) [1973c], pp. 583–94.

BROADBENT D. E. [1954] "The role of auditory localization in attention and memory", *Journal of Experimental Psychology*, *47*, pp. 191–6.

[1974] "Division of Function and Integration of Behaviour", in SCHMITT & WORDEN (eds) [1974], pp. 31–41.

BROADBENT D. E. & GREGORY M. [1965] "On the interaction of S–R compatibility with other variables affecting reaction time", *British Journal of Psychology*, London, *56*, pp. 61–7.

BROCA P. [1861] "Perte de la parole, ramollissement chronique et destruction partielle du lobe antérieur gauche du cerveau", *Bulletin de la Société Anthropologique*, Paris, *2*, p. 235.

BRODAL A. [1969] *Neurological Anatomy. In Relation to Clinical Medicine*, Oxford University Press, London.

[1973] "Self-observations and neuroanatomical considerations after a stroke", *Brain*, *96*, pp. 675–94.

BRONOWSKI J. & BELLUGI U. [1970] "Language, name, and concept", *Science*, *168*, pp. 669–73.

BUSER P. & RONGUEL-BUSER A. (eds) [1978] *Cerebral Correlates of Conscious Experience*, Elsevier, Amsterdam.

CAIRNS H. [1952] "Disturbances of consciousness with lesions of the brain stem and diencephalon", *Brain*, *75*, p. 109.

CHAPPELL V. C. (eds) [1962] *The Philosophy of Mind*, Prentice-Hall, Inc., Englewood Cliffs N. J.

CHOMSKY N. [1968] *Language and the Mind,* Harcourt Brace and World, New York.

COLONNIER M. L. [1966] "The Structural Design of the Neocortex", in ECCLES (eds) [1966], pp. 1 – 23.

[1968] "Synaptic patterns on different cell types in the different laminae of the cat visual cortex. An electron microsope study", *Brain Research, 9,* pp. 268 – 87.

COLONNIER M. L. & ROSSIGNOL S. [1969] "Heterogeneity of the Cerebral Cortex", in JASPER, WARD & POPE (eds) [1969], pp. 29 – 40.

CRAWFORD B. H. [1947] "Visual adaptation in relation to brief conditioning stimuli", *Proceedings of the Royal Society of London B, 134,* pp. 283 – 302.

CREUTZFELDT O., INNOCENTI G. M. & BROOKS D. [1974] "Vertical organization in the visual cortex (Area 17) in the cat", *Experimental Brain Research, 21,* pp. 315 – 336.

CREUTZFELDT O. & ITO M. [1968] "Functional synaptic organization of primary visual cortex neurones in the cat", *Experimental Brain Research, 6,* pp. 324 – 52.

CRITCHLEY M. [1953] *The Parietal Lobes,* Arnold, London.

CURTISS S., FROMKIN V., KRASHEN S., RIGLER D. & RIGLER M. [1974] "The linguistic development of Genie", *Language, 50,* pp. 528 – 55.

DARWIN C. J. [1969] "Laterality effects in the recall of steady-state and transient speech sounds", *Journal of the Acoustical Society of America, 35,* p. 114 (A).

DAVENPORT R. K. [1976] "Cross-modal Perception in Apes" in conference 'On origins and evolution of language and speech', Annals of New York *Academy of Sciences,* 280, 143–149.

DEECKE L., SCHEID P. & KORNHUBER H. H. [1969] "Distribution of readiness potential, pre-motion positivity and motor potential of the human cerebral cortex preceding volountary finger movements", *Experimental Brain Research, 7,* pp. 158 – 68.

DELAFRESNAYE J. F. (eds) [1954] *Brain Mechanisms and Consciousness,* Ist C.I.O.M.S. Conference. Blackwells Scientific Publications, Oxford.

(eds) [1961] *Brain Mechanisms and Learning,* Blackwell Scientific Publications, Oxford.

DELONG M. R. [1974] "Motor Functions of the Basal Ganglia: Single-unit Activity During Movement", in SCHMITT & WORDEN (eds) [1974], pp. 319 – 25.

DERFER G. [1974] "Science, poetry and 'human specificity' an interview with J. Bronowski", *The American Scholar, 43,* pp. 386 – 404.

DICHGANS J. & JUNG R. [1969] "Attention, Eye Movement and Motion Detection: Facilitation and Selection in Optokinetic Nystagmus and Railway Nystagmus", in EVANS & MULHOLLAND (eds) [1969], pp. 348 – 376.

DIMOND S. J. & BEAUMONT J. G. [1973 (a)] "Experimental Studies of Hemisphere Function in the Human Brain", in DIMOND & BEAUMONT (eds) [1973 (b)], pp. 48 – 88.

(eds) [1973 (b)] *Hemisphere Function in the Human Brain*, John Wiley & Sons, New York.

Doty R. W. [1975] "Consciousness from neurons", *Acta Neurobiologiae Experimentalis, 35*, pp. 791–804.

Eccles J. C. [1964] *The Physiology of Synapses*, Springer-Verlag, Berlin, Göttingen, Heidelberg.

[1965] *The Brain and the Unity of Conscious Experience*, Cambridge University Press, London.

[1966 (a)] "Conscious Experience and Memory", in Eccles (eds) [1966 (b)], pp. 314–44.

(eds) [1966 (b)] *Brain and Conscious Experience*, Springer-Verlag, Berlin, Heidelberg, New York.

Eccles J. C. [1969] "The Dynamic Loop Hypothesis of Movement Control", in Leibovic (eds) [1969], pp. 245–69.

[1970] *Facing Reality: Philosophical Adventures of a Brain Scientist*, Springer-Verlag, Berlin, Heidelberg, New York, p. 210.

[1972] "Possible Synaptic Mechanisms Subserving Learning", in Karczmar Eccles (eds) [1972], pp. 39–61.

[1973 a] "The cerebellum as a computer: Patterns in space and time", *Journal of Physiology, 229*, pp. 1–32.

[1973 b] *The Understanding of the Brain*, McGraw-Hill, New York, p. 238.

[1976] "The plasticity of the mammalian central nervous system with special reference to new growths in response to lesions", *Naturwissenschaften, 63*, pp. 8–15.

[1977 a] "An instruction-selection theory of learning in the cerebellar cortex", *Brain Research, 127*, pp. 327–352.

[1977 b] "An instruction-selection hypothesis of learning in the cerebrum" in P. Buser & A. Ronguel-Buser (eds) 1978.

[1977 c] *The Understanding of the Brain*, 2nd. edition, McGraw-Hill, New York.

Eccles J. C., Ito M. & Szentagothai J. [1967] *The Cerebellum as a Neuronal Machine*, Springer-Verlag, Berlin, Heidelberg, New York, p. 335.

Ettlinger G. & Blakemore C. B. [1969] "Cross-modal tranfer set in the monkey", *Neuropsychologia, 7*, pp. 41–47.

Evans C. R. & Mulholland T. B. (eds) [1969] *Attention in Neurophysiology*, Butterworths, London.

Evarts E. V. [1964] "Temporal patterns of discharge of pyramidal tract neurons during sleep and waking in the monkey", *Journal of Neurophysiology, 27*, pp. 152–71.

Feigl H. [1967] *The 'Mental' and the 'Physical'*, University of Minnesota Press, Minneapolis, p. 179.

Fouts R. S. [1973] "Capacities for Language in Great Apes", IXth International Congress of Anthropological and Ethnological Sciences.

FULTON J. F. (eds) [1943] *Physiology of the Nervous System,* 2nd edition, Oxford University Press.

GARDNER B. T. & GARDNER R. A. [1971] "Two-way Communication With an Infant Chimpanzee", in SCHRIER & STOLLMITZ (eds), volume IV ch.3, [1971].

GARDNER R. A. & GARDNER B. T. [1969] "Teaching sign language to a chimpanzee", *Science, 165,* pp. 664–72.

GARDNER W. J., KARNOSH L. J., McCLURE C. C. & GERDNER A. K. [1955] "Residual function following hemispherectomy for tumour and for infantile hemiplegia", *Brain, 78,* pp. 487–502.

GAZZANIGA M. S. [1970] *The Bisected Brain,* Appleton-Century-Crofts, New York.

GESCHWIND N. [1965 (a)] "Disconnection syndromes in animal and man", *Brain,* Part I, *88,* pp. 237–94.

[1965 (b)] "Disconnection syndromes in animal and man", *Brain,* Part II, *88,* pp. 585–644.

[1970] "The organisation of language and the brain", *Science, 170,* pp. 940–44.

[1972] "Language and the brain", *Scientific American, 226,* pp. 76–83.

[1973] "The Anatomical Basis of Hemispheric Differentiation", in DIMOND & BEAUMONT (eds) [1973], pp. 7–24.

GESCHWIND & LEVITSKY W. [1968] "Human brain: left-right asymmetries in temporal speech region", *Science, 161,* pp. 186–7.

GLOBUS G. G., MAXWELL G. & SAVODNIK I. [1975] *Mind and Brain: Philosophic and Scientific Strategies,* Plenum Publishing Corporation, New York.

GONSHOR A. & MELVILL JONES G. [1976 (a)] "Short-term adaptive changes in the human vestibulo-ocular reflex arc", *Journal of Physiology, 256,* pp. 361–79.

[1976 (b)] "Extreme vestibulo-ocular adaptation induced to prolonged optical reversal of vision", *Journal of Physiology, 256,* pp. 381–414.

GOTT P. S. [1973 (a)] "Cognitive abilities following right and left hemispherectomy", *Cortex, 9,* pp. 266–74.

[1973 (b)] "Language after dominant hemispherectomy", *Journal of Neurology Neurosurgery and Psychiatry, 36,* pp. 1082–8.

GROSS C. G. [1973] "Visual Functions of Inferotemporal Cortex", in JUNG (eds) [1973 c], pp. 451–82.

GROSS C. G., BENDER D. B. & ROCHA-MIRANDA C. E. [1974] "Inferotemporal Cortex: A Single-Unit Analysis", in SCHMITT & WORDEN (eds) [1974], pp. 229–38.

HASSLER R. [1967] "Funktionelle Neuroanatomie und Psychiatrie", in KISKER, MEYER, MÜLLER & STRÖMGREN (eds) [1967].

HÉCAEN H. [1967] "Brain Mechanisms Suggested by Studies of Parietal Lobes", in MILLIKAN & DARLEY (eds) [1967], pp. 146–66.

HEIMER L., EBNER F. F. & NAUTA W. J. H. [1967] "A note on the termination of commissural fibers in the neocortex", *Brain Research, 5,* pp. 171–7.

HELD R. & HEIN A. [1963] "Movement-produced stimulation in the development of visually guided behaviour", *Journal of Comparative and Physiological Psychology, 56,* pp. 872–6.

HILLIER W. F. [1954] "Total left hemispherectomy for malignant glioma", *Neurology, 4,* pp. 718–21.

HOLMES G. [1939] "The cerebellum of man", *Brain, 62,* pp. 21–30.

[1945] "The organization of the visual cortex in man", *Proceedings of the Royal Society, B 132,* pp. 348–61.

HOOK S. (eds) [1961] *Dimensions of Mind,* Collier-MacMillan Limited, London.

HUBEL D. H. [1967] "The Visual Cortex of the Brain", (Scientific American 1963) in *From Cell to Organism,* W. H. Freeman & Co., San Francisco, pp. 54–62.

[1971] "Specificity of responses of cells in the visual cortex", *Journal of Psychiatric Research, 8,* pp. 301–7.

HUBEL D. H. & WIESEL T. N. [1962] "Receptive fields, binocular interaction and functional architecture in the cat's visual cortex", *Journal of Physiology,* London, *160,* pp. 106–54.

[1963] "Shape and arrangement of columns in the cat's striate cortex", *Journal of Physiology,* London, *165,* pp. 559–68.

[1965] "Receptive fields and functional architecture in two nonstriate visual areas (18 and 19) of the cat", *Journal of Neurophysiology, 28,* pp. 229–89.

[1968] "Receptive fields and functional architecture of monkey striate cortex", *Journal of Physiology, 195,* pp. 215–43.

[1972] "Laminar and columnar distribution of geniculo-cortical fibers in the Macaque monkey", *Journal of Comparative Neurology, 146,* pp. 421–50.

[1974] "Sequence regularity and geometry of orientation columns in the monkey striate cortex", *Journal of Comparative Neurology, 158,* pp. 267–94.

HYDÉN H. [1965] "Activation of Nuclear RNA in Neurons and Glia in Learning", in Kimble (eds) [1965].

[1967] "Biochemical Changes Accompanying Learning", in QUARTON, MELNECHUK & SCHMITT (eds) [1967], pp. 765–71.

IGGO A. (eds) [1973] *Handbook of Sensory Physiology,* Vol. II, Springer-Verlag, Berlin, Heidelberg, New York.

INGVAR D. H. [1975] "Patterns of Brain Activity Revealed by Measurements of Regional Cerebral Blood Flow", in INGVAR & LASSEN (eds) [1975], pp. 397–413.

INGVAR D. H. & SCHWARTZ M. S. [1974] "Blood flow patterns induced in the dominant hemisphere by speech and reading", *Brain, 97,* pp. 273–88.

INGVAR D. H. & LASSEN N. A. (eds) [1975] *Brain Work: The Coupling of Function, Metabolism and Blood Flow in the Brain,* Munksgaard, Copenhagen.

ITO M. & MIYASHITA Y. [1975] "The effects of chronic destruction of the inferior olive upon visual modification of the horizontal vestibulo-ocular reflex of rabbits", *Proceedings of the Japanese Academy, 51,* pp. 716–20.

JACOBSEN C. F. [1936] "Studies on the cerebral function of primates: I. The functions of the cerebral association areas in monkeys", *Comparative Psychology Monographs, 13,* pp. 3–60.

JAKOBSEN C. F., WOLF J. B. & JACKSON T. [1935] "An experimental analysis of the functions of the frontal association areas in primates", *Journal of Nervous and Mental Disease, 82,* pp. 1–14.

JASPER H. H., WARD A. A. & POPE A. (eds) [1969] *Basic Mechanisms of the Epilepsies,* Little, Brown and Company, Boston.

JERNE N. K. [1967] "Antibodies and Learning: Selection versus Instruction", in QUARTON, MELNECHUK & SCHMITT (eds) [1967], pp. 200–05.

JONES E. G. [1974] "The Anatomy of Extrageniculostriate Visual Mechanisms" in SCHMITT & WORDEN (eds) [1974], pp. 215–27.

JONES E. G. & POWELL T. P. S. [1969] "Connexions of the somatic sensory cortex of the rhesus monkey. I. Ipsilateral cortical connexions", *Brain, 92,* pp. 477–502.

[1970] "An anatomical study of converging sensory pathways within the cerebral cortex of the monkey", *Brain, 93,* pp. 793–820.

[1973] "Anatomical Organization of the Somato-sensory Cortex", in IGGO (eds) [1973], pp. 579–620.

JUNG R. [1954] Correlations of bioelectrical and autonomic phenomena with alterations of consciousness and arousal in man in DELAFRESNAYE (eds) [1954] pp. 310–339.

[1967] "Neurophysiologie und Psychiatrie", in KISKER, MEYER, MÜLLER & STRÖMGREN (eds) [1967], pp. 328–928.

[1973 (a)] "Visual Perception and Neurophysiology" in JUNG (eds) [1973 (b)], pp. 1–152.

(eds) [1973 (b)] *Handbook of Sensory Physiology,* Volume VII/3A, Springer-Verlag, Berlin, Heidelberg, New York.

(eds) [1973 (c)] *Handbook of Sensory Physiology,* Volume VII/3 B, Springer-Verlag, Berlin, Heidelberg, New York.

[1974] "Neuropsychologie und Neurophysiologie des konturend Formsehens in Zeichnung und Malerei", in WIECK (eds) [1974], pp. 27–88.

KARCZMAR A. G. & ECCLES J. C. (eds) [1972] *Brain and Human Behaviour,* Springer-Verlag, Berlin, Heidelberg, New York.

KIMBLE D. P. (ed) [1965] *Anatomy of Memory,* Science and Behaviour Books, Inc., Palo Alto, California.

KIMURA D. [1963] "Right temporal lobe damage", *Archives de Neurologie,* Paris, *8,* pp. 264–71.

[1967] "Functional asymmetry of the brain in dichotic listening", *Cortex, 3,* pp. 163–78.

[1973] "The asymmetry of the human brain", *Scientific American, 228,* pp. 70–78.

KIMURA D. & DURNFORD M. [1973] "Normal Studies on the Function of the Right Hemisphere in Vision", in DIMOND & BEAUMONT (eds) [1973], pp. 25–47.

KISKER K. P., MEYER J.-E., MÜLLER M. & STRÖMGREN E. (eds) [1967] *Psychiatrie der Gegenwart. Forschung und Praxis,* Springer-Verlag, Berlin, Heidelberg, New York.

KOHLER I. [1951] "Über Aufbau und Wandlungen der Wahrnehmungswelt. S-B.", *Österreichische Akademie der Wissenschaften, phil.-historische Klasse, 227,* pp. 1–118.

KORNHUBER H. H. [1973] "Neural Control of Input Into Long Term Memory: Limbic System and Amnestic Syndrome in Man", in ZIPPEL (eds) [1973], pp. 1–22.

[1974] "Cerebral Cortex, Cerebellum and Basal Ganglia: An Introduction to Their Motor Functions", in SCHMITT & WORDEN (eds) [1974], pp. 267–80.

KRYNAUW R. A. [1950] "Infantile hemiplegia treated by removing one cerebral hemisphere", *Journal of Neurology, Neurosurgery and Psychiatry, 13,* pp. 243–67.

KUFFLER S. W. [1973] "The single-cell approach in the visual system and the study of receptive fields", *Investigative Opthalmology, 12,* pp. 794–813.

KUFFLER S. W. & NICHOLLS J. G. [1976] *From Neuron to Brain. A Cellular Approach to the Function of the Nervous System,* Sinauer Associates, Inc., Sunderland, Mass., p. 486.

LASHLEY K. S. [1950] "In search of the engram", *Symposia of the Society for Experimental Biology, 4,* pp. 454–82.

LASZLO E. [1972] *Introduction to Systems Philosophy,* Gordon and Breach, New York and London.

LEIBOVIC K. N. (eds) [1969] *Information Processing in the Nervous System,* Springer-Verlag, Berlin, Heidelberg, New York.

LENNEBERG E. H. [1975] In "A neuropsychological comparison between man, chimpanzee and monkey", *Neuropsychologica, 13,* p. 125.

LEVY J. [1973] "Psychobiological Implications of Bilateral Asymmetry", in DIMOND & BEAUMONT (eds) [1973], pp. 121–83.

LEVY-AGRESTI J. & SPERRY R. W. [1968] "Differential perceptual capacities in major and minor hemispheres", *Proceedings of the National Academy of Sciences,* Washington, *61,* p. 1151.

LEVY J., TREVARTHEN C. & SPERRY R. W. [1972] "Perception of bilateral chimeric figures following hemispheric deconnexion", *Brain, 95,* pp. 61–78.

LIBET B. [1973] "Electrical Stimulation of Cortex in Human Subjects, and Conscious Memory Aspects", in IGGO (eds) [1973], pp. 743–90.

LIBET B., KOBAYASHI H. & TANAKA T. [1975] "Synaptic coupling into the production and storage of a neuronal memory trace", *Nature, 258,* pp. 155–7.

LIBET B., WRIGHT E. W., FEINSTEIN B. [1977] "The physiological timing and the subjectively referred timing of a conscious sensory experience: A functional role for the somato-sensory specific projection system in man", (in course of publication).

LORENTE de NÓ R. [1943] "Cerebral Cortex: Architecture, Intracortical Connections, Motor Projections", FULTON (eds) [1943], pp. 274–301.

LUND J. S. [1973] "Organization of neurons in the visual cortex, Area 17, of the monkey (Macaca mulatta)", *Journal of Comparative Neurology, 147,* pp. 455–96.

LUND J. S. & BOOTHE R. G. [1975] "Interlaminar connections and pyramidal neuron organisation in the visual cortex, Area 17, of the macaque monkey", *Journal of Comparative Neurology, 159,* pp. 305–34.

MCFIE J. [1961] "The effects of hemispherectomy on intellectual functioning in cases of infantile hemiplegia", *Journal of Neurology, Neurosurgery and Psychiatry, 24,* pp. 240–9.

MCGAUGH J. L. [1969] "Facilitation of Memory Storage Processes", in BOGOCH (eds) [1969], pp. 355–70.

MACKAY D. M. & JEFFREYS D. A. [1973] "Visually Evoked Potentials and Visual Perception in Man", in JUNG (eds) [1973 (c)], pp. 647–678.

MACLEAN P. D. [1970] "The Triune Brain, Emotion, and Scientific Bias", in SCHMITT (eds) [1970], pp. 336–49.

MARIN-PADILLA M. [1969] "Origin of the pericellular baskets of the pyramidal cells of the human motor cortex: A Golgi study", *Brain Research, 14,* pp. 633–646.

[1970] "Prenatal and early postnatal ontogenesis of the human motor cortex: A Golgi study. II. The basket-pyramidal system", *Brain Research, 23,* pp. 185–92.

MARLEN-WILSON W. D. & TEUBER H. L. [1975] "Memory for remote events in anterograde amnesia: recognition of public figures from newsphotographs", *Neuropsychologia, 13,* pp. 353–364.

MARR D. [1969] "A theory of cerebellar cortex", *Journal of Physiology, 202,* pp. 437–70.

[1970] "A theory for cerebral neocortex", *Proceedings of the Royal Society,* B 176, pp. 161–234.

MAUSS T. [1911] "Die faserarchitektonische Gliederung der Großhirnrinde", *Journal für Psychologie und Neurologie,* Leipzig, *8,* pp. 410–467.

MILLIKAN C. H. & DARLEY F. L. (eds) [1967] *Brain Mechanisms Underlying Speech and Language,* Grune and Stratton, New York and London.

MILNER B. [1963] "Effects of different brain lesions on card sorting", *Archives de Neurologie,* Paris, *9,* pp. 90–100.

[1966] "Amnesia Following Operation on the Temporal Lobes", in WHITTY & ZANGWILL (eds) [1966], pp. 109–33.

[1967] "Brain Mechanisms Suggested by Studies of Temporal Lobes", in MILLIKAN & DARLEY (eds) [1967], pp. 122–45.

[1968] "Visual recognition and recall after right temporal lobe excision in man", *Neuropsychologia, 6,* pp. 192–209.

[1970] "Memory and the Medial Temporal Regions of the Brain", in PRIBRAM & BROADBENT (eds) [1970], pp. 29–50.

[1971] "Interhemispheric differences in the localization of psychological processes in man", *British Medical Bulletin, 27,* pp. 272–77.

[1972] "Disorders of learning and memory after temporal-lobe lesions in man", *Clinical Neurosurgery, 19,* pp. 421–446.

[1974] "Hemispheric Specialization: Scope and Limits", in SCHMITT & WORDEN (eds) [1974], pp. 75–89.

MILNER B., BRANCH C. & RASMUSSEN T. [1964] "Observations on Cerebral Dominance", in WOLSTENHOLME & O'CONNOR (eds) [1964], pp. 200–14.

MILNER B., TAYLOR L. & SPERRY R. W. [1968] "Lateralized suppression of dichotically-presented digits after commissural section in man", *Science, 161,* pp. 184–5.

MISHKIN M. [1957] "Effects of small frontal lesions on delayed alternation in monkeys", *Journal of Neurophysiology, 20,* pp. 615–22.

[1972] "Cortical Visual Areas and Their Interactions", in KARCZMER & ECCLES (eds) [1972], pp. 187–208.

MORUZZI G. [1966] "The Functional Significance of Sleep With Particular Regard to the Brain Mechanisms Underlying Consciousness", in ECCLES (eds) [1966], pp. 345–88.

MOUNTCASTLE V. B. [1957] "Modality and topographic properties of single neurones of cat's somatic sensory cortex", *Journal of Neurophysiology, 20,* pp. 408–34.

[1975] "The view from within: Pathways to the study of perception", *Johns Hopkins Medical Journal, 136,* pp. 109–31.

MOUNTCASTLE V. B. & POWELL T. P. S. [1959] "Neural mechanisms subserving cutaneous sensibility, with special reference to the role of afferent inhibition in sensory perception and discrimination", *Bulletin of Johns Hopkins Hospital, 105,* pp. 201–32.

MOUNTCASTLE V. B., LYNCH J. C., GEORGOPOLOUS A., SAKATA H. & ACUNA C. [1975] "Posterior parietal association cortex of the monkey: Command functions for operations within extrapersonal space", *Journal of Neurophysiology, 38,* pp. 871–908.

MYERS R. E. [1961] "Corpus Callosum and Visual Gnosis", in DELAFRESNAYE (eds) [1961], pp. 481–505.

NAUTA W. J. H. [1971] "The problem of the frontal lobe: a reinterpretation", *Journal of Psychiatric Research, 8,* pp. 167–87.

OBRADOR S. [1964] "Nervous Integration After Hemispherectomy in Man", in SCHALTENBRAND & WOOLSEY (eds) [1964], pp. 133–54.

PANDYA D. N. & KUYPERS H. G. J. M. [1969] "Cortico-cortical connexions in the rhesus monkey", *Brain Research, 13,* pp. 13–36.

PASCAL B. [1961] *Pensées,* tr. J. M. Cohen, Penguin Books Ltd., London.

PASCHAL F. C. [1941] "The trend in theories of attention", *Psychological Review, 48,* pp. 383–403.

PENFIELD W. [1966] "Speech and Perception – the Uncommitted Cortex", in ECCLES (eds) [1966].

PENFIELD W. & JASPER H. [1954] *Epilepsy and the Functional Anatomy of the Human Brain,* Little, Brown & Company, Boston, p. 896.

PENFIELD W. & ROBERTS L. [1959] *Speech and Brain Mechanisms,* Princeton University Press, Princeton N. J.

PENFIELD W. & PEROT P. [1963] "The brain's record of auditory and visual experience", *Brain, 86,* pp. 596–696.

PEPPER S. C. [1961] "A Neural-Identity Theory of Mind", in HOOK (eds) [1961], pp. 45–61.

PETSCHE H. & BRAZIER M. A. B. (eds) [1972] *Synchronization of EEG Activity in Epilepsies* (Symposium of the Austrian Academy of Sciences, Vienna, Austria, Sept. 12–13, 1971), Springer-Verlag, Berlin, Heidelberg, New York.

PHILLIPS C. G. [1973] "Cortical localization and 'sensorimotor processes' at the 'middle level' in primates", *Proceedings of the Royal Society of Medicine, 66,* pp. 987–1002.

PIERCY M. [1967] "Studies of the neurological basis of intellectual function", *Modern Trends in Neurology, 4,* pp. 106–24.

POLLEN D. A. & TAYLOR J. H. [1974] "The Striate Cortex and the Spatial Analysis of Visual Space", in SCHMITT & WORDEN (eds) [1974], pp. 239–47.

POLTEN E. P. [1973] *A Critique of the Psycho-physical Identity Theory,* Mouton Publishers, The Hague, p. 290.

POPPER K. R. [1945] *The Open Society and Its Enemies,* Princeton University Press, Princeton N.J.

[1972] *Objective Knowledge: An Evolutionary Approach,* Clarendon Press, Oxford.

PORTER R. [1973] "Functions of the mammalian cerebral cortex in movement", *Progress in Neurobiology, 1,* pp. 1–51.

PREMACK D. [1970] "The education of Sarah: a chimp learns the language", *Psychology Today, 4,* pp. 55–8.

PRIBRAM K. H. [1971] *Languages of the Brain,* Prentice-Hall, Inc., Englewood Cliffs N.J., p. 432.

PRIBRAM K. H. & BROADBENT D. E. (eds) [1970] *Biology of Memory,* Academic Press, New York, London.

PUCCETTI R. [1973] "Brain bisection and personal identity", *British Journal for the Philosophy of Science, 24,* pp. 339–55.

QUARTON G. C., MELNECHUK T. & SCHMITT F. O. (eds) [1967] *The Neurosciences,* The Rockefeller University Press New York.

RAMÓN y CAJAL S. [1911] *Histologie du Système Nerveux de l'Homme et des Vertébrés,* II., Maloine, Paris, p. 993.

RISBERG J. & INGVAR D. H. [1973] "Patterns of activation in the grey matter of the dominant hemisphere during memorization and reasoning", *Brain, 96,* pp. 737–756.

ROSADINI G. & ROSSI G. F. [1967] "On the suggested cerebral dominance for consciousness", *Brain, 90,* pp. 101–12.

SAUL R. & SPERRY R. W. [1968] "Absence of commissurotomy symptoms with agenesis of the corpus callosum", *Neurology, 18,* p. 307.

SAVAGE W. [1975] "An Old Ghost in a New Body", in GLOBUS, MAXWELL & SAVODNIK (eds) [1975].

SCHALTENBRAND G. & WOOLSEY C. N. (eds) [1964] *Cerebral Localization and Organization,* University of Wisconsin Press, Madison.

SCHEIBEL M. E. & SCHEIBEL A. B. [1970] "Elementary processes in selected thalamic and cortical subsystems: the structural substrates", in SCHMITT (ed.) [1970], pp. 443–57.

SCHEID P. & ECCLES J. C. [1975] "Music and speech: Artistic functions of the human brain", *Psychology of Music, 3,* pp. 21–35.

SCHMITT F. O. (ed.) [1970] *The Neurosciences Second Study Program,* The Rockefeller University Press, New York.

SCHMITT F. O. & WORDEN F. G. (eds) [1974] *The Neurosciences Third Study Programm,* M.I.T. Press, Cambridge Mass., London.

SCHRIER A. M. & STOLLNITZ F. (eds) [1971] *Behavior of Nonhuman Primates,* Vol. IV, Academic Press, New York.

SERAFETINIDES E. A., HOARE, R. D. AND DRIVER, M. V. [1965] "Intracarotid sodium amylobarbitone and cerebral dominance for speech and consciousness", *Brain, 88,* pp. 107–30.

SHANKWEILER D. P. [1966] "Effects of temporal-lobe damage on perception of dichotically presented melodies", *Journal of Comparative and Physiological Psychology, 62,* pp. 115–19.

SHERRINGTON C. S. [1906] *Integrative Action of the Nervous System,* Yale University Press, New Haven, London, p. 411.

[1940] *Man on His Nature,* Cambridge University Press, London, p. 413.

SMART J. J. C. [1962] "Sensations and Brain Processes", in CHAPPELL (ed.) [1962], pp. 160–72.

SMITH A. J. [1966] "Speech and other functions after left (dominant) hemispherectomy", *Journal of Neurology, Neurosurgery and Psychiatry, 29,* pp. 467–71.

SMITH L. (eds) [1972] *Cerebral Disconnection,* Chas. C. Thomas Inc., Springfield, III.

SOMJEN G. [1975] *Sensory Coding in the Mammalian Nervous System,* Plenum/Rosetta, New York.

SPARKS R. & GESCHWIND N. [1968] "Dichotic listening in man after section of neocortical commissures", *Cortex, 4,* pp. 3–16.

SPERRY R. W. [1964] "The great cerebral commissure", *Scientific American, 210,* pp. 42–52.

[1968] "Mental Unity Following Surgical Disconnection of the Cerebral Hemispheres", in *The Harvey Lectures,* Academic Press, New York, pp. 293–323.

[1969] "A modified concept of consciousness", *Psychological Review, 76,* pp. 532–6.

[1970] "Perception in the Absence of the Neocortical Commissures", in *Perception and Its Disorders,* Res. Publ. A.R.N.M.D. 48, pp. 123–138.

[1974] "Lateral Specialization in the Surgically Separated Hemispheres", in SCHMITT & WORDEN (eds) [1974], pp. 5 – 19.

SPERRY R. W., GAZZANIGA M. S. & BOGEN J. E. [1969] "Interhemispheric Relationships: the Neocortical Commissures: Syndromes of Hemisphere Deconnection", in VINKEN & BRUYN (eds) [1969], pp. 273 – 90.

SPRAGUE J. [1967 (a)] "The Effects of Chronic Brainstem Lesions on Wakefulness, Sleep and Behavior", in SPRAGUE [1967 (b)], pp. 148 – 94.

[1967 (b)] *Sleep and Altered States of Consciousness,* Williams and Wilkins Company, Baltimore.

STRATTON G. M. [1897] "Vision without inversion of retinal image", *Psychological Review, 4,* pp. 463 – 81.

STUDDERT-KENNEDY M. & SHANKWEILER D. [1970] "Hemispheric specialization for speech perception", *Journal of the Acoustical Society of American 48,* pp. 579 – 94.

SZENTÁGOTHAI J. [1968] "Structure-Functional Considerations of the Cerebellar Neuron Network", *Proc. of the I. E. E. E., 56,* pp. 960–8.

[1969] "Architecture of the Cerebral Cortex", in JASPER, WARD & POPE (eds) [1969], pp. 13 – 28.

[1970] "Les circuits neuronaux de l'écorce cérébrale", *Bulletin de l'Academie Royale de Medecine de Belgique,* pp. 475 – 92.

[1971] "Memory Functions and the Structural Organization of the Brain", in ADAM (ed.) [1971], pp. 21 – 25.

[1972] "The Basic Neuronal Circuit of the Neocortex", in PETSCHE & BRAZIER (eds) [1972], pp. 9 – 24.

[1973] "Synaptology of the Visual Cortex", in JUNG (ed.) [1973], pp. 269 – 324.

[1974] "A Structural Overview", in SZENTÁGOTHAI & ARBIB (eds) [1974], pp. 354 – 410.

[1975] "The 'module-concept' in cerebral cortex architecture", *Brain Research, 95,* 475–496.

SZENTÁGOTHAI, J. and ARBIB, M. A. [1974] *Conceptual Models of Neural Organization, Neurosciences Research Program Bulletin, 12.*

SZILARD L. [1964] "On memory and recall", *Proceedings of the National Academy of Sciences,* Washington, *51,* pp. 1092 – 9.

TANABE T., YARITA H., IINO M., OOSHIMA Y. & TAGAKI S. F. [1975] "An olfactory projection area in orbitofrontal cortex of the monkey", *Journal of Neurophysiology, 38,* pp. 1269 – 83.

TEUBER H.-L. [1964] "The Riddle of Frontal Lobe Function in Man", in WARREN & AKERT (eds) [1964], pp. 410 – 44.

[1967] "Lacunae and Research Approaches to Them", in MILLIKAN & DARLEY (eds) [1967], pp. 204 – 16.

[1972] "Unity and diversity of frontal lobe functions", *Acta Neurobiol. Exp. Neurobiol., 32,* pp. 615 – 56.

[1974] "Why Two Brains?", in SCHMITT & WORDEN (eds) [1974], pp. 71–4.

TEUBER H.-L., BATTERSBY W. S. & BENDER M. B. [1960] *Visual Field Defects After Penetrating Missile Wounds of the Brain*, Harvard University Press, Cambridge, Mass., p. 143.

TOYAMA K., MATSUNAMI K., OHNO T. & TOKASHIKI S. [1974] "An intracellular study of neuronal organization in the visual cortex", *Experimental Brain Research, 21*, pp. 45–66.

TREVARTHEN C. [1973] "Analysis of Cerebral Activities That Generate and Regulate Consciousness in Commissurotomy Patients", in DIMOND & BEAUMONT (eds) [1973], pp. 235–63.

TREVARTHEN C. B. & SPERRY R. W. [1973] "Perceptual unity of the ambient visual field in human commissurotomy patients", *Brain, 96*, pp. 547–70.

DE VALOIS R. L. [1973] "Central Mechanisms of Color Vision", in JUNG (ed.) [1973 a].

VALVERDE F. [1967] "Apical dendritic spines of the visual cortex and light deprivation in the mouse", *Experimental Brain Research, 3*, pp. 337–52.

[1968] "Structural changes in the area striate of the mouse after enucleation", *Experimental Brain Research, 5*, pp. 274–92.

VICTOR M., ADAMS R. D. & COLLINS G. H. [1971] *The Wernicke-Korsakoff-Syndrome*, Blackwell Scientific Publications, Oxford.

VINKEN P. J. & BRUYN G. W. (eds) [1969] *Handbook of Clinical Neurology*, Vol. 4, North Holland Publishing Company, Amsterdam.

VOGT C. & VOGT O. [1919] "Allgemeine Ergebnisse unserer Hirnforschung", *Journal für Psychologie und Neurologie*, Leipzig, *25*, pp. 277–462.

WADA J. A., CLARKE R. J. & HAMM A. E. [1973] "Morphological Asymmetry of Temporal and Frontal Speech Zones in Human Cerebral Hemispheres: Observation on 100 Adult and 100 Infant Brains", Xth International Congress of Neurology, Barcelona.

WARREN J. M. & AKERT K. (eds) [1964] *The Frontal Granular Cortex and Behaviour*, McGraw-Hill, New York.

WEISKRANTZ L. [1968] "Experiments on the r.n.s. (real nervous system) and monkey memory", *Proceedings of the Royal Society, B 171*, pp. 335–52.

[1974] "The Interaction Between Occipital and Temporal Cortex in Vision: an Overview", in SCHMITT & WORDEN (eds) [1974], pp. 189–204.

WERNER G. [1974] "Neural Information Processing with Stimulus Feature Extractors", in SCHMITT & WORDEN (eds) [1974], pp. 171–83.

WERNICKE C. [1874] *Der aphasiche Symptomencomplex: Eine psychologische Studie auf anatomischer Basis*, Cohn and Weigert, Breslau.

WHITE H. H. [1961] "Cerebral hemispherectomy in the treatment of infantile hemiplegia. Review of the literature and report of two cases", *Confinia Neurologica*, Basel, *21*, pp. 1–50.

WHITTAKER V. P. & GRAY E. G. [1962] "The synapse: Biology and Morphology", *British Medical Bulletin, 18*, pp. 223–28.

WHITTY C. W. M. & ZANGWILL O. L. (eds) [1966] *Amnesia,* Butterworths, London.

WIECK H. H. (eds) [1974] *Psychopathologie musischer Gestaltungen,* F. K. Schattauer Verlag, Stuttgart, New York.

WIESEL T. N. & HUBEL D. H. [1963] "Single-cell responses in striate cortex of kittens deprived of vision in one eye", *Journal of Neurophysiology, 26,* pp. 1003 – 1017.

WIESENDANGER M. [1969] "The pyramidal tract. Recent investigations on its morphology and function", *Ergebnisse der Physiologie, Biologischen Chemie und Experimentellen Pharmakologie, 61,* pp. 72 – 136.

WOLSTENHOLME D. W. & O'CONNOR M. [1964] *Disorders of Language, Ciba Symposium on Disorders of Language,* J. and A. Churchill, London.

ZAIDEL E. [1973] Linguistic competence and related functions in the right cerebral hemisphere of man following commissurotomy and hemispherectomy. California Institute of Technology, Pasadena, California, Thesis.

[1976] "Auditory Language Comprehension in The Right Hemisphere Following Cerebral Commissurotomy and Hemispherectomy: A Comparison With Child Language and Aphasia", in ZURIF & CARAMAZZA (eds) [1976].

ZAIDEL E. & SPERRY R. W. [1972 (a)] "Functional reorganization following commissurotomy in man", Biol. Ann. Rep., *California Institute of Technology,* p. 80.

[1972 (b)] "Memory following commissurotomy", Biol. Ann. Rep. California Institute of Technology, p. 79.

ZANGWILL O. L. [1960] *Cerebral Dominance and Its Relation to Psychological Function,* Oliver & Boyd, Edinburgh, p. 31.

[1973] "Consciousness and the Cerebral Hemispheres", in DIMOND & BEAUMONT (eds) [1973], pp. 264 – 78.

ZIPPEL H. P. (eds) [1973] *Memory and Transfer of Information,* Plenum Publishing Corporation, New York.

ZURIF E. & CARAMAZZA A. (eds) [1976] *The Acquisition and Break-down of Language: Parallels and Divergencies,* Johns Hopkins University Press, Baltimore.

Part III

Dialogues Between the Two Authors

Dialogue I

10 a. m., 20 September, 1974

E: Karl, could you start our discussion with a short statement on epistemology?

P: The usual view of knowledge is that it originates with observations. We may replace this by the view that knowledge is always a modification of earlier knowledge.[1] This view seems at first sight to lead to an infinite regress. I don't think that it really does so in a dangerous way, any more than does the riddle of life itself, which, in a sense, also leads to an infinite regress. Knowledge goes back, ultimately, to inborn knowledge, and to animal knowledge in the sense of expectations. Observations are always already interpreted in terms of previous knowledge; that is to say, the observations themselves would not even exist if there was no previous knowledge which they could modify; for example, which they could falsify. That is the main epistemological point I wanted to make. So far as I know, I think you would be ready to accept it.

E: Yes, I would be happy with those ideas. I have some modifications to suggest because I always think of what is going on in the brain under all these conditions. How in fact are our sensory perceptions given? You would agree, I think, that in our experience of the world everything comes to us through the senses in the manner described in chapter E2. It is transposed upon our inborn dispositions that derive from genetic instructions in the building of the brain and upon the stored memories whereby our brains have become more and more gifted in their interpretation of the input. All of life is learning. We are learning to make the most subtle interpretations of what is given us by our

[1] See my [1963(a)], p. 23, and my section 34.

sense organs. We have to realize that these ideas are implicit in an evolutionary origin. Genetic coding is essentially an evolutionary concept. Evolution in fact can be most simply thought of as a wonderful biological process for creating the genetic coding that is most appropriate for the conditions of the ecological niche that we happen to be in.

Perhaps we differ in the following respects. I am always thinking of myself as central in the first place to my perceptions, my imaginations, my environment. Everything comes to me in the first place. Then from all that is inborn in my brain and all that is built in my brain by experiences, I proceed to interpret so that I can act most appropriately in the various situations, and of course assimilate the new knowledge into all the experiential remembrances that I have already accumulated. And so I have the belief that I am central to my own experiences and interpretations. I escape from solipsism by utilizing these experiences in order to understand other persons and the world around me. I feel, though, that I have first of all to be primary in this whole action so far as I myself am concerned. I readily give to each experiencing self the same prerogative of being primary to its whole sensory experience, the whole tremendous incoming load of information that is pouring in by its sense organs and that has to be interpreted in the light of memory (cp. chapter E8). Our wonderful memory has given each of us wisdom and understanding at each stage of our life. It relates to the immediate sensory experiences, but, more importantly, it is modified by and developed by the whole of our past experiences. This is essentially the position of a person of civilization and culture.

P: I think our disagreement is mainly about your use of certain stock phrases, if I may so call them; for example: "everything comes to me in the first place" and "central to my own experiences". These expressions, and the view that everybody is primary to their whole sensory experience, seem to me uncritical. What really happens is, I suggest, this. *After* I am established, so to speak, as a self-conscious person, things look as these phrases suggest; but the word "primary" carries with it the mistaken suggestion that the ego is, in time, or logically, the first thing. But in time, or logically, I am, first of all, an organism not fully conscious of myself – when I am a small baby. I have, however, already at this stage, expectations or inborn knowledge, which consist of theory-like dispositions to interpret what reaches me through my senses, and without which the incoming sensory data would never begin to crystallize into perceptions, experience and knowledge. I suppose that the incoming sensory data in the very first days of life are pretty chaotic, and that they are only gradually organized and interpreted.

I think that this is also true of the working of the brain. Stimulated or, if you like, challenged by sense stimuli, the brain has to begin to do its work, which, with respect to the senses, is mainly that of interpretation. This work must be very largely predisposed; and *it* must be "primary" to experiencing either the external world or the ego. I would therefore suggest that it is incorrect to say that primarily everything comes to *me*, or that in the first place everything comes to *me*, through the senses. Rather, what is "primary" is the inborn disposition to sense, and the inborn disposition to interpret what arrives through the senses. Thus, if you say that I am central to my experience, then I accept that, but only after I am constituted as a person or a self; which in itself is the result of learning. I think, however, that you are absolutely right to say that "all of life is learning". Learning is interpretation and the formation of new theories, new expectations, and new skills. I have first of all to learn to be myself; and I learn to be myself in contrast to learning what is not myself. By this process I can ultimately establish myself, by degrees. It does not happen all at once – it will probably take weeks; I don't mean weeks from birth, but, say, weeks from the moment that this particular process, the process of becoming oneself, gets started: it will probably take weeks before this process is more or less crystallized. From then on, I am central to my experiences; but if what I have here suggested is correct, we should see this not as something primary, but as something which is itself the result of learning.

E: I think that we are not in disagreement in this respect but we have different perspectives about it. I would readily agree that the newborn baby is acting with the few primitive instincts that a newborn child has in the way of suckling and crying and so on, but it is learning quite fast. In a few days it learns to follow with its eyes, and it even learns its mother's voice, and also it is orienting itself. Of course it is acting in accordance with the instinctive drives of a primitive organism though it is rapidly outgrowing these. It is learning very fast indeed I think, much more than we can imagine. It is relating vision to movement of its hands, all the time watching and touching, relating touch and vision, touch and hearing, and so on. There is an intensive learning process going on. Now of course I don't know how to decide which is primary and which is not. I don't think the question can be well phrased at this stage. I think we have simply here an organism with immense potentialities and drives to learn, to develop, and gradually to find out that it is an independent existence by discovering what it is and what it is not; that is, environment: what belongs to it as hands and feet, and what does not belong as shoes and socks and so on. It is learning gradually to strip itself down to essentials and it is learning how it can act and how it can bring about happenings by movement under visual control and so on. It is learning how it can auditorily command. All of this is going on through the first year of life. All of this time it is deficient in the performances of other young mammals, namely all the skilled instinctive performances — to be able to stand and run and leap as the young herbivores can do for example. It is initially quite helpless, but it is learning rapidly and being very flexible. I think this is the essence of babyhood in the first year or so until with its developing language it comes more and more to realize its own selfhood.

Then I think there is a change to quite a different story with the developing linguistic efforts of a young child. Despite all that is written I think we still underestimate the immense linguistic striving that there is. A 2-year-old child already has a feeling of language with meaning and intention. We are apt to think that you learn your first language easily. I think, on the other hand, we underestimate the immense experimental effort and the intensity of the effort being made by a young child in learning how to use the language, to learn how to name things, to learn how to describe experiences. Furthermore it has to relate itself as an individual against the other individuals which already, at one to two years old, it is recognizing as beings like itself.

There are ways in which I think we should consider the use of the word primary. We have hitherto restricted ourselves to the newborn baby and its first year or two when it is developing its knowledge of the world and of itself in an experimental manner, utilizing its brain and sense organs and a whole sensory structure which is built in the most designed manner. For example its job is to relate its visual perceptions to its tactual perceptions and to its kinaesthetic perceptions. It makes some unified world out of sight, touch and movement. That is a simple way of looking at it. We have the explanation developed by Held and Hein with the kittens (cp. chapter E8, Fig. 12) to illustrate the importance of what I call participation learning. It is sometimes called perceptual learning. Babies are learning all the time on that level. I think we don't disagree.

Where I think we might disagree is about the use of the word primary. In the ordinary adult life, where we can now consider some new experience, we have to see how we achieve some understanding and interpretation of this new experience. I give as an example a kind of thought experiment. Supposing that we were suddenly transported to the moon as one of those observers. We are suddenly confronted with a strange landscape, where the atmosphere is infinitely clear and we have not got the ordinary criteria for telling us of dimensions or of distances. We don't know sizes and everything is strange. We have then to set about working out how to interpret our experiences. They come to us primarily through vision and we have other tricks like parallax and so on in order to use this for the interpretation. I would say that in the first place our moon observer has his own experiences and from that he tries to use all kinds of skilled techniques to build up an understanding of the spatial relationships of what is giving him his experiences of the external world. The external world, or the moon world in this case, is to him secondary to the way he comes to knowledge about it from his primary experiences which are delivered by his sense organs.

P: I do not agree. I think that if we were taken to the moon and left only with vision, we would be lost. Only if we could somehow or other engage in activities, move about, and so on, could we ever really establish ourselves on, say, a strange planet or in completely strange surroundings. So, you see, I give much more weight to the part played in interpretation by activity: both to the activities of our limbs and to the activities of our brain. These are active processes, and so is the process of making and matching in the brain. That I lay such weight on active processes is based on the fact that there can be people like Helen Keller, who are defective in all the (for us) most important senses like sight and hearing, and are still able to achieve a complete interpretation, and in the main a correct interpretation, of the world. This has happened with people who are both blind and deaf and dumb.

I do not, of course, want to deny that the senses are immensely important, and, as you have mentioned, this will be particularly true if an adult is suddenly placed in completely new surroundings. But even here I would wish to claim that we would first make a hypothesis as to where we were, and then try to test that hypothesis. In other words, we would use a trial and error, a making-and-matching, process: a process of conjecture and refutation.

This is why I think that the old story that the senses are primary in learning is wrong (especially in learning something new, i. e. in discovering). I believe that, in learning, hypotheses have a primary role; that making comes before matching.[2] The senses have two roles: first, they challenge us to *make* our hypotheses; second, they help us to *match* our hypotheses – by assisting in the process of refutation, or selection.

E: Yes, I agree of course that we are never presented with a clean slate with no past experiences, no past understandings on which to interpret a fresh lot of sensory data. What I was trying to say was that, when we are confronted

[2] This is Ernst Gombrich's phrase: see, for references, the index of his *Art and Illusion* [1960].

with new sensory data, then that is primary to the interpretations. I admit that the interpretations are built upon all of our experiences, inborn and learned, but, on the other hand, I think we have to say that in any one instance we are all the time acting on the basis of the immense information input from our sense organs — interpreting it, rejecting it, modifying it, correlating it. I have immediately to say all this depends upon a brain which has learnt the whole wonderfully subtle means of sensory interpretation from the past. You say that we are always trying to make before matching. In making and matching are we trying to get our sensory experience related to and matched with earlier sensory experiences? Is that what you mean?

P: I shall try to formulate this again, since it is important; I think it contains one of the key elements of my epistemology. I can, perhaps, put it like this. There are no sensory "data". Rather, there is an incoming challenge from the sensed world which then puts the brain, or ourselves, to work on it, to try to interpret it. Thus, at first, there are no data: there is, rather, a challenge to do something; namely, to interpret. Then we try to match the so-called sense data. I say "so-called" because I don't think there are sense "data". What most people hold to be a simple sense "datum" is in fact the outcome of a most elaborate process. Nothing is directly "given" to us: perception is arrived at only as a result of many steps involving interaction between the stimuli which reach the senses, the interpreting apparatus of the senses, and the structure of the brain. So, while the term "sense datum" suggests primacy in the first step, I would suggest that, before I can realize what is a sense datum for me (before it is ever "given" to me), there are a hundred steps of give and take which result from the challenge presented to our senses and our brain.

My epistemology arises in the following way. I try to show first what one would expect to happen on more or less logical grounds and then suggest that things actually do happen like this in reality.[3] All I have learned from you about the brain supports the view that this *is* really the case. I have, for example, learned that there are certain cells which react only to inclined lines of light, or only to edges or something like that (chapter E2, Fig. 6). This we take it, is the result of evolution; in the course of evolution, perhaps, there emerged the theory that there are inclined lines of light and parallel lines, and that the distance between these lines was somehow important for our interpretation of visual challenges.

---

[3] It is not suggested that as, say, induction is logically invalid we can tell *a priori* that it does not exist in psychology, but just that we should *try* to see if psychology will work without induction.

E: Yes, I think I am beginning to see your point now. I think there is a misunderstanding. This is a mistake that people make when they don't appreciate fully the immense complexity of the handling of sensory data. One is apt to think that a visual experience is actually a perfect replica of the retinal image. This is of course not true. There are immense complications of interactions starting in the retina, and, as I have written in chapter E2 on sensory experiences, the visual data goes through stage after stage in the visual cortex, where it is being processed and relayed. At one stage there is the tendency of cells to be optimally excited by bright lines in one or other orientation. Then it gets more complicated and it gradually builds in complexity so that we can imagine in principle how simple geometrical shapes can have cells specially relating to them, as happens in the inferotemporal lobe (cp. chapter E2). This is still not the stage of conscious perception.

All of this comes before you actually have the experience, so in a sense when you get the experience, you can say it is not primary. It is based upon all of this immense patterned development that is a necessary prelude to a conscious experience. Having this experience, we have then to interpret it. It may be an illusion. It may result from all kinds of strange misunderstandings and misinterpretations of sensory data. We may be looking in a mirror, for example, and see the perceived object the wrong way around. We have to do all interpretations from past knowledge and so gain from it our knowledge of what is giving rise to this experience. At the practical, survival level it isn't important if you enjoy your experiences. What you have to do is to use your experiences to understand the world you are in and to act appropriately in this world.

P: Now I think we are very near to complete agreement; and I hope to be able to show you the beauty of this way of looking at things.

All experience is already interpreted by the nervous system a hundredfold – or a thousandfold – before it becomes conscious experience. When it does become conscious experience then it can be interpreted, more or less consciously, as a theory: we may formulate a hypothesis – a linguistic statement of a theory – to explain these experiences. This statement can then be publicly criticized – a discussion may start about it. That is, we may use language to select the best interpretation from the various alternatives that have been put forward.

Now, the thing to note is that the process at the last and highest stage – the World 3 process of critical discussion – uses in effect the same mechanism of elimination, of trial and error, of making and matching, that occurs at the lower levels. The same mechanism is used on the lower levels and then on the higher levels of the nervous system, and ultimately, at the scientific or logical level. This mechanism becomes objectivized – linguistically formulated, and incorporated into our institutions – and becomes, as it were, public property.

This is an application of the heuristic idea that the same thing that happens on the logical level will have happened on all levels of the organism.

You will now see why I think that it is better not to speak of sense data as being primary. I think that we get a really beautiful picture of the organism and of the working of the mind if we see both as involving a hierarchy of levels at which these operations take place. These levels or layers are probably at the same time very largely evolutionary layers. The highest interpretative layers in the brain are followed by still higher interpretative layers which transcend the organism and which belong to the objective World 3; and the same process is continued there. You can approach this the other way round if you study the process of theory-making in World 3. For it involves essentially the same process which the organism applies in a comparatively mechanical way – instinctively or automatically, or as a result of its structure or its genetic instructions. Or, rather, the process is in part the same – it is less and less mechanical the higher we go in the hierarchy of controls and revisions.

E: I should now make a final comment about the brain and the way it has come to give us this marvellous performance. Up to a certain stage we can explain what is going on, particularly in the *visual system*, where we can see the way in which the retinal picture is converted first of all into a punctate mosaic. That is the way it has to be transmitted to the brain by something like 10^8 sense cells to 10^6 nerve fibres in the optic nerve, and this is again punctate action. Then it has got to be brought together again in the light of and on the basis of the neuronal connectivities built in the brain and the learned modifications of these through life, as we learn to interpret more and more subtly the sensory data given to us through the visual or the somaesthetic sense for example.

Another point is that it has to be not only handled as pure visual data, but it has to be blended with the data from the other sense organs (the other modalities) so that we are now beginning to have a real world such as we know with colour and shape and sound and form and dimension and even with smell. This is the world we know, but we are a tremendously long way from being able to give an account of how that world is built out of the data provided by our sense organs. I want to go back to our original point. It concerns this building from moment to moment of the pictured world that we experience. This is dependent on an immense learning performance as well as the structure that was originally built by genetic instructions. This great learning performance was a trial-and-error learning so that we became more subtle and more sophisticated and more clever. Also there is another side to it all. When we are dealing with the human brain we have to think that pictures are not just patterned experiences for action. They are also for enjoying, for appreciating, for understanding at higher levels than the ordinary mere reactions for immediate survival. Reactions for immediate survival occur in the wonderful performance of our brain, driving a car in traffic or being a pedestrian in traffic or what you will. That is a survival operation and we tend to think of the sense organs as giving us mere survival under these conditions, but they give us much more, they make life worthwhile, and this we are far from understanding.

P: I think that we are now largely in agreement. What I feel is important about this in relation to our book is that the epistemology fits together well with our present knowledge of brain physiology, so that both things mutually support each other. Of course, it is all conjectural: everything is conjectural, and we must not be dogmatic. But when you speak about the huge task before the brain physiologists in finding out more about, for example, the visual cortex (and the decoding in the visual cortex of the point action code which is delivered to the visual cortex by the retina via the optic nerve) I would suggest that a good conjecture and working hypothesis – a sweeping hypothesis – would be that all the integration processes or decoding processes are of the critical or trial-and-error type. That is to say, that each of them, so to speak, comes with its hypothesis and sees whether it works. The nerve cell which reacts to an inclined line is actually ready to fire or tries to fire; or it actually fires, and, if the matching is successful, it fires more, or better, or whatever it is. There is a difference if the action matches, or if it finds out that the action does not match. How this works in detail of course I, who am not a physiologist, would not dare to say. But I would say that it is a good working hypothesis that each of these integrative stages is essentially a stage of action, of actually doing something. Thus, if we were not moving about and moving our limbs, then our various senses would never integrate and constitute a reality. What we do with touch is to control our vision and what we do with our vision is to control our touch. That is to say, the different senses mutually control each other, and quite obviously, if a man is deficient in a sense, then he is deficient in some controls, and to that extent may be more dependent on his fellow men for controls, as was Helen Keller.

E: It is important now that we have got to this stage to refine our concepts of what sensory experiences give us. For example, I am looking out on a beautiful garden. As you look out and see the flowers, you can identify the plants if you are a good botanist. You would find an immense wealth of interest there if you were taken around by a good botanist. This would show you how subtly you can interpret your visual experiences to give you some newer and deeper understanding of some botanical life with leaves and stalks and flower forms and bud forms and so on. It is true of our understanding of the whole of the animal world. I can suggest other examples. Just think of the way in which we judge movement and action in watching skilled games. There we can participate in a way with the game because we have had our own experiences. You can't look at a skilled game with a proper appreciation if you haven't been trained to do this. American football looks like nonsense to me. I never know anything about it. I know other forms of football and tennis. I am not deficient in my understanding of some games, but I am ignorant about many others. This is just to give you an indication of how we train and learn to interpret our sensory data in terms of reaction or excitement or skills of performance in a way which I think is absolutely remarkable. You have to realize just what we are deriving by our learned experiences in the way of new interpretations transcending the mere sensory data that we are provided with.

P: But that action or participation is required is shown in the experiments with the gondola kitten, for example, as illustrated in chapter E8, Figure 12.

E: Yes, that is true. This beautifully simple and revealing experiment done by Held and Hein shows how participation learning is required in order to appreciate the simplest things about the sensory data. I believe very much that we should through all our lives be active in exploring and sensing and testing. Moreover the message from such experiments is very important from Karl's point of view, that we have been discussing. You cannot, for example, learn to appreciate pictures of one period or another by just looking at them yourself. You have either to discuss with people or read the critical and evaluative literature. You have to enter into the World 3 relationship with everything you see in order to become a human appreciator of it. The whole of life I think has to be enriched in this way so that we are not just simply naive experiencers of visual or tactual or auditory data, but that all the time we are challenged by it to become more and more able to see the more subtle relationships in space and time of form, colour, pattern, melody, harmony, etc. This is the essence of art.

P: I think that it is terribly important that, throughout our whole life, we should avoid being mere passive receivers of information. There is a special danger in childhood: that our schools may treat children like the gondola kitten. This was especially true when children had to sit in a confining form – a form which was made so as to reduce the possibility for the children to move, in order that they shouldn't disturb other children and, especially, the teacher. In other words, our children were once gondola kittens. While it would not matter so much if people our age spent their time staring at television screens, I think it is very undesirable if television or teaching machines are used as a medium of instruction in such a way that the children play a passive role: that they just sit and learn. I don't deny that television has its good sides if used very sparingly, but a growing young person should be stimulated to have problems and then to try to solve these problems, and should be helped in solving these problems only if help is needed. He should not be indoctrinated, and should not be fed with answers where no questions were asked: where the problems did not come from the inside.

E: Yes, I think there is something in that. On the other hand, I do think that we have to talk. If we are trying to train our children to be good at some sophisticated game or dancing or skiing or skating, then it is silly to sit them on a form and talk about skiing. They should do it and they should dance, and so on. But if on the other hand you want to train them in mathematics or train them in a language, in linguistic expression, they might as well give up moving around and concentrate on the task in hand. They get their activity then by trying to solve problems in mathematics or by expressing their ideas in sentences. To be critical about their performance is in this way to be active again.

P: I would like to add to what we have said by referring to a passage from pages 47 and 48 of my *Conjectures and Refutations* [1963(a)].

The point I make there is that, for logical reasons, the hypothesis must come before the observation; and I suggest that what is true for logical reasons is actually true for the organism – both for its nervous system and for its psychology.

I might add that I think that the integration of the different senses and their mutual cooperation is very largely a matter of the mutual checking and mutual criticism, as it were, of one set of interpretations by another. I would suggest that the various messages coming from the various senses – the interpreted messages – are revised in the light of how far they agree and give the same results.

E: A point that we have to realize is that sense impressions, the total perceptual input that we have, is a call for action. Under most cases it is an action to explore, an action to gain a better understanding, an action to avoid something. We are all the time using all these inputs in order to bring about movements of one kind or another, and of course we delight in this. We can think of the small child where it is simply having the most wonderful experiences in movements with somersaults and swings and so on studying and experiencing everything. Later on we take to sophisticated ball games, and to games of dancing, skiing, skating, sailing, and so on. All these are wonderful experiences where we are challenging one sense against another: the movements and stresses of our limbs, the senses of our vestibular orienting mechanisms, the senses of touch, the senses of vision and so on. Life is amazingly rich because in this way we can use the tremendous range of our sensory experiences, organizing them and acting on them and so enjoying some delightful harmony of space and time.

P: I would certainly agree with that. And, although I am not a brain physiologist, I would like to add that in my view these challenges happen only within the brain. However, my hypothesis is that not only are practically all interpretations which are brain-dependent performed in the manner of a mechanism, as it were, but that they are supported by a built-in need or drive, a need to be active, and to experience the enjoyment of performing the action.[4] In this connection, I have a hypothesis about colour blindness and the need to interpret in terms of colour. My hypothesis is that we may give children who are colour blind some sense of colour vision if we give them coloured glasses with, let us say, the left eye containing a red glass and the right eye a green glass, so that they get different inputs from the two eyes. I think that they may learn to interpret these in a two-coloured manner.

---

[4] Karl Bühler used to speak of the "enjoyment of action (or of functioning)" *("Funktionslust")*.

Dialogue II

5:15 p.m., 20 September 1974

E: We turn to the discussion of the very controversial question: how did consciousness come into the biological world? I think for a start most would agree that animals differ from plants or, shall we say, higher animals differ from plants in that they have a nervous system which is a highly specialized part of the organism that is concerned with picking up information and reacting to it. This gives animals a performance quite different from that of plants, which are essentially organisms that have a much more passive role in their whole existence, sessile and not as a rule evincing any responses except those of growth and turgor. When we come to survey the whole sequence of biological evolution of animal forms and behaviours, then if you wish you can see all kinds of purposive actions in primitive organisms, even in protozoa such as amoeba or paramoecium. If you examine the higher animal level, the multicellular organism, you can see, as in coelenterates, a primitive nervous system that develops appropriate reflex reactions in response to stimuli. So it goes on in the whole of the invertebrate story into quite complex forms with complex reactions as, for example, in the higher insects. We are all familiar with the bee's ability to learn its environment so that when its hive is changed, it can do a few circuits around and learn the way home when it goes out on its flights. That is a learning response and then of course we are familiar with the information given symbolically in the dance of the bees. Finally at the top of the invertebrate tree there are the still more highly developed nervous systems of the higher molluscs. The octopus for example has been studied in detail by J. Z. Young, who has shown that it has a highly developed brain with most complex responses to signals, and the ability to learn. Now, that is the summit of the invertebrate story and I think we could now question and ask: is there evidence that invertebrates have some kind of responses of their brain which could be classed as giving conscious experiences?

P: The question of how consciousness came into life is of course an incredibly difficult one because the evidence is almost nil. Just as is the evidence of how life came into the world. The situation is very similar, and I think perhaps the best one can say is that if the evolutionary story applies to life and to consciousness, then there ought to be degrees of life and degrees of consciousness. When we look for evidence as to whether there are degrees of life and consciousness, I do think we find reasonably good evidence for both, but I am afraid it is too difficult a question to go into deeply just now.

I might mention, however, the fact that we can, on the basis of self-observation, find that we are sometimes on the border of being not conscious. And there is also the very important fact that we quite normally have a loss of full consciousness in sleep; and in very deep sleep there is a pretty severe loss of consciousness. Indeed, this kind of evidence is practically all the evidence we have for the existence of degrees of consciousness, and therefore, all the evidence we have about the possible emergence of consciousness.

Some people have found the idea of the emergence of consciousness incredible and ununderstandable. It is a miracle, but it may not be a far greater miracle than that we can wake up in the morning and recreate full self-consciousness out of more or less nothing. Against this, it might be said that the process of waking up consists of making a link, within our brain, with memories of previous periods; and that this is more understandable than the creation of consciousness from nothing – at any rate, nothing like memory. Here, however, we might consider the case of the newly-born child. Although it probably has nothing which we would call memory, it does of course have some sort of knowledge or information or expectations, and it has to synthesize consciousness out of what is certainly not consciousness. Although the re-creation of consciousness happens every day, I think that this is probably as miraculous as the first occurrence of consciousness and that it is almost as difficult to understand – if we *really* want to understand it.

How did consciousness come to exist? I think that the main answer which we can give, and which has some evidence in its favour, though not very much, is the answer "by degrees". I would say that anything like conscious awareness – not self-consciousness; rather, anything resembling our own conscious awareness of a lower degree, let us say, the conscious awareness which we attribute to a child before it has learned to speak – can probably only be attributed to animals with a central nervous system. But something resembling consciousness in some way can probably be attributed to an earlier stage of evolution. Of course, it is most unlikely that we shall ever obtain evidence for or against this conjecture, and even if we have evidence, it itself is obviously all highly conjectural. I agree with you, Jack, that the evidence that other people have minds is infinitely better than the evidence we have that animals have minds, but I do think that the evolutionary hypothesis more or less forces us to attribute lower degrees of consciousness to animals. My conjecture has what one may call a partly evidential and a partly intuitive basis. Now the intuitive basis is difficult to spell out, but the evidential basis consists not only of what I have just mentioned — including the child before it speaks — but also of the evidence with respect to the minor hemisphere and its functions. That is to say, I agree with you, Jack, that the minor hemisphere may be characterized as being something like an excellent animal brain. I would say that it was still an animal brain — or related to an animal brain — in that it is cut off from full self-consciousness. But I think that the achievements of this minor hemisphere (although it is comparable to the animal brain) are so high that we have to attribute to it not only memory, which is a kind of prerequisite of consciousness, but a certain degree of creativity. There is also the ability to solve pretty abstract problems. Thus take for example the case of the ordering of those strip cartoons which you describe in chapter E5. This ordering of the strip cartoons did more or less convince me that we have to accept Sperry's conjecture concerning the minor hemisphere.

Now, all this seems to me to make it at least possible to attribute to animals with a well developed central nervous system something like consciousness. But it is very important to note that while we have every reason to say that they have a sense of time, they are probably not fully conscious of time: they do not have even the rudiments of a theory of the regular progression of time (such as that yesterday is followed by today, and today is followed by tomorrow). Full consciousness depends on having an abstract theory which is linguistically formulated. It would, incidentally, be interesting to check the minor hemisphere for an understanding of progress in time in this sense. The comic strip assemblage has established that the minor hemisphere can order pictures according to a time sequence, but this does not mean that the minor hemisphere has a consciousness of the difference between yesterday, today, and tomorrow, and it would be most interesting to find out whether it has.

E: The subject under discussion has moved on to higher animal brains, their performance, and the possibility that there is something like an awareness, a consciousness associated with some of the activities going on in the brains of these animals; and via higher animals, I will go all the way up to the anthropoid apes. Now I would say that we don't have any proper tests for this. I don't want to put myself on record as denying the evidence of something which could deserve a name of consciousness because it has something of the same attributes or experiences that occur with us when we are self-conscious. The self-conscious mind is something we know about. We don't have to test for it. We experience it, and we can talk about it to others and soon learn through linguistic and other communications that other people have this same inner illumination or self-consciousness that we have, and that this is carrying on continuously through our waking day and is interrupted during sleep and on other occasions of unconsciousness and resumed again. That this is a universal human experience is realized by communications at higher levels of symbolism.

This brings us to inquire what do we imagine can be happening to an animal during its waking life. We will take a domestic animal or an anthropoid ape. Then I think we have to be very careful because we will start to anthropomorphize the situation and think they are more like ourselves than in fact is the case. Karl, you made one very good point there that they do not have a proper sense of time, that they live in the present. Of course their actions are modified by past happening. They learn from experience. They are constantly inquiring and learning and give evidence of a great many purposive performances. I readily agree, but I am not sure that this should be taken as a certain test that they have some consciousness. I think at best it is only an indication. This is where I would have to put it. If we look at their intelligence, their purpose, their memory, their ability to learn, and all the most delightful performances of the animals, the mother with the young, the mating and the organization of animals into flocks and so on, we have to say that they have some kind of social life. All of this we can agree is making us biased towards thinking that they have some consciousness. Then you can think that they give evidence of pain when injured, and this we think is like the pain we suffer, and they give evidence of happiness and anticipation as with a dog going for a walk with its master, and so on. I am aware of all that.

I feel embarrassed to point out that nice as it would be to believe that they were having experiences just like ours, this is far from being certain. For example, take the reactions to pain, which is the commonest example given. You can have a decorticate animal with its whole cerebral hemispheres removed and it would still react to pain and show rage and fear, in fact the whole range of basic adversive reactions. You don't have to have, nor do we have to have the higher levels of the cerebral cortex in the performance of reacting to injury. This can all be done when you are unconscious.

I would rather think that we had to base our possibility of consciousness in animals upon more subtle things such as their performances in the ordinary life in their relationship to one another and to human beings and so on.

Nevertheless there are certain things at that level we have to be careful about. The point I wanted to make about animals is that it is nice to see how they get on together as living beings in company with one another and with other species of animals, and so on, but one of the questions that I ask is: how do they care for their sick and their dead? Professor Washburn of Berkeley has described the case of a pack of monkeys going through the forest climbing and jumping and so on, while the sick monkeys, one or two of them, who can't keep up with the pack, struggle along doing their best but falling, and eventually the pack goes on and leaves them behind to die. It takes no cognizance of them whatsoever. In the monkey, therefore, there appears to be no feeling of compassion. It is doubtful even that Jane Goodall has described so much of this at the chimpanzee level. I am not speaking of course at any level about the maternal affection of mother and child. This is something which is instinctive and inborn and can happen in quite lowly organized animals. I am speaking about the care that animals have for the sick and for the dead. Do they in fact just reject their dead or do they begin to take some cognizance that this dead animal is like themselves and that they too may die? I have seen no evidence of this in any of the recorded cases of animals in the wild. It of course is generally recognized by ethologists that you shouldn't use anecdotal data from domesticated animals. Because of their imitative abilities you are never sure how much they are imitating without understanding in their relationship to, say, a dead animal or a dead master. This whole question is very important. I venture to suggest that, if animals have consciousness, they don't have self-consciousness even at a minor level.

That brings me to the most important of all of these stories of evolution. How did self-consciousness come to man? That I think will be a later story for discussion, but at this time it is important for me to review this question of animal consciousness. I will say that, if one wanted to be difficult about it, one could perfectly well be a reductionist, identity theorist, or what you will, saying that all the performance of animals of every kind you can imagine is simply the performance of its neural machinery and that there is no need to be superimposed upon this something which is a spinoff from the brain action. Thus I think with animals we may become parallelists, stating that their conscious experiences are a spinoff from the neural actions, but in fact cannot act back and cause any change in the operations of the neural machinery. Here is a question to be debated, and I think, Karl, you might like to take that up. Do animals give any evidence that their conscious experiences act back upon and change their behaviour?

P: I readily agree that there is no evidence at all that animals have experiences just like ours, except the evolutionary hypothesis and also the degrees of consciousness which we find in ourselves. Thus there is no direct evidence, and I would therefore describe the problem of the consciousness of animals as a kind of metaphysical problem, in the sense that any hypothesis, any conjecture about it, is not falsifiable – at any rate not at present. And since it is not falsifiable or testable, it is metaphysical.

But metaphysical hypotheses are important for science in at least two ways. First of all, in order to have a general picture of the world we need metaphysical hypotheses. Secondly, in the actual preparation of our research we are guided by what I have called "metaphysical research programmes".

So at the outset I would grant that the theory that animals have consciousness is untestable, and thus metaphysical (in my terminology), and that it would certainly not be unreasonable for someone to deny this theory. However, I do think that it is worthwhile to consider whether any other view of animal consciousness would fit better into our general scheme or view of the world. As to the *self*-consciousness of man, I am inclined to think that the most adequate metaphysical hypothesis is that it only arises with World 3: indeed, my suggestion is that it arises together with World 3, and in interaction with World 3. It seems to me that self-consciousness, or the self-conscious mind, has a definite biological function, namely to build up World 3, to understand World 3, and to anchor our selves in World 3.

I also think that one can consider the possible functions of the lower levels of consciousness which may exist in animals, and that these may have definite tasks. They may make possible certain interpretations of perceptions which may not be made by the brain alone. That is to say, the brain may deliver to the animal consciousness an uncertain or unclear perception, and then the animal may experiment with various interpretations of it, just as we do, trying out different interpretations of this in the first instance far from unambiguous perception. That would be one possible function for the lower levels of consciousness. In other words, I do think that we have every reason to believe that animals have perceptions. And we can find from our own experience that the process of perception only takes place partly in the appropriate sense organ: that it partly occurs in the conscious mind. (I do not wish to imply that the *self*-conscious mind is needed for it.) I also think that there are other functions which we can attribute to consciousness. You tell me, Jack, that all the symptoms of pain may arise without consciousness, and I accept what you have told me about this. But I am not quite clear about this point. I would like to ask you whether human beings who are not conscious show symptoms of pain. I think that that would be a very important piece of evidence. Perhaps you could say something about it.

E: With regard to human beings and their symptoms of pain, it of course is well known that, when the anaesthetic in an operation gets a little too light, the subject will react and scream and struggle, yet, when he comes out of the anaesthetic, he has no memory of this and therefore you could argue that he never felt the pain at all. He was reacting without feeling; that is the usual interpretation. On the other hand, you could argue that he felt it and reacted, but had lost his memory of it. We are always up against this problem in answering that question with human beings. If they are reacting to a pain and then reporting later that they don't feel it, you could always argue that they had felt the pain but not remembered. So I can't answer that question with any assurance.

P: I think that this is very important and interesting. For I think that we can actually argue that if memory is interrupted in the sense of being cut into short pieces sufficiently often and to a sufficient degree, then consciousness would no longer exist. Perhaps if the memory is interrupted there may at first be episodes of awareness, but, if the atomization goes far enough, there would be no consciousness at all. (See my section 19.) There will probably also be intermittent stages of a very low degree of consciousness; these may border on unconsciousness. It has been suggested that some, or even all, general anaesthetics work in this way by more or less atomizing consciousness or by interrupting its temporal coherence. An important point here would be whether, if the anaesthetic is a little less deep, a human being could still answer questions but afterwards forget the episode completely. It would be quite interesting to know about this. It would represent an intermediate stage; intermediate, but only at a slightly higher level than complete unconsciousness.[1]

I think the fact that we have some evidence in this direction shows just how we might, with the help of our metaphysical hypothesis, get nearer and nearer to something like real evidence — which at present is out of sight for us. The evidence we could arrive at would be analogical evidence, but still, we may accept analogical evidence for other minds without getting too deeply involved in the "problem of other minds" as some philosophers call it. It may be similar with animals.

You mentioned earlier the question of compassion. Again there is no real evidence, but when I was a child I had a big dog who, when I was ill, showed every sign of compassion. Now you can of course say that this was only a kind

---

[1] Note that something like this may happen when children, especially, answer questions and hold conversations when they are asleep.

of imitation, but actually he showed much more compassion than did my relations, so whom did he imitate? Of course, all these things are very far from real evidence – I am quite clear about that. But they *are* indications, and more than that we cannot get at present, and I suspect that we will not get more than indications until we know very much more. I should say that it is conceivable that we could advance our knowledge of animal consciousness if we knew more about the relationship of human consciousness to the human brain; that is to say, more about the brain-mind problem. As we learn more about that, we may get, by analogical reasoning, more information about the possibility of animal consciousness. Once we have a theory about the brain-mind liaison it might possibly lead us on to a theory of liaison at the lower levels of consciousness. And this might possibly lead further to a theory about animal consciousness.

However, I agree that the question is metaphysical at present; but I propose that the more satisfactory metaphysical hypothesis, especially in view of the evolutionary story, is that animals have some sort of awareness based on memory. It is not based on abstract theories. These lead to the human consciousness of self which, I would suggest, evolves together with the evolution of World 3.

E: Let me back-track a little. At the beginning I went through the whole invertebrate sequence up to the octopus that has the most complex brain structures. I should have asked the question there. I think that we would be dubious about putting anything comparable with conscious experience at the level of the invertebrate, even the mollusc or the insect. We certainly don't treat them as if they could suffer pain or were in any way like ourselves in having some conscious awareness apart from their ordinary reactions.

Now we advance into the vertebrates and we come, in a first step to the fish. When you look at their brains, you find out they are very primitive indeed in respect of brain levels which we would associate with consciousness at higher levels of vertebrates. We do know from human experiments that the pain comes only when the impulses from the sense organs come up to the higher levels of the cerebral cortex or at least to the thalamus. Now, in the evolutionary story, such levels of the brain had not evolved in the fish where the forebrain is the smell brain. You could wonder whether there was any part of the brain in which there could be a performance that gave rise to any conscious awareness. As you know, the common sense attitude is to treat the fish as if they did not have any consciousness! This goes on through the amphibia, where a frog or any urodele can be again regarded as interesting, but having no more self-awareness or conscious experiences than the fish.

I think it is really only when we get up to the mammals and the birds that we would have some kind of feeling about there being a consciousness in certain levels of their experience. This is particularly true of course when we come to the higher mammals, the cat and the dog, these great companions of man. But there are many mammals with larger and more complex brains. The elephants, for example, have obviously high intelligence and there is some evidence that they do care for their dead, although this may be imitative. There is anecdotal evidence that when an elephant dies, other elephants cover the body with leaves and even care for elephant bones! Then the very interesting animals, the dolphins, have a brain at least as large as man's, and, so far as they have been studied, apparently do show some feeling for one another. There is the help when the mother gives birth to the baby. This could be ordinary instinctive animal actions, but it's nice to read into their actions some kind of human qualities because they have such large brains, and they quite clearly have very complex performances. In fact, though, when you come to study their brains anatomically as Jansen of Oslo has done, a great deal of their cerebral hemispheres would appear to be used in auditory localization. The very big auditory cortices are apparently related to the sensing of their position relative to sound waves in the water, reflections from rocks, etc. This gives apparently an orientation to environment which is obviously very important for them, and they probably also get signals from fish they are catching. This auditory sensing may be at such a complex and subtle level that it requires a great deal of their cerebral cortex. We are not sure how much cerebral cortex they have left over to function as does the human cerebral cortex for speech (cp. chapter E4) and other subtle expressions related to higher nervous activities.

Finally we of course come to the anthropoid apes who have smaller brains than elephants and dolphins, only about 500 ccm or so, and we have of course all the examples of the efforts to train them in linguistic performance, but that's another story. I'll leave that aside for the present. The evidence that they are tool makers and can construct a primitive World 3 is, I think, very dubious. I would say they are no better at this than other orders of lower mammals, or even the birds. After you have commented on this, I would like to raise the question of evolution and consciousness, and in fact, self-consciousness. How did consciousness come to man? That, I think, is the ultimate question that we have to face, and we can talk about that.

P: I completely agree that the care for the dead is an immensely important point in the story of the evolution of consciousness (see my section 45), and I also agree that we can look at the care for the dead as being one of the main evidences for higher self-consciousness, for reasons which are pretty obvious. That is to say, the conscious awareness of the self goes, as it were, hand in hand with the idea that I — the self — will die; and in the light of this we can understand better the idea of the care for the dead. As to the existence of lower forms of consciousness, I think we have some evidence from ourselves that they exist. And with respect to the question with which we started — how consciousness came into life — I want to formulate some metaphysical conjectures.

I would say that the first beginning, or some very early intermediate stage of consciousness may actually be a sense of curiosity, a feeling or a wish to know. This hypothesis is suggested by the tremendous importance which the intellectual aspect of our consciousness has for the whole evolution of consciousness and especially of higher consciousness. Strangely enough there is hardly any advantage from an evolutionary point of view in making some kinds of pain conscious. Or at least while there is some advantage in pain, in so far as it is a warning, there is hardly any biological advantage in having a toothache conscious; rather, there was only a biological disadvantage, at least until the invention of dentists. Before the invention of dentists, which was certainly a World 3 affair, there was certainly no advantage in having a conscious toothache. On the other hand, the invention of dentists is a consequence of toothache.

I wanted to formulate two hypotheses which are closely related and both somewhat bold. The first I have already mentioned — that curiosity is the beginning of consciousness. The second is that, in the evolutionary story, young animals become conscious before old animals. That is to say, consciousness may be connected with the exploratory period in the evolution of animals. If animals have consciousness, as I propose we assume, then it is very possible that animals lose this consciousness as they grow older and that they grow more and more like automata. One actually has a kind of intuitive impression that old animals become less and less conscious: this is especially noticeable when compared with the behaviour of young animals, which shows many more signs of consciousness. The distinctive evolution of consciousness in man may then be linked with the delayed maturing and the somewhat delayed ageing in man — or at least in some men. My two hypotheses are, of course, both metaphysical in character. Jack, what is your impression about this suggestion?

E: I would agree. Put it this way. I want to take this suggestion and use it only for the origin of the self-consciousness of man which I think is of supreme interest. The other is more dubious. The questions that interest me are: How did self-consciousness come to primitive hominids? What were in fact the conditions, the situations that gave rise to it? We can say that these hominids were more exploratory than their forebears. They were more imaginative. They were, in some incredible way, moving into new levels of association with their environment. Undoubtedly curiosity and the exploratory sense were high with them. This I think could have been one of the triggers to bring about the gradual beginning of self-consciousness. My own belief is that the most important factor there was the beginning of linguistic communication on a sophisticated level. It was this that lifted up the primitive hominids.

P: Of course, but my metaphysical conjecture was meant to apply to the pre-human stage, to the beginning of consciousness. As a metaphysical conjecture I was attributing consciousness to higher animals, and my suggestion was that the function of consciousness may be to extend a state of curiosity beyond the sensory stimuli which bring it about – to a lasting curiosity, which leads to exploration. What I have in mind is not merely that something which happens in our field of sensation may challenge us, but rather that it may lead to curiosity which in its turn leads to exploratory activity: to active exploration. Now the feeling of curiosity need not of course go with exploratory activity in animals. That it does is an untestable hypothesis – a metaphysical hypothesis. But if you observe the behaviour of young animals then while young animals at play are very largely unconscious – that is one of the charming things about them – when in their play what one interprets as curiosity is aroused, one has the feeling that the play may be conscious. There is something a little more than unconscious play about it. There is a transition from play to something a little more earnest, and it was this that suggested to me my metaphysical hypothesis. On the human level the hypothesis need not even be metaphysical, in that there is possibly some evidence for it.

I would like to add something to the suggestion I made a little earlier: that young animals are more conscious than older ones. I want only to refer to a conjecture which I think may be testable, and which has often been remarked on: namely, that the older we get the faster time goes. One could put it like this: the older we get the less we can do in a given stretch of time. Measured in terms of what we do in a given stretch of time, the given stretch of time seems to move faster. I think we have good reasons to attribute to young children extremely slow-moving time; that is to say, for a child (I remember it myself) a day may be a tremendous period in every sense. First of all, it is very much more real as a unit than for adults; and secondly, a child experiences so very much during a day that it works extremely hard at acquiring its experiences. If this is correct, it might provide some slight evidential support for my general metaphysical hypothesis that young animals are more conscious than older ones. By conscious I of course mean conscious in an entirely different way from humans. I fully agree with you, Jack, that what we call the full consciousness of self cannot be attributed to animals. There is, incidentally, also reason to think that self-consciousness is not something simple. It is something highly complex, and comes comparatively late in the life of a child; that is to say, only after perhaps a year or so. So there is a tremendous period of time to which we have to attribute something like a forerunner of self-consciousness; in which we may assume that there is a lower degree of consciousness. This is in itself an almost necessary conjecture from the point of view of our experience, so it is necessary to postulate that there exists a form of consciousness different from self-consciousness. It is then not difficult to attribute this to animals. Not full self-consciousness: no, we agree on that; but there is no difficulty in our attributing to animals non-self-conscious awareness. That is my opinion, at least.

E: When we go on to the question of self-consciousness, we have to take as an important sign or test of this, how consciousness came not to man as a whole, but to each individual man in his own lifetime from babyhood up. In a way there is something parallel with this. The two of them are related in that they both come through World 3. I think that this must be one of our major discussions about World 3 and consciousness. Furthermore I think we will be able to say something much more important on this problem of self-consciousness when we are looking at it at that level. Maybe we can then look back at the animals who don't have this incredible experience of living in a World 3, growing up in a World 3, assimilating it to themselves. By contrast human beings live in this other dimension given by World 2 and World 3 in interaction. That is I think the really important position.

P: I do not think we have reached full agreement. That is to say, my impression is that for me the metaphysical hypothesis of animal consciousness is more important than for you, Jack, who probably do not so much like metaphysical hypotheses, and especially not this particular one. But there does not seem to be any difference between us concerning the specifically human character of the consciousness of self, if we forget about such things as the case of elephants looking after their dead.

Dialogue III

10 a. m., 21 September 1974

E: Karl, could you start our discussion by saying a little about World 3?

P: World 3 is the world of the products of the human mind. These products, in the course of evolution, were first probably encoded only in the human brain and even there only in a fleeting way. That is to say, if an early man told a story of a hunt, or something like that, then the story would be both encoded· in his brain and in the brains of his listeners, but it would soon be forgotten and in a sense disappear. The more characteristic objects of World 3 are objects which are more lasting. They are, for example, early works of art, cave paintings, decorated instruments, decorated tools, boats, and similar World 1 objects. At that stage there is perhaps not yet a need to postulate a separate World 3. The need arises, however, when it comes to such things as works of literature, theories, problems, and, most clearly of all, such things as, for example, musical compositions. A musical composition has a very strange sort of existence. Certainly it at first exists encoded in the musican's head, but it will probably not even exist there as a totality, but, rather, as a sequence of efforts or attempts; and whether the composer does or does not retain a total score of the composition in his memory is in a sense not really essential to the question of the existence of the composition once it has been written down. But the written-down encoding is not identical with the composition – say, a symphony. For the symphony is something acoustic and the written-down encoding is obviously merely conventionally and arbitrarily related to the acoustic ideas which this written-down encoding tries to incorporate and to bring into a more stable and lasting form. So here there already arises a problem. Let us pose the problem in the following way. Clearly, Mozart's Jupiter Symphony is neither the score he wrote, which is only a kind of conventional and arbitrarily coded statement of the symphony;

nor is it the sum total of the imagined acoustic experiences Mozart had while writing the symphony. Nor is it any of the performances. Nor is it all performances together, nor the class of all possible performances. This is seen from the fact that performances may be good or less good, but that no performance can really be described as ideal. In a way, the symphony is the thing which can be interpreted in performances – it is something which has the possibility of being interpreted in a performance. One may even say that the whole depth of this World 3 object cannot be captured by any single performance, but only by hearing it again and again, in different interpretations. In that sense the World 3 object is a real ideal object which exists, but exists nowhere, and whose existence is somehow the potentiality of its being reinterpreted by human minds. So it is first the work of a human mind or of human minds, the product of human minds; and secondly it is endowed with the potentiality of being recaptured, perhaps only partly, by human minds again. In a sense World 3 is a kind of Platonic world of ideas, a world which exists nowhere but which does have an existence and which does interact, especially, with human minds – on the basis, of course, of human activity. It can also interact with physical things, for example, if a musical score is duplicated, or if a record is made. And a record may operate directly on a loudspeaker without a human being intervening. However, while World 3 is perhaps best conceived along Platonic lines, there are, of course, very considerable differences between the Platonic world of ideas and World 3 as I conceive it. First of all, my World 3 has a history; this is not the case for the Platonic world. Second, it does not consist, as would the Platonic ideal world, of concepts, but mainly of theories and problems, and not only of true theories but also of tentative theories and indeed false theories. However, I will not go into this now because I have done so on other occasions.[1]

E: Karl, you have done a remarkable exposition upon World 3 in some of its highest manifestations, but I'd like to go back and retrace our steps to its very origin. How far back in the human prehistory can we recognize the beginning, the origin, the most primitive World 3 existences? As I look at the prehistory of mankind, I would say that we have it in tool culture. The first primitive hominids who were shaping pebble tools for a purpose had some idea of design, some idea of technique.

This illustrates that probably in the design, in the purpose and in the instructions of one to the other in carrying on the tool culture, one can think that the beginnings of language had come. This I suppose is the most impor-

---

[1] Cp., for example, the discussion in chapters 3 and 4 of my [1972(a)], and my section 13.

tant World 3 development – the development of linguistic performance where thoughts and experiences can be coded in some form. The survival from generation to generation would be in the remembered verbal form that is ensured by endless verbal repetition.

P: While I agree with what you say, I nevertheless prefer to regard the beginning of World 3 as having come with the development of *language*, rather than *tools*. The reason is that it is here that World 3 may become both external to us and an object of *criticism* and of deliberate improvement. It seems to me improbable that before language existed, tools would be subject to criticism or anything really like it. It is perfectly true that they might be thrown away as not very useful, but one can hardly describe that as a form of criticism – although it is perhaps a forerunner of criticism. Real criticism – the criticism of ideas, of theories – arises, I think, only with language, and it seems to me that this is really one of the most important aspects of language. I want here to draw attention to that little step between thinking a certain thought in one's head as it were, and speaking it out. As long as the thought is not formulated, it is more or less part of ourselves.[2] Only if it is formulated in language does it become an object which is different from ourselves, and towards which we can adopt a critical attitude. So the very small difference between *thinking* (in the sense of *acting on the assumption*) "today is Saturday" and *saying* "today is Saturday" makes a tremendous difference from the point of view of the possibility of criticism. Although there is often not much of a gap between thinking and speaking, from the point of view of criticism (and of sharpening our thought) the difference can be very great. Of course, once language is established, we can actually formulate a thought in our minds *and* criticize it; but that is only after language itself has been established objectively, so to speak, as a social institution: after the possibility of objectivization has been established. Only after that can we really have a critical attitude towards the products of our own minds. However, I quite agree with you that one can of course probably trace World 3 back to earlier stages, but these are not the same thing as the criticizable World 3.

On the other hand, one can consider tool-making as being a higher stage of something which goes back to the very beginning of life, namely that living organisms in a sense select and fashion their own environment. One can even say that the environment of a naked gene somehow or other consists of the enzymes produced by that gene and that these enzymes are something

[2] The first step is objectivization in physical terms. Cp., however, my discussion of Euclid's theorem (dialogue XI) for a much later stage, after much feedback has taken place.

vaguely analogous to tools produced by the human brain. I quite see that this is carrying the analogy a very long way, but I do think that in a sense these enzymes are almost like tools; they are actually a self-created artificial environment. The strange thing is that these artificial environments grow and grow and become more and more complicated; and ultimately they become criticizable. That is the great step which I think is really achieved only with language.

I may perhaps add here that two things seem to me decisively important about language. One is that it allows for criticizability; the other is that it gives rise to the need to criticize because of story-telling. With the invention of language there also comes the invention of excuses, of false excuses, and of false explanations produced in order to cover up something not quite right that one has done, and so on; and with this arises the need to distinguish between truth and falsity. Thus with story-telling there arises the need to distinguish between truth and falsity, and this, I think, is how criticism actually arose originally in the development of language and of World 3.

E: I am challenged to criticize after this exposition of yours, Karl and I want to do it quite strongly now because I think that very much confusion can be introduced by using the word "tool" as foreshadowed by ordinary biological processes such as the DNA, messenger RNA, enzyme building, and so on. I think something quite other came in with tools. I want to suggest that we can greatly underestimate the skill required to make even a simple stone tool such as early man was making half a million years ago. The primitive man had primitive instruments to make tools. He didn't have the machine tools that we are gifted with now. He had only what he made from stones in order to work with stones. I think the full implication of this comes out in an interesting archaeology class that Prof. Washburn has at Berkeley. The students have a whole semester to try to make a stone tool matching some exemplars that are there, using only the tools available to primitive man. The stones are chosen carefully to be similar to those that primitive man had. In this class for many years the students have struggled hard with lots of language and lots of instruction about how to hit the stone so as to make the flakes come off in this way and that way; but in a whole semester not one has succeeded in making what you might call an acceptable stone axe. They have only made objects that primitive man would have thrown away. However, a teacher in the class, Dr Desmond Clark, can do it. So it is possible to learn. I instance this because it gives an example of intelligent action in the skills, in the controls of movement and in the use of critical ability and judgment. How to flake the stone, where to hit and with how much strength are questions to be debated and decided in order to make even such a primitive tool. This is something quite other than any animal can ever do, and this I think required a language and critical ability. We have to be careful that we don't write off this tool culture of primitive man as being simply at a level of a very unskilled human performance. It was a skilled human performance considering the environment and the means of action that they had available.

P: This is of course immensely interesting and completely acceptable to me because you say that this kind of higher tool-making or human tool-making *presupposes language.* My point was only that the kind of tool-making which does not presuppose language does not seem to me to be on the same level as the kind of tool-making which does presuppose language. As to the question at which moment this higher tool-making appeared, I am not sufficiently informed; and as to when language appeared, probably nobody is sufficiently informed. I suppose we have to assume that language starts from very small beginnings and actually that it is the interaction between the need to speak and the abilities of the brain which provided the challenge and the stimulus for the brain to develop as it did over the past one or two million years. So I conjecture that the very beginnings of language were probably connected with the not yet enlarged brain; but that language led very soon to an increase in the size of the brain. I do not think that there is a difference of opinion here. I was actually previously speaking about tools prior to language. Tools prior to language, I should say, must be more primitive than the ones you have described and which have been investigated in Washburn's class.

E: It is quite clear that we can only imagine and try to reconstruct the past from what is available to us now. I think there are two lines of evidence available from these earlier days. One is the rate of growth of the brain. We have to think of the very nice endocranial casts being made by Holloway and described by him in a recent *Scientific American* article. This gives you some idea of the form of the brain with the associated growth in weight and also the growth of the various lobes. I personally think that they rather overdo the interpretation of the lobes in relationship to speaking. There is a tendency to think that if you get an enlargement in the area of the temporal and parietal lobes, that there is an associated growth of language. I would in general agree with that, but, when you consider all the hazards of making the cranial reconstructions in the first place and then casting from them, it is of course only suggestive evidence. The other evidence we have for the growth of language comes really from the development of cultures. There is firstly the development of tools and finally with Neanderthal man there are the ceremonial burial customs, which as Dobzhansky very rightly points out give us the first clear indication that this primitive man had now developed some spirituality, some self-consciousness which he was not only experiencing in himself but also recognizing in his fellow beings. Hence ceremonial burial gives evidence that primitive man thought "death comes to this person, this creature like myself, it will come to me and I would therefore do all honour to him so that it may be done when I too die".

These, then, are the signs that language had come to man at quite a high level; and still much later of course we have the beautiful art forms, say in the Lascaux caves, which I think is a sign that there was a primitive art school there, groups of men painting, criticizing, assessing and instructing each other. This could only have happened when language was very highly developed. Unfortunately, when it comes to the linguistic art forms as distinct from plastic art forms, we have no record until we get much further on in prehistory, or protohistory, as it may be called. Before the language was written down, we have the evidence from the repetition of tales by singers which eventually, as in the Homeric epics, became written down after some hundreds of years of repetition by bards who made a profession of the repetition of the heroic deeds of the past. This long oral tradition certainly obtained with the Epic of Gilgamesh which was the first great epic of which we have knowledge. It eventually achieved a linguistic form in Babylonian times although the epic itself had a long Sumerian existence before the first written form at something about 2000 B. C.

The point of all this discussion and illustration is its relation to the growth of the brain and the development of special performances of different zones of the brain that I have described in chapters E1, E2, E3, E4, E6. I believe that this growth did not arise spontaneously in some kind of uncaused manner, but that it arose in response to the needs, the demanding needs, of the linguistic developments and all of the associated creative aspects required in thought, in discursive thought, in critical thought and so on.

So we now come full circle to the story that the evidences that we have for World 3 developing in the early human existence can be linked with the growth of the brain at that same time. It is remarkable that they appear to be not in phase, as you may at first think. Surely the human brain developed far ahead of the World 3 that it was required to handle. This is one of the mysteries of human existence. In Sumerian or early Egyptian times I would say that the human brain had the full performance of modern man's brain, and had still done very little in the abstract sciences and not so much even in the creative arts, particularly in music. This was all to come. One can wonder what was the evolutionary survival value for example in Neolithic times of a mathematical genius or of people having great ranges of conceptual thought or of artistic imagination. Yet in two or three thousand years the first great civilizations (Sumerian and Egyptian) were created from the Neolithic progenitors. That is I think a mystery because we don't have enough imagination to realize in thought the conditions of life under which primitive man was struggling upwards for survival using the intellectual and the critical abilities of imagination in a crude and rough world. It is certain that the growth of the brain came on amazingly fast in the million or two years of the Paleolithic Age, developing in Neanderthal man a brain as big as ours and which, as I already mentioned, was associated with some cognizance of primitive spirituality.

P: Yes, I agree. But I should like to add to something I said before. It seems to me that the function that led to this whole development is *the descriptive function* of human language (see my section 17), as opposed to such things as mere name-giving. What characterizes a descriptive statement is that it can be true or false, and therefore also that it can be used for different purposes: for the purpose of telling the truth — that is to say, for conveying information — or for the purpose of lying; for example, for making certain excuses acceptable, or for covering up failure, and so on. I think story-telling emerges directly from these descriptive reports, from the telling of lies, or from both. Both descriptive reports and lies fulfil a kind of explanatory function. Story-telling is in the main no doubt stimulated by the need to explain certain ununderstood events in life of all kinds, and it then leads to the development of an enjoyment of story-telling, which I think we can assume developed at a fairly primitive stage, long before the very important myths described in Gilgamesh and the Homeric epics. Practically all primitive people known have fairy tales, and fairy tales all have a complex structure. Most of them can be regarded as explanatory; they can also be regarded as having in them a frightening element and a comforting element and so on. Now I think that the really important aspect of all this is that it leads to something which is certainly only possible on this level of human development, namely the development of human imagination, of fantasy, and of inventiveness. I don't think that there is anything comparable to this on the animal level at all. That is to say, animals may do something new, but they can hardly have flights of the imagination and of fantasy. These flights of the imagination seem to me incredibly important in connection with the development of higher civilization or material culture or whatever one wants to call it, and for obvious reasons. These things led to the pluralism of human tool making, to the many-sidedness of even very primitive civilizations, and then to the fact that great inventions were made, not only once or twice, but continuously, again and again, from very early days. It is really this which makes me feel that the tools you have described, which are such real works of art, and which are so difficult to make, are likely not to have emerged prior to the beginnings of language.

So much for the descriptive function of language. However, the interesting thing is that the descriptive function of language brings with it the basis for the argumentative function of language, and for a critical attitude towards language. Just the very fact that lying becomes possible means that for obvious practical and adaptational reasons it is important for men to distinguish between truth and falsehood. It is just for this very reason that we have built into us the need to develop criticism and the need to develop a critical attitude towards a report, and with it, the need to develop an argumentative language – a language in which the truth of a report can be criticized or attacked, or in which it can be defended by supplementary reports. That, I think, marks the beginning of argument in human language. I would say that everything speaks in favour of the view that these two functions of language, the descriptive and the argumentative functions, are the most characteristic aspects of *human language* as distinct from animal languages and other means of social communication.

I should like to add the following conjecture: it may be that this tension between *description* and *the need to criticize description* is the basis of the important intellectual problem which the invention of descriptive language puts before man, and this intellectual struggle stimulated the unprecedentedly fast growth of everything which follows – namely, the growth of language itself, of the brain, and of civilization.

E: There is an aspect of World 3 that I think deserves further consideration. In the first place, there is a tendency to consider World 3 as information, ideas, concepts, and so on, that are encoded upon some material base and so assume a public character available for all to see and read out if they have the appropriate abilities of interpretation or decoding. This is the way you can look at all of the art forms, plastic art forms, tools, sculptures, technical developments like the wheel as well as all the linguistic written down texts that we inherit from the past. But there's another side that has been touched on and this is important. I think that, right through from its beginning, World 3 has had a component of memory storage. The storage is not on some external medium, metal, stone, paper or what you will, but it is storage also in the brains of subjects who have memorized creative ideas, imaginative thoughts, artistic stories and so on and then have handed them on. This was the way in which earlier literature in fact was preserved before it could be written down. The verbally transmitted folklore that went on through countless ages must have been one of the principal means of growth of civilization in these peoples. You can see all this in an intelligent people before they learnt writing. I instance for example the Maoris you and I were both in New Zealand and we are familiar with the stories of Maori history and of their heroic exploits in finding their way across thousands of miles of ocean to New Zealand (identified from afar as the Long White Cloud) and returning and bringing more of their peoples there. All of this was told in remembered epics which were handed on and recited and repeated and no doubt modified and enhanced. Nevertheless that history bears up pretty well with tests giving the dating of their time of arrival and where they came from.

This tribal memory in the form of a verbal tradition has gone on through all ages, in what we may call oral narrative poetry. In the last few decades Professor A. B. Lord has made visits to Yugoslavia and Bulgaria where in remote areas there is a relatively illiterate population. The book he wrote is called *The Singer of Tales.* He finds many similarities between the way in which the tales are sung in certain rhythms and verse forms and repeated, and the way in which the Homeric poems, the classical works of the great past, were handed on probably for hundreds of years before being written down.

So this now brings me to the next development — it is that we are doing the same thing all the time today. We do not immediately have to encode in print or tape or in some other permanent form our thoughts and ideas. We are also holding them in memory. I instance for example that, if I am going to lecture somewhere, I have a few notes and slides to work from, but I am mostly using my own memories from which I can retrieve my ideas for presentation to the audience. I think that we are always working in some fluid manner between our memories and what we permanently store in codes in written and diagrammatic texts.

P: I don't think I have anything important to add to this, but I should like to say that early poetry — the early epic — may be an indication of the *need* for something like writing, long before writing actually developed. One could almost say that the unfulfilled need for written records is the beginning of poetry: that the use of spoken rhythm to support the memory led to what we would now call the poetic art.

E: I regard this whole development of ideas relating to World 3 as being one of the great illuminating and synthesizing concepts that we have because it does link together such a diversity of human performance that has so much in common. In a sense I look on World 3 as having what you might say is an anatomy and a physiology and a history. It is an evolutionary story. It is the story of the cultural evolution of man, and I think it has to be put in perspective that way – that man developed as a result of two interacting but quite different evolutions. One is the biological evolution by the ordinary chance and necessity with mutations and survival on the terms of natural selection; and the second way is with his development of the thought processes leading to creativity in a wide range of cultural performance; artistic, literary, critical, scientific, technological and so on. Finally we come up to the level at which man is not only trying to make life more acceptable, more sure, but at the same time where he is trying to struggle with the immense problems of the meaning of life: what is it all for? What is the nature of my existence? How can I face up not only to self-awareness but to death-awareness?

All of this has come in the story of the development of World 3 and of course this whole question of the meaning of life has given us wonderful performances in literature and art and music. You might say it is the creative cry of mankind in his loneliness and also in his fear of the world that he finds himself in, but of course it also portrays his intense enjoyment and appreciation of his existence in the world. All of these experiences have come through the development of man's culture in World 3, with of course the refinement of feeling and of sensibility and of artistic creativity. All of this has come with the growth of the brain. The two come together. It wasn't as if the brain grew first and then man suddenly found that he had a brain capable of all this performance. We have to imagine that the growth of the brain, which is a biological process giving survival value, entailed not only better survival, but also entailed the immense range of human performances, which attains of course its full expression in World 3. And so the great philosophical advantage given by this clear concept of World 3 is that it sharpens the distinction between biological evolution on the one hand and cultural evolution on the other. The biological evolution gives man his World 1 body and brain, and the World 1 body and brain makes it possible for the development of World 3 and World 2 in locked interaction. I think therefore World 3 is a great illuminating concept making clear what often had been rather confused and cloudy.

P: I should like to comment on the two methods of evolution which you have mentioned. The first method of evolution is, in brief, that of introducing some novelty, anatomical or physiological or behavioural, and having it tested by natural selection. The second method of evolution introduces something new in place of natural selection, namely, conscious critical rejection, and that, I think, is the really fundamental difference between natural evolution and cultural evolution. Some people have said that the difference is that natural evolution is Darwinian in character, but that cultural evolution is Lamarckian and proceeds by induction. This I think is a mistake. Cultural evolution is also Darwinian; the difference is only that, in place of natural selection, we ourselves begin in part to take responsibility by way of the critical elimination of our efforts. In this connection I would like to say something about novelty in evolution and invention. I suggest that much, although not all, novelty in evolution can be interpreted as being the result of a kind of invention, by the organism, of a new environment: of a new ecological niche. (See my section 6.)

Now that incredible thing, the invention of language amounts to a completely new kind of change of the ecology. For example, with the invention of language, sounds become divided into meaningless and meaningful sounds. We are led to attempt to interpret even natural sounds, the sounds of birds and so on, to try to see whether they are not meaningful; whether thunder is not, perhaps, some sound, made by a god, which has a definite meaning. In this way, our whole ecology becomes animated and is in need of a new kind of interpretation, interpretation on a conscious, or rather self-conscious, linguistic level; and this results in a need to interpret our perceptions not only *qua* perceptions but *qua* perceptions which may express a certain hidden meaning which is behind them. In other words, it led to the invention of a kind of metaphysical world behind a world. This is one of the greatest challenges which language presents to man, and this challenge in the end leads to science, which is an attempt to discover a world behind the comparatively immediate world of perception (which, of course, is also not really immediate but is interpreted). This brings into being a new level of interpretation, and this, I think, is one of the great challenges which probably led to the kind of natural selection which then led to the growth of the brain.

E: Yes, I agree that we have to think that creative imagination came quite early to mankind. When, as Dobzhansky says, the first self-awareness came to mankind it was linked with death-awareness. With that was linked the terror of existence, not only the wonder but the terror and awe. The creative minds in those primitive times must have struggled with this new illumination developing the myths of origin of which we have many records. At a later time came myths of explanation by another unseen world in which all were participating, so giving some kind of greater meaning, a cosmic meaning, to the whole life of the primitive society and to the world around them. We can conjecture that this religious insight must have given rise to the first artistic, imaginative, creative thinking. There is no doubt that primitive man must have needed something of this kind. However the only evidence we have from very early times is the burial customs where we can see something organized was being done for the dead bodies, but this must have been simply the final result. Before that ceremony there must have been a great deal of talking, of thinking, of imagining, of myth making, and so on.

I think we agree that myth making was one of the big incentives to man and of course the myths required better human performances. With the myth making and the better human performances came the better survival value of the primitive man with the brain capable of all of this new, imaginative, creative thinking. Tribes with leaders of this kind would be more effective in hunting, in social cohesion and in war than tribes which were not unified or brought together by this kind of creative thought. This again is a challenge to the brain in its evolutionary story with natural selection playing its role in the characteristic manner, but of course at the same time cultural development was built upon the brain that had grown by biological means and selection. These two, biological evolution and cultural evolution, act together in a way because the culture gives you the natural selection that selects for the better brain.

P: Language produces its own problems and its own strains and its own challenges, and thereby its own selection, both natural and critical.

E: How can we go back and discover more from this past? I think one of the most important problems confronting man in coming to terms with his present existence is to know more about how he came to be in his present state and what was the past, what were the challenges of the past and how did primitive man rise to these challenges. I would think therefore that one of the great contributions to the future of mankind would come from the archaeologists who are studying and making more vivid, and more intensely understood the past history of mankind. I further think that we need a detailed assessment pushing the story of burial customs of a hundred thousand years ago back into earlier times with more primitive burial customs. Many valuable new discoveries undoubtedly will come with the excavations in archaeological sites. We have to remember that the whole of the archaeology that we think so much of is only a hundred odd years old in its detailed discoveries and interpretations and explanations.

Dialogue IV

3:50 p. m., 21 September 1974

P: There are various distinctions or divisions to be made within World 3; for example, the division between the products of our mind as such, which are there in some sense (such as a well-known theorem, say, or a well-known song) and the unintended and as yet unknown consequences of these products which may be discovered. But there is another question which we should perhaps mention first, namely, the question of the actual process of discovery. The process of discovery can, I think, be described by an elaboration of and, in a way, a deviation from, the Platonic doctrine that we see the ideas or forms with an inner eye: the Platonic forms of World 3. (See my section 13.)

If we want to understand a theory, then I think just staring at the theory, as it were, gets us nowhere, and to this extent the Platonic theory of ideas and of our way of grasping them is unsatisfactory and has to be reconsidered. What I suggest is that we can grasp a theory only by trying to reinvent it or to reconstruct it, and by trying out, with the help of our imagination, all the consequences of the theory which seem to us to be interesting and important.

Understanding is an active process, not just a process of merely staring at a thing and waiting for enlightenment. One could say that the process of understanding and the process of the actual production or discovery of World 3 objects are very much alike. Both are making and matching processes.[1]

Ordinary seeing (and the "grasping" of a visual object) is also not just simply a kind of photographic process, but a process of interpretation, and as such undoubtedly a trial and error affair. It should not be compared too

[1] The matching aspect is that it has to fit into a framework, and that framework is what I call World 3.

closely to colour photography, for it is a dynamic process. It is a process of interaction – a process of give and take – similar to that by which we discover World 3 objects. Actually, I would say that the way in which we discover World 3 objects or "see" World 3 objects (to use a Platonic term) is a kind of slow-motion picture of the way in which seeing or perceiving happens in the brain. I have now reached a point which I am not very clear about, but which fascinates me: namely, that the whole relation between ourselves – our conscious selves – and World 3 is altogether something which definitely goes on at a somewhat slower speed than does the normal process of interpretation in the brain. This may happen because more things are going on in the brain, but my feeling is that there is more to it than that: that it may be due to the fact that the work is really more difficult, rather more abstract, and not so closely related to the stimuli as is the normal work of interpretation. I think that if my conjecture about the existence of a lower form of consciousness were developed, we might find that the lower consciousness is also connected with a time delay,[2] though perhaps with a shorter time delay than the higher consciousness. It may be part of the biological function of the lower consciousness to intervene between perception and motor action and somehow delay the motor action.

E: I like the idea that you have developed that there are gradations in the times at which cerebral processes happen. There is quite a lot of evidence on this now. Work has been going on in several laboratories of a high quality. I've given instances in the chapter (E2) on conscious perception, but I might mention some additional examples now. In the first place we do know that you get a quicker judgment about the recognition of a face which has already been presented and which can later be picked out from an ensemble of faces by the *Gestalt*-like mechanisms of the right temporal lobe. This is much quicker than the more verbal analytical operations on the left side, so this is a sign that there is some specially organized, very efficient machinery in parts of the brain just to get out quick picture recognition in a *Gestalt* manner.

There are ways of demonstrating this. For example, if there is a complete section of the corpus callosum, this right hemisphere function is put out of action for the visual field coming in from the right side (chapter E5). Face recognition can still be done but takes longer. The subject has to analyse the picture into pieces in order to see whether this face is the same as the one he remembers. He looks at the ears, the eyebrows, the nose, and so on in pieces and talks to himself all the time it's going on, so revealing that the left

---

[2] Cp. chapter E2, Figs. 2 and 3.

hemisphere is using a verbal tag mechanism and not at all the *Gestalt* mechanism that the right hemisphere uses. I think that we have all kinds of levels of this happening.

I think we cannot overestimate the wonder and complexity of performance of the brain when it is engaged in operations based often upon a large amount of technical know-how in mathematics, in linguistic or in spatial thinking, and developments built upon them. That is the way we have to think of our brains; and in the World 3 level of operation of course we are testing them to the utmost. The very dedicated struggle along and accept all of the various meanderings of thought and branchings of thought. Their criticisms may lead them to reject some theory that they have put a great deal of mental effort into. They have to recognize that failure and try with creative imagination to develop and formulate new and better explanations and theories. These are the levels of high intellectual and artistic performance because great art is achieved in this same manner as well as great science.

P: I have two points to make on this theme. First of all, about long time-spans of sustained problem solving; in other words, real brain activity and mind activity. These depend, I think, essentially on World 3. I even think that they depend on our experiencing the objects of World 3 as if they were things: we experience them more or less on the model of material things. This partly explains the Platonic metaphor of looking at and seeing World 3 objects and why these were regarded as analogous to things, because things are our standard metaphor for something which has duration. It is the enduring character of World 3 objects, the objects in which our interest is anchored, which underlies the coherence between our various efforts, especially between our various attempts at solving a problem. During these attempts, there is something which we experience as being an object of thought. And this object, the problem which we study, has to be experienced as enduring in time, like a material thing. I think that this is the root of what is called hypostatization. That is to say, I think that we have somehow to hypostatize all our abstract ideas because otherwise we cannot come back to them again and again; and we need that kind of endurance in time.

The second point which I wanted to make here is that, when I say that the self is anchored in World 3, then I mean something similar; namely, that it is in fact anchored in a World 3 theory in which we visualize, so to speak, ourselves as something enduring: almost, as it were, like a piece of metal. We visualize ourselves as being there yesterday, the day before yesterday, and, providentially, we may be there tomorrow . . . unless something serious happens to us. This is a kind of hypostatization of the self which helps us in our self-understanding. We know very well that the self is not a material substance, but, so to speak, the non-material ghost in the machine is not a bad hypothesis with the aid of which the self may reach an understanding of the self. In other words, I think that such an idea is an almost necessary stage – the ghost stage – in understanding ourselves as selves, although it is, of course, a very naive and crude stage. But we never get rid of it entirely, just as we practically never get rid of our hypostatization.

E: You raise this question of the ghost in the machine and Gilbert Ryle. I gave the Waynflete Lectures right at the summit of the influence of *The Concept of Mind.* I claimed there in the Preface, that adequate justice was not done to the present understanding of the brain as a neuronal machine, but we were still talking about the Cartesian brain with pumps and valves and pipes and with fluid flowing in them. I went on to say that the new subtleties and complexities still only dimly understood did look more like the kind of machine that a ghost could inhabit and effectively work! It wasn't meant too seriously, but I just thought that I should raise it now as you mention this very idea, whatever the word ghost is meant to be. Of course it was derisory in the sense used by Ryle, but in a way I accepted it partly with my own interpretation because it's not altogether bad, this idea of a ghost.

P: You told me that you afterwards said to Ryle (and I think it is also in your book[3]): Let us first see what the machine is like before we decide on the role of the ghost.

I have a similar story. Shortly after Ryle's book was published, I gave a lecture to a student society in Oxford, in which I criticized Ryle's book, and tried to give an alternative outline of the body-mind problem. The students were apparently very much impressed by Ryle, but they said all the time, about what I was saying, that it was exactly what Ryle would say. So, in despair, I said: all right, I'll make a confession, I believe in the ghost in the machine. You cannot say that *that* is exactly what Ryle has said.

E: Karl, when you were talking about the kind of way we thought of ourselves, thought of our problems, and of our attempts to solve problems, I thought of some other attitude. I am a practical scientist in a not yet too sophisticated field with no high-power mathematics. When I am trying to formulate a theory or a new way of critically looking at a whole field of results, I'm all the time thinking in terms of diagrams, often with dynamic

---

[3] J. C. Eccles, *The Neurophysiological Basis of Mind* [1953]; see p. vi.

properties. That is to say I conjure up in my imagination dynamic pictures or models of the events. Of course they will be crude models, but still I have to construct something in thought in order to try to come to terms with the experimental results that I am trying to explain. I start to draw diagrams to see how it would go, and I put up theories with some diagrammatic base, admittedly imperfect. These simplified models enable me to develop my conceptual thinking and so develop further testing experiments.

P: This diagrammatic method of framing hypotheses can perhaps be subsumed under the term model-making. And the method of constructing simplified models is a quite well known method. Indeed, it is perhaps the most widespread method of forming theories, but it is certainly not the only one. Einstein, for instance, describes a procedure of handling symbols; not words, but symbols, which are related to each other in a way which is quite indistinct at first, but in which they become gradually more and more closely related.[4] This method may also have a diagrammatic element, but I think that from his description of it one would say that the diagrammatic element is comparatively unimportant in this way of thinking. But diagrams are, of course, particularly helpful where the question is in part an anatomical one.

E: Of course I agree naturally that these are models that I am constructing and thinking in terms of. Some of course are more anatomical than others, some of them are more dynamic with flow pathways or with gradients. You have to model nature to get some kind of understanding with our efforts within the scope of World 3 creativity.

P: One needs models together with animating laws which indicate how the models operate. Together, these make up a theory and give an explanation and, almost, as it were, a copy of the natural process.

E: One point that I think I should bring in now because we are getting around to the brain and this is part of our central theme. Karl, you mentioned about anatomical models – that of course is what they are. I wanted to say that is what they should be because, at all the levels of understanding possible to us now, we have to be heavily building upon an anatomical base. What we know about the nervous system is that it is built up of units, neurones, with stereotyped properties. There are the excitatory neurones and inhibitory neurones as described in chapter E1. They are hooked up with synaptic

---

[4] See Hadamard [1954], pp. 142f.

mechanisms working one way or the other according as they are excitatory or inhibitory, and they have of course both convergent lines and divergent lines. It is a numbers game. You count them and see how they all are in some kind of a network, if you like, which in the end will have to be put into an n-dimensional network for the purpose of computation. If each cell, shall we say, connects to ten other cells and so on through a serial array of perhaps 100 connectivities, you are into enormous numbers of structural elements in a network which would be in our particular model calculated in ten dimensions. This is I think a really fruitful field for the application of n-dimensional geometry.

I am sure there is much more to come from this change of model from anatomical to geometrical. Anatomy leads the geometry. Neuronal connections are all in form and structure and pattern. In trying to derive some kind of theoretical understanding at the World 3 level of the nervous system we have to develop enormously our concept of patterns in space and time because the basic constructs upon which the whole nervous system works are patterns. We can think of the immense complexity and of the immense number of possibilities of permutations and combinations of cell associations. There are a relatively limited number of cells in the brain, but the opportunities for pattern, the potentialities for pattern are enormously greater than the cell numbers. Theories of pattern will have to be developed especially for this purpose.

P: I would like to make one further remark about the way in which the self is anchored in World 3. I think that the most simple and primitive way of putting the point which I wish to make is to point out that without some conscious theory about sleep and the interruption of our consciousness by sleep, we cannot have self-consciousness. I also think it is here that another remark may be made about Dobzhansky's emphasis on death; namely, that our idea of the relationship between sleep and death is quite clearly dependent on a World 3 theory which plays a very considerable role in our consciousness of death. The theory is that death is somehow related to sleep, or somehow similar to sleep, because it involves a loss of consciousness in some sense, yet that it is different: in a way final, though possibly in another way not final. These things are, I think, at the very root of any theory of death, of sleep, and of self-consciousness; and here, of course, a theory of time also enters the field. Whorf, the famous linguist, has asserted that the Hopi Indians actually have no idea or model of time as we have it; that is to say, of time as in some way similar to a spatial co-ordinate. I think that there is certainly something in what Whorf says, but I doubt whether the Hopi

Indians have no abstract theory of time (Whorf denies that the Hopis have an abstract idea of time at all). I think that they must have an idea of sleep, of falling asleep, of coming awake again, and of the repetition of these processes, and such abstract ideas are, I should say, fundamental both to our sense of time and to theirs. Anyway, however it may be with the Hopis according to Whorf, these ideas are anchored in language, and our Western languages have tenses, and the idea of time is of course involved in the idea of tenses.

E: I would like to talk a little on the role of imagination in our development of theories, in our explanation of phenomena, in our building up of World 3. Imagination seems to be some active thought process exploring, rejecting, exploring again, all the time trying to create some new synthesis, some new understanding, some breakthrough in our concepts. There seem to be various ways leading to success. The way I would place the greatest store by is to fill the mind with all of the stories, the ideas, the results, the experiments, the explanations. Somehow or other you feel tension building up, and, if you start to write, you begin to find new ideas coming out for expression. They may of course have to be rejected, if they are refuted by existing knowledge. Nevertheless you have the feeling that there is something happening at a certain stage of thought about a subject – intense thought about it – and that your imagination will win through and get at some new level of understanding.

At the present time I am struggling in this respect with this great problem of the self and its brain. I have the feeling of the tension in my mind. I have read a great deal now on the neurological side and much on the anthropological side and on the philosophical side and we have had all these discussions and all the time I have the feeling that something may break. I mean that some little light at the end of the tunnel may be sensed or some flash of insight may come. I of course know very well that there's no guarantee it will come, but I have already got myself into this state of expectancy that something will come to my imagination which has some germ of truth about it in this most difficult field. Of course I know that there won't be any ultimate solution on this deep problem, and that we have to be modest about our expectations. If we can only get some little insight, some edge on the big problem, some little handhold somewhere to grasp, to get some understanding of, then that is encouraging and we may go on in these directions from one position to another.

You see I have the feeling that there are some very challenging discoveries that we haven't assimilated fully yet. There is the commissurotomy problem of Sperry and how this right hemisphere can do such very sophisticated and clever things as described in chapter E5. Of course it couldn't have done them if it hadn't been originally hooked up to the whole brain in all the learned procedures of the past. When the commissurotomy is done, the right hemisphere is on its own, you might say, as far as the cerebral connections are concerned, but it does carry with it all of the remembered skills that can be deployed in the building up of the strip cartoon that you were so impressed with. This wouldn't have happened, I am quite confident, if that brain had been split in very early childhood before the subject ever had any of this experience of strip cartoons. Then that right brain would have been forever a naive brain, but before the commissurotomy it had become a sophisticated adult human brain. I think it was adolescent in this case, 14 years old, when the commissurotomy was performed. It carries all its past with it and that is why it also carries some primitive linguistic abilities. Some of the very challenging aspects of this problem of how the cerebral events give us self-consciousness come when we are handling events at a more sophisticated level.

For example, take the following situation. We are listening to music. As I have described (cp. chapters E2, E4, E6), this is coming in by the auditory machinery and being handled in the first instance in the right temporal lobe. One can imagine that a great deal of experience is used from all of our long knowledge and our learnt skills in bringing us the full analysis and synthesis, the full sense of the perfection of the performance, the time sequences, the melodies, the harmonies, and all the rest of it, sequential in time. One would very much like consciousness to be associated with the actual sites where all of the incredibly complex neuronal operations are going on with all their base in the learning of the past with the memories and all of the structure that is built into that area genetically, giving the initial abilities to appreciate music. The right temporal lobe is this area, and yet, according to the results from the Sperry operation of cutting the corpus callosum, self-consciousness of the subject is found only in the left dominant hemisphere. One assumes that under these conditions these unfortunate commissurotomy subjects will have lost virtually all of their appreciation and judgment and evaluation of music. Maybe they have. It's hard to judge because in the cases I have known there probably was very little musical ability to start with, and to my knowledge they haven't been tested for this yet.

P: What about applying the Wada technique to some musicians?

E: You ask whether we can test this with the Wada injection technique into the left or right carotid arteries, in which case we are with some luck able to put out of action one or other hemisphere for a certain limited time. That again hasn't been tested yet so far as I know. The trouble with the Wada test is that there is considerable risk attached. You don't want to use it indiscriminately. These tests are practically only used now where it is necessary to discover if there is speech in the left or the right hemisphere because this guides the surgeon as to what parts of the cerebral hemisphere he can remove. The Wada test could be used more I suppose. When it's given to subjects there could be a more searching examination during the few seconds of its action. They would have to be very well designed experiments.

P: Jack, you have just mentioned the importance of imagination, and I think you are quite right. It cannot be over-estimated how important imagination is. Now I think that the beginning of imagination is almost certainly due to language. Of course, there is also the imagination shown, for example, by the painter, but I think that painting is very largely illustrative, at least in its beginnings. It is still very largely so even with highly evolved painting, like the work of the great masters, and in the beginning it probably originated in diagrams drawn at times to illustrate a story. It may be worth recollecting my earlier suggestion that the beginning of imagination probably goes back to the origin of descriptive language and to lying. From the tests on apes made by Köhler it emerges that the imagination even of apes is extremely weak. I think it is for this reason rather unlikely that apes have a descriptive language.

E: In reference to this question of animal imagination, I can describe how imagination can be tested at a very simple level. I am referring to experiments on what is called cross-modal transfer. That is to say you can test whether an object seen with vision alone and then in the dark felt by the hand can be recognized as the same object. This could be say a tetrahedron or some other geometrical form or it could be a banana, but it must be something with a simple recognizable shape. The seen and the felt are identified precisely by even quite young children. Now in experiments on cross-modal transfer in monkeys, Ettlinger and Blakemore had practically no success at all (cp. chapter E6). The monkeys could be trained to respond in an appropriate manner to a seen object, being conditioned to make the appropriate response when they saw it, but they were not able to make this response when they were not seeing it, but were merely feeling it. The felt object to them didn't give the signal that the seen object did. These animals are notoriously well endowed with sensibilities in these two respects, so you are not working upon weak senses. This cross-modal testing is to my mind a test for imagination because the subject seeing an object has to imagine it in order to identify it from touch. Of course it is a very low level of imagination. It's the only level you can try with animals and even that might be too hard for them. I think we have to try to think of tests for imagination which start off at a simple level and which can become more sophisticated.

Dialogue V

10 a. m., 22 September 1974

E: You will remember that last night, Karl, when we were on our peripatetic discussion, you raised a very important criticism of the story I was there developing. Briefly my story was that we had to consider the brain events as giving a complete integrated response to the whole of the sensory input and of all the remembered past; and in this integrated complexity we had, as it were, the whole of the human performance. My next point was that the self-conscious mind was merely reading out from this neurally integrated ensemble. It was rather passive in this, not actively concerned in modifying it, but taking it as it was presented by the neuronal machinery in the spatio-temporal patterned operation. This warning of yours that I would be trapped in parallelism by such a view really worried me because I could see that, if the self-conscious mind was doing no more than give a readout of the neuronal machinery's performance, it would certainly be a parallelistic position. Of course I could save it a bit by saying that, in the action of voluntary will, one can have an action back from the self-conscious mind onto the neural machinery, but that seems to me to be a quite inadequate way out.

Therefore I rethought the story in the light of this criticism and came to the conclusion that I had been misled in trying to account for the whole integrational performance in terms of neural machinery. I realized that this was not a necessity. We have in fact two levels of integration in the ordinary performance we ourselves experience. The first is the integration given by our actions in movements, the movements of a whole organism correlated and organized to give appropriate responses. There is a unity of expression. That we are familiar with. On the materialist-monist concept this can be a complete explanation, a behavioural explanation, of the operational unity of a living person. As against that we have the other unity which is our experiential unity, and there I see the dichotomy.

Let us think then of the hypothesis that the self-conscious mind is not just engaged passively in a reading out the operation of neural events, but that it is an actively searching operation. There is displayed or portrayed before it from instant to instant the whole of the complex neural processes, and according to attention and choice and interest or drive, it can select from this ensemble of performances in the liaison brain, searching now this now that and blending together the results of readouts of many different areas in the liaison brain. In that way the self-conscious mind achieves a unity of experience. You see that this hypothesis gives a prime role to the action of the self-conscious mind, an action of choice and searching and discovering and integrating. The neural machinery is there as the medium that is ever-changing and multi-complex in space and time. It is there for all operations of the self-consious mind. I think that is the essence of my story. There are many further developments from it, but I wanted to tell you that your criticism of me in our peripatetic discussion led me to rethink the story out in this way. I think it is a radical departure from anything that has been defined precisely in the past and one that lends itself now even to experimental investigation, as I shall later on talk about.

P: I am greatly interested in what you say. I do think that the limits to parallelism, if I may so call them, are very interesting. Certain aspects of parallelism are undoubtedly valid; but parallelism has its very severe limits, and it is there that interaction takes place — that something totally different from the physical system acts in some way on the physical system. There is no doubt that this is connected with the problem of integration.

I was also very happy about your stress on activity because, as you know from my interest in the gondola kitten story in Held and Hein's experiment (cp. chapter E8), I also feel that activity is very important and that the conscious self is highly active. Even if it is merely contemplating, it contemplates actively. I think that this emphasis on action is very important. I might also refer to the idea of the searchlight theory of the mind.[1]

I would also like to add another point, namely, that in a way the self-conscious mind has a personality, something like an ethos or a moral character and that this personality is itself partly the product of actions done in the past. To a certain degree the personality somehow really does form itself actively. Admittedly, it may be partly pre-formed by its genetics. But I think that we both believe that this is not the whole story, and that a great part of the formation is really achieved by the free actions of the person himself. The

---

[1] See my [1972 (a)], *Appendix.*

personality is partly a product of its own free actions in the past. Now this is an important but very difficult idea. Perhaps one could try to understand it if one thinks that the brain is actually partly formed by these actions of the personality and the self. That is to say, the memory part of the brain, especially, can be said to be partly the product of the self. It is in part because of this idea that I suggest that we should replace as the title of our book *The Self and The Brain* by *The Self and Its Brain.*

E: There is a very important concept coming from these new developments. Not only have we got the self-conscious mind actively reading out from the great display of neuronal performance in the liaison areas, but we also have to recognize that this activity has a feedback and that it isn't just receiving. It is also giving or acting. I would like to think in a way that there is a give and take all the time in this active process, this selection process. Karl, I would like to take your concept of the physical world being open in certain sites and to think that we can propose that in certain unique locations of the brain you have the physical world open. We can conjecture that these brain areas have this property of openness because of subtle design and poise in their operating features. Now this interaction is a two-way process, the self-conscious mind receives and develops its experiences in all of its wide-ranging searching and selecting from the liaison brain. But also it acts back; and as it receives, so it gives. In this way it will produce changes in the performance of the brain, and, as it blends and moves and harmonizes these performances in the brain, they will eventually become, if they are played enough, stabilized in neuronal circuits which can be related to memories as described in chapter E8. So you could say that the self-conscious mind is in fact helping to mould the memory circuits, the memory stores of the brain. These memory stores are not simply at the disposal of all of the immediate perceptual input. At the same time they are at the disposal of the whole of the perceived world and the world of thought and imagination which is our self, the world of the self-conscious mind.

I think it is most important that we have this feedback. If I were to continue on this theme for a moment, we might say that one small element in this feedback from the self-conscious mind to the brain is effective in bringing about mechanical events in the external world by muscles moving joints and/or by causing speech and so on as described in chapters E3 and E4. However I would say that we have to think of voluntary movement as only a small component, a specialized component, of the total performance of the self-conscious mind in working back and controlling the brain processes.

We conjecture that all the intellectual, artistic, creative, imaginative performances of the self-conscious mind are not just passively read out from the brain events. The self-conscious mind is actively engaged in the tremendously subtle and transcendent operation of organizing, selecting and integrating its read out. It is the instigator of the brain processes which are necessary for the readout. The brain processes in turn may become stabilized in some memory process to be recovered as a memory on demand by the self-conscious mind. I think we are all the time doing that. When we think of something, saying to ourselves we must remember that, we are acting on the brain so that the neuronal circuits can be built that will enable retrieval at a later stage. Furthermore you may have some kind of associative rememberings which will enable you to effect the appropriate retrieval.

So we are now giving the self-conscious mind an immense range of actions, really effective actions, not passive as in parallelism and epiphenomenalism and all the other similar theories – psychoneural identity, biperspectivism, double aspect, etc. By contrast we are now giving the self-conscious mind a master role in its relationship to the brain. Sperry has in several recent publications expressed a similar idea, namely that the mental events are actively engaged in giving to and receiving from the brain. Further he goes on to say that this gives the reason for conscious mind having evolved.

P: Let me add something to this. I think it is altogether wrong to think of memory as a kind of cinematographic or television film about perceptual experiences. Action is quite obviously very important for memory. If for example we remember how we learned to play the piano, then this is entirely the learning of a certain way of acting. And the learning of this way of acting is a typical achievement of the memory, just as, for example, if we play a piece on the piano and can then repeat it without any help, just from memory. Thus the action element seems extremely important in memory, and, since action is a matter of the moral character and of its will, it is pretty clear that our brain is in part at least the product of our mind.

E: I can go still further into this interaction of the self-conscious mind and the neuronal machinery. In the parallelist view there is the completely rigid relationship of the purely passive readout. I would say that we have to be much more open now in our concepts. There is coherency, that is to say the operations of the neural machinery are coherent with what the self-conscious mind finds here or there, but the self-conscious mind is not just limited to some restricted zone or to the whole zone. It has the choice. It selects at will, shall we say, from the total display of neural machinery from moment to moment. You may think that this is very wasteful, that you've got a tremendous amount of action going on in the brain that never comes through to be experienced in consciousness and is not stored in memory. It is lost irretrievably; but that is of course extremely important. The self-conscious mind has to select. We'd be overloaded by information if at any moment we had to take notice of everything that was poured into all our senses. This is perhaps one of the very important reasons for the operation of the self-conscious mind and its evolution, if there is consciousness in animals. It gives a selection or a preference from the total operative performance of the neural machinery.

Now another point that I wanted to deal with here is that in this interplay between the self-conscious mind and the cerebral events we have an enormously rich field for new thinking and new experimental investigations. We have also to imagine that we are able to play forwards and backwards in time. The self-consious mind isn't clamped to the immediate events going on in the brain, but it is all the time judging them and thinking of them in relationship to past events and to anticipated future events. One of the simplest examples of that I can think of is in relationship to music. When you are listening to some music that you know, you not only are blending the immediately perceived notes or harmonies with the past, which is still held in your memory to give you some unity of melody, but you are also anticipating the future, and all of this gives you some unique experiences which couldn't possibly have happened on the basis of the neural machinery alone. The self-conscious mind is in this way exhibiting its ability to lift itself out of strict coherence with the neural patterns as they are at any one instant. I think that again gives us a flexibility in handling the brain operations by the way in which our mind can range over them and can draw on its resources of the past and build into the future.

P: I was very interested in what you said about music. It is important, for example, in learning to play the piano or in learning to play a piece on the piano that the conscious process of training in time becomes unconscious. The self-conscious mind is relieved by a skilled memory on a completely physiological level which is not any longer in need of conscious attention but which may be badly interfered with if we suddenly attend to it consciously. Sometimes it is interfered with positively by conscious attention but sometimes negatively. I want to stress the great significance of the memory of actions and of skills.[2] One of the most important parts of the memory storage (of acquired memory), is the memory of actions exemplifying acquired skills, the memory of knowing how, rather than merely the memory of knowing

[2] See also my section 41.

that. We have, as it were, a completely different apparatus for a skill which has been acquired and for a skill as it is in the process of being acquired with the help of conscious attention to certain actions. This is the process by which we impress our activities on our brain, and amongst these activities are, of course, our personality traits which are also impressed on the brain.

E: There is something very important in the timing relationships of the self-conscious mind in relationship to neural events. Already I have described in chapter E2 an experiment of Libet's which caused him to develop the hypothesis of antedating. The cortical activities evoked by some sharp stimulus to the hand in conscious human subjects took as long as half a second to build up to the level for giving consciousness; yet the subject antedated it in his experience to a time which was the time of arrival of the message from the periphery onto the cerebral cortex, which may be almost half a second earlier. This is an extraordinary happening, and there is no way in which this can be explained by the operations of the neural machinery. It simply has to be explained by the manner in which the self-conscious mind becomes cognizant of the peripheral event by reading out from the neural machinery when its responses had developed to the necessary level of size and of action.

The second point is that we know now from studies by Kornhuber and others (chapter E3) that, when you are willing an action, you don't immediately trigger off the action; but in this case, too, the self-conscious mind is working upon the neural machinery in wide ranging parts of the brain and gradually is moulding the patterns there, actively changing them. So eventually the patterned neuronal operation homes in on the correct pyramidal cells in the motor cortex in order to bring about the desired action. This whole process takes about 0.8 of a second and therefore you can think of the incredible complexity of the events going on. This is again an active influence of the self-conscious mind upon neuronal machinery.

From these findings I develop the conjecture that there isn't any simple unitary relationship between neural events and the self-conscious mind. The self-conscious mind is only effective on the brain when the brain is in special states of very highly integrated dynamic activity, and of course this leads on to the question of unconsciousness and sleep, coma, convulsions. Under these conditions there is no self-consciousness. It can be conjectured that the neuronal machinery is not working at a level in which the self-conscious mind can get into liaison with it. This will be the theme of a later discussion, and is also considered in chapter E7.

P: In a way, one could say that the mind not only decodes the coded information, for example about the visual field, received from the retina and so on, but that it tries to read immediately from it the state of the world in so far as it bears on the organism in question. I think that in this sense there is something in naive realism or, if you don't want to call it naive realism, you could call it direct realism. That is to say, the brain tries to obtain directly a view of the situation in the external world relevant to the organism. Further, this is not merely a perception of a *Gestalt* or anything of that sort: it is itself an *activity* and it is in a sense part of the preparation for further action, both for the movements it is just about to make, and also for that kind of action which consists of developing expectations about the future, more particularly about the future development of the organism's situation in the external world.

E: I am very much in agreement that our self-conscious mind is reading out from the brain nothing simple or unitary. I am sure that the task is one of lifting out an immense integrated performance of the brain. If we were to take it to the other extreme, it would be quite absurd to think that the self-conscious mind was paying any attention to the firing of any particular nerve cell. There is almost no interest in this because there is almost no information in the firing of one cell. It's the collective communal operation of a large number of neurones that has to be the basis of the readout.

P: I think you have to distinguish this from field theory.

E: I agree completely. This is something quite other than the field theory of the *Gestalt* or the micro-field theory of Pribram. Now we are talking not of fields but of new operational developments in what we may call the modules. Szentágothai has recognized that the organization of the cerebral cortex is in multitudes of vertically oriented modules, each with a complexly organized assemblage of some thousands of neurones (chapter E1). He has thought of the module as being like an integrated micro-circuit of electronics, only very much more complicated. It is this kind of integrated complex neuronal assemblage in dynamic operation that is I think giving something of interest to the self-conscious mind. But a problem still arises: What is in fact the self-conscious mind listening in to? What is the nature of the neuronal activities? Is it the firing of some nerve cells, or the whole collusive action of the nerve cells? This is something that we have further to discuss.

P: You have spoken quite rightly about what the mind reads out of the activity of the nervous system. I would like to take this word "reads" further.

When we read a book, we very soon become quite unconscious of the letters and even of the shapes of the words which we see, and the mind begins to read the meaning directly; the meaning as such. Of course, we do also read the words, but only in context and as carriers of a meaning. I think that this is probably very similar to the process you describe. In perception we read the meaning of the neuronal firing pattern of the brain and the meaning of the neuronal firing pattern is, as it were, the situation in the outside world which we try to perceive.

E: When we are thinking furthermore about what the self-conscious mind is reading out, we can think of the module with its integrated micro-performance of neuronal patterns. That is something about which we are still very ignorant, but we can use our imagination in that respect (cp. chapter E1). We can conjecture that the module with 10,000 nerve cells is not a simple structure. It has an intense inner active life with mixtures of excitatory and inhibitory neurones. It has two levels of operation, a much more subtle superficial level (laminae I and II), and a deeper level (laminae III to VI), more strongly operating. The module could be an especially designed structure whereby the physical world, World 1, achieves an openness to the world of mind, to World 2. I think this is implicit in our hypothesis. There must be some special neuronal structure and action which allows this liaison to occur and there is operation both ways. If we were to stretch the analogy very far, we could liken the module to a radio transmitter-receiver, so that it functions not only for transmitting to the mind, the self-conscious mind, but also for receiving from it. I think this concept is valuable because I believe, as we have said earlier, that we have to stress that the action is both ways all the time. I think the self-conscious mind isn't just passively receiving, it is actively working. In receiving it is active. When it receives, it achieves more action in controlling the performance of the neuronal machinery.

There is an on-going ever-changing operation of the mind upon the brain, and therefore we have to think that there is a very remarkable openness of the physical system of the brain. We shall, I assume, go on considering this in reductionist terms as a purely physical system, a physical system though with the openness to the self-conscious mind – at least open when in certain special states, but not always open. When you're asleep, it isn't open. When you have an anaesthetic, it's not open. When you're in deep coma or hit on the head, there is no openness; but under normal waking conditions, it is open, and there lies the whole problem of our book you might say.

P: I have quite a number of questions that I want to ask. First, a question about the present state of this hypothesis which we are discussing. You would I suppose now reject completely the idea that there is, in the visual centre, a region upon which visual pictures are, as it were, projected in a topologically correct way if not a metrically correct way. That is to say, you would reject the theory that there is projection from the retina to the centre. This theory is a typically parallelistic idea, and if accepted it would lead to a new problem, namely, how is *this* picture now interpreted. And this would, so to speak, merely have shifted the original problem one stage further back. Now I suppose that fundamentally the coding is a coding in time; that it is similar to the coding received by a television receiver, which receives a picture as a purely temporal succession of signals.[3] So perhaps the coding reaching the conscious self is a coding essentially in time, and perhaps not at all in space. All of these questions are of course rather crude, but I think they should be asked. Are my questions clear?

E: The question is formulated with respect to the perception of some picture that we're looking at, some landscape, or what you will: how is it put together after the way in which it has been taken apart in the retina? There is the projected image on the retina, but for transmission and handling it all has to be made into a mosaic arrangement coded in the firing frequencies of the million or so optic nerve fibres. We have traced in chapter E2 of this book the elements of the way in which the picture starts to be reassembled. For example it is put together into directionality (orientation), into length of line, into angle of line, and finally, in the infratemporal cortex, into more complex shapes, so there are some cells with reactions to circles rather than squares and so on. This is alright as far as it goes, but, as you will stress, it hasn't shown us at all how we see a picture, how this is all put together to give us the visual experience that we all enjoy. That is where this new hypothesis becomes important.

The question now asked is: How is the picture put together? It may be that we never will find cells with truly specialized triggering imagery. That is to say we don't find cells that would respond to something, shall we say a whole face. This idea is often bandied about, and such cells are ironically referred to as "grandmother cells". Yet we have to explain how we can in some global manner identify a face in a flash from another face. Do we then have to imagine that, in the areas where this is accomplished, some cells are specialized for one kind of face and another kind of cell for another kind of

[3] For what we experience is not merely the picture but the fact that, for example, one physical body stands in front of another.

face, and that we have thousands of cells like this each one tuned to be triggered by a particular face? Then we have to think that this gets very complicated because it isn't just a face at a given distance in a given illumination, a given profile relationship and so on. It's that human face in the most varied situations, and we still can accomplish the identification. It becomes a tremendous challenge for the neural machinery to accomplish such a discriminative task, because it is unbelievably discriminative. We tell one face from another face from another face and so on. Testing procedures show that we have great ability in this respect.

Perhaps the situation may now be lifted to a different level when we think of our self-conscious mind as scanning over the whole wealth of data in the liaison modules and selecting in some holistic manner in relationship to a life-time of remembered experiences. Of course I am picking out from this immense diversity the correct interpretation of the visual experience presented there. That's just an example. I think that all of these are challenges to further thinking, but I should point out that, as stated in chapter E2, in the present theories of neuronal machinery there is no explanation whatsoever of our ability to integrate into a coherent picture the disparate neuronal events arising in the visual centres as a consequence of a retinal input. According to our hypothesis it is the self-conscious mind which accomplishes this incredible reassemblage into a consciously observed picture. But also we can make a coherent image of polymodal inputs of great complexity. For example visual, auditory and tactual inputs can be assembled to give the experience of a musical instrument being played.

P: It may not be quite uninteresting to mention in this connection a speculation by Hobbes. In a way Hobbes might be said to be the inventor of the wave theory of light, or rather, of the vibration theory of light. His discussion was interesting, although he had no theory of light propagation. Hobbes's argument is best understood as a refinement of an argument of Descartes's. Descartes thought that, in effect, we see in the same way in which a blind man feels with a stick as he goes along. Hobbes made a kind of variation on this theme by saying that the blind man would have constantly to feel and feel again, renewing the pressure all the time as it were, in order to be sure that nothing had changed. In consequence, even if nothing changes at all, and we just see one colour, the colour must consist of a constant vibration of pressure on our eyes. That was Hobbes's idea. It was a completely speculative argument, derived only from the fact that the stimulus of seeing a colour persists in time.

I think that one might extend this most interesting speculative thought of

Hobbes's by saying that in general it is an essentially temporal succession of signals that acts upon us, in a way similar to that in which a television receiver is acted on by a one-dimensional succession of signals in the form of vibrations, and that this is really what works upon us and what we interpret and read off when we decode. Now if I may mention another point in connection with this business of "reading off", just as when we read a book we try to penetrate, so to speak, through all the sensory elements of reading to the World 3 meaning which is intended by the writer, so I think that in a similar way we – the selves – read the message of the brain by penetrating through it to World 1, and by reconstructing the relevant structure of World 1 (including its situational significance for us),[4] just as we try in the other case to reconstruct the relevant structure of World 3. I think it is again very important that in all this the mind is very active. That is to say, it is not just passively receiving these temporal signals as Hobbes thought, but it is actually constantly trying to interpret them. There is a kind of resonance to this: that is to say the mind is constantly trying to put forth actively what the next messages might be, and then to compare these anticipations of the messages with the incoming messages to see if they will fit. It is a process of making and matching, and one might actually work with the hypothesis that making and matching involve, from the brain's point of view, a message which is essentially temporal, as I suggested before. Of course, there will be many places in the brain where these temporal messages play a role. One could think of the mind as actively manipulating the brain in the process of perception: as being similar to a doctor who taps a patient, actively, instead of merely listening passively (he auscultates and palpates the patient). The doctor tries actively to test his various conjectural diagnoses by pressing various places on the patients' body and in the end he may get an integrated picture of the situation within the patient. In a way, all scientific discovery proceeds like this.

---

[4] From the point of view of development, significance seems to be the earliest element in interpretation. The baby smiles and reacts to smiles by smiling at a very early age: it somehow registers the significance of smiles. (See my section 31.) After all, the so-called imitative contraptions (cp. my [1963(a)], p. 381) to which babies and birds react, as Konrad Lorenz discovered, are probably not so much simplified shapes (of the mother bird for example) as release signals for biologically highly significant reactions. That is to say, the little bird recognizes in these shapes not so much its mother – that is, a certain physical body – but the carrier of food. Thus the significance of a visual signal seems to be prior to its physical interpretation. And we may perhaps wonder whether something analogous does not happen when we read: the meaning of a word in a sense may have priority over its spelling (which partly explains spelling mistakes).

E: I want to raise a further problem. Although, when you cut the corpus callosum, you completely prevent the access of the self-conscious mind to the neural events in the right hemisphere, are we justified in thinking that it does not have any access to these events when the corpus callosum is intact? Or is the corpus callosum some channel the self-conscious mind may work along, and by the section we have prevented its normal access route to events in the minor hemisphere? We may conjecture that the access is from open to closed modules, and even that, when the corpus callosum is intact, the callosal influence may cause modules of the minor hemisphere to be directly open to the self-conscious mind (cp. chapter E7; Fig. 5).

P: When the corpus callosum is intact, probably everything that happens in the minor hemisphere leads to a kind of reverberation in the major hemisphere, so that if the mind had access only to the major hemisphere, it would nevertheless have indirect access to practically all the interesting information from the minor hemisphere. In fact we do know that if the corpus callosum is cut the patient does get some such indirect information via repercussions upon the right hand side of his body from movements of his left limbs. We must not forget that even if the coded signals are very incomplete, the action of interpretation may complete the message. The supply of missing parts of the incoming information is one of the most important functions on every level of interpretation, and especially on the highest level.

E: I agree that it would do it that way. What worries me is just this. That we have in the minor hemisphere, I take it, wonderful neural machinery in all the subtlety and learnt performance to handle for example a musical experience, even the complexity of musical experience in all of its detail. How can this come through in the corpus callosum to some unknown receiving area for the self-conscious mind to read it out? Maybe it comes that way. I have a feeling though that the self-conscious mind, knowing what's going on, may be able to "sneak" over to the minor hemisphere and have a look there, where the really subtle integrational, global, operational aspects of this musical appreciation is going on! I raise these questions. I think it is still possible that we may have to change our hypothesis a bit and give the self-conscious mind the ability to move under conditions where the corpus callosum is intact, and it recognizes that there is something of high interest going on in the other side, so it scans the appropriate modules there. Of course it's normally "fluttering" around, scanning the dominant hemisphere, and if the corpus callosum is intact, it may often assume that there is nothing of interest going on in the minor hemisphere to bother about. Well this is I think all very crude analogical talking, but, if we can't talk better, we have to talk the way we can!

P: I would like to ask whether there is evidence that musical appreciation is so completely confined to the minor hemisphere. That is to say, a lot of evidence would be needed to show that the dominant hemisphere does not cooperate in real musical appreciation. The minor hemisphere may be a necessary condition for being able to appreciate music but it may not be sufficient for a full appreciation. I think that this is probably the case, and that we must work with this conjecture unless you have real evidence to the contrary. One reason is that music very often consists of words which are sung: an ordinary song is one of the simplest forms of music. May I also refer to what you said yesterday about the origin of the epic. The epic is apparently sung in order to obtain, with the participation of the minor hemisphere, an easy way of memorizing words, for both rhythm and melody help. I think these are some *a priori* reasons why one must be very careful before one says that the working of the minor hemisphere is a sufficient condition for the full appreciation of music.

E: I think that's a very good point that you have made. I have to confess that the investigations so far made upon the musical appreciation of the brain are at a very elementary level, a crude level. It is difficult to develop sufficiently discriminative and sophisticated testing of musical appreciation; and many of the subjects that come along with some kind of neurological lesion are musically illiterate. There is little to work with. There are rare cases of much more interest. I know of one that I just heard of by accident. A distinguished musician went to his doctor saying, "Doctor, I've had something wrong in my brain because now I've lost all appreciation of music. I can still play the piano, but it means nothing to me. I have no thrill, no emotion, no feeling. I've lost the sense of beauty, of value." It was discovered that he had a vascular lesion in his superior temporal lobe on the right side. He lost everything of his artistic life with one not very extensive vascular lesion.

P: This only shows that these parts of the brain are needed. Indeed, the very fact that he was missing it shows that there is normally a cooperation between the left and the right sides. Otherwise he might not have missed it so badly.

E: Yes, I agree with that. I of course would like to put as much as possible of the mind-brain liaison onto the dominant hemisphere because that simplifies our hypothesis. But it is hard for me to think that you can have in the right temporal lobe the full neuronal performance for giving musical appreciation and bringing in all the memory, all the subtlety, the immense stored performance that is there and that this is then somehow shot across in encoded form to the dominant hemisphere to be read out.

P: I can't help feeling that there is, to put it again very crudely, a structure in self-consciousness; that self-consciousness is somehow a higher development of consciousness, and possibly that the right hemisphere is conscious but not self-conscious, but that the left hemisphere is both conscious and self-conscious. It is possible that the main function of the corpus callosum is, so to speak, to transfer the conscious – but not self-conscious – interpretations of the right hemisphere to the left, and of course, to transfer something in the other direction too. This possibility really has, I think, to be taken very seriously. We know so little about these things that one has to consider some sort of structural development of self-consciousness from a lower level of consciousness.

E: I come at the end to say that this problem of commissural transfer should be looked at also in the pictorial sense. In the split brain patients of Sperry and Bogen there is a very complete examination of the performances of the right hemisphere, that is the minor hemisphere, and of the left hemisphere, contrasting the two in respect of copying pictures and also in recognizing pictures. The minor hemisphere comes out superior to the dominant hemisphere. So you have in this respect to admit that machinery for doing all this detailed evaluation of pattern and picture, of perspective, of meaning of forms and landscapes, and so on, all of this is processed in the neural machinery of the minor hemisphere. If the corpus callosum is cut, the dominant hemisphere fails abysmally in these respects. Presumably it could perform well if it gets the messages through, and it would be the simplest form of our hypothesis for us to say that all of the neuronal processing involved in pattern and picture, all of the detailed neurological machinery is working in special places in the minor hemisphere, and then the integrated result is transmitted through the corpus callosum. Of course it is transmitted through all the time, as we know, and we conjecture that for conscious recognition there is transmission to special liaison sites which we still haven't even located in the dominant hemisphere. These would be the scanning sites, if you would like to call them that, for the self-conscious mind. I think that there are a great many unknowns in the whole detailed brain performance and many challenging problems could certainly arise in this connection. However I do think there is hope because these new hypotheses are so fertile in problems for the future. Further treatment of this theme of the functional performances of the dominant and minor hemispheres is given in chapters E5 and E6.

Dialogue VI

10:15 a.m., 23 September 1974

P: There is a great problem concerning the way in which we may conceive of interaction between the self and the brain and, indeed, a wider question as to whether two entirely different worlds can be open to each other and interact with each other. I have discussed this question in my historical chapter P5, but only in a negative way; namely, by saying that the usual way of posing the question is really illegitimate because it is based on a view of causality which has been superseded by the development of physics. The Cartesian model of interaction between extended bodies which gave rise to this problem has certainly broken down completely: it is inapplicable to modern physics.

However, the question remains a very interesting and very deep one. I suggest that we actually have in our immediate experience, in so far as immediate experiences exist at all, a sort of model of the way in which the self may interact with the brain; and this model is really our experience of the way in which the self interacts with the memory. (I am thinking mainly of a task such as recalling a name.) There can be very little doubt that memory is essentially physiological and brain-based. There can also be little doubt that, like general brain activity, memory is one of the prerequisites of consciousness. However that may be, memory undoubtedly has a conscious aspect. That is to say, we can rack our brains in order to remember something, and in doing so we are actually actively engaged, actively interfering as it were, with (if we may say so) the clockwork of memory, or the telephone exchange of memory. (Whether this is a good metaphor doesn't matter for my purpose.) Now, if we look at the ways in which we interfere with memory, we discover that there is something which is intuitively accessible to us and sometimes something which is intuitively inaccessible to us. That is to say, we somehow know how to press the trigger of our memory and at the same time we somehow don't know how we do it. My suggestion is that when we search our memory, we feel that we are sitting in the driver's seat of our car, as it were, and doing certain things which have certain effects. Like a driver we have at best partial knowledge of what we are doing — of the causal chains we are setting in motion. The combination between the feeling that we operate a known mechanism and the other feeling that we do not know how the effects of our actions are actually brought about can be taken as a model of the way in which the self interacts with the brain. That is to say, the working of the brain is partly accessible and partly inaccessible to the self.

All the feelings I have just described lie within our conscious experience and therefore within *one* world, namely, World 2. This model, the model of a driver in a car or, in Ryle's terminology, the ghost in the machine, is very rough, but it may be taken as a model for the interaction between two worlds, namely, World 1 and World 2.

It is generally assumed that it isn't very difficult to understand interaction within one world. But what I have described are experiences within World 2, and I think that we find, firstly, that it isn't true that interaction within one world is quite so generally understandable: not only within World 1 — after Descartes — but also within World 2. Secondly, there is apparently not much greater difficulty in understanding interaction between two worlds than interaction within one world.

I wonder whether one can make anything of the fact that there is something intermediate, as it were, namely the memory, which has its conscious aspects and its unconscious aspects; but about this one would need a separate study. I would just like to add that I think that the interaction between the self and the memory may not only be similar or analogous to, but may possibly actually be the same as, the interaction between the self and the brain. I think that this has at least to be explored.

E: That's a very stimulating and exciting introduction that you have given this morning. I can see many important and difficult problems ahead. I think in the first place we have to realize that, insofar as the self-conscious mind and memory are concerned, we have interaction with the brain which plays both ways. That is, I regard the self-conscious mind as deliberately operating upon the brain, trying to recover brain actions which lead in turn to the experiences that the self-conscious mind desires. We may be doing something very simple. To take an example, we may be searching for a word or a phrase or a sentence, searching for some simple memory of this kind; but I think the self-conscious mind can't do it alone because it requires the brain to deliver the memory to it and so it is searching and probing and eventually accepting the answer. If we are looking, for example, for a synonym, for a better word to express some thought we have, that again has to be played into the brain and received from the brain. Perhaps we may repeatedly play it backwards and forwards evaluating and judging. Here we have then a very strong dualism involved in something which is amongst our commonest experiences.

I would like to say further that a great deal of intense learning is required for the efficient operation of this interplay, that is for the self-conscious mind to work effectively with the brain and to interact with the brain. This is of course what comes with the skilled use of language, ideas being expressed in words and sentences, checking backwards and forwards. I think here we have to realize that this is no simple mechanical process of the self-conscious mind, just simply pulling out some stops in the brain and getting a message back just as you would out of some pigeon hole or computer memory! It is infinitely more complicated than that. The self-conscious mind has to play upon the very complex machinery of the brain, which is turning over and is all the time playing and receiving and interacting. It isn't just a sort of staccato process, pressing a key and getting an immediate and final answer back. In the generation of sentences there is the continual moulding and modification forwards and backwards that I think is the essence of the interacting game played between the self-conscious mind on the one hand and the higher cerebral centres on the other.

While I am talking about this, I am of course questioning. Can we go further on and ask whether the self-conscious mind has its own internal question and answer machinery or whether it is tied to the brain for this, being only able to question and to receive answers and to question again? There is what you might call a vertical level of communication both ways between World 2 and World 1. Is there also a horizontal level of communication? We know that there is such a horizontal level in World 1 in the brain. We have an immense amount of neurophysiological and anatomical evidence for this, as is described in chapters E1 and E2 for example. You might say that the whole brain is an immense horizontally operating complex machine. But now we come to the question: are there also some horizontal operations going on in World 2 within the self-conscious mind, or has it always to interact with the liaison brain in order to get the requisite horizontality of performance?

P: What I have to say more or less fits in with the question that you have just raised. In the process of racking our brains and ultimately getting the goods delivered by our memory, the self remains outside as it were, and it remains for the time being as a spectator, almost as a recipient of these delivered goods. That is to say, it is just in such moments that we see very clearly that we must distinguish the conscious self from its experiences.

One might be tempted, under the indirect influence of Hume, to think of the self as the sum total of its experiences. (Cp. my section 53.) But it seems to me that this theory is directly refuted by the memory experiences to which I have referred. At the actual moment at which the memory delivers something to us, neither the delivering memory nor the object that it delivers to us is part of our selves; rather, they are outside of our selves, and we look at them as spectators (though we may be active immediately before and after the delivery) and, as it were, watch the delivery with astonishment. We can therefore separate our conscious experiences as such from our selves. To me this doesn't look so much a vertical as a kind of horizontal distinction within consciousness, with the self on a higher level than certain other regions — almost at a higher logical level than the sum total of experiences. This idea of the self as a spectator is also very clearly and vividly described by Penfield (see my sections 18 and 37). Penfield, of course, discusses a highly artificial situation in which the brain is electrically stimulated. I would say that in normal circumstances the self is only a spectator for rare moments, and that as a rule it is highly active. It may be perhaps a spectator just at the moment at which its activity leads to a success. Using Ryle's terms, "remembering" (in the sense in which it is the result of an effort) may be described as a "success word". "I remember" is equivalent to "I succeed in remembering". So only at the moment at which its activity leads to a success is the self really a spectator. Otherwise it is constantly, or almost constantly, active.

E: Yes, I think that's a very good comment on the question of verticality and horizontality — that there are within the World 2 these differences and that in a way we can think of the self-conscious mind as superior to all of the experiences and memories that are presented to it. This relationship is illustrated in Figure E7 – 2 in chapter E7, where the self is distinguished from its experiences in the outer sense and inner sense categories.

All the time when we are searching for a memory, searching for a word, searching for something from the past storage in our brains, we are searching and receiving and judging and evaluating with this conscious self. It is superior to its objects which are delivered, and it is superior in that it can accept or reject them and use them or modify them and put them into the brain storage. That is certainly an important concept. We have to realize that there is an active interplay. The self-conscious mind is in fact probing always into the brain in some manner to retrieve from there or to attempt to retrieve something which it wants back, some desired input from the brain. Now this must involve an immense learned performance. You have to conceive that the whole of our civilized development, of our cultural development, consists not in having a brain with all of this storage, but in having a self-conscious mind that can retrieve and know how to retrieve subtly and effectively from this storage. It has some way of playing into this immense store of memory that is in the spatio-temporal patterns of connectivity in the neural coding, and of receiving back from that – not perhaps the first time; but it has strategies and tricks of retrieval.

I know myself that I have difficulties in retrieving some names of people and names of places, but I have tricks to try to get hold of these names. Some memories I can recover immediately in a kind of global manner and be confident I can always do it. Other ones I know I have more trouble with. This is something I think we all experience, namely that we have to have tricks of memory retrieval or strategies of memory retrieval, and this is all part of how we can manage to supervise and to read out at will from the tremendous store of information that is coded in our brains. If we try to think of the kind of card index system we would require in order adequately to give us the full human performance of a highly trained brain, it would be beyond any imagination. Of course we use all kinds of strategies based on indexing. That's why we write books and index them, why we keep card indices, and so on. We have all kinds of devices in order to lighten the immense loading of memory.

When you come think of it, that was essentially what written language was developed for. The writing of language was invented in Sumer when oral memory was proving quite inadequate for storage of business transactions, of economic affairs, of decrees of state, and so on. In the operation of the first big cities, cities with more than a hundred thousand inhabitants, written language was necessary because the complexities could no longer be stored and retrieved in the minds of the men who were involved for the first time in running a large civilized community.

P: I should like to say something which is not important, and which concerns terminology. I prefer our terms "the self-conscious mind" or "self-consciousness" or "the higher consciousness" to the term "the pure ego", because, even though such terms as "the pure ego" were intended by their authors to refer to the same kind of object as we refer to when we speak of the self-conscious mind, these terms are heavily loaded with philosophical theories which in my opinion are not really acceptable. (See my section 31.)

Another point occurred to me when we were talking about the incredible retrieval system which we have with respect to our memory. (In my case, owing somehow to my age, it is beginning to fail; and I experience its failure very strongly and feel it as a very considerable loss, if not to my personality, at least to, let us say, the intellectual aspect of my personality.) What I wanted to say about this retrieval system which you describe so beautifully is this. We spoke a day or two ago about the astonishingly fast evolutionary development of the increase in size of the human brain, and we discussed the possible challenges, the possible needs, which may up to a point explain the kind of selection pressure which may have led to this very fast development. Now I actually think that it is quite clear that animals would not have this conscious retrieval system. That is to say, I think that we have to distinguish two kinds of memory or two kinds of relationship between the conscious self and the memory. One is the *implicit memory* and the other is the *explicit memory.*[1] The implicit memory is, as it were, all present in us. As long as we are awake there are lots and lots of things which are implicitly just simply there, available, determining in part what we do and influencing us all the time. But there is also the explicit memory which you described when you spoke about the retrieval system. Now I wish to offer a hypothesis; namely, that the explicit memory is specifically human, and that it arises together with human language; that is to say, that the retrieval system develops together with human language.

Quite a lot could be said concerning this hypothesis, but among other things it would explain the incredible demand made on the brain and accordingly the incredible selection pressure which would be exerted on the evolution of the brain owing to the emergence of language. It isn't only that we have to learn to speak, which is one thing; it is actually that we have to learn to use our language not only unconsciously (as does a babbling baby) but, in certain cases, when necessary, in a conscious way, which really means that the retrieval system must be available to us. So my hypothesis is that the big size of the brain results from demands made on the retrieval system owing to the evolution of language. The distinction between implicit and explicit memory is pretty important (and should be investigated by us further, especially by you, for example in the light of Brenda Milner's work, in which there are described certain failures of both implicit and explicit memory) but the two are very clearly distinguishable. Also, incidentally, explicit memory may in time become more and more implicit, as does, for example, the ability to speak and to tell stories of the man, HM, in Brenda Milner's account of his attempt to fall back on old stories. The old stories were apparently both implicit and explicit and for that reason were very easily available, while there was, in other respects, a failure of explicit memory. (See chapter E8.)

---

[1] For other distinctions concerning memory, see my section 41.

E: I like that distinction of memory in two categories. I might even go further though. I perhaps rather naughtily would like to think that a great many human beings, although they use language, use it in an implicit manner. It is some kind of ongoing stream which they immerse themselves in without any thought – the idle chatter, the repetition of stories, the repetition of events, the immense descriptions of trivialities with no judgment, no critical judgment, no mercy for their hearers. This is I suppose what you would call implicit memory, as I gather from your description.

P: It may be a third, a kind of intermediate stage. We really should work this out more carefully. What is said here is all only a suggestion.

E: Yes, maybe there's a spectrum. But I rather feel myself that the concept of explicit memory should be explored further. You see this is where in linguistic expression the brain is used at its highest levels. It involves a long and arduous training and it involves also the whole of the growth of World 3. I think this occurs by the use of explicit memory with all the range of problems and discussions, and with the evaluations of any overt performances, such as in the arts, crafts, technologies, sciences, etc. All of this involves the critical judgments that come with the use of language and explicit memory at that level. Furthermore I suppose we could say the whole of mathematics is a kind of explicit memory. So now there appears to be some sharp distinction evolving. We have conjectured that World 2 grows because of World 3. They interact, each helping the other, but is it not possible that we could say it is the explicit memory category of World 2 that is involved in this symbiotic relationship with World 3, both in its growth, and at any one time in its utilization?

We have to think of World 3 in two ways: that we are utilizing it in all of our civilized and skilled actions, the scientific, the artistic, the creative; and secondly we are also adding to it and therefore having a positive feedback to World 3, adding something to the great and wonderful storage of human creativity which we call World 3. Your description of the memory spectrum I think is undoubtedly valid, and there is even within the explicit memory, a kind of spectrum.

P: I would suggest that the implicit memory is perhaps the strongest factor which forms our personalities when they are seen, as it were, as developing through time; and even here World 3 elements undoubtedly have an effect. You once told me that as a little boy you were surrounded by reproductions of famous classical pictures. Now this has no doubt somehow influenced your whole personality, your way of looking at a landscape, and your way of enjoying life. In my case, it is similar with music. I have very deep personal relationships with certain pieces of music, which, in a way, are there implicitly, and give, so to speak, a kind of rhythm to my life. In the case of Brenda Milner's subject, HM, one actually gets from her description an impression of his personality, which is a charming, innocent personality, but which seems very largely to be formed by the implicit memories he still has of the time before his anterograde amnesia developed. Generally speaking, the aims and plans we have, our conception of our self and of our status, are all very largely determined by our past interactions with World 3. These, and therefore indirectly World 3 elements themselves, have formed our personality, and form part of our implicit memory.

E: Karl, could you please say some more about what you actually mean by implicit memory. What does it cover? For I am a little confused about that end of the spectrum. At the other end I think I have no difficulty, but at what levels are you talking about memory when you speak of implicit memory?

P: By implicit memory I mean all sorts of things which were our past experiences, which, although they are not explicitly before our consciousness, are nevertheless there, influencing our actions, and which *may* possibly become available to us. But there are also things which are there and are not available, and which I would be inclined also to call implicit memory as long as they do not become explicit. This includes things which are quite forgotten but which are possibly retrievable, and capable of being made explicit. (I therefore suggest that we make many subdivisions within the implicit memory.) My main idea is that our ability to speak is a result of our early experiences of our earlier attempts to speak; we do not explicitly remember them, but they have left a kind of trait, a kind of constant feature of our self and of our personality, which constantly moulds us and which of course in its turn is constantly further developed by our actions, our thoughts and our activities.

E: I understand this now and in a way I think you are also including what is usually called subconscious memories, memories which are not overt but perhaps can be retrieved under special conditions and of course in a sense we can agree with Freud that our characters themselves are moulded a great deal by influences that we have accepted in the past and now do not often recognize. This is all a part of life, of a normal life, and we can take all this as part of the given. It moulded our selves and our characters. It means that we have certain attitudes, certain fears, certain beliefs, certain terrors, certain prejudices and so on which we can't explain. These are perhaps results of unremembered incidents of past times. Obsessions come into this same category. Normally we can handle all this, but on the other hand they sometimes escape control and destroy or greatly injure personalities. This is the way in which I suppose psychiatry has had a good therapeutic influence. I don't say it's all good, but I think it is good in the sense that it does recognize these influences and tries to help the patient to handle them in some rational manner by exposing them and in that way perhaps helping to immunize against them.

P: In connection with what you said about psychiatry, I would like to refer to section 6 of chapter 1 of my [1963(a)], pp. 49–50.

You were also talking about the relation between explicit memory and World 3. Now, in the sense in which World 3 is encoded in the brain, I suppose it is mainly encoded in the explicit memory, but I just wanted to indicate that, in so far as World 3 has a strong bearing on the framing or moulding of our personalities, it is also probably encoded in the implicit memory.

As to the question of the unity of the self, there are, in my opinion, various "unities". One is the self as the subject of action, of activity, and as a subject which receives information and so on. That is one kind of unity which is very important. But there is also another kind of unity, that is, the unity of our personality, which is somehow or other engraved into our memory – probably the implicit memory – and which is very largely the result of our previous actions. Up to a point one can even say that this engraved personality, so far as it exists, belongs as such, in a sense, to World 3. It is really, in a way, the product of our mind, the product of our self, and, being a product of our self, it is a kind of World 3 object. (The self as a World 3 object includes our expectations of what we shall be tomorrow, and, as Dobzhansky emphasizes, of our death. In this sense, the self is a theoretical object, as I have said before, and its "unity" is a theory.)

I may perhaps refer here to a question which was once put to me, namely, if we consciously breed certain races of animals, whether these are not then World 3 objects. My answer was: Yes, up to a point they are World 3 objects, much as works of art are; and indeed, there is a very old theory which says that our own life is a work of art. Now I would say that this theory is also true of our selves, in so far as our own selves are, up to a point, World 3 objects which are encoded in our memory and in the personality traits which our memory has established. There is both a kind of unity and also something which is comparable to World 3 and in which the other World 3, the non-personality World 3, has in my opinion played a very decisive role. So I would say that it is important to distinguish various "unities"; but you were in the main speaking of the unity of the self as the subject of activity and the centre of information.

E: I would like to comment on that very interesting and important remark you made that in a way each human self is a World 3 object. I think this is a terribly important concept. You can say that this is immediately recognized when you think of a biography. A biography is a work of art or of scholarship or a history about a World 3 object, namely a living being – an autobiography is even more intimately so. And even if people don't have long biographies, they at least have stories and memories and reminiscences and obituary notices and so on, which show that they belong to the whole stream of civilization and culture in their own particular way. We must recognize that individuals are living exemplars of a cultured and civilized and moral life and in that respect are World 3 objects having a message for humanity.

P: That is exactly what I intended to say, and I completely agree with you in your interpretation.

E: We can turn now to other aspects of the basis for our strong dualistic hypothesis. I want to mention just briefly that we have to assume that our self-conscious mind has some coherence with the neuronal operations of the brain, but we have furthermore to recognize that it is not in a passive relationship. It is an active relationship searching and also modifying the neuronal operations. So this is a very strong dualism and it separates completely our theory from any parallelistic views where the self-conscious mind is passive. That is the essence of the parallelistic hypothesis. All varieties of identity theories imply that the mind's conscious experiences have merely a passive relationship as a spin-off from the operations of the neural machinery, which themselves are self-sufficient. These operations give the whole motor performance, and in addition give all conscious experiences and memory retrievals. Thus on the parallelistic hypotheses the operations of the neural machinery provide a necessary and sufficient explanation of all human actions.

P: That is exactly what I tried to express when, with a feeling of despair, I said in Oxford in 1950 that I believe in the ghost in the machine. That is to say, I think that the self in a sense plays on the brain, as a pianist plays on a piano or as a driver plays on the controls of a car.

E: As a challenge, I will present a very brief summary or outline of the theory as I see it. Here it is. The self-conscious mind is actively engaged in reading out from the multitude of active centres at the highest level of brain activity, namely in the liaison brain. The self-conscious mind selects from these centres according to attention and interest and from moment to moment integrates its selection to give unity even to the most transient conscious experiences. Furthermore, the self-conscious mind acts upon these neural centres, modifying the dynamic spatio-temporal patterns of the neural events. Thus in agreement with Sperry (1969), it is postulated that the self-conscious mind exercises a superior interpretative and controlling role upon the neural events.

P: I think that is very good. The only place where perhaps one should seek to make it even stronger is where you speak of the liaison brain; namely, we could make it stronger by making clear that the liaison brain is, as it were, almost an object of choice of the self-conscious mind. That is to say, if a certain part of the brain is not available, the self-conscious mind will seek another part as substitute. I think that in view of the fact that after certain operations or injuries the liaison brain will, as far as we know, actually change its position, we should not look at the liaison brain as something which is physically given. Rather, we should see it as being something like the result of co-operation and interaction between the brain and the self. So I go even a little further than you in my interactionism, in that I look at the very location of the liaison brain as being the result of interaction between the brain and the self-conscious mind. But on other points I would agree with you fully.

E: Also relevant to this discussion there is an account of what happens in sleep and dreams in chapter E7. I can imagine that in normal waking life the self-conscious mind is all the time scanning and probing over all the modules of those parts of the brain that we may think are accessible to it or those parts of the brain which are of interest to it. I think in many ways it doesn't bother about the ordinary low level processing areas of the cerebral cortex where there is only one modality (as illustrated in chapter E1, Figs. 7 and 8) and where there are early stages of the assemblage into meaningful features. The modules of these areas would be permanently closed. These are of no interest to the self-conscious mind. The self-conscious mind wants to read out from, perhaps by choice, perhaps by experience, the cortical areas where there are events happening which are of interest to it, because you have to think it is always provoking interest by means of its attention. It isn't just taking anything that's happening in the brain, but it is selecting from the happenings according to choice or interest. I believe we must incorporate this into the theory.

Sleep is a natural, repeated unconsciousness that we do not even know the reason for. It's obviously related to our theme now because it is related to the self-conscious mind and the activity of the brain as described in chapter E7. We do know furthermore that dreaming is good for us. If subjects are wakened just at the beginning of a dream cycle which can be seen in the electroencephalogram and this is repeated for each dream cycle night after night, the subjects become quite psychotic in about 2 or 3 days. This strange, bizarre activity of the brain which does get read out by the self-conscious mind, has some salutary value for us perhaps because of the immense, intense operation of the brain during waking hours. There is some cleansing process, some discarding of the immense store of data which the brain gets each day, and so it comes out in dreams. I don't know how this relates to the read-out by the self-conscious mind. Is it necessary that it should have also this read-out or will it be enough if the neural events went on as if there were a dream, but not giving a dream?

P: What you have suggested almost involves the hypothesis that the dream has a healing function, and that this function consists of purging the memory of unneeded or unwanted memory material that has, so to speak, accumulated. I think that this idea could be used in a kind of anti-Freudian theory of dreams.

E: The only dreams we do remember the next day are the dreams which wake us up. We were awakened by the dream and experienced it in retrospect, in memory, having recalled the dream in all its bizarre character and then maybe we sleep again, and the next day we may recall it more or less. Of course, the way to recall a dream most effectively is, when you waken from it, to go over and over it, analysing it in detail and organizing it and relating it perhaps to other remembered events and so on. Then you may really recover and remember it. In this respect there is of course the remarkable story of Otto Loewi who in a dream got in a clear vision of how to do a fundamental experiment on the chemical transmission from the vagus nerve to the frog heart. He had been worrying about this problem, and in his dream saw the way to accomplish this experiment. He awakened the next morning realizing he had had a dream, and it was important, and could remember no details.

The next night, to be sure, he put a paper and pencil by his bed, and, as he anticipated, the dream came again to him, he wakened up, remembered the dream, and wrote up with pencil and paper what the dream was about. Next morning he remembered he had written it and anxiously grabbed the paper and looked at it, but alas couldn't interpret it at all. So the final solution was of course not to trust paper and pencil. On the third night he fully awakened himself and made a full plan of the experiment. The dream experiment was immediately carried out in his laboratory. It was successful and for this discovery Loewi was awarded the Nobel Prize in 1936, sharing it with Sir Henry Dale who many years later told me the full account of this sequence of the three dreams. Later in his life Loewi greatly simplified the story, eliminating the first two nights. The final erroneous legend was reported knowingly by Dale in his biography of Loewi in the Obituary notices of the Royal Society!

P: You have put in a very beautiful way how the self-conscious mind has in these cases to be very active indeed, in order to impress the dream on the memory. That is to say, the normal thing is obviously to forget a dream and the extraordinary thing is to remember or reconstruct the dream, and to do something to impress it on the memory. This again shows how active the self-conscious mind is, and in the partial consciousness of dreaming it is obviously very much less active.

One could perhaps even propose a biological conjecture why it is that we forget our dreams so easily and so quickly. It is because the self-conscious mind actively dismisses the dream as some kind of disturbance or chimera; as something which does not fit into the world of purposes which is described to the self-conscious mind by its theories about the world. From the fact that we cannot fit the dream into the world of wakefulness, we discover that it cannot be matched. It thus belongs to the many things made by us which we unsuccessfully try to match and therefore eliminate. I am of course speaking of ordinary people, not of neurotic people who may be very deeply disturbed by many of their dreams, especially if their attention is drawn to them.

Dialogue VII

10:45 a.m., 25 September 1974

P: We all have certain needs, and one of the strongest needs which concerns the self is that of integration: the need for the self to establish its genidentity (to use Kurt Lewin's term [1922]). An example of this is the constant turning back by Brenda Milner's subject HM to his past experiences because this provided the only point of integration for his self. This need for integration is no doubt one of the things which makes the self act on the brain. That is to say, the self has the drive or the need or the tendency to unify and bring together the various activities of the brain.

I would propose the following hypothesis concerning animal consciousness. Wherever we have both wakefulness and sleep and a periodic change between one and the other, there we also in fact have consciousness, possibly of a fairly low level; that is to say, without any trace of explicit memory; consciousness which is, so to speak, completely unconscious of self, but which has implicit memory. It also seems to me that if we give up parallelism, and give up with it, with respect to the human brain, looking for integration in the brain itself, then we will have to do something similar also for the animal brain.

E: I am of course prepared to agree with these concepts, Karl, that you have about the animal brain and consciousness. I would point out that, if we are going to give it on the input side from brain to some animal consciousness, then we have also to propose that there is a reverse action and that the animal consciousness is not some entity that has been evolved for no purpose except perhaps to give some kind of enjoyment or suffering to animals. Animal consciousness would then have a real biological survival value in that it would organize the performance of the whole animal and effectively control its reactions to situations. That means to say that just as with the self-consciousness of humans, we would have to think that the animal consciousness had both an input and an output.

P: This also bears on the problem of the possibility of two worlds interacting and on my historical description of Descartes's physical theory of action, the theory of push. (See my section 48.) I think it is very important to notice that there is also, dating from the same period as Descartes's theory, a similar theory of interaction within the mind – the theory of the association of ideas (see my section 52).

I have for many years held the following view in connection with the learning of something new, with the development of a new *skill*, or with the discovery of a new hypothesis: as long as the things to be learned or the hypotheses to be discovered (which shade into one another and are more or less the same) are new to us, we have to concentrate upon them and pay them full *conscious attention*. Take, for example, piano playing. Piano playing is actually a very good case, for here the development of a new skill in a way goes together with the development of new hypotheses as to how we should play. That is to say, one tries out various hypotheses: can it be done this way? No; but it can be done that way, and so on. We operate with both hypotheses and skill. My suggestion here is similar to, but not quite the same as, an hypothesis of Schrödinger's. (See my section 36.)

E: This is quite in line with my own thinking on the learning of movements and of how we learn a new movement which we have to take thought about. You express this as an hypothesis concerning how to play the piano, and you preprogram your movements. There are several circuits we now know about in this preprogramming of a movement as described in chapter E3, Figures E3 – 6 and 7. You go over in thought what you want to do and how you can do it, and this involves circuits going from the cerebral cortex to the hemispheres of the cerebellum and coming back again by the thalamus. It also involves circuits probably going to the basal ganglia. So not only are we involved in cerebral circuits, but we are involved in a great deal of subcortical activity where skills are organized; and eventually when the movement has been carried out, there are all kinds of feedback arrangements to control it and put it back onto the desired pattern. Of course when you carry out some action repeatedly, you gradually learn the whole correct sequence of muscular contractions and feedback and all of that. It can then become automatic. It no longer needs to be programmed in the way that was done originally. Perhaps in those cases you keep the program for the overall performance. For example, the pianist is no longer thinking of every little sequence of hand movements and the phrasing of each piano piece. He is getting a wider view, a more detached view of the whole artistic creativity of his performance now. And that is the way I think we learn high skills. We gradually relegate to the automatic level the carrying out of more simple performances, and keep ourselves, our consciousness, our self-conscious mind open for the more highly evolved, integrative, creative side of our actions.

P: I should like to make a remark about induction. The fact that we can learn by repetition has been misunderstood by some people, and has been used as an argument in favour of a theory of induction. But (as I say in my section 39) I think that learning by repetition means relegating something from consciousness to the subconscious or to memory and making it unproblematic (this means making it subjectively secure, but this is quite distinct from making it fit the world, or objectively true). As distinct from this, the problem of induction is the discovery of something new (of, for example, a new theory). That is done not by repetition but by making and matching. We produce a hypothesis from, so to speak, inside us, and we then try out the hypothesis—that is to say, we test it and try to falsify it, and in the event of that happening, we try to produce a new hypothesis, and so on. This making and matching process seems to operate very fast. It even operates in perception.

E: What I want to talk about now is how we can lay down a memory trace or what happens when we are recalling some event into conscious experience once more—that is the sequence from a consciously experienced event through some storage process to the eventual recovery again. We'll consider some simple but unique perceptual experience.

Let us take a most simple example. You suddenly have seen the use of a new word that you never had used before and you would like to use it, say the words "paradigm" or "algorism" or "phoneme". Now the first thing is that it comes to consciousness, being read out by the self-conscious mind. At that level it is held in memory by verbal repetition for as long as you want it to go on as described in chapter E8. You could use the word in one way or another and keep going on with it and playing with it. While you are doing that, you have what is called short-term memory of the usage of this word. You can do the same with a telephone number you want to remember. You keep on rehearsing it. This is verbal rehearsal. But it could be a picture that you've just seen. While that activity is going on, there is no need to think of more than a continual neuronal machine of great complexity carrying in its spatio-temporal operations the memory which can be read out at any moment by the self-conscious mind in the usual manner of the first experience. That is to say, this is a continual experience of the same kind as the initial one. This seems to be all that happens. For example, we know this very well in cases of total hippocampectomy, when the whole hippocampus has been removed on both sides, the patients have no more than this brief verbal recall, a few seconds of memory (chapter E8). The interesting finding is that they lose the memory as soon as their attention is distracted. As soon as this continuous verbal recall operation is switched to some other neuronal pattern, it cannot be recovered.

In ordinary life how much do we carry in our verbal rehearsal and our pictorial rehearsal operations in our brain! That's my first point. There are other levels of memory, but in the light of this hippocampal story, we have to consider that if anything longer than that is to be recalled, the hippocampus has to be brought into the operation. It has been shown that on the left side, hippocampectomy results in a failure of verbal recall. The time course of the loss has been plotted on subjects, and by about 20 sec. you get failure (chapter E6).

P: May I just ask: you say verbal recall, but that means, I suppose, that verbal facility or verbal skill is not affected. Or is verbal skill affected? That is to say, is the Broca area affected?

E: No. These subjects can use language in accordance with their old memory store. There's no problem there. The defect is not in the use or interpretation of language. The defect is only in their consolidation of new verbal experiences. The subjects are in fact given a sequence of numbers or words to remember and this has gone in 20 sec. The rate of this loss even can be graphically plotted.

P: I would like to mention something else. It is to do with how we impress things on our memory. I may perhaps mention an experience of my own, about telephone numbers. I try to remember telephone numbers with the help of diagrams. There is, for example, one number I often want to recall—the telephone number of my sister. In my sister's telephone number there occur the figures 35—37—02. Now I had a certain difficulty in remembering whether it was 35—37—02 or 37—35—02, so I impressed it into my memory with the help of a diagram which has the shape of a pointed roof—it indicates that you start from a small thing then go to a big thing and then go back to something small:

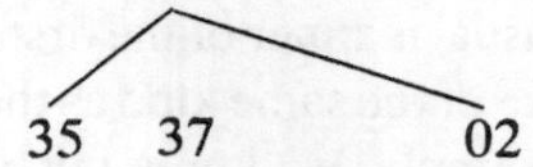

This diagram has helped me to distinguish between 37−35−02 and 35−37−02. This is just one example, but I do think that the use of such diagrams is a very characteristic mnemonic device, and also characteristic for theory construction. Jack, you yourself said that in thinking about theories, you work out a diagram. And this, I think, was just such a diagram. In other words, there is a very similar mental operation involved in trying to impress something new on your mind and in trying to find something new.

E: This is of course quite true. All the time this is what your self-conscious mind is doing. The self-conscious mind isn't passive, it's active. The important message I've got through to myself in the last few days is to take full account of the activity of the self-conscious mind on the brain, not just in some voluntary action but in the ordinary, moment-to-moment operations going through the whole of our lives where thought leads to other thoughts, and where memories are recalled and replayed in our mental life and so on—recalling and remembering and acting and developing. All that is very important.

P: What you said about action reminded me of the gondola kitten. It is, as it were, a schematic symbol for me of the significance of activity in all learning processes and in all conscious processes.

E: Now to return to the hippocampus. It is an extraordinary hypothesis in a way that we have to think of the hippocampus being brought in so early and so effectively, so that even after a very few seconds it helps us to recall a memory. This is shown of course by the lesional work I mentioned (cp. chapter E8).

I think we should propose that the self-conscious mind acts upon the open modules of the neocortex because it is enough for us to think that in these special places in the brain and under special circumstances World 1 is open to World 2 (chapter E7). We don't want it to be opening up everywhere! I think that an economy is required. In the first place, we have to think of the minimum zones for opening and see if we can explain all the phenomena in that manner. My first conjecture is that we can.

P: This is a very important point of method, and it can be formulated in this way: so far as parallelism *can* be achieved, we should try to get parallelism between mind and matter; only it breaks down somewhere, and interaction has to come in. Of course, we should at first operate with a kind of minimum interaction.

Here I should perhaps also mention, tentatively, an idea I had many years ago, namely, that conditioned reflexes really don't exist. What Pavlov called the conditioned reflex is the hypothesis-making of the dog. (See my section 40.) I think that the idea of conditioned reflex goes back to Lockean association psychology. In other words, the conditioned reflex was intended as the physiological side of association. But I think that association psychology is completely mistaken, and therefore that one should give up talking about conditioned reflexes.

E: Well, let's not be too dogmatic about this because the conditioned reflex is of course a misnomer. I readily agree, and furthermore, the investigative experimental work shows that it does normally involve cortical action, and so it is in fact an extremely complicated series of events. The mistake was to give it the name reflex in the first place. It's not a reflex at all. Sherrington would never believe it was a reflex. He thought that it was the whole complicated behavioural pattern of the dog and that it was learned experience with, as you say, anticipation and memory built into it. It's had an unfortunate result in being called a reflex, namely that it has given rise I think to a very limiting behaviourism. A behaviouristic attitude to man and animals is all the time thinking in terms of an absurdly simple reflex performance with stimulus-response and then with operant conditioning coming in with its caricature of how the nervous system works.

P: This is so, and it's not only the word "reflex" that is a caricature, but also the word "conditioned". My theory is that we do not condition anything at all from the outside, but we challenge the brain to produce from the inside, so to speak, expectations, or hypotheses, or theories, and then they are tried out. Of course, if these expectations are tried out and operate well, they will, as we have mentioned before, sink into the unconscious part of the brain, into the lower level, by repetition, and will operate more or less automatically. So both words "conditioned" *and* "reflex" are actually misnomers and together they lead to the behaviourist approach, which I regard as totally mistaken.

E: I agree with these criticisms. I think we cannot overestimate the transactional relationship across the interface between the liaison brain and the self-conscious mind (cp. chapters E7, E8).

Now I next ask how do we retrieve memories? I think that is indeed a very important functional activity of the self-conscious mind. I believe that in this retrieving the self-conscious mind is continuously searching to recover memories of words, phrases, pictures by an action which is not just a mere scanning over the modular array, but it is probing into the modular array in order to evoke responses from it and in order to try to discover the preferred modules, the ones which are related to the memory by their patterned organization. In that way the self-conscious mind is, as it were, taking a very active role in recovering memories which it regards as being desirable at that time. It is I think all the time scanning over the cerebral liaison areas by a trial and error process. We are all familiar with the ease and difficulty of recall of one or another memory, and we have many tricks about it. Some come always easily, we can always get some word or phrase; others are more difficult, and these are all problems for the self-conscious mind and a continuous challenge for it in order to recall the desired memory by this scanning and probing operation on the modular patterns. I think this is something which is tremendously important in the whole of our cultural performance.

P: May I just add something perhaps rather trivial about culture and memory. Very often we remember only that we have read something in a book, that the book is located in a certain place, and how to find it in the book. There is a give and take between brain-stored culture and the external World 3 culture, and it useful to develop the technique of putting as much as possible into the external World 3.[1] That is why we are taking notes and why we have a tape recorder. There is also a further point. Namely, that if we are ourselves active and producing something, then it is quite insufficient just to work it out in our minds: although this is a very important stage, it is insufficient. We have to write our ideas down, and by writing them down we typically find problems which we had previously overlooked and which we can then think about. In other words, the activity of the self-conscious mind relative to a sheet of paper and a pencil has a definite similarity to the activity of the self-conscious mind relative to the brain. And both involve a kind of trial and error operation.

E: In our scholarly life we would be completely defeated if all that we could use was what we had remembered and had nothing written down. Of course, there was a stage when this was so and very little was written. I suppose Socrates never wrote anything, but Socrates was fortunate in having a lot of

[1] Cp. Auguste Forel's (autobiographical) remark: "What we can put on our shelves we should not put into our brains."

people around him whom he could probe for memories. There was an atmosphere of cultured discussion and inquiry and argument with questions and problems being raised and answered and criticized. This can be done up to a certain level with very favourable conditions without committing it all to the written mode; but then Plato and others came along of course and wrote it down. It is exactly the same with the New Testament. Nothing was written at the time; it was written from memory many years later for us all to read. Some of the greatest periods of human creativity at the highest levels didn't have the advantage of books, but I don't want to discredit books, not even for a moment! I believe that we are now at levels of complexity of knowledge that have far outgrown anything that could be handled in the old schools of disputation. Furthermore, I think that we have become sophisticated in writing so that we can now be more self-critical and critical of others in terms of original expressions and ideas than we can in the spoken form. So I have learned quite a lot myself from writing my thoughts down or by diagramming them.

P: Let us consider the retrieval problem. I do think that, if we want to retrieve, let us say, a name or a word or something like that from our memory store, then we have a kind of diagrammatic representation of the thing we wish to find before we really go into the storage, as it were, and try to find it. I think that there is something very important and very interesting about the process of retrieval, namely, that we try out and reject various solutions to our problems. We somehow compare what we come up with with our vaguely conceived aim and say: No, No, it isn't this; but when we really find it, then we are usually quite certain that we have reached what we were looking for. But sometimes an intermediate stage is reached. That is to say, sometimes we get to a name and say: Oh, Yes, Yes, it could be this; but apparently it is only something very much like it, and we later may reach the complete assurance of having really got to what we were looking for, which was a bit different from the intermediate thing. So here we operate, so to speak, with a diagrammatic idea of an aim; with a certain point in a diagram which we can reach, which we can come nearer to, or be further removed from; and with the help of this diagram we can say whether or not our aim has been reached.

E: Another problem arises when we consider if there are memories not retrievable in the ordinary manner by the scanning technique of the self-conscious mind that we deliberately can instigate for recall. Is there a great memory storage that is not so recoverable at will? I think there is evidence that these memories can be recalled under special conditions, and we have of course the example of Penfield's stimulation of the temporal lobe (cp. Fig. 10 of chapter E8).

P: Quite apart from Penfield's experiments, I suggest that a great deal which is stored but not retrievable actually consists of skills and ways of doing things. This may even include recapturing certain emotive overtones which certain situations have for us – say, reciting. On the other hand, certain smells may have certain emotive overtones, and this is something which can hardly be retrieved at will; something which is not open to retrieval, but which nevertheless does exist.

E: I agree of course that memories can be stored as skills. When you have thoroughly learnt some action, some performance, in games or in music or in dance, then you can enjoy the overall effects and not be bothered with the detailed controls which run in the subconscious manner by all kinds of circuits that we know about in principle. I think one of the delightful things about our control of movement is that we can learn to do this subconsciously and automatically and with beauty and style and skill. We can greatly enjoy watching our performance which is often better than we thought we could do! This is one of the joys of life. Young children have it very early in all of their play and games and of course young animals give you the feeling that they have the same enjoyment in play. In all learning we have to use the self-conscious mind in the earlier stages, but later we can graduate to the level of an automatic performance. I think that the same thing can happen at other levels of conscious experience. For example on the sensory-perceptual level we can learn a great many skills of synthesis so that we can get some kind of holistic or *Gestalt* impression which originally had to be built up from piecemeal components; but now we can take one glance and the whole of this synthesis is given to us by some deep-down, learned skill. I am sure we are not born with this global memory of our pictorial imagery. Similarly with music we can imagine the learned skills where you have to try to understand the sequences in melody and the notes in harmony and all of the phrasing and so on at higher and higher levels. This is all part of the learning process. In the end you can enjoy the whole ensemble, or can listen to any instrumental piece you wish, picking it out at will, then blending it all into some lovely aesthetic appreciation. In fact, I think all aesthetic appreciation comes to us in this way. It has to be learned in bits and gradually with more and more skills we can attain to synthesis with transcendent levels of enjoyment. So this automatic synthesis happens both on the motor side and on the sensory side, and I think it happens at a still higher level in the imagination, where there are the levels of creativity, creativity of thought and of idea and so on. This is again the life of World 2 in relationship to World 3.

P: I still would like to hear more about memory—especially about the various distinctions with respect to memory, like the memory of skills and the memory of knowledge, and how explicit and implicit memory are related to these two distinctions. If short-term retrieval is not, as you say, related to the hippocampus, then it is likely that the physiology of, say, implicit memory, of long-term memory, and of skills will be differently located. For example, speaking skill (I mean the knowledge of how to speak, not the knowledge of what to say) is apparently located in the Broca area.

E: Possibly quite other processes are concerned for learnt motor skills as distinct from the retrieval of sensory experiences, perceptions, and ideas (cp. chapter E8). I am sure that we need a great deal more investigation on possible differences as with motor and sensory memory. I wonder, too, whether the attempt to store in memory all the stages of some logical argument or of some mathematical proof requires the hippocampus at all. I don't think that this has been tested. The hippocampal learning process is concerned with the recall of ordinary day to day events, what have you just been saying, what have you done, how did you get here, what happened yesterday, and all those sort of things in the ordinary life performance.

P: I would like to make a remark about the problem of the unity of the self-conscious mind and parallelism, namely, that we should not expect to find too much of a parallelistic basis for that unity in the brain. That is to say, we might go so far as to say that the self-conscious mind appears to concentrate on one half of the brain for achieving its particular unity. How far is it able, especially in childhood, to choose, as it were, the part of the brain, left or right, on which it will ultimately concentrate for self-conscious unity? This is a very interesting question. How far is this physiological and how far is it actually psychological? That is to say, how far does activity play a role?

E: I think you've raised a transcendent problem. It's one that's teasing me all the time. Firstly I had to make the break from the position where I assumed that the unity of all experiences was built in the nervous system, and was read out more or less passively as a unity by the self-conscious mind. Then came the new concept that the nervous system works in all its multiple disparity of widely dispersed modular activity over an immense area of the liaison brain, and that all its diversity is read out and unified in some transcendent process by the self-conscious mind. This is quite a staggering hypothesis. My mind reels at the thought of it! We've never conceived of this wide diversity of operation of the self-conscious mind upon all of this pattern of World 1 events involving hundreds of thousands of independent units. The self-conscious mind is probing on to that great diversity and synthesizing it and making it into a unity from moment to moment. This is happening within fractions of seconds as our self-conscious mind plays over our brain activities making our world picture from moment to moment in consciousness. We are now beyond any process that could have some physical basis in World 1, and this is why we have to introduce something quite other, namely the self-conscious mind in World 2. This is where this idea of interaction will meet with such incredulity from people who are used to living flat-footed on World 1! How can they school themselves at all to accept the kind of ideas that we are now developing for the actual way in which we receive consciousness and in which the self-conscious mind plays and interplays over the cerebral cortices.

I would suggest, that the self-conscious mind is scanning all kinds of modules. It is scanning everywhere and it finds that it can communicate with only some modules, both in giving to and in receiving from. These are the open modules. The closed modules it can just pass over, just like a bee finding flowers that have nothing, and it just flies by to the others. You don't have to think that there is any blockage of activity in closed modules. It is just that there is no reaction to the self-conscious mind, nothing coming back, and therefore nothing given to these closed modules. The self-conscious mind treats such modules just like any other bit of World 1. It is only in liaison to the very special open modules and then only during special states of these modules. This idea has been suggested above in relation to sleep. When you're in a deep sleep, the self-conscious mind is scanning and finding no reacting modules at all. That is when you are unconscious. Then some modules will come to react a bit, developing some coherent activity. That gives a dream read out by the self-conscious mind. You know we can have great fun in playing with imagination on these new ideas!

P: I think that that brought out very well what I was trying to suggest. There is still of course a great problem, namely, how much is physically predetermined—obviously there is quite a lot that is genetically predetermined in the difference between the dominant and the minor hemisphere. That is obvious, because otherwise it would be a 50:50 affair rather than a 90:10 affair. Nevertheless, it is not fully predetermined, as we know from cases of lesions, and it apparently demands the cooperation of the self-conscious mind to bring out fully the dominance of the left side of the brain.

I would also like to make some remarks on the various aspects of memory. First of all, there is a spectrum which has as its extremes explicit and implicit memory. Secondly, there are distinctions according to the way in which memory was acquired. Here I want to mention three points. (1) Memory acquired by a learning process starting from a problem which leads to a trial and error method of discovering a solution; the discovered solution; and then the practical repetition which leads to a skill. (2) A learning process which does not start from a conscious solution, such as when the problem took only the form of a vague irritation. (3) Memory due to a process that recalls our actions and active choices in an unconscious manner and thus forms our personality. (See also my section 41.)

Dialogue VIII

10:40 a.m., 26 September 1974

P: In my sections 48 – 56 I have given a history of the body-mind problem since Descartes and especially of the steps which led to parallelism – the parallelism of Geulincx, of Malebranche, of Spinoza, and of Leibniz. I have tried to show that the emergence of parallelism is almost completely based on the view that we have a valid theory of causation in World 1 – that bodies behave just as if pushing each other and so causing one another to move (which is the Cartesian theory of causation). There was also a theory of causation in World 2, namely that one idea is associated with another and therefore that the recalling of one idea, a, brings about as a sequel the appearance in the consciousness of the idea, b. *So there are two simple theories of causation, one for World 1 and one for World 2*; and given these theories it appears to be completely ununderstandable that World 1 and World 2 can interact. This apparent impossibility of interaction leads to the parallelism of Geulincx, Malebranche, Spinoza and Leibniz.

I have criticized this kind of justification of parallelism by pointing out that the theories of causation on which it is based have been completely superseded, and that we have, within physics, a pluralism of different kinds of causes, namely of forces (at least four different kinds of forces), and that within World 2 or the subjective mind, we also have theories which are totally different from the theory of association. I have, especially, attacked the theory of conditioned reflex which is the brain analogue of Locke's theory of association. The theory of association does not even hold in a case which is, as it were, pure memory; namely, the case of memory recall. For in the case of memory recall, far from just waiting for the working of the association of ideas, we are intensely active, operating with all sorts of means to get the key to open the door, as it were, of that particular part of the memory in which we are interested. Dynamic elements in our thought and in our thought processes are also not associationist. Something like association does of course exist, but it does not play the role of an elementary mechanism which the association theorists attributed to it. And, especially, it is uncharacteristic of the mind, because associationism has a kind of "passive spectator" aspect with respect to the mind while in fact almost all the time we are conscious the mind is active—it searches actively, trying to operate with models, with diagrams, and with schemata, and it is constantly making and remaking and changing, and trying out, again and again, the adequacy of its constructions. Thus both the theory of causality in the physical World 1 and the theory of causality in the psychological World 2 on which parallelism was based are completely unacceptable today.

This, of course, does not mean that parallelism is refuted. It only means that the *a priori* arguments—which looked like *a posteriori* arguments—on which parallelism was based, are invalid. But parallelism in itself may pose simply as a conjecture about the relationship between body and mind, and it may still be a valid conjecture even though the arguments leading to it have been refuted. I think we should today make an attempt to criticize parallelism not from the point of view of whether it is demonstrable or can be justified by deductive arguments, but from the point of view of whether its *consequences* are acceptable. In other words, we should try to criticize parallelism not as a *conclusion* but rather as a *premise*—as an hypothesis from which certain consequences follow.

E: Karl, I like that very much. I like particularly the way in which you stress the active relationship of the self-conscious mind to the brain and therefore criticize the passivity that is implied in parallelism. I myself believe that that is the principal trouble with parallelism. It fails in this essential manner, and I can instance several examples from the way we think of the brain-mind problem. In the first place, it isn't just in voluntary action that we have to think of the self-conscious mind working upon the brain. This is of course the most overt of all examples of mind acting upon matter or thought bringing about action. We have dealt with that in another dialogue and in chapter E3. But it is, as you say, that we are all the time trying to recover memories, to develop ideas, to play, as it were, with our concepts and play with our theories and to imagine actively. In this way we go far beyond the data presented in our sensory experiences, acting with interpretation and with judgment and with criticism. All of this involves an active side to the mental processes or the self-conscious mind; and it is quite clear that we have to think of this activity as being exerted upon brain events and changing them in order to bring about the desired effects. For example, to recover the memory that is under interest at the moment, we have to probe and try all manner of strategies. I think it is a tremendously complex active process by which the self-conscious mind works upon the immensity of neural actions going on in the cerebral cortex and selects from them in a very specific way—in a way which certainly is not automatic. We have developed wonderful skills in our handling by our mental processes of the events in the brain to which they are related, so that they can bring about the desired readouts from the cerebral events and modify the readouts and so on. That is the principal point I would make about the way in which parallelism fails completely to account for the phenomena of experience.

Now, a second failure of parallelism is to my mind somewhat related to the first, but it is simpler to express. It concerns the unity of conscious experience that we have from moment to moment. Attention flits from one thing to another. At any moment we are oriented with special relationship to an element of the perceptual world, ignoring an enormous amount of what is pouring in by our sense organs. Then we can flit over to some other feature of interest in a moment and so on. Now this operation of our self-conscious mind giving this unity from moment to moment seems to be quite an outstanding performance. It never has been possible in neurophysiological theory to develop any plausible explanation of how unity can be created out of the immense diversity. It is beyond comprehension how immense is this diversity of the neuronal events. How can this diversity be unified in experience? We don't know any neurophysiological means except for feature recognition neurones, which give but small fragments of a perceived picture. There has to be some overall scanning mechanism such as we postulate for the self-conscious mind in order to give us that unity. There is nothing in the material description of the brain actions which at all accounts for this. I reject, as we've said already, the *Gestalt* theory about fields or the micro-potential field theory of Pribram (cp. chapter E7); because in these cases apparently you have to have an homunculus to read out the picture! You have lost the essential materialist purity of parallelism by inserting an homunculus as an active agent. In our theory of dualism the self-conscious mind accomplishes this incredible, unimaginable performance in its relationship with the cerebral events as described in chapter E7. That it does so is evidenced by the unity of experience from moment to moment. We cannot account for this integration by any material theory of the nervous system, and therefore the parallelistic theory fails because it cannot give us the experienced unity.

P: I agree that it is this activity of the mind which is incompatible with parallelism with a physicalist emphasis—a parallelism which stresses the physical mechanism of the brain.

What I should like to say to start with is that we should try to give parallelism its due. I would say that there are cases where there is a direct dependence of the experiences of the self-conscious mind on what is delivered to it by the physical brain. This, I think, would especially be the case for *optical illusions.* It is very interesting that we cannot get rid of a typical illusion *qua* optical experience even if we are quite sure that it is an illusion and we actively try to see the thing in its non-illusional significance. Consider, for example, the Müller-Lyer illusion.[1] We can measure how far we are out and can see how we measure it, but we will still be unable, even with all that knowledge and all that conscious interpretation in our minds, really to get rid of the impression, the visual experience, which is delivered to us by our brain. That is to say, dualism can in this case be actually experienced: I mean, on the one hand, the dependence and inactivity of the perception, the visual experience; its dependence on higher (but nevertheless, compared to the ultimate interpretation, lower) brain functions; and on the other hand our knowledge that this experience is not to be trusted. (One might be tempted to explain this "dualism" as one between two mechanisms of decoding or interpreting; however, we do not feel a double personality while we take note of this dualism.)

This puts the active aspect of the mind in a very interesting light. We can see here that we may experience the passivity of the mind, and *therefore* the dependence of the mind on the brain. So we may describe this optical illusion as really, so to speak, an epiphenomenalistic experience, and we can contrast our experience of such illusions with our activistic experiences and see how different they are and how little parallelism can take account of this difference.[2]

E: The optical illusion story that you mentioned is a very interesting and important one. The fact is of course that we are not saying as dualists that the self-conscious mind cannot rise superior to what is going on in the brain.

---

[1] Müller-Lyer illusion. The vertical lines are the same length. (Compare also the Figures in my section 18, pp. 63–65, above.)

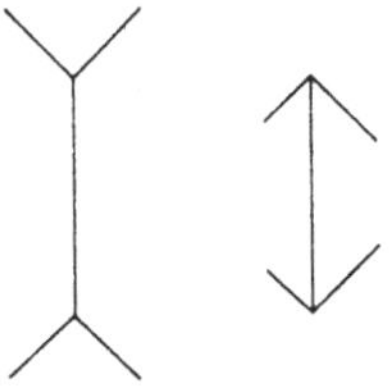

[2] J. J. C. Smart [1959] has made out an excellent case for his identity theory by referring to a weak after-image. In this case, there is really no urgent reason to deny that some brain event is experienced (so that the brain event and the experience are parallel – and I do not much object even to his claim that they are perhaps identical). But far more typical and important are examples which, rather, fit the opposite case: the case of dualistic interaction.

P: Yes. But sometimes it doesn't!

E: The self-conscious mind is always as it were working backwards and forwards, and we could even say that in all of its perceptual processes it is moulding or modifying the modular activities in the brain in order to get back from them what it wants. This is a deliberate control one might say of cerebral events. That makes it quite distinct from parallelism. It will get back from them what they are at that moment reporting, but it will be deviating it all the time into another mode and searching for experiences that are more in tune with what its interests are at that time.

But I want to go further into this illusion story. Some illusions are created as we now know in principle by the processing of information at various stages in the cerebral cortex. For example you can so explain the Mach phenomena, the Müller-Lyer illusions, and the after-images. You have to remember that all the time we are making good use of illusions. For example, parallax due to the difference between images in the two eyes is transmitted selectively to the modules of the visual cortex (Fig. E2 – 7) and is interpreted to give us depth perception. There is a fusion of two different pictures into a picture of another kind with depth. When we have that ability, it can also be made the theme of most beautiful and exciting demonstrations. I can instance those random dot stereograms that are designed by Bela Julesz [1971] and that show incredible illusions in three dimensional experience.

Here again there is the active intervention of the self-conscious mind upon the brain events. I believe there are a lot of illusions in which we can do that. Of course there are some illusions that you know to be an illusion, yet you cannot voluntarily modify them. Presumably this is so because the self-conscious mind is very weak in its influence on the brain, as has been proposed in chapters E3 and E7. Thus there are severe limitations to its effectiveness. It also takes time and with the more subtle and perplexing inputs to the brain, like the one I have just mentioned, it takes a very long time.

Thus it is shown that the relationship between the mind and the brain is not something instantaneous and automatic as in parallelistic theory. It involves a whole process of slow and gradual modification and of sculpturing, you might say, with backwards and forwards interaction. I think this has got to be recognized and with that recognition there is a rejection of parallelism.

P: The question you have raised concerning the comparatively weak action of the mind on the brain can be explained biologically. That is to say, there are two kinds of illusions – illusions delivered to us or imposed upon us by the brain, and illusions which have a mental origin like, let us say, wish-fulfilment. It is apparently built into our organism and into the whole "mechanism of interaction" between the brain and the mind that the mind should be in very many respects dependent on the brain, in order not to fall too easily into that kind of illusion which we experience in fantasy.

I would say that this whole field can be used to show at the same time a kind of gulf and also a kind of dependence between the self-conscious mind and the brain. The main point here that shows the gulf is that we can be highly critical of an optical illusion and yet nevertheless experience it. It is the self which is critical of the optical illusion. And it is a kind of lower level of the self which experiences it (cp. chapter E7, Fig. 2), in conformity with what the brain delivers to it. The question may be raised whether this kind of gulf or split between a critical apparatus and a non-critical part of the self may not be imitated by a computer. I think it probably can be. We could build a computer so that it critically revised its input, but if we did so, we would have in fact to distinguish sharply between *two parts* of the computer. It is this dualism which shows the point we are trying to make. There would have to be, in the computer, a kind of split between first-order results, and second-order results which are the result of a critical review of the first order results. It is this kind of split which we could build into a computer on the basis of our own criticism, using the difference between our own first-order results and their critical review as our model. Built into our brain itself there are, superimposed, several such hierarchies of controls, but nevertheless, the final result of the brain's activities can be distinguished from the self in the case of an illusion, in so far as we can assume that the illusion which we know to be an illusion but nevertheless see, can be taken to result from the interpretations of the decoding mechanism of the brain. It may well be a parallelistic effect. It can be clearly distinguished from our active critical attitude towards it. This, I think, has no complete physical basis. It may, of course, have some basis in the brain, but I do not think that it can be fully reduced to the sifting mechanisms of the brain. So far as I know, these things have never been discussed. Psychologists have been very interested in optical illusions, but I don't think that they have ever discussed the hierarchical structure arising from the fact that there can be a self which observes the optical illusion and which is critically aware of the fact that it "has" an illusion, and which can critically discuss the illusion as such.

I should now like to refer to the Necker cube. (See note 1 to my section 24.) The very interesting thing is that up to a point we can make the Necker cube submit to our will, as it were, and switch, when we want to switch it, to one side; and switch, when we want to switch it, to the other side. (See also my section 18.) If we can see one of the two inside corners of the cube as being in front, this brings the switch about, and one can learn to bring the switch about in this way. I suggest that we might try to train ourselves and then make an experiment like the one with the movement with the finger; that is to say, to discover whether we can find that the efforts needed to change the interpretation can be neurologically recognized. Of course, we would need a trained subject who has the thing in his grip, otherwise a subject would experience involuntary switches from one interpretation to the other.

E: I agree with the necessity for a highly trained subject. That is necessary even for the much simpler task of moving the finger in Kornhuber's experiments (chapter E3). I have the feeling that parallelism gives us a very uninteresting and flat explanation of experience which not at all relates to the rich, vivid, controlling experience that each of us recognizes in ourselves. Parallelism fails completely in its explanatory effort to account for this, and what does it offer us instead? It offers us merely the belief that these neural events can somehow give rise to the experiences, but the experiences themselves have no way back to the brain. Operationally they are merely a spinoff. It's this passivity that defeats me. But a final criticism is this. It's such a simple criticism, and it's never mentioned by the parallelists, and it is this: there is on the parallelist view no biological reason whatsoever why the self-conscious mind should have evolved at all. If it can do nothing, what is the evolutionary meaning of it? After all, I think parallelists will agree that the self-conscious mind is in some incredible manner a result of evolution, so it has some survival value; yet it can only have survival value if it can do things. To have it in the role of a passive experience just for our enjoyment or for our suffering is an absurd notion biologically. We have to think that it was developed because of selection pressure, and so has survival value built into it. This does demand that the self-conscious mind is able to bring about changes in the brain and hence in the world. In its experiences it would have a controlling influence upon the brain, and hence on the organism, the hominid or the man who has it. This idea of effective control is contrary to the parallelistic view which in every version is dedicated to a purely passive relationship.

P: I agree with almost everything you have just said, except that it is implicitly answered by some parallelists with the theory of panpsychism. If you are an evolutionist and cannot attribute a special function to the mind (say, because you are a parallelist), then panpsychism may seem to offer a way out of the difficulty. Panpsychism is the theory that the ultimate nature of the world is dualistic; not, of course, interactionist-dualistic but parallelist-dualistic. On this view, consciousness need not be looked upon as something which has a special biological significance. Of course, panpsychism can be criticized for other reasons. (See my section 19.)

However, I completely agree with your biological argument, and I find it very significant. (In this context, we should mention Sherrington's book *Man on his Nature* [1940], pp. 273–5.)

I also think that in this context we could refer, as a criticism of association psychology, to Freud's so-called free association experiments. These experiments show in two ways that associationism is wrong. First of all, the experiments show that if you allow association to work, then the resulting flow of ideas is very different to what we may call the "normal" flow of ideas. The latter is much more purposeful and is partly directed by World 3 problems and purposes. And secondly, Freudian "free association" is of course not a free flow either, but, as Freud himself points out, is determined by something like *hidden* problems and purposes (by what Freud called a "complex"). All this suggests that association is not really the main or even a very important way of, let us say, forming, unifying, or organizing what has been called "the stream of consciousness"; that is to say, the way our subjective experiences are linked (or "causally connected").

Incidentally, this theory of *"the stream of consciousness"* is an idea which has had a very dubious effect on the theory of consciousness and also on novelists like James Joyce. Quite obviously, it results from a completely passivist way of looking at the mind. In dreams we are perhaps less active than in a state of full awareness and wakefulness; and perhaps there is something more or less like a "stream of consciousness" going on in dreams; though I doubt it. I think that the description "stream of consciousness", which I believe is due to William James, is a description of a very artificial situation: a description of the artificial situation created when we just watch ourselves and try to do nothing. Then, when we – actively – try to be passive, there may be something like a stream of consciousness; but normally we are active, and then there is nothing like a stream of consciousness but, rather, organized procedures of problem-solving.

E: I wanted now to make some comment with respect to that earlier statement of yours, Karl, about panpsychism being the only way out. I think that is quite correct. The only way out for the parallelists is to adopt panpsychism, and this has to be accepted all the way down through not only the biosphere but also in the material inorganic world. You can think of mineral souls and biological souls and human souls and so on! It is a completely silly idea I think, but it shows the poverty of parallelism. I regard the espousal of panpsychism as a most desperate effort to save the parallelist theory beyond all reason; and to my mind it is completely unacceptable. The alternative is to imagine that at some time during the evolutionary development of man, or animals shall we say, there came to be developed certain special structures in the brain which are open to World 2, that is where World 1 is not any more closed. This gives rise to immense and very worrying problems of course, but we have the problems anyway in one way or other, and the heroic way I think is to face up to the full immensity of the problem of thinking that the World 1 is open to World 2 in extremely special situations and that this openness was eventually discovered in the evolutionary process and exploited. This must have been done by the designing of what we can only regard as World 1 structures of transcendent sensitivity, with their dynamic poise, if you like, so that they were open now in a way which hitherto had not been possible. I think we wouldn't want to accept the idea that the physical world under all conditions is open all the way down. This is panpsychism – some version of it anyway. What we have to think is that at high levels of biological development central nervous systems were constructed which had these special properties. We can readily imagine what is involved in this because the performance of the nervous system of higher animals and, in particular, of man shows that something of quite a different order has entered in. In particular, of course, I want to stress that this is true of man where, with linguistic development and the growth of World 3, cultural evolution has taken over from biological evolution. All of this results from the fact that the World 1 structures in the brains of men had become open to World 2 interaction; and hence came about the ability of man in creating World 3 and in interacting with World 3. This is the story of man. I am sure that this is a story much more acceptable when looked at critically than the panpsychism story.

P: I would like to make the perhaps fairly obvious remark that it looks as if this process of becoming open to World 2 took place in stages. That is to say, there was at first probably very little openness and only in time more and more. That is really the reason why I think that one should not deny consciousness to animals even though, of course, self-consciousness does not seem to be within the scope of animals.

E: We are now back on the question of animal consciousness and I can only reiterate my agnostic view. The problem that I am particularly interested in concerns the growth of self-consciousness, and how self-consciousness came to man at some early hominid stage back in the Australopithecines when they were creating simple pebble tools and making the first tentative steps into

World 3; but World 3 developed ever so slowly with technical and art discoveries and no doubt linguistic counterparts of this. This development continued through the era of hominid man to the Homo Erectus stage and so through the whole Paleolithic era. This is the most wonderful creative story whereby from World 3 came World 2, the self-consciousness of man. We would conjecture the dawning of self-consciousness that was due to brains developing some new properties related to language. Maybe the coming of consciousness is foreshadowed in the brains of higher mammals. Yet it is important to realize that we cannot as yet point to some special structures. In the best electron-microscope studies that have yet been made, there are no special structures in man's brain matching speech development, in contrast say to the anthropoid ape brain (cp. chapter E4). This is where we are at the present time. I have no doubt that, with still more refined methods, there will be found special properties of the brain, particularly in those areas specialized for speech, the planum temporale and Brodmann areas 39 and 40 as described in chapter E4. Yet we are not yet able to know what detailed structures to look for. We still lack the imaginative understanding of the degrees of functional refinement that are exhibited by the open modules at these high levels of development of the wonderful human cerebral cortex.

P: We do not seem likely to agree on the question of animal consciousness. About the question of self-consciousness and on the fact that it seems only to appear with man I think we do agree. I think I can now show better what I mean about the lower forms of consciousness and higher forms of consciousness, again with the help of optical illusions. An optical illusion itself is, of course, a conscious experience, but it does not belong to the highest and most critical part of our consciousness, because we can be well aware that it is an illusion and yet, as it were, we can't get rid of it. Now I think it is possible to make a quite fair conjecture that under certain circumstances animals also suffer from optical illusions, but that we can be pretty sure that animals cannot be critical of their optical illusions. Here, I think, we get both animal consciousness and a lack of self-consciousness.

I would also like to mention something in connection with eidetic memory. There we may really again be faced with one of those effects which have a parallelistic look about them. Just as we said before that illusions have a parallelistic look, so eidetic memory seems to have a parallelistic look. And characteristically it is not the normal functioning of the brain to have eidetic memory. One could also put it like this: the associationist model is really one of association between eidetic ideas, and this is not a realistic description of memory at all.

E: Eidetic memory carries some remarkable problems deriving from this very accurate readout by memory of past experiences. It carries more accuracy than we usually are associating with the recovery of memory, but I think it is still all accountable to special brain events of a very selective, highly sensitive kind. That is to say, if it isn't this, what is it? It must be that in the brain there is a much more reliable and rigorous recovery of the spatio-temporal patterns that match those of the remembered experience. I think no explanation can overlook that. The only point we then make is that this brain performance can be read out by the self-conscious mind. Eidetic memory is no problem I think for dualism. Rather it is a problem for the cerebral machinery to perform this very accurate repetition of patterned performance.

P: I believe that there *is* a problem for an interactionist or dualist here. What I mean is that we ought actually to be on the look-out for experiences which seem to be parallelistic in character, as opposed to normal experiences which are so clearly non-parallelistic, because it is in this way that we really bring out the character of non-parallelism much more clearly. The eidetic memory seems, from all I have read about it, to be much more passive than the normal memory. I don't mean the original first impression on the memory. I don't know whether this is more active or more passive. But the recall seems to be something in which the self is really very much more a spectator than the actor that it is in normal memory processes. Anyway, even if this particular interpretation is incorrect, I think we should be on the look-out for parallelisms (in the plural) – I think that there are several different sorts of parallelism. However, the important thing for our present discussion is that interactionist dualism is compatible with the existence of parallelistic cases but any parallelistic theory of the body-mind problem is incompatible with the existence of interactionist cases. Thus, for our problem the existence of interactionist cases is the important thing.

E: I agree that the eidetic memory is much more passive. It's as if the subject is scanning some recovered visual field and able to read out from it. Now this is interesting because it shows that the self-conscious mind is able to recover so completely the original experience.

Dialogue IX

4:15 p.m., 27 September 1974

E: We may open with a discussion on illusions because I believe that there is a great range of phenomena that are interpretable in terms of new ideas on the interaction of the self-conscious mind with the brain. It occurs to me that this is particularly well exhibited by the unity of experience in looking at one of the ambiguous figures. For example, I refer to the figure on p. 276 of Sherrington's book, *Man on His Nature,* where you have a drawing that can be interpreted either as a staircase or as an overhanging cornice. (See note 1, below.) What we notice when we look at this is that it is quite a unitary experience. We hold it in one interpretation for the moment, that is the self-conscious mind assembling the whole modular performance into a meaningful picture. Then at a time when a slight movement occurs, it will be transformed to an overhanging cornice. The point of great interest is that you cannot get a partial interpretation. It is globally one or the other and in the switch there may be a slight white-out as the new interpretation comes about. I would suggest that this is an example of the self-conscious mind interacting with the brain and reading out from it. Admittedly there are extensive brain patterns for the experienced interpretation, but to my mind the interesting thing is the global nature of the interpretation. The self-conscious mind is doing its usual job of trying to extract a meaning from the total cerebral performance that relates to its present interests.

P: There is no doubt that in this case, in the original learning, the self-conscious mind is engaged in interpreting the perspective figure, and that the experience of a cornice, especially, is essential to the establishment of the interpretation.[1] In other words, I don't think that an animal, or a very young

---

[1] Sherrington describes the figure on the next page as "a set of steps" which "suddenly

baby, or somebody who had never seen a cornice, would be able to interpret this figure.[2] So I agree that the self-conscious mind was involved in it. (Though it is not my contention that it is involved in all cases of perception or illusion – compare my remarks in dialogue VIII and dialogue X.) However, I suggest that the learning of the interpretation of perspective drawings has become so well-established in us that it has sunk from our psychology into the physiology of the brain, and that it is no longer really subject to our will and to our conscious interpretation. I, for example, can hold the picture in the staircase form for as long as I like, but not in the cornice form. From the cornice form it switches automatically over into the staircase form after a comparatively short interval. Even if I wish to hold it and to impose the cornice form onto the picture, the stairs will win in the end, and they do not spontaneously switch back into the cornice, while the cornice can only be held with a willed effort. I think that this shows, in one picture, both interaction and parallelism. (Compare also our discussion of the Müller-Lyer illusion in dialogue VIII.) That is to say, where we are dependent on our physiology, there I think we can speak of some sort of parallelistic effect, but where our will interferes, there is clearly interaction.

E: You have made I think, Karl, a good point there, but the point to me does suggest that the will is weak. The self-conscious mind is not a powerful operator upon the brain, it is an interpreter, attempting to get meaning out of it and gradually to modify it, as we know when we are actively searching for meaning, or searching for words, or causing actions. It is not power that distinguishes the mind-brain action, but the fact that we can operate it

---

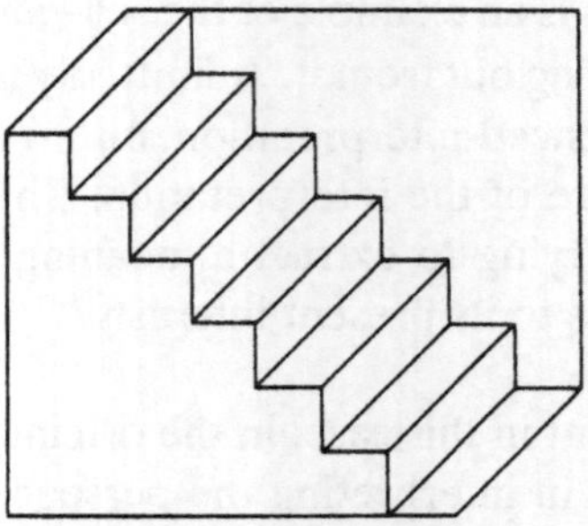

without warning becomes an overhanging cornice". See *Man on his Nature* [1940], p. 276; Penguin books edition, pp. 226f.

[2] This remark will have to be reconsidered in the light of an experiment of Tinbergen's with a kitten, reported in W. H. Thorpe [1974], pp. 134f.; see especially Figure 41. For the influence of World 3 on optical illusions, see R. Gregory [1966], pp. 160–2, and J. B. Deregowski [1973].

voluntarily by taking thought. I think that the point I want to make is that, even though there is a brain machine behind the whole of this interpretation, yet the interpretation itself in a meaningful manner as a staircase or as a cornice is an integrated achievement by the self-conscious mind.

P: The integration is an achievement of the mind; and actually a World 3 achievement. The reading of perspective drawings, like the invention of perspective itself, is a World 3 achievement, and I would say that it is one of the World 3 achievements which are partly encoded in the brain; and, if the encoding in the brain is effective, then this effect may *become* parallelistic, although it was first *established* by interaction.

E: Another point for discussion is depth perception and parallax. I think again we have no brain processes that give us the final clue in explaining the depth perception of a picture. We have of course the differential pictures coming from the two eyes and going by separate pathways to separate levels in the lateral geniculate nucleus (Fig. E2 – 7) and thence to adjacent modules in the visual cortex and eventually at a further stage converging on single cells in the visual cortex. After that the interpretation gets a little obscure, but at this level or a further level this disparity between the two images of the left and right eye is recognized by special neurones (disparity recognition cells) and eventually is subsumed in the higher perceptual synthesis of depth stereopsis, which is a global interpretation. It seems to come in a flash for the whole visual image through the self-conscious mind interacting with the brain. This of course leads on to what I was mentioning yesterday, the designs by Bela Julesz of random dot stereograms that provide all levels of challenge to stereopsis.

P: I think that it is important clearly to distinguish between the ego or the self on the one side, and the perception on the other side. This is just what is, for example, denied by Schrödinger on the last page of his *What is Life?*:[3]

> ". . . *What is this 'I'?*
> If you analyse it closely you will, I think, find that it is just a little bit more than a collection of single data (experiences and memories), namely the canvas *upon which* they are collected. And you will, on close introspection, find that what you really mean by 'I' is that ground-stuff upon which they are collected."

Now in my view the self is *not* just the canvas on which our perceptions are painted. I can struggle with a perception, as I do when I try to hold the cornice

[3] Cp. E. Schrödinger [1967], p. 96.

interpretation or the Necker cube and don't succeed. Here, in this case of a willed effort, there is quite obviously a real clash between the self and the perceiving apparatus. It seems to me that one may read off, from these cases, that the self sometimes has a hierarchical structure – that it is experienced as a hierarchy of controls of different heights or depths. Also, that there are different ways in which we may experience our selves. Thus, if I remember my struggling to "hold" a picture, then I am again only an observer of a past experience, but if I am actually struggling to "hold" the picture, then I am more myself than in any of the other cases of perceiving or remembering.

E: I have one other alternative to offer for what the self-conscious mind is doing when it is reading out from the brain performance the immensely varied patterns that are presented from moment to moment. Perhaps it is trying to secure a unified interpretation. That's another way of describing its actions. Some of the fascinating designs by Escher are constructed in order to defeat attempts at a unified interpretation.

P: I think that the term "unified interpretation" is very useful, and it covers the whole series of coherence, significance and meaning. They are all unified interpretations. That is to say, they are the results of efforts at unified interpretation.

E: This is a very important statement because it stresses the active role of the self-conscious mind rather than the purely parallelistic passive role, and we struggle for this unified interpretation all the time. There is tremendous pragmatic value in our efforts to interpret what the meaning or significance is of all the varied data pouring in through our senses.

P: That is precisely why I stressed the willed effort in holding the picture. It was an active attempt to impose a particular unified interpretation, a particular significance, on the picture; and there one can see, so to speak, the struggling, active self working – and failing because of the deeper impression made on the brain by our sensory experiences.

E: I would like to go on to a slightly different field now and that is the whole of colour interpretation. We of course derive our colour essentially from a three colour process with the appropriate cones with selective colour appreciation in the retina and these have independent transmitting lines. So it is a three-colour process that runs right through to the visual cortex. Now the interesting thing is that you find out that these are sorted into special areas.

Zeki has discovered that there are special areas to which the colour specific lines come, after many sequences of transmission. Then Sherrington noted that you do in fact blend the colours that are coming in by two eyes. If you have one eye green and one eye red in their fields, you get the bronze illusion from fusing the two retinal images.

It looks as if you have again modules activated in the special colour-sensing areas of the visual cortex, and these are read out by the self-conscious mind to give some colour which is a hue, a blend. It has all the subtleties of interpretation. In fact you can realize the interpretative character by the learning that is involved. There is a very active remembering, learning, assessing, and naming job by the self-conscious mind in all of its skills in colour perception. Then you have to think furthermore of all the subtleties of colour when it is blended into contrasts and shadows and so on.

P: I would like to raise the question of the validity or invalidity of Land's paper [1959], about which we had an argument before starting the recorded discussion. Why did I like Land's paper so much? Of course, I do not know whether what Land says is true; I haven't made the experiments. But I liked his paper so much because it falls in extremely well with the point of view we have developed here.

The interesting point is Land's thesis that two colours are enough to obtain the same result as is obtained from the standard three-colour process. The brain and the conscious self which interpret are so active that they replace, as it were, the missing colour. The decisive thing is that the experiments are not about abstract diagrams but about pictures of real-life situations. The pictures he uses are partly coloured in one colour, and partly in tones of grey, and what Land says is that we experience these pictures as if they were in full colour.

I must say that I don't really expect that his reports are faulty. If what he says is true, it would really not be surprising, from our point of view, that our experience and our learning or interpreting overshoot, as it were, in a full picture of, let us say, a landscape, a rose, and so on; that they overshoot the mark – in the sense of what is given – and aim at a full interpretation. I think that it is even possible that with Land's method – if his results are correct – one might obtain a situation similar to that of the staircase, so that we could switch from one interpretation of the colour to another interpretation of the colour. So that, for example, if red were given, that we might switch from yellow to blue and from blue back to yellow. This, of course, would have to be tried out, but certainly there is nothing in the theory of colour vision which would prevent it.

E: I have not seen the Land experiments. I have heard them described, and I always have the feeling that it has more or less all been done before. If you go back through the old German literature of last century from Helmholtz on, you will see there is an immense range of colour illusional work shown. It is quite easy to get complementary colours with one colour and surrounding gray. Then you make the complementary colour. Isn't that what we are doing in the Land story? It is just further development of this very simple colour contrast. I don't see anything specially new in it only, shall we say, much ingenuity in giving a striking illustration.

P: That is only one interpretation of it, namely the interpretation in terms of contrast and the effect of complementary colours. But the real thing that, in my opinion, Land asserts (though he does not put it in our terms) is that we actively interpret the picture in a realistic fashion, and that this is not just dependent on a (so to speak) mechanical complementary colour effect, but on an active addition or supplementation made by ourselves, merely utilizing the contrasts in the picture. In other words, we try to give a unified interpretation (or, in your terminology, a coherent interpretation) in terms of colour and our experiences of colour vision. It is important to try the experiment again, and see whether it is based on the mechanics of contrast and complement, or whether it is mainly based on our efforts at a unified interpretation.

E: It is certainly interesting. I have only heard second-hand reports. I now want to come to another phenomenon, namely the completion phenomenon with line drawings. I refer particularly to the very interesting discussions in Ernst Gombrich's book *Art and Illusion.* Completion is the basis of so much graphic art. The artist seems intuitively to know to what degree he can rely upon the observer for filling in. In a subtle way you are reconstructing out of his drawings figures of the kind that he has presented. I think this is a very interesting example of the self-conscious mind's unified interpretation. It takes the drawings and tries to make an interpretation of them. I think that Gombrich would be most interested in thinking about our new theories of this.

P: Yes, this is the same kind of unified interpretation which plays such a great role in art, and which makes art interesting to us.

E: What is very striking is the chimera phenomenon described in chapter E5 (Fig. E5 – 5). I think this again is an experiment on mind-brain interaction and completion in an effort always to complete the picture and to make a unified perceptual image.

P: This clearly raises a problem for our view that the self-conscious mind has no direct access to the right hemisphere. I wonder whether the phenomenon you have described may be part of the tendency, perhaps innate, of seeing faces and especially eyes in rather arbitrary compositions of lines or dots.

E: Similarly we are very skilful in the efforts to extract a portrait from blocks of different colours of a very crude grain and still be able to recognize the portrait. Of course the standard portrait, as you know, is of Lincoln. But there is a long history of this phenomenon, as is illustrated for example by the mosaic portraits of classical times. I would like to refer to the question of global recognition, spatial and pictorial, by the right hemisphere. This theme is fully developed in chapter E7 (cp. Fig. E7–5).

P: There are actually two different hypotheses to consider here. Yours is one of these. I am led by my belief in animal consciousness to a different hypothesis, namely, that the right hemisphere has a kind of higher level of animal consciousness that does the interpreting on its own, and only gives its results to the self-conscious mind, which, as we know, is sometimes really dependent in a parallelistic way upon what is delivered to it by lower interpreting mechanisms or a lower interpreting consciousness. Thus, there are two competing hypotheses here. I think that it is important that we have more than one hypothesis. It may lead to experiments, for example of the Sperry type (experiments with the "split brain"), which possibly may help us to judge between them.

E: At this stage of our discussion I think it is important to consider music. As we know, the interpretation of music in all of the ways that it is possible yet to investigate goes on in the right temporal lobe, and lesions there lead to failure in the various Seashore and other tests and loss of musical sense and appreciation.

Now the case of the musician Ravel is of interest. We have the evidence from Dr. Alajouanine ([1948]; see chapter E6) that late in his life Ravel was suffering from a cerebral lesion with severe aphasia and that this was a disease that involved both sides of his brain, not only the speech centres on the left side but also the musical centres on the right side (cp. chapter E6). It was a very complicated picture that Dr. Alajouanine described in his Harvey Lectures. It is quite unique to have an account of a famous artist detailed in this manner by his doctor. The report discloses that Ravel had lost completely his ability to compose music, and he had lost his ability to learn new musical pieces on the piano but he could still play those that he had known before, fairly well anyway. The other point was that he could still recognize and criticize what he heard and pick up defects in the performance and make some amazing comments on the details of playing of his own works. All of this was possible. Yet, on the other hand, he had no sense for creating music and for appreciating music that he hadn't heard before. It was a limited loss and interesting, but I think not of great importance to us for our present discussion because the brain lesion itself was so diffuse. It wasn't restricted to any one area. At the most, I think you could say it was remarkable in that it showed how widely dispersed the musical performance can be over the surface of the cerebral hemisphere, and this could be particularly so in the right hemisphere.

P: Was the lesion mainly in the right hemisphere?

E: No, it was in both hemispheres because he had a quite severe aphasia. It could have been as much in the left as in the right. It was a kind of overall spotty lesion which picked out certain of the musical abilities of Ravel but didn't deprive him of his musical appreciation or criticism of what he remembered from the past.

The other point I would like to make is with regard to automatic movements and the dominant hemisphere. It is a mistake to think that every movement that is initiated by the dominant hemisphere is some deliberately planned action operated by the self-conscious mind upon the open modules. This is the case when we are beginning to learn a new movement. We are doing it with mental concentration and checking it, observing the actions getting better and better. Once they have been learned, they are relegated down to the automatic mode.

We should also mention musical instruments, because performance with musical instruments is one of the most exacting of all possible controls of movement. In the playing of a piano with very fast movements, one has to recognize that one is at the limit of what can be controlled. In fact you can't control by feedback circuitry from the periphery the individual finger movements at seven a second, which I understand is about the highest frequency possible. This has to be done in phrases sequentially. The control is automatic in the sense that one phrase leads to another to another, and even the controlling mechanisms of your movements are working in phrases in modifying them, working in pieces, as it were, and putting the phrases together and not the individual units of movement. That is happening too fast to be individually controlled.

P: The learning of the piano is a very strange affair. It may be imagination, but I think that there is something which one may call touch. This must be an incredibly finely balanced affair from the point of view of the motor mechanism and its controls, and it goes with the personality and the self-conscious mind. I actually have here a rather nice story.

I am a friend of the great pianist, Rudolf Serkin, and I know his touch very well. The following thing happened to me after a meeting with him in Interlaken. Each of us went to his car, and we went away in different directions. It was late at night, and one couldn't see anything — or only very little. Later, I passed a car — one of very many — and heard its horn, and I knew at once that it was Serkin's touch. The horn of the car was played pianissimo. I was concentrating on driving and was not expecting that I should meet him; I just recognized his personality in this pianissimo touch on the horn — and it was an electric horn.

E: I want to raise the question of the experience of time. We are all conscious that sometimes time seems to run slowly and sometimes quickly, and there is a belief among some people that it runs faster and faster as you get older, but for me it doesn't, you know. I feel time is still very full and each day is a good day. However, apart from that, we recognize that under certain conditions, under very attractive conditions, for example, say a very nice dinner party, the time for the whole meal has gone without us appreciating even perhaps the food too much! We have been so busily engaged in attractive conversation. On other occasions you can feel a dinner party lasts a very long time because no one talks to you, and if they do talk to you, it is without interest, even boring, and you are there left counting the time until you can escape.

Now there is one particular aspect of time that is of greatest interest and that everybody has experienced. It occurs in emergencies. When acute emergencies arise, time seems to run in slow motion. This must be an arrangement for the self-conscious mind reading out from the modules where they are under all of this acute input relating to the emergency and the self-conscious mind is now able to slow down the time so that it apparently has more time to make decisions in the emergency. It has refined the experience of time into smaller pieces, you might say, for its actions, so that it has the best opportunity of countering this emergency.

My own experience of this in an intense form has only come once. It was a very acute emergency when I thought I was going to be killed in a road crossing in Switzerland. We were doing a left turn into a main traffic road with nothing in sight, but it so happened that the low sun was in our eyes, and the road was heavily covered in trees. Down that dark road there was a dark red truck hurtling at perhaps 80 mph down the hill. My wife and I didn't see it until it flashed out of the darkness into the light. It was too late to stop so that all we could do was to try to accelerate to get out, and we were moving slowly because we had just come off a standing start! As I watched this truck coming closer and closer, time seemed to go on forever. I could watch it, thinking now I am past it, it won't hit me directly. We can get the front of the car out. It was getting closer and closer and then I thought it would hit the back of the car only, and then I thought, if it was the back of the car, we shall be spun around and perhaps crushed. Then in the end miraculously, I found out that the back of the car even wasn't hit and the truck moved past, but all in slow motion. It was the most incredible experience, and my wife had the same experience that time had almost come to a stop in this emergency. And so we drove on without ever daring to look back. The truck driver didn't seem to have seen us and made no attempt at braking. We had to do it all on our own.

This was the self-conscious mind making in the emergency the very remarkable performance of steering and accelerating so as to get across.

The point I would further like to make is that, when you have a severe impression of this kind, you have not only this slow motion experience at the time, but you also have it in memory. Deeply embedded in your memory is this terror of the emergency, of this red monstrosity hurtling at you, and you dream of it at night, and at times during the day it keeps on recurring. Of course I shall never forget it, but this is part of my theory of memory, namely that we remember instances that happen in a brief flash because we are replaying them again and again and again and so lay down our memory traces for permanent enjoyment or, in this case, for terror!

P: I have had some similar experiences, and even also some of actual car crashes. They all support this view that time slows down in a critical situation.

E: This is very important evidence though on our problem of interaction. You just can't explain how this can be done purely by brain action. The cerebral events, per se, cannot be changed in their time courses. It is the interaction of mind on brain that is giving this effect with the self-conscious mind receiving and giving in this intense emergency. So here is a final comment. Not only do we have to think of the self-conscious mind reading out in a kind of linear manner the happenings of the open modules and all the performance of interacting modules and so on, and giving us these experiences, but it plays tricks with time. Already in chapter E2 we have seen in the experiments of Libet that the self-conscious mind influences the time for the sensing of stimuli applied to the periphery. It takes, for example, half a second before a very weak electric shock to the hand actually evokes the sensation in conscious experience. That is the time it takes to get through to the self-conscious mind, but the self-conscious mind actually antedates it back approximately to the time at which the impulses arrive at the cerebral cortex. The ingenious and complex experiments of Libet are described in chapter E2, Figures 2 and 3. The self-conscious mind is, as it were, influencing the temporal sequences for its own purposes of making everything come out in the right way.

P: Just as in optical illusions a mechanism is at work adjusting the interpretation to normal reality, so it is with these temporal illusions. Interpretation takes account, so to speak, of a temporal perspective: it makes us refer the event in our intuitive experience to a moment of time at which it ought to have taken place in the real world according to our canons of interpreting the world realistically.

E: Another example of the self-conscious mind reading out with a temporal correction is known to occur with speech. We hear the individual words in a spoken discourse, but no gaps in time can be detected in the encoded message actually present in a taped recording.

Dialogue X

10:30 a. m. 28 September 1974

P: Jack, you thought that nothing quite like our criticism of parallelism had been made before. In a way this isn't quite correct. There was a German discussion which may be interpreted as a forerunner of our discussion.

The background of this was the parallelistic doctrine of Wilhelm Wundt, which was incredibly influential, not only in Germany, but also in America and in England too. Wundt's psychology was consciously parallelistic. Now Wundt's ideas were criticized by Carl Stumpf, who laid stress on the holistic or *Gestalt* character of our mental experiences, especially of certain mental perceptions. (As far as I know he did not use the term *Gestalt* in the early part of the discussion; it was Christian von Ehrenfels who was really the man who (in [1890]) first brought in the concept of the *Gestalt*, and applied it, especially, to melodies and tonal *Gestalten* and to the possibility of melodies' being transposed into a different key.)

Stumpf's argument was that nothing of this kind can be found in the physical world, and therefore that nothing of this kind can be found in the brain. Now, the interesting point is that this argument (which is in some ways similar to our argument, in so far as it points out the difficulties of parallelism) was answered very well, in 1920, by Wolfgang Köhler in his very interesting and very well informed – but essentially parallelist – book *Die physischen Gestalten in Ruhe und im stationären Zustand* [1920] both on the psychological and on the physiological side. (See also my section 8.) In his book, dedicated by the parallelist Köhler to the interactionist Stumpf, Köhler pointed out that there *do* exist *Gestalten,* not only in the mental world, but also in the physical world. Perhaps the simplest and most typical example is a soap bubble: if we blow a little more air into a soap bubble it becomes larger, but essentially retains its global shape. Of course, even a drop of water can be described as a physical *Gestalt,* and what leads to its shape, as in the case of the soap bubble, is surface tension. A particularly nice example is a soap film, held by a frame with a thin piece of thread tied in a loop dropped into it. If you puncture the film inside the loop, then the thread will always take up a circular shape, again due to surface tension and to the fact that the circle is the figure of greatest area for a given circumference.

Now Köhler's conjecture, and it was supported by some quite good conjectures about the brain, was that whenever we perceive a *Gestalt*, a *Gestalt* is also impressed on the brain: that there is a parallel *Gestalt* in the working of the brain. I think that, in so far as such a theory can be refuted at all, everything speaks in favour of the view that Köhler's theory has been refuted by more recent investigations of the brain. (I have, of course, especially in mind the disruption of the visual picture in the retina and its translation into very many point-events in the brain, and the fact that these point-events are not apparently fully integrated again by purely physiological activity. Here *we* actually bring in the activity of the conscious mind, and the experiments about the random dots which you mentioned yesterday are quite important in this connection.) So I think that Köhler's very beautiful hypothesis is wrong; anyway, it is not tenable in its original form.

Our criticism points out two further difficulties about parallelism, just as Stumpf pointed out the difficulties in parallelism before. However, we do not emphasize particularly strongly, as did Stumpf, the holistic character of mental experiences, but instead some other characteristics of mental experiences. So our criticism can be said to be a new challenge which a new Köhler might be able to answer from the parallelistic side. And if such an answer does come forward, we shall in any case have learned a lot.

E: Furthermore, we shall probably be able to develop our own theory in a more embracing manner in order to account for whatever the new findings are, because I think that is the way we have to venture. My own very strong belief is that the whole neurophysiological discoveries of the past and right up to the present and on into the future, as far as we can anticipate them, are all in a particular mode (cp. chapter E2). At the end of some remarkable new achievement in the feature recognition properties of neurones in the visual centres, we find statements that the physiological work seems to lead on indefinitely. There is no answer in sight if you do demand an ultimate interpretation of how visual pictures are experienced in their range and complexity. For example David Hubel will say he feels that all the time we are learning more and more about feature extraction neurones and how they come to make more and more complex patterns but never does it get beyond the stage of showing us more than little flashes of simple geometrical fragments to which each cell is responding specifically. How the whole great picture comes to be represented in the brain is quite another matter.

You will remember, Karl, we were talking about that when we were up at the castle looking up to the beautiful view of the head of Lake Como with the mountains, with the boats in the water, with all the villages around the lakeside, to the mountains rising up on all sides. Here is a wonderful picture of the most varied kind, all in the most incredibly fine detail, all in the clear air. Somehow from the fine punctate picture in our retina an integrated picture is eventually experienced as a result of all the processing in the brain of the coded transmission from the retina. It comes to us in this picture of vivid delight, and it seems to me that never can we get this completion on the neurophysiological level.

All we were working with there are patterns of impulses signalling progressively more complex features. There has to be an interpretational read-out. This is what we believe to give us a unified picture and it is a picture involving all kinds of features such as light and colour and depth and form. You see what we are up against. The retinal mosaic is made into codes of impulses in optic nerve fibres and in cells of the visual cortex, simple, complex and hypercomplex, and then you have to put it together again. The best we can do in neurophysiology is the feature extraction performance observed in neurones of the inferotemporal lobe as described in chapter E2. Cell after cell can be discovered with selective response at this level of simple geometrical features. This performance is tremendously remote from the vivid picture that was impressed on our retina and which we experience at the end of all of this cerebral processing.

The only way I believe we can explain the picture is that the cerebral action has to be converted into a mental experience, which of course is what eventually it is in its recognition. It isn't assembled together by the brain and read out as a single unitary phenomenon of the mental experience by the self-conscious mind, but in our hypothesis the self-conscious mind is in fact doing all the putting together. It is reading out the diversity, the immense complexity of the neuronal responses and it is creating the picture (cp. chapter E7). This is of course possible only when we have spent a lot of our lifetime learning to interpret cerebral activities as pictures. Our visual experience of the external world is delivered to us in our imaginative interpretation of the immense and complex pattern of brain events that derive from the retinal discharges.

P: There is one thing which I would like to question. For it seems to me quite possible, and even likely, that perception is the activity and the function of some lower part of consciousness and not of that kind of higher consciousness which we have decided to call the self-conscious mind. That is to say, perception may occur without our being fully conscious or fully self-conscious, as it may actually be there already on the animal level. The only question which I would raise in this connection is that you refer perception directly to the activity of the self-conscious mind. It is certainly a mental activity, but I think it is an open question whether the highest function is necessary for perception. I think that it is certainly necessary, for example, for the full enjoyment and the aesthetic appreciation of a scenic view. For that, certainly, the self-conscious mind is needed, but that is partly due to the fact that the aesthetic appreciation of a view is something which is almost a World 3 affair, and not merely a matter of perception for biological purposes. I would say that perceptions – integrated perceptions – have a biological purpose: the finding out of what is out there – the finding out of what is threatening me out there, or something like that. *That* does not, I would conjecture, require the self-conscious mind, but full aesthetic appreciation comes only with the self-conscious mind.

E: I see your point and of course I agree. We have mentioned before the role of attention. Attention comes when we are deliberately turning to some particular aspect of neural events that have been triggered off in some way, and when we are concentrating on these with the forward and backward interaction that the self-conscious mind has with the open modules and indirectly on all the other modules.

P: You have told me that the right hemisphere is able to read pictures, and in so far to do quite a bit, but I think that it is the left hemisphere which draws our attention – that is to say, the attention of the self – to an object. Or, let us say, it is the self-conscious mind interacting with the left hemisphere which draws the attention of our selves to certain aspects that are, perhaps, biologically quite irrelevant but aesthetically significant and important in a picture. I feel that there are two aspects to attention: biological attention and willed attention. Katz says (see my section 24) that an animal in flight sees only ways of escape and an animal that is hungry sees only possible opportunities to find some food. In other words, the attention of the animal is determined here by its physiological and biological situation. As opposed to this, the attention characteristic of the self-conscious mind is an act of the will. We consciously concentrate our will on some aspect of the situation or the picture or whatever it may be. So I think the distinction between these two kinds of attention speaks very strongly for a distinction between a higher and a lower form of integrating consciousness.

E: I agree of course. There is some kind of holistic interpretation or meaningful interpretation of pictures by the right hemisphere after commissurotomy (cp. chapter E5). This is unknown to the conscious subject, so the self-conscious mind is not concerned in this holistic interpretation. In these subjects who were doing this, putting together the strip cartoon, for example, you have to remember that before the commissurotomy they had a long history of doing that interpretation and experiencing it. Their right hemisphere had been part of a normal brain or a more or less normal brain for many years with all the experiences of conjoint interaction. When it is cut off from the self-conscious left hemisphere, it retains all the performances that it normally exercised in conjunction with the left hemisphere. I would like to suggest that in the right hemisphere there would be a very remarkable modular interacting operation which normally would be played upon by the open modules of the left hemisphere. In that way in this interaction between the left and the right hemispheres, backwards and forwards, we have the self-conscious mind able to get into very close relationship with all that is going on in the special areas of the right hemisphere that are in the picture mode, and the same could be true of the musical mode.

I am attracted by the idea that the right hemisphere gives a unified action because it has all of these memories or laid down reaction patterns. Furthermore, it is acting out in the motor mode as a unitary organized agent, using the left hand. There could be some overriding integrating conscious experience that doesn't give self-consciousness to the right hemisphere, but that is working like the self-consciousness of the left hemisphere in unifying and making some kind of overall picture of what is presented in all the vast array of activity in the coded information of the modules.

P: The question of the uniqueness of the self in the particular form raised by Jennings (in his Terry Lectures [1933]), and also by you, Jack, may possibly be a pseudoproblem. The self is, partly through our theories of the self, linked to its body, and just as our bodies are not identical with any other bodies, our selves are not identical with any other selves. Thus, the question can be raised whether the minds of identical twins are similar, just as their bodies are similar, but *not* the question whether their minds might be identical, because their bodies, similar though they may be, cannot be identical.

May I in this context criticize a very widespread approach to selfhood, to be found for example in Hume. I mean, thinking of oneself as a perceiving self or as an observer. I think that perception or observation is a very special kind of activity, and one in which the self is comparatively less active than in other activities, while the brain is doing the main job of interpretation.

E: We are now going to have some discussion on "Indeterminism is Not Enough", a paper published in *Encounter* by Karl [1973(a)]. The first point I wanted to make is with regard to the relationship of World 1, World 2 and World 3. I agree completely with the statement that there must be causal openness of World 1 towards World 2, but I rather feel that a misunderstanding can arise if we speak about the causal openness of World 2 to World 3 by direct action. I would like to suggest that in between there is always inserted a step via World 1. This of course is obvious enough if one is deriving one's conscious experiences from the coded representation of World 3 on some material object. Then it is clear that it has to be perceived through the senses going through all World 1 stages of reception and transmission. On the other hand, there is the more subtle condition where World 3 is coded in neuronal networks by some memory processes in the brain in special areas. Even there I emphasize that you have to get it out from the World 1 encoding in the neuronal connectivities.

P: I would suggest that instead of saying that World 3 is encoded in the brain, we say that certain World 3 objects are recorded in the brain and thus, as it were, incarnated. The whole of World 3 is nowhere; it is only certain individual World 3 objects which are sometimes incarnated and thus localizable.

E: They can be retrieved as memories and expressed. However, even there, the World 3 objects are as it were coded onto the neuronal machinery and have to be extracted from that by the action of the self-conscious mind. So in a sense there is still World 1 entering into the relationship. I think this is quite a small matter, but I just wanted to mention it because some critics may point out that there would seem to be some direct relationship (clairvoyance) between the self-conscious mind, World 2, and the information (World 3) coded on objects either in the external world or in the brain. In effect, of course, the story as told in "Indeterminism is Not Enough" is acceptable. It is just that minor criticism that I would like to make.

P: It is very important that you stress this point. However, I do not fully agree with your criticism. It is perfectly true that in many of the interactions between World 2 and World 3, the brain is involved, and with it, World 1. But, especially in many creative acts involving World 2 and World 3, I think that World 1 is *not* necessarily involved, or that World 1 is involved as an epiphenomenon of World 2. That is, something is going on in World 1, but it depends partly on World 2. (This is the idea of interaction.) By "creative acts" I mean such things as the discovery of new problems or the discovery of new solutions to our problems. It is perfectly true that this process of discovery is likely to have World 1 processes going on alongside it; but not, I would stress, in parallel to it, because the discovery of something new is a unique process, and I do not think that one can speak of a parallelism between two unique processes which are not analysable into standard elementary processes.[1] (This is one of the cases, alluded to above, where World 1 processes may be epiphenomenal with respect to what is going on in World 2.)

But quite apart from this, I think it is most important to realize that, when we have the feeling that there is some as yet not fully formulated problem in World 3 to be discovered and to be formulated, then in these cases we, or more precisely our World 2, deal essentially with World 3, without World 1 being involved in every step. World 1 gives a general background; no doubt that is true. Without World 1 memory we could not do what we are doing; but the particular new problem which we wish to bring out is conceived by World 2 directly in World 3. (See my section 13, and dialogue XI.)

The grasping of a World 3 object is, above all, an *active* process. Indeed, I want to conjecture that selves are the only active agents in the universe: the only agents to whom the term activity can properly be applied. (See also my section 32.) But since animals are active, they must have something like selves – they must be conscious, although not reflectively conscious of the fact that they have selves. Being conscious of this fact presupposes theory and therefore descriptive or human language. An automaton cannot be active or take action, and it does not seem compatible with evolutionary theory to regard animals, especially higher animals, as automata. They certainly seem to take purposeful actions.

I think that human achievements, that is to say, those of World 3, are unique, and that this makes our selves and our minds unique. I don't think that we need, for the uniqueness of man, a thesis of the genetic uniqueness of man. Admittedly, the evolution of the human brain was incredibly fast. But it was not one unique jump: it, like all evolution, consisted of many smallish steps.

---

[1] To put it more fully, any analysis into standard elements of the World 1 process which we may produce will fail to correspond to an analysis of the unique World 2 process because World 2 cannot be fully analysed into standard elements (such as ideas, representations, feelings, or anything else). Incidentally, it may be suggested that in the hope of producing such an analysis lies perhaps the deepest motive of those who speak of a "stream of consciousness" or a "stream of ideas". The impossibility of such a complete analysis becomes particularly obvious in the light of the role played in World 2 by unconscious processes which interrupt and intercept the sequence of conscious World 2 processes.

E: I now turn to a page of your article in *Encounter* which deals with the question of the openness of World 1 to World 2. You say, for example, "But nothing is gained for us if this World 1 is completely closed to what I have called World 2 and World 3." I think that it is very important to discuss this issue because I am sure that the principal criticism of our dualism will be that we are proposing that the physical world, World 1, is open to influences of some other unimaginable kind, a self-conscious mind's influences with forwards and backwards communication. For that we have to propose that the World 1 of certain speech areas and related regions in the brain, what I have been calling open modules, is open to these influences from World 2. We have to recognize that this is a quite revolutionary concept in terms of modern science.

P: I completely agree with what you say. It is of course only in the brain that there can be interaction between World 1 and World 2, and in this we must really say that Descartes was our forerunner. Even though it may be revolutionary for modern science, we are only in one way or another bringing back Descartes's fundamental idea that World 1 (which was for Descartes the mechanical world) is open, in the brain, to World 2.

E: I would like you, Karl, to comment further on this question of the openness of World 1 to World 2. You see, there are fundamental principles of physics that seem to be outraged by this because it is not possible I think to utilize quantum indeterminacy for this purpose. This gives random chance events and is of no use in accounting for the very precisely causal events that are in the relationship between World 2 and World 1 in these very special areas of the brain. Of course I realize that we have to protect ourselves from too severe criticism by pointing out that this postulate of openness occurs only in relationship to certain very highly sophisticated and highly designed structures that are built biologically and endowed with incredible properties in their dynamic activity, namely the modules in the cerebral cortex (cp. chapter E1) and only some of these modules would have the property of being open to World 2, and then only in special states of these modules (cp. chapter E7). We have already dealt with that, for example, in the question of sleep and the unconsciousness accompanying various depressed cerebral states as well as the hyperactive cerebral states in convulsive seizures. In those cases the modules are not open. Furthermore, one would think that the openness varies from time to time according to the heightened consciousness or to the dullness of the subject. So there we have our problem told. But how do we formulate it? We still have before us this incredible hypothesis that, there are structures existing in World 1 which we are proposing to have a relationship with World 2, a two-way relationship, of being influenced by World 2 and of influencing World 2. That is the problem that I would like you to talk more about.

P: Of course, it is a very difficult problem. I have quite a number of ideas in connection with it, but they are far from being mature.

First of all, I do of course agree that quantum theoretical indeterminacy in a sense cannot help, because this leads merely to probabilistic laws, and we do not wish to say that such things as free decisions are just probabilistic affairs.

The trouble with quantum mechanical indeterminacy is twofold. First, it is probabilistic, and this doesn't help us much with the free-will problem, which is not just a chance affair. Second, it only gives us indeterminism, not openness to World 2. However, in a roundabout way I do think that one may make use of quantum theoretical indeterminacy without committing oneself to the thesis that free-will decisions are probabilistic affairs. In this context I may just mention one point. New ideas have a striking similarity to genetic mutations. Now, let us look for a moment at genetic mutations. Mutations are, it seems, brought about by quantum theoretical indeterminacy (including radiation effects). Accordingly, they are also probabilistic and not in themselves originally selected or adequate, but on them there subsequently operates natural selection which eliminates inappropriate mutations. Now we could conceive of a similar process with respect to new ideas and to free-will decisions, and similar things. That is to say, a range of possibilities is brought about by a probabilistic and quantum mechanically characterized set of proposals, as it were – of possibilities brought forward by the brain. On these there then operates a kind of selective procedure which eliminates those proposals and those possibilities which are not acceptable to the mind, anchored in World 3, which tries them out in World 3 and checks them by World 3 standards. This may perhaps be the way in which these things take place, and it was for this reason that I so much liked the suggestion about the inhibitory neurones working like a sculptor who cuts away and discards part of the stone in order to form his statue.

Thus, what I am here suggesting is that we might conceive of the openness of World 1 to World 2 somewhat on the lines of the impact of selection pressures on mutations. The mutations themselves can be considered as quantum effects; as fluctuations. Such fluctuations may occur, for example, in the brain. In the brain there may at first arise purely probabilistic or chaotic changes, and some of these fluctuations may be purposefully selected in the light of World 3 in a way similar to that in which natural selection quasi-purposefully selects mutations. I don't say that these analogies can be easily accepted, but they are at least worth speculating about. (The all-or-nothing principle of the firing of nerves may indeed be interpreted as a mechanism which would allow arbitrarily small fluctuations to have macroscopic effects.) The action of the mind on the brain may consist in allowing certain fluctuations to lead to the firing of neurones while others would merely lead to a slight rise in the temperature of the brain. This is one of the possible ways to "sculpture" (and to save the law of the conservation of energy).

This brings me to my next question: does all this really clash with some of the fundamental laws of physics, and particularly, with the laws of thermodynamics?

I do not think that we have to worry about the second law of thermodynamics at all. We have only to assume that the brain gets tired under mental activity and that this tiredness is in some way or other equivalent to heat production, and so to a degradation of energy, and that the second law is thus preserved. There is just a lot of heat produced by all these processes: one gets, so to speak, a hot brain.

The problem is perhaps different with respect to the first law, the law of the conservation of energy. Here there are various possibilities.

One possibility that would suit us extremely well would be that the law of the conservation of energy would turn out to be valid only statistically. If this is the case, it might be that we have to wait for a physical fluctuation of energy before World 2 can act on World 1, and the time-span in which we prepare for the "free-will movement of the finger" may easily be long enough to allow for such fluctuations to occur. In fact, some physicists have proposed theories in which the conservation of energy is only statistically valid. There was, for example, the theory due to Bohr, Kramers and Slater [1925]. But this was later rejected; it was really superseded by quantum mechanics, in which the first law of thermodynamics is not statistically valid but strictly valid. However, Schrödinger made later [1952] another interesting suggestion about the possibility that, on a still deeper level, the first law may only be statistically valid. He pointed out that energy is $h\nu$. That is to say, it is proportional to ν – to the frequency – and frequencies have statistical averages. Thus, in the frequencies of the light waves we may have before us a statistical element. (For another possibility – that slight deviations from the first law may be compensated for – see my section 48, and also dialogue XII.)

I may perhaps say a little more about the openness of a physical world (more precisely, the world of mechanics) to another world. (This would be also an alternative to the approach sketched above, which uses the statistical interpretation of the law of the conservation of energy.)

At the time of Oersted, the basis of physics was still circumscribed by Newton's mechanics. Oersted's experiment (in which a wire carrying an electric current is held along a magnetic needle, and in which the needle is deflected as long as the current is switched on) seemed to violate – and did violate – Newtonian mechanics. That is to say, it turned out that the world of mechanics: of push, gravitational attraction and elastic repulsion, and especially also of conservation of (mechanical) energy, was suddenly discovered to be open – open to a new world, namely the world of electricity. This openness of the mechanical world to the world of electricity was the main challenge which led to a new reconstruction of physics in which electricity became basic and mechanics derivative with respect to electricity. We had a theory allowing the reduction of the mechanics of push to electrical phenomena, such as the repulsion of negatively charged electrons. This reduction was very successful, and for a time it looked as if an electrical monism had been established. However, this was not so. There is no monistic physical world of electricity. There are forces other than the electrical forces; forces such as nuclear forces and weak interactional forces in addition to gravitational forces. Accordingly, we can say that each of the two physical worlds, the mechanical world and the electrical world, is, on our current understanding, "open" to at least one other physical world which somehow or other interacts with the mechanical and the electrical world. In other words, modern physics is pluralistic (and the law of the conservation of energy had constantly to be generalized whenever the physical world was enlarged). Thus, we should not be too worried about a *prima facie* violation of this law: somehow we may be able to smooth it all out. (The real difficulty was the generalization of the highly intuitive mechanistic world picture.) This situation makes it very much easier to assume the possibility of interference from outside – from something as yet unknown which, if we want physics to be complete, would have to be added to the physical world.

However, I am not necessarily in favour of the metaphysical research programme of completing physics (but I have no *a priori* axe to grind here). I am, rather, in favour of saying that physics is open. There are two ways of going about this matter of openness, as Wigner has somewhere pointed out. Wigner also believes that physics is incomplete, but he thinks that physics may possibly be completed by adding certain novel laws to it. I think that this is only to say, in a different way, that physics is open to something as yet unknown. (And I am inclined at the moment to say that it is open to World 2 rather than to other physical laws, for, as far as we know, only World 2 can interact with World 3. That it does so interact, of this we have much experience, as do we of the fact that World 2 interacts with World 1; especially of the fact that it does so in such a way as to allow World 3 plans and theories to enact great changes in World 1. It is for these very strong reasons that we have, I think, in any case to postulate the openness of World 1 to World 2, while the mere openness of the known World 1 to an unknown part of World 1 would not help in solving the great problem that World 3 plans and theories bring about changes in World 1.)

E: In my discussions with Eugene Wigner, I get the impression that he feels a complete transformation of physics is required, not just an addition to some aspect of physical law but that the very basis of physics has to be reconstructed with a revolution that would transform the existing physics more than occurred with the earlier physics under the influence of Einsteinian relativity and Planck's quantum theory.

P: I myself hope for a revolution in physics because I feel that the present state of physics is unsatisfactory, but this is a different issue. I mean, we can't know what will actually happen. Even in a revolution in physics, the present physics will have to be valid as a first approximation because our present physics is extremely well corroborated; so in the first approximation our present physics will have to continue to exist. But that it will not be fully satisfactory from the point of view of a new physics is, I think, also clear. I am not terribly troubled by the openness of World 1 to World 2, but I would agree with you that from the point of view of present physics it is certainly a revolutionary step. Perhaps I may just add in conclusion, concerning the second law of thermodynamics, that the second law is in any case only statistical, and is already known to be violated, in a sense, in the small. That is to say, Brownian motion can be said to violate the second law in the small at every moment, only these violations are then amply compensated for by what happens in neighbouring parts of the system (of the gas or the fluid) and in the preceding and succeeding moments. Anyway, the idea that the brain gets hot in connection with every creative thought is quite sufficient to make sure that there would be no problem in connection with the second law.

E: At this stage I will add two quotations, one from Wigner and one from Schrödinger giving a brief statement of their views on the necessity for the reconstruction of physics.

Schrödinger [1967] "The impasse *is* an impasse. Are we thus not the doers of our deeds? Yet we feel responsible for them, we are punished or praised for them, as the case may be. It is a horrible antinomy. I maintain that it cannot be solved on the level of present-day science which is still entirely engulfed in the 'exclusion principle' – without knowing it – hence the antinomy. To realize this is valuable, but it does not solve the problem. You cannot remove the 'exclusion principle' by act of parliament as it were. Scientific attitude would have to be rebuilt, science must be made anew. Care is needed."

Eugene Wigner [1969] has demonstrated the fallacy in postulating "that life is a physicochemical process which can be explained on the basis of the ordinary laws of physics and chemistry." He goes on to predict "that in order to deal with the phenomenon of life, the laws of physics will have to be changed, not only reinterpreted."

P: The fundamental argument in favour of the openness of World 1 through World 2 to World 3 is simply that our culture makes changes in World 1. If a sculptor makes a statue, then he makes a fundamental change in World 1, and we cannot assume that it is a completely World 1 affair. That is to say, to assume that Michelangelo's works are simply the result of molecular movements and nothing else seems to me very much more absurd than the assumption of some slight and probably unmeasurable violation of the first law of thermodynamics.[2]

E: Here is something very much to the point from p. 25 of your *Encounter* article, "Indeterminism is Not Enough." It goes on like this: "Thus indeterminism is necessary but insufficient to allow for human freedom and especially for creativity. What we really need is the thesis that World 1 is incomplete; that it can be influenced by World 2, that it can interact with World 2; or that it is causally open towards World 2, and hence, further, towards World 3. We thus come back to our central point: we must demand that World 1 is not

[2] A materialist might try to explain all this as the result of natural selection. However, I think that *natural* selection is not enough, and that we also have Michelangelo exercising *critical* selection (with respect to certain World 3 principles). Moreover, even the theory of natural selection presents a problem for the materialist.

One of my main points about the body-mind problem is this. Even though World 2 may have emerged from World 1, it must have become to a considerable extent independent of World 1, for in a critical discussion it must orientate itself on World 3 standards – say, on logic – rather than on World 1. If it were only an epiphenomenon of World 1, then our beliefs would all be illusions and on equal terms with other illusions; and this would hold for all "isms", including epiphenomenalism and the theory of natural selection. It thus turns out that materialism reinforced by the theory of natural selection is a metaphysical theory which cannot be refuted; but it also cannot be rationally upheld because, from its own point of view, all such metaphysical views are epiphenomenal illusions and thus equivalent. Unless we assume that (say by natural selection) there has emerged an autonomous World 3 of autonomous standards of critical discussion, all theories are equally epiphenomenal illusions (including, of course, the theory of natural selection). See my section 21.

self-contained or 'closed', but open towards World 2; that it can be influenced by World 2, just as World 2 can be influenced by World 3."

P: In view of your previous criticism of what I said about the relationship between World 2 and World 3, and of your argument that World 1 always intervenes in any interaction between World 2 and World 3, I am quite ready to assume that there may always be some World 1 processes going on whenever any World 2 process is going on, and thus whenever World 2 is in contact with World 3. There may also be any amount of energetically excessively wasteful processes in the brain. That is to say, the brain may consume more nourishment than we should otherwise expect, if it is in contact with World 2. Actually, that is probably the case because the brain has to be extremely active in order to be in contact with World 2. I must say that I think that it is even possible to conceive of a view in which the first law of thermodynamics, the law of energy conservation, is satisfied and in which there is still an influence exerted from World 2 on World 1. I think that this is a possible theory, but it is necessary to think more about it.

E: The trouble about more energy for the brain under certain conditions is that overall measurements show that, in mental activity of a quite severe kind, there is very little more oxygen consumption. That is of course with measurements for the whole brain made by Seymour Kety and others. Then there are the measurements of discharge frequencies of cerebral neurones recording from single neurones by Evarts, for example. There are different patterns of performance by nerve cells and you do have large cells and small cells varying in activity, one going up and the other going down under special states of activity or in sleep, but again it is hard to make any clear rules about it (see chapter E7).

P: I may perhaps mention again that in processes in which World 2 acts upon World 1 we do not need to assume any more than that the physical magnitudes involved are as small as you like – that is, vanishingly small (remember the all-or-nothing principle); thus they may possibly be below any measurement. What bears on our problem is the general idea that only a highly active and agitated brain is open to World 2.

E: I'm going to give you a little surprising information deriving from experiments recently done by Professor David Ingvar [1975] of Lund. He has been using radioactive xenon injected into the carotid artery in order to discover the circulation of the cerebral cortex and he actually is able to put 32 recording windows over the cerebral hemisphere of that side so that he can evaluate the circulation through these different areas. This is of course done in relationship to clinical investigations on psychiatric patients and chronic alcoholics. It is important therapeutically to know about the circulation through the cerebral cortex from one area to another. He has been able to discover what happens when patients are using in a specific way one or other part of their speech areas. The production of spoken language increases the circulation through the Broca area and to a less extent Wernicke's area and also the motor areas involved in speaking. In reading there was a flow increase in addition in the occipital lobe, which would relate to the visual involvement. With linguistic performance there was no flow increase over the minor hemisphere. Finally abstract thinking such as silent problem solving resulted in an increased circulation in the frontal, parietal and occipital association areas. So there is under these conditions a circulation change of a specific kind. He does the same with manual activity which brings up circulation to and complex neuronal activity in the sensori-motor cortex of the brain matching what the theories would suggest about the areas involved. I think these results are important because they indicate increased activity in cortical areas that have been associated with these specific functions. Ingvar is a master in this field, and he realizes the philosophical implications of his discoveries.

I would like to add a comment about determinism. If physical determinism is true, then that is the end of all discussion or argument; everything is finished. There is no philosophy. All human persons are caught up in this inexorable web of circumstances and cannot break out of it. Everything that we think we are doing is an illusion and that is that. Will anybody live up to this situation? It even comes to this, that the laws of physics and all our understanding of physics is the result of the same inexorable web of circumstances. It isn't a matter any more of our struggling for truth to understand what this natural world is and how it came to be and what are the springs of its operation. All of this is illusion. If we want to have that purely deterministic physical world, then we should remain silent. Alternatively if we believe in an open world, then we have all the world of adventure using our minds, using our understanding, in order to develop more and more subtle and creative ideas, that is to develop World 3. Our relationship to World 3 becomes distinctively a willed human performance. In the ultimate world of human existence we are using this openness of World 1 in these very special areas of our brains.

P: That's a very good statement. But again I want to suggest a very small correction. Fundamentally, our relationship to World 3 is certainly a "willed human performance"; but it has unintended consequences built into it, in addition to those which are consciously willed.

E: I would agree and furthermore it's like some great symphony with different instruments playing different parts and the whole is blended into some incredible synthesized performance, some harmony. This is the way individual persons by their creativity can construct a civilization and a great culture. It is not just a single individual deliberately acting in isolation. It is the whole immense performance of human beings that builds our World 3 and with that the World 2 of each of us.

Dialogue XI

5 p.m. 29 September 1974

E: Karl could you please talk of the idea you have about a direct relationship between World 3 and World 2 by the reference to Euclid's theorem that you have just told me.

P: I think that this problem is very important. Although, of course, there are some World 1 brain processes going on all the time while World 2 is awake, and especially when it is busy in solving problems or in formulating problems, my thesis is not only that World 2 can grasp World 3 objects, but that it can do so directly; that is to say, although World 1 processes may be going on (in an epiphenomenal manner) at the same time, they do not constitute a physical or World 1 representation of those World 3 objects which we try to grasp.

Let me illustrate this by discussing Euclid's theorem, that for every natural number, however large, there exists a greater one which is a prime number; or in other words, that there are infinitely many primes. Certainly, Euclid had impressed upon his memory (and thus presumably upon his brain) some facts about prime numbers, especially facts about their fundamental properties. But there can, I think, be little doubt about what must have happened. What Euclid did, and what went far beyond World 1 memory recordings in the brain, was that he visualized the (potentially) infinite sequence of natural numbers – he saw them before his mind, going on and on; and he saw that in the sequence of all the natural numbers the prime numbers get less and less frequent as we proceed. The distances between the prime numbers get, in general, wider and wider (although this has exceptions; for example it seems that however far we go, there are still so-called twin primes which are separated just by one even number; but these twin primes get rarer too).

Now, looking at this sequence of numbers intuitively, which is not a memory affair, he discovered that there was a problem: the problem whether or not the prime numbers peter out in the end – whether there is a greatest prime number and then no further ones – or whether the prime numbers go on for ever. And Euclid *solved* this problem. Neither the formulation of the problem nor the solution of the problem was based on, or could be read off from, encoded World 3 material. They were based directly on an intuitive grasp of the World 3 situation: of the infinite sequence of natural numbers.

The solution of the problem is that, if we assume that there is a greatest prime number, then, with the help of this alleged "greatest prime number" *we can construct a greater one.* We can take all the prime numbers up to the "greatest", multiply them all, including the "greatest", and then add the number *one.* Let us call the number so produced *N.* We can then show that *N* must be a prime number, under the assumption that the factors of *N*–1 were all the primes in existence. For if we divide *N* by any of these factors, the remainder is *one.* Thus if *N* is not prime, it can have only divisors which are greater than that number which we assumed to be the greatest prime.

The problem whether there exists a greatest prime is thus solved, negatively. The related problem whether there exists a greatest pair of twin primes has not, to my knowledge, been solved so far.

Euclid's proof operates with the following ideas: (1) A potentially infinite sequence of natural numbers. (2) A finite sequence (of any length) of prime numbers. (3) A possibly infinite sequence of prime numbers. Euclid *discovered the problem* whether the sequence of prime numbers is *finite* or *infinite*; and he solved the problem by discovering that the first of these alternatives leads to the second, and thus to an absurdity. No doubt, he operated with intuitive symbolic representations and diagrams. But these were merely a help. They neither constituted the problem nor its solution. We may say that the very idea of infinity – a World 3 idea – cannot have a direct brain representation, although the *word* "infinite" may of course have one. The problem is read off from an intuition of the World 3 situation. This can, of course, be achieved only by becoming familiar with the World 3 situation and its various aspects.

My point here is that there need not be a World 1 representation of a World 3 idea (for example, a model in terms of brain elements) in order that we can grasp the World 3 idea in question.[1] I regard the thesis of the possibility of a direct grasp of World 3 objects by World 2 as generally valid (and not only for infinite World 3 objects like infinite sequences); yet the example of infinite objects makes it, I think, quite clear that no World 1

[1] In connection with the problem of grasping World 3 objects, see also my section 13 above.

representation of the World 3 object need be involved. We could, of course, build a computer programmed for an operation (such as adding 1 to any intermediate result) which goes on for ever. But (1) the computer will not in fact go on for ever but will wear out (or absorb all the available energy) in a finite time and (2) it will, if so programmed, deliver a sequence of intermediate results but not a final result; it is *we* who interpret the *sequence* of intermediate results as an infinite sequence, and understand what this means. (There are no (finite) physical models or representations of the World 3 idea of potential infinity.[2])

The argument for the direct grasp of World 3 objects does not depend on the non-existence of World 1 representations of infinity. The decisive point seems to me this: in the process of discovering a World 3 problem – say a mathematical problem – we at first vaguely "sense" the problem before it is formulated either in spoken or in written language. We first suspect its existence; then we may give some verbal or written indications (epiphenomena, as it were); then we may put it more clearly; and then we may put it sharply. (Only in this last stage do we represent the problem in language.) It is a process of making and matching, and making again.

The completed World 3 proof must be critically checked for validity, and for this purpose it must be put into a World 1 representation – into language, preferably into written language. But the invention of the proof was a direct operation of World 2 upon World 3 – certainly with the help of the brain, but without any reading off of problems or results from brain-encoded representations or from other incarnations of World 3 objects.

This suggests that all, or most, creative acts of World 2 which produce new World 3 objects, whether problems or new proofs or anything of that kind, even though accompanied by World 1 processes, must be other than readings out of memory and encoded World 3 objects. Now this is very important, because I think that this kind of direct contact is also the way in which World 2 uses encoded or incarnate World 3 objects to see directly their World 3 aspects, as opposed to their encoding. This is the way in which, in reading a book, we transcend the encoding on the page and get directly to the meaning.

The centre in the brain which grasps linguistic meaning (the Wernicke centre) must somehow be in direct contact with World 3. There is something going on in World 1, but this process of grasping goes beyond what is going on in World 1; and this may perhaps be a reason to suppose that it is really the

[2] A materialistic metaphysics would thus quite consistently lead to a finitistic mathematics, in which Euclid's problem would become meaningless.

Wernicke centre which contains some open modules; an opening of World 1 to World 2.

E: Yes, I am convinced that the Euclidean story indicates a direct relationship between World 3 and World 2. Now that I have fully understood it, it is very convincing indeed. It leads to many other ideas which I'll briefly mention, but I wanted to say first of all that I wouldn't restrict the open modules to the Wernicke centre. The ideational areas are more than that, involving all kinds of experiences: pictorial, musical and emotional, and so on. I have a final comment that I believe is important. The conclusion that you have drawn and the belief that you have now given me may be formulated as follows. In the operations of the creative imagination, when something original is conceived that has never before been expressed in any way, World 2 is interacting with World 3 directly. This is the operation of the creative imagination. It is the highest level of the human performance. As a World 2 – World 3 interaction it is happening independently of the brain and then gets coded back on the brain. I think it first is the self-conscious mind exploring into its own resources, the immense potentialities that are available to it.

P: I should like to add something about the relationship between the components of World 1 in which World 3 objects are encoded, and World 2 and World 3. I think that, if we look at a sculpture by Michelangelo, then what we see is, on the one hand, of course, a World 1 object in so far as it is a piece of marble. On the other hand, even the material aspects of this, such as the hardness of the marble, may not be irrelevant to the World 2 appreciation of this World 3 object encoded in a World 1 substrate because it is the artist's struggling with the material, and the artist's overcoming of the difficulties of the material, which is part of the charm and the significance of the World 3 object. So I do not want generally to relegate the World 1 aspect of an encoded World 3 object to an epiphenomenon – but sometimes it is. If we have a book which is moderately well printed but not very well printed – not, say, a special edition – then the World 1 aspect of the book may be utterly irrelevant, and in a sense no more than an epiphenomenon, a sort of uninteresting appendix to the World 3 content of the book. However, both in the case of the Michelangelo statue and in the case of the book, what we – what our World 2, our conscious self – really gets in touch with is the World 3 object. In the case of the statue the World 1 aspect is important; but it is important only because of the World 3 achievement which consists in changing and modelling the World 1 object. In all cases, what we really look at and admire and understand is not so much the materialized World 3 object as the various World 3 aspects regardless of their materialization. For example, an old edition of a book is admired because of its historical significance – again a World 3 aspect. And it is important to note that the World 2 enjoyment of the materialized World 3 object – such as the connoisseur's enjoyment in handling a very rare edition of Dante – is based very largely on his *theoretical knowledge* of these things, which means that, again, World 3 aspects play a major role.

E: Karl, we have developed and clarified the concepts of the self-conscious mind. Never before has it been so clear to me, and not only so clear, but we can now recognize its manifold properties. It comes in much more now into the total human performance than I had ever dared to think. The self-conscious mind is responsible for the act of attention, selecting from all the immense activities of our brain, the neural bases of our experiences from moment to moment. The unity of conscious experience with all its perceptual qualities is also there in memory and in the other higher aspects of mental activity. But the self-conscious mind is not just there receiving. In all these respects, both in the perceptual side and in the higher intellectual side, it is actively engaged in modifying the brain. So it is in a dynamically active relationship with the brain and undoubtedly has a position of superiority (cp. chapter E7). As we have developed our hypothesis, we have returned to the views of past philosophies that the mental phenomena now are ascendent again over the material phenomena.

Finally, we have come just now to recognize that, in the creative imagination, the self-conscious mind is actively engaged in the World 2 – World 3 interchange in bringing about new, completely new, concepts or ideas or problems or proofs or theories. The creative imagination is being driven by the self-conscious mind into flights of imagination which of course are the greatest achievements of humanity. We can look back in the past and think of the great flights of imagination in all the creativeness of art and science and literature and philosophy and ethics, etc. that have made humanity what it is and given us our civilization. Now this achievement again we are crediting to the self-conscious mind in the first place. Of course eventually it is played down through the brain and encoded there, and also it is expressed as World 3 objects; nevertheless it is in the first place the activity of the self-conscious mind.

I wanted to stress this pre-eminence of the self-conscious mind because now I raise the questions: What is the self-conscious mind? How does it come to exist? How is it attached to the brain in all its intimate relationships of give and take? How does it come to be? And in the end, not only how does it come to be, but what is its ultimate fate when, in due course, the brain disintegrates?

P: I am glad that you have laid so much stress on the human imagination. This is one of the reasons why I think that the origin of the self-conscious mind somehow goes together with the origin of language, as I have mentioned earlier.

As to the question of *what is* the self-conscious mind, I think that these "what is" questions are not in general really very important, and that they are really not very good questions to ask. They are of such a form that no really enlightening answers can be given to them. Thus, to the question what is life, you can give the unsatisfactory answer that life is a chemical process. This answer is unsatisfactory because there are lots and lots of chemical processes apart from living processes. We *may* indeed find some interest in saying that life is a chemical process; but mainly because it may suggest some interesting metaphors. If we say that life has some similarity with the chemical processes of a flame, that it is a kind of open system like the flame of a candle, then this may indeed be a striking metaphor, but it isn't really very valuable.

Now, in connection with the question "What is the self-conscious mind?" I might say first, as a preliminary answer (always bearing in mind what I have just said against all "what is" questions): "It is something utterly different from anything which, to our knowledge, has previously existed in the world." This is an answer to the question, but it is a negative answer. It just stresses the difference between the mind and anything that has gone before. If you then ask: is it really so totally different, then I can only say: Oh, it may have some sort of forerunner in the not self-conscious but perhaps conscious perception of animals. There may be some sort of forerunner of the human mind in the experience of pleasure and pain by animals, but it is, of course, completely different from these animal experiences because it can be self-reflexive; that is to say, the ego can be conscious of itself. That is what we mean by the self-conscious mind. And if we ask how that is possible, then I think that the answer is that it is only possible via language and via the development of imagination in that language. That is to say, only if we can imagine ourselves as acting bodies, and as acting bodies somehow inspired by mind, that is to say, by our selves, only then, by way of all this reflexiveness – by way of what could be called liaison reflexiveness – can we really speak of a self.

E: I am very interested indeed in what you have said and I wanted to just mention the light that we can have upon this in man's evolutionary origin. I will quote from my book *Facing Reality* [1970], p. 62: "Certainly one of the poignant problems confronting each man in his life is his attempt to become reconciled with his inevitable end in death. This of course is relatable to his evolutionary origin. He dies as do other animals, but the inevitability of death affects man alone because man in his development gained self-consciousness."

P: From an evolutionary point of view, I regard the self-conscious mind as an emergent product of the brain; emergent in a way similar to that in which World 3 is an emergent product of the mind. World 3 emerges together with the mind, but nevertheless it emerges as a product of the mind, by mutual interaction with it. Now I want to emphasize how little is said by saying that the mind is an emergent product of the brain. It has practically no explanatory value, and it hardly amounts to more than putting a question mark at a certain place in human evolution. Nevertheless, I think that this is all which, from a Darwinian point of view, we can say about it.

I am quite sure that you and Dobzhansky are right in stressing that the realization of death – of the danger of death and of the inevitability of death – is one of the great discoveries which led to full self-consciousness. But, if that is so, then we can say that self-consciousness arises to full self-consciousness only slowly in a child, because I don't think that children are fully self-conscious before they are fully conscious of death.

In connection with these questions which we are now discussing, it is extremely important to realize that explanation is never ultimate. That is to say, all explanation is in some sense intellectually unsatisfactory because all explanation has to start out from certain definite conjectures, and these conjectures themselves are used as unexplained assumptions for the purpose of explanation. As to these unexplained assumptions, we may always become conscious of a need or a wish to explain them in their turn. But of course this leads to the same problem again. So we find that we have to stop somewhere. In this way we arrive at the doctrine of the non-existence of ultimate explanations. And evolution certainly cannot be taken in any sense as an ultimate explanation. We must come to terms with the fact that we live in a world in which almost everything which is very important is left essentially unexplained. We try our best to give explanations and we penetrate deeper and deeper into the really incredible secrets of the world with the help of the method of conjectural explanation. Still, we should always be aware that this is only in a sense scratching the surface, and that ultimately everything is left unexplained, especially everything in connection with existence. Newton, the first man to produce a really satisfying explanatory theory of the universe, was also perhaps the first to realize this fully. (See my sections 47 and 51.) I wish to add to this that I do not necessarily take existence in the sense of the existentialists, but that I have in mind simply the fact that the world exists, and of course also that *we* exist in this world. This is of course ultimately inexplicable; and it seems to be so also from the point of view of modern evolutionary theory, in which the existence of life is something which becomes a scientific problem. The origin of life may have happened only once, and it may be essentially improbable, and if so it would not be subject to what we normally call explanation; for explanation in probabilistic terms is always an explanation that, under given conditions, an event is highly probable.

E: I have something in my book, *Facing Reality,* appropriate to this stage of the present discussion and I will read just a paragraph (page 83). "I believe that there is a fundamental mystery in my existence, transcending any biological account of the development of my body (including my brain) with its genetic inheritance and its evolutionary origin; and, that being so, I must believe similarly for each human being. And just as I can't give a scientific account of my personal origin — I woke up in life as it were to find myself existing as an embodied self with this body and brain — so I cannot believe that this wonderful gift of a conscious existence has no further future, no possibility of another existence under some other unimaginable conditions." I quote this now because this is taking us perhaps further than you would like, Karl, but it is where I want to go in considering the implications of the self-conscious mind that we have been discussing over these last few days. I try, as it were, to face up fully to the wonder, to the terror, and to the adventure of my self-conscious life. All of these words can be used, but ultimately it's beyond my imagination or power of expression.

I think, Karl, you implied that also; that there is something inexplicable, some mystery about the existence of each one of us. This is necessarily so because it's beyond any explanation, scientific or otherwise at the present time. We can recognize that this World 2 existence came to primitive man with his developing linguistic accomplishment. Language enabled him to grow in World 3 creativities and so further to develop his own World 2. These two together, World 2 and World 3, have given rise to this refined self-consciousness that we now have and which you might say is at the ultimate of man's efforts in his creative thinking. And so through the ages men have asked: What does this personal conscious life mean? How can I make the best of my life? What might I expect ultimately after death?

P: I think that we agree on all these points. Where we may perhaps disagree is on another point which I will now put forward – with a certain hesitancy. It concerns the question of survival. First of all, I don't look forward to an eternity of survival. On the contrary, the idea of going on for ever seems to me utterly frightening. Anybody who has sufficient imagination to deal with the idea of infinity would, I think, agree – well, perhaps not everybody, but at least some people. On the other hand, I do feel that even death is a positively valuable element in life. I think that we should value life and our own lives very highly, but that we should in some way come to terms with the fact that we have to die; and that we should see that it is the practical certainty of death which contributes much that gives value to our lives, and especially to the value of the life of another person. I think we really couldn't value life if life were bound to go on for ever. It is just the fact that it is precarious, the fact that it is finite and limited, the fact that we have to face its end which, I think, adds to the value of life and so even to the value of ultimately suffering death. This is one point that I wanted to make about death.

I may perhaps say also that all attempts to imagine an eternal life seem to me to have failed completely to make this idea in any way attractive. I need not go into details, and far be it from me to ridicule these attempts, but perhaps I might just mention that the Islamic heaven, especially, seems to me particularly intolerable as an ideal of eternal life. But most terrible of all prospects appears to be the prospect which the people who believe in psychical research and spiritualism seem to offer. That is to say, a kind of ghostly semi-existence after death, and one which is not only ghostly but which seems to be intellectually on a particularly low level – on a lower level than the normal level of human affairs. This form of semi-survival is probably the most unpleasant form which has so far been conceived. I do think that if there is anything in the idea of survival, then it would have to be different from anything we can imagine in order to be tolerable, and therefore to be nothing which is really comparable to life, and thus to survival. There are people who have to believe in survival to find life bearable; and it is the thought of these people, and my sympathy with them, which makes me somewhat reluctant to publish anything along the lines that I have here indicated. But if we do publish anything, then I want at least to say one thing which I find very comforting with respect to the certainty of death. This is the fact that death gives value, and in a sense an almost infinite value, to our lives, and makes more urgent and attractive the task of using our lives to achieve something for others, and to be co-workers in this World 3, which apparently embodies more or less what is called the meaning of life.

E: I think that, Karl, you are put off by all the very crude attempts to describe life after death. I am put off by them too. But I believe that there is some incredible mystery about it. What does this life mean: firstly coming-to-be, then finally ceasing-to-be? We find ourselves here in this wonderful rich and vivid conscious experience and it goes on through life, but is that the end? This self-conscious mind of ours has this mysterious relationship with the brain and as a consequence achieves experiences of human love and friendship, of the wonderful natural beauties, and of the intellectual excitement and joy given by appreciation and understanding of our cultural heritages. Is this present life all to finish in death or can we have hope that there will be further meaning to be discovered? I don't want to define anything there. I think there is complete oblivion about the future, but we came from oblivion. Is it that this life of ours is simply an episode of consciousness between two oblivions, or is there some further transcendent experience of which we know nothing? I think I'd leave these questions open at this time.

The self-conscious mind is to my way of thinking in a position of superiority over the brain in World 1. It is intimately associated with it and of course it is dependent on the brain for all detailed memories, but in its essential being it may rise superior to the brain as we have proposed in creative imagination. Thus there may be some central core, the inmost self, that survives the death of the brain to achieve some other existence which is quite beyond anything we can imagine. The uniqueness of the individuality that I experience myself to have cannot be attributed to the uniqueness of my DNA inheritance, as I have already argued in my Eddington Lecture (1965) that was reprinted in my *Facing Reality,* chapter 5. Our coming-to-be is as mysterious as our ceasing-to-be at death. Can we therefore not derive hope because our ignorance about our origin matches our ignorance about our destiny? Cannot life be lived as a challenging and wonderful adventure that has meaning to be discovered?

P: Of course, this is really the decisive thing. If we find that life is worth living, and I think it is very much worth living, then it is the fact that we will die which gives, in part, value to life. If life is worth living, then we may live with the hope that we have not done too badly; and this may, somehow or other, be a fulfilment in itself. I would like to stress here the word hope, which may be interpreted as a reference to the future (but not a future beyond this life).

If there is anything in the idea of survival, then I think that those who say that this cannot be just in space and time, and that it cannot be just a temporal eternity, have to be taken very seriously.

E: I would like to add a quotation from Wilder Penfield [1969] the great neuroscientist and neurosurgeon. "The physical basis of the mind is the brain action in each individual; it accompanies the activity of his spirit, but the spirit is free; it is capable of some degree of initiative." Penfield goes on to say: "The spirit *is* the man one knows. He must have continuity through periods of sleep and coma. I assume, then, that this spirit must live on somehow after death. I cannot doubt that many make contact with God and have guidance from a greater spirit. But these are personal beliefs that every man must adopt for himself. If he had only a brain and not a mind, this difficult decision would not be his." Sherrington in his *Man on His Nature* [1940] wrote against immortality despite his advocacy of dualism. As I wrote on page 174 of my book, *Facing Reality,* he gave me to understand just before his death in 1952 that he had perhaps changed his mind on this, stating "For me now the only reality is the human soul."

P: I am happy to add as a last word on this topic that while Jack and I seem partly to disagree on this question — as I think becomes clear from our discussion — I think I may speak for both of us in saying that in spite of disagreeing we take seriously and respect each other's views on this matter. A disrespect for someone's attitude on these very important matters is something which I think we would both stand against.

E: I would further like to say that man has lost his way these days — what we may call the predicament of mankind. He needs some new message whereby he may live with hope and meaning. I think that science has gone too far in breaking down man's belief in his spiritual greatness and in giving him the idea that he is merely an insignificant material being in the frigid cosmic immensity. Now this strong dualistic-interactionist hypothesis we are here putting forward certainly implies that man is much more than is given by this purely materialistic explanation. I think there is mystery in man, and I am sure that at least it is wonderful for man to get the feeling that he isn't just a hastily made-over ape, and that there is something much more wonderful in his nature and in his destiny.

P: As a kind of anticlimax after the very good things that Jack has said, I would just mention that I also think that there is a danger in science, in that it may perhaps make life too easy for us. Life is a struggle for something; not just for self-assertion, but for the realization of certain values in our life. I think that it is essential for life that there should be obstacles to be overcome. A life without obstacles to overcome would be almost as bad as a life with only obstacles which could not be overcome. (See also my section 42.)

Next Morning 10:30 a.m. 30 September 1974

P: Concerning the vastness of our ignorance, I would like to make a reference to the Introduction to my *Conjectures and Refutations* [1963(a)], section x, page 16. In this section there are allusions to Nicolas of Cusa's *De Docta Ignorantia – On Learned Ignorance.*

E: Karl, I'd like to raise some discussion and criticism of the position we finished at last night. I have been thinking more about it and I feel that something is not explained by the ideas you put forward. It concerns the origin of the self. This after all is what the book is about, The Self and Its Brain. I think that there is an absolutely key problem raised by this because we know the uniqueness of the self, each of us for ourselves, and we assume that this is true for other people. It is a uniqueness that goes continuously through our whole life time, being strung together with all our memory sequences. So this is an experience that I think we can all share. Now you were mentioning its evolutionary origin and that in some way it emerged in relationship to the brain, some kind of emergent evolutionary process. I feel that, if in its origin it is a derivative of the brain even in this emergent or, if you like, transcendent way, then in the end we are becoming somewhat allied to the monist-materialists. You may have David Armstrong saying this is a development of his materialist theory of the mind. Will he not be justified in pointing that out? If it is an emergent derivative of simply a brain developed in the highest level in the evolutionary process, then I think, we give way finally to a view that makes the self-conscious mind simply a spin-off from the highly developed brain. Then we use it to act on the brain in all the ways that we have been talking about.

My position is this. I believe that my personal uniqueness, that is my own experienced self-consciousness, is not accounted for by this emergent explanation of the coming-to-be of my own self. It is the experienced uniqueness that is not so explained. Genetic uniqueness will not do. It can be asserted that I have my experienced uniqueness because my brain is built by the genetic instructions of a quite unique genetic code, my genome with its 30,000 or so genes (Dobzhansky, personal communication) strung along the immense double helix of the human DNA with its 3.5×10^9 nucleotide pairs. It has to be recognized that with 30,000 genes there is a chance of $10^{10,000}$ against that uniqueness being achieved. That is, if my uniqueness of self is tied to the genetic uniqueness that built my brain, then the odds against myself existing in my experienced uniqueness are $10^{10,000}$ against.

So I am constrained to believe that there is what we might call a supernatural origin of my unique self-conscious mind or my unique selfhood or soul; and that gives rise of course to a whole new set of problems. How does my soul come to be in liaison with my brain that has an evolutionary origin? By this idea of a supernatural creation I escape from the incredible improbability that the uniqueness of my own self is genetically determined. There is no problem about the genetic uniqueness of my brain. It is the uniqueness of the experienced self that requires this hypothesis of an independent origin of the self or soul, which is then associated with a brain, that so becomes my brain. That is how the self comes to act as a self-conscious mind, working with the brain in all the ways that we have been discussing, receiving and giving to it and doing a marvellous integrating and driving and controlling job on the neural machinery of the brain.

There are deep problems of how this liaison of self with brain comes to be and how it will cease to be. These are a new set of problems; but on the other hand I believe that these problems derive from a more realistic hypothesis than the one which could assume that my self is in a transcendent emergent relationship with my brain, and therefore in that explanation completely derived from a material structure in World 1.

P: I would like to stress, in case I have not done so before, that evolutionary theory never gives us a full explanation of anything's coming into being in the course of evolution. We may say that in the course of evolution birds, for example, have developed from reptiles; but, of course, this isn't an explanation. We don't know how birds developed from reptiles, nor really why birds developed from reptiles. In a sense, evolutionary theory is terribly weak as an explanatory theory, and we should be conscious of this. But in the sense in which, according to evolutionary theory, the archaeopteryx developed from reptiles, in that sense I think man, for all we know, developed from a cousin of an ape. This is a conjecture, but it is pretty well founded.

I think that with respect to consciousness, we have to assume that animal consciousness has developed out of non-consciousness – we don't know more about it. At some stage this incredible invention was made. This is much more incredible even than, for example, the invention of flight, which in itself is really sufficiently strange that we should be deeply struck by it. Now the self-conscious mind (as opposed to animal consciousness, which possibly may even go back to pre-brain forms) seems to me to be very clearly a product of the human brain. But in saying this I know very well that I am saying very little; and I am anxious to stress that we cannot say much beyond it. It is not an explanation, and it must not be taken as an explanation.

We have the same situation with the emergence of life from something non-living. It is incredibly improbable that life ever emerged; but it *did* emerge. Since it is incredibly improbable, it cannot be an explanation to say that it emerged because, as I have said before, an explanation in probabilistic terms is always an explanation in terms of a high probability: that under such and such conditions it is *very* probable that such and such happens. That is an explanation, but we do not have such an explanation for the emergence of life, or for the emergence of the human brain.

Dialogue XII

11 a. m. 30 September 1974

E: We agree in general in our thinking on all these immense problems of biological evolution. I now want to consider further the problems of evolution in relation to the evolutionary origin of self-consciousness. How far back in the hominid line did primitive man gain self-consciousness? We know that it is at least back to Neanderthal Man, and we can imagine that, paralleling the linguistic development, self-consciousness gradually came at much earlier evolutionary stages. It raises problems for both your view and my view, as to how something of this transcendent kind (I am following Dobzhansky in calling it the transcendent emergent) came to be grafted on to a brain which hitherto had not delivered self-consciousness to its owner.

Now, there is a complementary way of looking at this problem. Let us consider this from the point of view of a child in the way that ontogony recapitulates phylogeny. I think the most important work has yet to be done on this development of the child mind and of the child's knowledge of itself. I am aware that Piaget has pioneered work of this kind, but I think his work is too dogmatic and a little too unimaginative. I'd like to see investigators who are inspired by a full appreciation of the wonder and mystery of human self-consciousness engaged in this study on the developing child. They should do it with many series of children, particularly highly skilled and imaginative children. I think these are the ones most valuable to study. This whole mystery of the self and the uniqueness of the self was revealed to me quite early in my life when I was a teenager, but I wasn't able to get anybody to listen to me!

I am concerned then that we envisage in our hypothesis of the self-brain problem, the supremacy of the self, World 2, over the brain in World 1, particularly in its control and in its synthetic power. To me the conscious self is quite other than the brain in these respects, and I refer with approval to

Sperry's statement that the new ideas that he develops "restore to mind its old prestigious position over matter." So I am left in the perplexing position of knowing that the brain has become associated in its evolutionary development with the self-conscious mind.

P: I have no doubt that you have touched here on certain ultimate questions, but they are also questions which, I have no doubt, we *cannot* answer, at least not at present. However, I do think that there is something like a possible approach towards deriving an answer through World 3. World 3 transcends World 2. I think that that is very important, and that it is very important that we establish this point fully. There is an interaction between World 3 and World 2, which somehow is within the scope of reason. World 3 transcends not only World 1 but also World 2. It really does exist; and not only does it exist, but it is active; it acts upon us (only, of course, by way of interaction). I conceive the relationship between World 1 and World 2 as being similar. (See my section 15.) What I say is not very much, and I don't feel at all that this is an explanation. It is no explanation, but it is an attempt to penetrate into these mysteries by means of reason. I am quite ready to say that we have made some progress with this, but this is just about as far as I think we have been able to get. There is much left unsolved, and there is very much left open. I fully agree that we know very little.

I think that in this context, it is important to remember the limitations of explanation: the fact that we can never achieve explanations which are fully satisfactory in the sense of being ultimate (see dialogue XI, and my sections 47 and 51).

There are also the particular limitations of evolutionary explanation, which I discussed at the end of dialogue XI (see also my [1972(a)], chapter 7, and my [1976(g)], section 37). I am therefore far from any kind of assurance that we have solved these difficult problems.

For this reason, I don't take your criticism that I am saying something similar to Armstrong [1968] very seriously. However, I do think that we have to be clear about our present limitations, and that there are certain things which at least look now as if they are eternal mysteries. Further than that I am not really willing to go, except by pointing to the relationship between World 2 and World 3, and by pointing out that the relationship between World 1 and World 2 is similar. But beyond that I can't see that we can go at present. This of course does not mean that I do not respect the wish to go further, or that I belittle the problems. On the contrary, the problems are too big for us at present – which adds to their challenge.

E: I would like to comment on several points, Karl, in that very fine summing up you gave of these immense problems we have. I would agree with you of course about the mysteries we cannot solve. We try to solve them with reason but we only can go a very little way in these successes. I agree also with you that we should all the time be raising problems instead of trying to cover them up. That I think is what happens with all the parallelistic explanations. They are covering up all these problems of brain-mind interaction and there is in fact nothing left except the dogmatic statement that everything that we are talking about is simply a spin-off of brain events and that everything is determined and we are committed simply to be viewers of a parallelistic canvas or screen, if you like, where in a passive manner the mental happenings are read out from brain events and so experienced. There is no further problem at all. I want to make the point clear that I didn't say I believed you to be in line with the materialistic explanation of the mind in the Armstrong manner. However, I thought Armstrong might claim that you had come to join him, perhaps not directly, but in a roundabout way and no doubt at a more subtle level; nevertheless that you were in his way of thinking. Your last statements have been quite clear that you are not. So I think that this might be a good point to summarize this discussion.

We are agreed that with our puny intelligence and understanding we can only venture so far in the great mysteries that confront us on all sides in trying to account for everything in existence and experience. Science is very successful in its limited field of problems; but the great problems, the *mysterium tremendum,* in the existence of everything we know, this is not accountable for in any scientific manner. So we leave it with that. We live with mysteries which we must realize if we're going to be civilized beings facing up to our existence. Of course I like particularly your introducing World 3 into the problem because I believe too that it is only through World 3 coming that World 2 came. These two are linked together. If you have no World 3, there is no World 2. I think it is well illustrated by the case of a tragically deprived girl in Los Angeles that is described in chapter E4. For $13^1/_2$ years she had no World 3 and she had no World 2 either.

4 p. m. 30 September 1974

P: In connection with the open modules and the openness of World 1 to World 2 influences, I only want to say again that I am not really in the least impressed by the danger, as it were, of falling foul of the first law of thermodynamics, to say nothing of the possibility that the first law of thermodynamics may on this level be valid only statistically. (Any violation in one direction may be statistically levelled out by one in the opposite direction.) My main point is that there is, from the point of view of energy, a great deal going on in the brain and it is going on at all levels; and the levels are open systems. No doubt the brain is an open system of open systems. Any energetic loss or gain in one place could easily be stabilized by the gain or loss in its neighbourhood, and the deviation, if any, from the first law would be of a character which could never be ascertained by measurements. Thus we could not even say whether the deviation (if any) is statistical or not.

E: At the micro-level of operation, it can hardly be imagined at the present time. Furthermore we have to think that it isn't as if the self-conscious mind comes in with a powerful action with cells immediately firing in response to its action. Its action is very weak and slow. It may take, for example, hundreds of milliseconds for an effect to be registered, that is for the self-conscious mind to get a message through from the operations in the modules. This timing we know from Libet's work (chapter E2); and again with action in the other direction, as in Kornhuber's work (chapter E3), it takes up to 800 ms to initiate an action. This means that the self-conscious mind is not bashing certain modules heavily, the open ones, but that it is slightly deviating their action and this has to be built up by modular interaction so that the very slight influences statistically spread over the open modules are lifted up gradually by modular interaction. I think it requires a statistical operation for the finest changes to be lifted out of noise by virtue of an intense ongoing modular interaction. There are hundreds of milliseconds of time to play with, and each synaptic connection only takes about 1 ms. There are levels of subtlety of performance both for receiving and giving, which would be quite in line with your point that it is all at a level far below anything that is measurable.

P: I would like to compare the situation with that of an electric organ or, if you like, an electric typewriter. You can in principle so adjust the relays of such an instrument that the instrument becomes more and more sensitive to the slightest touch, so that, in the end, it becomes sensitive to Brownian motion (moreover, we must not forget the all-or-nothing principle which may apply to such an instrument). Now, roughly at this stage, we achieve a kind of situation in which the first law of thermodynamics can no longer be checked; and there is thus no real reason for saying that it has been violated. On the contrary, I think that we know that such a stage can be technically achieved and therefore that a stage very little removed from it would be practically indistinguishable from the point of view of measurement; yet it may still be "open" to the self and the self may be working on it; and, if it is interfered with by any unexpected motion (let us say by Brownian motion), the self may correct it.

A final remark on evolution. I am somewhat critical of evolutionary theory and of its explanatory power, and especially of the explanatory power of natural selection. However, in spite of this criticism, I think that we should try to see how far one can go within the theory of natural selection. I may mention again the theory of organic evolution (see my section 6, Sir Alister Hardy's *The Living Stream* [1965], and Ernst Mayr [1963], [1976]). It stresses that the choices of the animal are a causal factor in the establishment of its environment, thus leading to a certain type of selection. We may say that the animal is creative in an almost Bergsonian sense or in a more or less Lamarckian sense, even though we may remain completely within the theory of natural selection.

Whether the theory of natural selection is sufficient is a different question, but I think that the importance of this point which I have just mentioned was, for example, missed by Darwin himself (to say nothing of his acceptance of the theory that acquired characteristics may be inherited[1]). In a sense one could say that animals partly create themselves: certainly partly, not wholly; and that man has created himself, by the creation of descriptive language and, with it, of World 3.

[1] Cp. Darwin's *The Variation of Animals and Plants Under Domestication*, second edition [1875], volume i, pp. 466–70.

Bibliography to Part III

ALAJOUANINE T. [1948] "Aphasia and artistic realization", *Brain, 71*, pp. 229–41.

ARMSTRONG D. M. [1968] *A Materialist Theory of the Mind*, Routledge & Kegan Paul, London.

BOHR N., KRAMERS H. A. & SLATER J. C [1924] "The quantum theory of radiation", *Philosophical Magazine, 47*, pp. 785–802.

DARWIN C. [1875] *The Variation of Animals and Plants Under Domestication*, second edition, John Murray, London.

DEREGOWSKI J. B. [1973] "Illusion and Culture", in Gregory & Gombrich (eds) [1973], pp. 161–91.

DOBZHANSKY T. [1967] *The Biology of Ultimate Concern*, The New American Library Inc., New York.

ECCLES J. C. [1953] *The Neurophysiological Basis of Mind*, Clarendon Press, Oxford.

[1970] *Facing Reality*, Springer Verlag, New York, Heidelberg, Berlin.

EHRENFELS C. von [1890] "Über Gestaltqualitäten", *Vierteljahrschrift für wissenschaftliche Philosophie, 14*.

GOMBRICH E. [1960] *Art and Illusion*, Phaedon, London.

GREGORY R. C. [1966] *Eye and Brain*, Weidenfeld & Nicolson, London.

GREGORY R. C. & GOMBRICH E. (eds) [1973] *Illusion in Nature and Art*, Duckworth, London.

HADAMARD J. [1954] *The Psychology of Invention in the Mathematical Field*, Dover, New York.

HARDY A. [1965] *The Living Stream*, Collins, London.

HOLLOWAY R. L. [1974] "The casts of fossil hominid brains", *Scientific American, 231*, July, pp. 106–115.

INGVAR D. H. [1975] "Patterns of Brain Activity Revealed by Measurements of Regional Blood Flow", in *Brain Work*, ed. D. H. Ingvar and N. A. Lasser, Munksgaard, Copenhagen, pp. 397–413.

JENNINGS H. S. [1933] *The Universe and Life*, Yale University Press, New Haven and Oxford University Press, London.

JULESZ B. [1971] *Foundations of Cyclopean Perception*, University of Chicago Press, Chicago.

KÖHLER W. [1920] *Die physischen Gestalten in Ruhe und im stationären Zustand*, Vieweg, Braunschweig.

LAND E. H. [1959] "Experiments in Colour Vision", *Scientific American*, May, 1959.

LEWIN K. [1922] *Die Begriffe der Genese in Physik, Biologie und Entwicklungsgeschichte*, J. Springer, Berlin.

LORD A. B. [1960] *The Singer of Tales*, Harvard University Press, Cambridge, Mass.

MAYR E. [1963] *Animal Species and Evolution,* The Belknap Press, Harvard University Press, Cambridge, Mass.

[1976] *Evolution and the Diversity of Life,* The Belknap Press, Harvard University Press, Cambridge, Mass.

PENFIELD W. [1969] "Science, the arts and the spirit", *Trans. Royal Society of Canada, 7,* pp. 73–83.

PLACE U. T. [1956] "Is consciousness a brain process?", *British Journal of Psychology, 47,* pp. 44–51.

PLATO *The Laws*
Timaeus

POPPER K. R. [1963(a)] *Conjectures and Refutations,* Routledge & Kegan Paul, London.

[1972(a)] *Objective Knowledge: An Evolutionary Approach,* Clarendon Press, Oxford.

[1973(a)] "Indeterminism is Not Enough", *Encounter, 40,* No. 4, pp. 20–6.

[1976(g)] *Unended Quest,* Fontana/Collins, London.

RYLE G. [1949] *The Concept of Mind,* Hutchinson, London.

SCHRÖDINGER E. [1952] "Are there quantum jumps?", *British Journal for the Philosophy of Science, 3,* pp. 109–23. and 233–42.

[1967] *What is Life? & Mind and Matter,* Cambridge University Press, Cambridge.

SHERRINGTON C. [1940] *Man on His Nature,* Cambridge University Press, Cambridge.

SMART J. J. C. [1959] "Sensations and brain processes", *Philosophical Review,* LXVIII, pp. 141–56.

THORPE W. H. [1974] *Animal Nature and Human Nature,* Methuen, London.

WIGNER E. P. [1969] "Are we Machines?", *Proceedings of the American Philosophical Society, 113,* pp. 95–101.

Index of Names

Page numbers in *italics* refer to the bibliography

Index of Subjects

Nn denotes footnote reference